Ultrasound of the Thyroid and Parathyroid Glands

Robert A. Sofferman • Anil T. Ahuja
Editors

Ultrasound of the Thyroid and Parathyroid Glands

Springer

Editors
Robert A. Sofferman, MD, FACS
Division of Otolaryngology-Head and Neck Surgery
University of Vermont School of Medicine
Burlington, Vermont, USA
robert.sofferman@vtmednet.org

Anil T. Ahuja, MD, FRCR, FHKCR, FHKAM
Department of Imaging and Interventional Radiology
The Chinese University of Hong Kong
Prince of Wales Hospital
Shatin (NT), Hong Kong (SAR), China
aniltahuja@cuhk.edu.hk

Please note that additional images for this book can be downloaded from
http://www.springerimages.com/videos/978-1-4614-0973-1

ISBN 978-1-4614-0973-1 e-ISBN 978-1-4614-0974-8
DOI 10.1007/978-1-4614-0974-8
Springer New York Dordrecht Heidelberg London

Library of Congress Control Number: 2011941798

Printed on acid-free paper

Springer is part of Springer Science+Business Media (www.springer.com)

I wish to take an unusual precedent to dedicate this textbook to my co-author and editor, Dr. Anil T. Ahuja, who has been my ultrasound mentor, academic colleague, and special family friend for the past several years. He has a remarkable clinical knowledge of conditions of the head and neck and is perhaps the foremost comprehensive imaging expert of this special region of human anatomy. He has understood the relevance of ultrasound to the daily interpretation and management of diseases of the thyroid and parathyroid glands and in particular its office use by endocrinologists and surgeons to the benefit of their patients. It is his unselfish interest in educating me as a head and neck surgeon that has resulted in this collaborative effort. I hope that we are able to transfer this information to others with a similar passion for ultrasound through the text and electronic access to relevant cine loops.

– Robert A. Sofferman, MD, FACS

Preface

This textbook is devoted to comprehensive portrayal of high resolution ultrasound of the thyroid and parathyroid glands. This goal cannot be accomplished without addressing the entire cervical lymph node basins as well as other clinical conditions and anatomical areas which may be misinterpreted as being of thyroid origin. Ultrasound technology is not specific to any single medical discipline and as such the authors represent an objective merger of both radiologic and clinical specialties devoted to study of this fascinating endocrine region. In fact, the text attempts to extend beyond the simple dry presentation of groups of images to apply sufficient clinical information concerning function of the thyroid and parathyroid glands in a variety of disease states. The reader may recognize some redundancy in discussion of ultrasound physics, scanning techniques, and application of fine needle aspiration. By design, this concept emphasizes certain important details and illustrates that there are multiple ways to apply variations in technology to arrive at the same endpoint. The images included in the text are a result of decades of experience with head and neck imaging and frequently both CT and MRI are included in parallel with ultrasound to enhance the presentation. The one process which cannot be demonstrated in a written text is dynamic cine loop imaging. Thus, an on-line link to a variety of carefully selected cine loops is included as an adjunct to provide the reader with the most comprehensive understanding of this technology and its relevance to radiologists, endocrinologists, endocrine, and head and neck surgeons. In fact, the cine loop may be the most important tool to adequately portray the pathology of interest and to allow sharing of imagery with other clinicians in a simple and brief overview. This concept is analogous to the realm of photography where black and white, color, and movie renditions all have a creative role in properly capturing a scene.

In discussion of the history of ultrasound and its modern day application, several American societies which have a vested interest in clinical ultrasound of the thyroid and parathyroid glands are mentioned to barely scratch the surface of modern day issues. It is apparent that there will be omissions from various parts of the world where ultrasound is the primary imaging tool and is performed to excellent clinical advantage. These countries from Asia, Europe, South America, Australia, and Africa each have their own specialty societies and contributions to the understanding of this marvelous imaging tool. Finally, with the advent of both changes in technology, reduction in its market cost, and clinical relevance ultrasound has in part become an office-based procedure. This has allowed clinicians to serve their patients with efficiency and convenience and to become more involved in the direct observation of the anatomy and pathology of the condition under study. In fact, it has presented the clinician with an opportunity to better enjoy the outpatient experience since so much detailed information can be accrued simply and beautifully in the examining room. There are a few economic and political hurdles to overcome, but establishment of an office-based use of ultrasound can easily be accomplished if the commitment is present on the clinical side [1]. The authors hope that this comprehensive investigation of cervical ultrasound will both assist the clinician to better understand images of interest and develop new initiatives in its use.

Internet Access To Cine Loops

Cine loops are dynamic movie clips which compliment the static text images and explanations. During routine ultrasound examination of the thyroid and parathyroid glands it is necessary to evaluate the entire cervical lymph node basins. In the process of this examination, salivary glands, muscles, vessels, nerves and potential congenital abnormalities may be encountered. For this reason, no discussion of the thyroid and parathyroid glands would be complete without addressing in some way these other relevant areas and structures. Although a single ultrasound image transfers some information, the cine loop is a more complete rendition of the pathologic condition under study. These dynamic movies are collated into the following categories: 1-general 2-lymph nodes 3-parathyroid glands 4-thyroid gland 5- FNA and sampling. The owner of this text will be able to access these cine loops through Springer with the following Internet link: http://www.springerimages.com/videos/978-1-4614-0973-1.

Burlington, VT, USA Robert A. Sofferman, MD
Shatin, Hong Kong Anil T. Ahuja, MD

Reference

1. Nagarkatti S, Mekel M, Sofferman R, Parangi S. Overcoming obstacles to setting up office-based ultrasound for evaluation of thyroid and parathyroid disorders. Laryngoscope. 2011;121:1–7.

Contents

Contributors

Anil T. Ahuja, MD, FRCR, FHKCR, FHKAM
Department of Imaging and Interventional Radiology, The Chinese University of Hong Kong, Prince of Wales Hospital, Shatin (NT), Hong Kong (SAR), China

Kunwar S.S. Bhatia, B Med Sci, MBBS, MRCS DLO, FRCR Department of Imaging and Interventional Radiology, Prince of Wales Hospital, The Chinese University of Hong Kong, Shatin, NT, Hong Kong, People's Republic of China

Carmen C.M. Cho, MBBS, FRCR Department of Imaging and Interventional Radiology, Prince of Wales Hospital, The Chinese University of Hong Kong, Shatin, NT, Hong Kong, People's Republic of China

Daniel S. Duick, MD, FACE, FACP Staff Physician, Endocrinology Associates, Phoenix, PA, Arizona

Clinical Professor of Medicine, College of Medicine, University of Arizona, Phoenix, Arizona

Yolanda Y.P. Lee, MBChB, FRCR, FHKCR, FHKAM
Department of Imaging & Interventional Radiology, Prince of Wales Hospital, The Chinese University of Hong Kong, Shatin, NT, Hong Kong

Darshana Dattatray Rasalkar, MBBS, DMRD, DNB, FRCR
Department of Radiology, Kokilaben Dhirubhai Ambani Hospital, Mumbai, Maharashtra, India

Robert A. Sofferman, MD, FACS Division of Otolaryngology-Head and Neck Surgery, University of Vermont School of Medicine, Burlington, VT, USA

Cina Shin-Loong Tong, MBChB, FRCR Department of Imaging & Interventional Radiology, Prince of Wales Hospital, The Chinese University of Hong Kong, Shatin, NT, Hong Kong

Ka Tak Wong, MBChB, FRCR, FHKCR, FHKAM
Department of Imaging and Interventional Radiology, Prince of Wales Hospital, The Chinese University of Hong Kong, Shatin, NT, Hong Kong SAR, People's Republic of China

Michael T.C. Ying, PhD, MPhil, PDip (DR) Department of Health Technology and Informatics, The Hong Kong Polytechnic University, Hung Hom, Kowloon, Hong Kong, People's Republic of China

Hok Yuen Yuen, MBChB, FRCR, FHKCR, FHKAM
Department of Imaging and Interventional Radiology, Prince of Wales Hospital, The Chinese University of Hong Kong, Shatin, NT, Hong Kong

Section I

History and Basic Concepts

The History of Clinical Ultrasound

1

Robert A. Sofferman

Introduction

No text devoted to the application of ultrasound to medicine would be complete without at least a brief review of the remarkable events which have preceded its current uses. In fact, one review of musculoskeletal ultrasound includes "From bats and ships to babies and hips" in its formal title [1]. Although this is clearly an oversimplification, it emphasizes the presence of ultrahigh-frequency sound in our natural environment and its scientific adaptation to more practical matters.

Perhaps the earliest documented experiments concerning sound waves about our audible registry did occur with bats during the lifetime of an Italian priest and physiologist, Lazzaro Spallanzani who lived from 1729 to 1799 [2]. He was fascinated by the ability of bats to navigate in complete darkness. He proved that these animals could continue to fly effectively while being blindfolded but could not do so when their ears were occluded. In spite of the fact that this suggested that audition is critical to the bat in its rapid flight maneuvers, the true foundation of these special navigational aptitudes remained elusive until 1938. Two Harvard students, Donald Griffin and Robert Galambos, recorded directional ultrasonic noises emitted from bats during flight, and the theory of echolocalization was confirmed [3].

Of course, clinical ultrasound is intimately connected to an understanding of the physics of sound transmission. Jean Colladon was a Swiss mathematician and scientist who fortunately redirected his interests from law. In 1826, he designed a clever experiment to determine the relative ability of air and water to support sound waves [4]. With the help of another co-scientist positioned in a boat exactly 10 miles away, he struck a church bell underwater at the same time a gunpowder explosion was initiated above the water surface. The distant boat was equipped with a trumpet-type instrument to receive sound waves placed beneath the boat. The bell sound was subsequently appreciated well in advance of the recognition of the gunpowder report which proved that sound waves travel more efficiently in a fluid medium. In addition, he calculated the velocity of sound in water during the experiment and arrived at a value of 1,435 m/s which is remarkably close to the modern accepted standard in spite of the relative simplicity of the experimental design.

Perhaps no greater advance in the development of ultrasound can be argued above the identification of the piezoelectric effect. In 1881, the physicist Gabriel Lippmann deduced mathematically that an electric charge could produce a mechanical stress [5]. Pierre Curie and his brother Jacques began to study various crystals concurrent to the work of Lippmann [6]. They demonstrated that

R.A. Sofferman (✉)
Division of Otolaryngology-Head and Neck Surgery, Fletcher Allen Health Care, University of Vermont School of Medicine, 111 Colchester Ave., Burlington, VT 05401, USA
e-mail: robert.sofferman@vtmednet.org

R.A. Sofferman and A.T. Ahuja (eds.), *Ultrasound of the Thyroid and Parathyroid Glands*,
DOI 10.1007/978-1-4614-0974-8_1, © Springer Science+Business Media, LLC 2012

several crystals (quartz, tourmaline, topaz, cane sugar, and Rochelle salt) emitted an electrical charge when subjected to mechanical deformation. This was the inverse of the practical application of Lippmann, and together, these are fundamental to transducer transmission and reception of ultrasound waves. Synthetic piezoelectric crystals (lead zirconate titanate (PZT) were developed in 1954 and serve as the most widely used materials for sound transduction [5, 6].

Echolocalization (the application of directional sound and reflection to detect objects and measure distances to them) is the term initially applied to nautical circumstances. When the Titanic sank in the northern Atlantic Ocean, a Canadian inventor submitted a patent in 1912 for devices to locate icebergs. Reginald A. Fessenden thus developed the first sonar apparatus (the acronym SONAR from "SOund NAvigation and Ranging" immediately evolved), and it was put to practical use 2 years later with the ability to detect an iceberg 2 miles away [7]. Since this occurred in the midst of World War I with threats to Allied shipping from German submarines, the adaptation of this technology to its military advantage became a pressing necessity. Paul Langevin and Constantin Chilowsky developed an underwater quartz generator sandwiched between two steel plates, which is credited as the first modern ultrasound transducer prototype [7].

The very first recorded successful sinking of a German U-boat using this echolocalization was on April 23, 1916, and refinements of the device became widely employed during World War II for protection of North Atlantic convoys [4]. In fact, in conjunction with the use of depth charges, these sonar devices were responsible for leveling the playing field in the deterrence of submarine effectiveness. Further applied use of ultrasound in the shipping and aeronautical industry occurred after World War II for the detection of flaws in metal. These reflectoscopes were the indirect precursors of diagnostic ultrasound in medicine [8].

Karl Dussik, a neurologist at the University of Vienna, is credited with the first medical use of diagnostic ultrasound in the attempt to use transcranial ultrasound beams to locate and characterize brain tumors and adjacent ventricles [9]. In the late 1940s, George Ludwig was enrolled at the Naval Medical Research Institute in Bethesda and applied his experiments to detect foreign bodies in animal tissues and to study gallstone reflectance using pulse-echo principles [10–13]. He explored the attenuation of ultrasound in tissues, the concepts of impedance mismatch, and the ideal frequencies to allow penetration of sound waves into tissues without producing excessive heat and injury. His insight was one of the important foundations for future clinical use of ultrasound.

A University of Colorado radiologist, Douglas Howry, became interested in the development of B-mode ultrasound to allow interpretation of cross-sectional anatomy [14]. He was one of the earliest radiologists to embrace ultrasound and its imaging capabilities, performing a significant amount of his research in the basement of his home. A University of Cambridge student, John Julian Wild, reported on the use of A-mode ultrasound in the examination of malignancies of the breast and intestinal tract and the development of a linear handheld device which was B-mode in design [15]. He also described A-mode ultrasound for transvaginal and transrectal scanning. Wild then met Professor Ian Donald, who was working at the Hammersmith Hospital in London, and a natural cross-fertilization of mutual interests evolved. Donald had experience with sonar techniques while serving in the Royal Air Force during World War II and became very enthusiastic about the application of ultrasound to obstetrics and gynecology. In collaboration with an English engineering firm, his group developed instrumentation which allowed the differentiation of cystic from solid abdominal masses [16]. Perhaps the sentinel ultrasound event at that time surrounded a patient with a pelvic mass presumed to be inoperable cancer on clinical grounds. Ultrasound suggested that it was a cyst, and this fortunate pathology was eventually confirmed at successful surgery. This event was published in a 1958 edition of Lancet and marked a major success for diagnostic ultrasound [16]. Subsequent development of an "automatic" scanner in 1960 led to several clinically relevant advances in obstetrics: (1) first antepartum diagnosis of placenta previa using ultrasound, (2) measurement of biparietal diameter of the fetal head, and (3) utilization of the full bladder transmission to allow detection of early pregnancy at 6–7 weeks gestation in 1963 [17].

In spite of these selected diagnostic processes concerning ultrasound, in fact, its initial uses for medicine were in the realm of therapeutics. The destructive qualities of high-intensity ultrasound were recognized in the 1920s to the point where it was used therapeutically in neurosurgery. At the Universities of Iowa and Illinois, during craniotomy, ultrasound was employed to ablate parts of the basal ganglia in patients with Parkinson's disease [18].

It was employed extensively for physical therapy and rehabilitation medicine for its ability to produce deep heat in tissues of patients with rheumatoid arthritis [14]. In fact, during the 1940s, it became a panacea for many conditions without good controlled evidence-based studies with conditions such as arthritic pain, gastric ulcers, eczema, asthma, thyrotoxicosis, hemorrhoids, urinary incontinence, elephantiasis, and even angina. In fact, its tissue-disruptive qualities were of such concern that the evolution of diagnostic ultrasound was curtailed for several years.

B-mode ultrasound continued with examination of the heart. Helmuth Hertz, a physicist at the University of Lund, Sweden, and Inge Edler, a cardiologist, allegedly met over a lunch in 1953 and decided to pursue the development of echocardiography [14]. In the United States 3 years later, Robert Rushmer, pediatrician and physiologist, and two engineers collaborated to design instruments which allowed the examination of the dog's cardiovascular system in the conscious state. Their work allowed the development of handheld Doppler devices [14].

Several relevant historical elements about modern thyroid ultrasound are nicely reviewed by Robert A. Levine in the text by Baskin, Duick, and Levine entitled "Thyroid Ultrasound and Ultrasound-Guided FNA" [19]. Thyroid ultrasound received its impetus with a study in 1967 by Fujimoto of 184 patients [20]. The B-mode ultrasound required that the patient be immersed in water bath and examined the characteristic echoes within the thyroid gland and contained nodules. Although the thrust of this paper was to demonstrate that ultrasound was capable of differentiating benign from malignant lesions, 25–35% of nodules were incorrectly classified [28].

A 1971 paper by Blum described the ability of A-mode ultrasound to distinguish cystic from solid thyroid nodules [21]. A 1974 paper by Ernest Crocker described the findings of "low-amplitude, sparse, and disordered echoes" seen in thyroid cancer which, in today's descriptive terminology, would be hypoechoic and heterogeneous in pattern [22]. In their series, all six definitive preoperative cancer diagnoses anticipated on ultrasound were confirmed at surgery.

In 1977, Wallfish reported on experience with ultrasound-guided fine needle aspiration [23]. Although cytology was not as well developed and accepted as it is today, this concept set the stage for providing more accuracy in sampling specific lesions within the thyroid gland. In fact, there is no current ultrasonographic characteristic which determines malignancy with certainty, but the addition of guided aspiration cytology comes the closest. This early paper was prophetic in its message.

Advances in ultrasound technology continued to receive major contributions from Austria, Germany, Japan, United States, Denmark, Finland, Italy, Hungary, Spain, Belgium, Union of Soviet Socialist Republics, China, England, France, Poland, Holland, and Australia. In 1972, Kossoff and Garrett from Australia employed gray scale imaging for the differentiation of tissue type and density by combining A-scan sonography with B-mode display [24]. The fine single echoes of A-scan ultrasonography were combined sequentially side by side to arrive at a composite gray scale image.

Christian Doppler was a mathematician and physicist at the University of Vienna and published a paper at the Royal Bohemian Society in Prague in 1841 entitled "On the coloured light of double stars and certain other stars of the heaven" [25]. The astronomical principles in that publication were said to be the foundation for certain wave principles, most notably, that wave frequencies change as moving objects approach and depart from a static point of reception [26, 27]. Since those early theoretical interests in the alteration of sound waves with movement, Doppler principles have been applied in virtually every area of clinical medicine. The development of color flow imaging has been a critical element in interpretation of the character of lymph nodes of the head and neck and identification of vascular structures. A paper by Lagalla and coworkers in 1992 was one of the initial attempts to differentiate benign from malignant thyroid nodules [28]. They demonstrated that absence of flow (type I) within a nodule is useful in identifying the innocent nodule. Type II with perinodular flow is generally an indicator of the benign lesion, whereas type III with chaotic intranodular flow is usually associated with malignancy. These findings have been consistently similar to modern thyroid ultrasound interpretation.

In fact, Doppler has become so sophisticated in its anatomical performance that the typical color Doppler techniques employed to assess blood flow velocity and volume in large vessel assessment are not as preferred as its related methodology, power Doppler. Because neither the direction of flow or volume is critical to thyroid, parathyroid, and lymph node assessment, power Doppler was recognized as a better tool as it demonstrates less distortion and shows small vessels with low flow to better advantage [29].

The development of the transistor and integrated circuitry allowed miniaturization of electronics and thus smaller consoles. Probes then became smaller, and the era of portability of equipment became a reality. The larger expensive consoles continued to reside within radiology departments in hospitals and universities, and the resolution evolved slowly but progressively through the 1990s. With the portability of ultrasound units and their accessibility to Emergency Room physicians and surgeons, abdominal ultrasound became a convenient method of determining cavitary hemorrhage. The clinical development of determining cholelithiasis and the assessment of breast masses are but a few examples of the transition of ultrasound to an office-based procedure in general surgery. As well, ultrasound-guided fine needle aspiration cytology has become as much a clinician-associated office procedure as one performed by radiologists. Endocrinologists, otolaryngologists, and surgeons interested in thyroid disorders have embraced the technology in spite of its potential conflict with the efficiencies of office scheduling.

Ultrasound Education and Administration

As ultrasound advanced and became a commonly performed procedure in radiology departments, technicians performed most of the actual examinations and were supervised by radiologists and residents. Striving to achieve recognition, in 1970 the sonographers organized, and this group eventually became the Society of Diagnostic Medical Sonography [14]. 3 years later, the US Office of Education determined that ultrasonography should be worthy of an occupational designation. This membership has grown significantly to the point where 20,000 members were listed as of 2007 [14].

While these sonographers represent the nucleus of the American Institute of Ultrasound in Medicine, there are now 54 professional societies represented in the AIUM from a broad segment of medical, radiological, surgical, and allied health-care disciplines.

The American Association of Clinical Endocrinologists has developed a training/credentialing postgraduate program for its members, which allows clinicians to perform office-based ultrasound and FNA of requisite lesions [Baskin, Jack. Personal communication, 2010]. The first course on ultrasound for endocrinologists was established in 1998 under the direction of Jack Baskin, M.D., who became the undisputed father of ultrasound education for his specialty. In fact, he was instrumental in developing and maintaining the Endocrine University devoted in large measure to the further development of ultrasound for endocrinology fellows. A special certificate of excellence has been developed by AACE, which requires individuals who are interested to prove significant experience by submission of cases to a panel of experts, take a written examination, and accommodate to recertification every 10 years (Endocrinology Certification of Neck Ultrasound). To date, approximately 150 endocrinologists have completed full validation through this process [30].

The American College of Surgeons has developed postgraduate ultrasound courses in multiple surgical disciplines. The history of this development and the breadth of this educational project have been elucidated in a manuscript published by the surgeon leaders who have been instrumental in the application of ultrasound to clinical surgical practice [31]. Breast, abdominal, thyroid and parathyroid, biliary, vascular, and FAST examinations are areas covered at the Annual Congress in these courses. These consist of didactic lectures, hands-on skill sessions with formal ultrasound examination of patient volunteers, practice FNA on phantoms, and faculty observation and written examination. The ACS has developed a mechanism for these courses to be exported to sites outside of the Annual Congress. In fact, the American Academy of Otolaryngology–Head and Neck Surgery has been the recipient of this opportunity such that each year, interested head and neck surgeons can receive identical training and certification to that presented at the ACS Congress.

In 1984, Wolfgang Mann published the first textbook in Germany devoted to clinical ultrasound of the head and neck [32]. In fact, by the mid-1990s, ultrasound experience was a requirement for board certification for otolaryngology in Germany [32]. While ultrasound education can be obtained through postgraduate courses, the foundation for the future will be in the development of formal residency training in ultrasound history, physics, and hands-on experience. Whereas general surgical training encompasses the use of ultrasound in central line placement, FAST examination in trauma, assessment of both gallbladder and appendix in abdominal pain, and breast examination and biopsy, to mention a few areas of interest, other specialties have been slower to become formally aligned with this technology. With the profusion of exposure to thyroid and parathyroid surgery, otolaryngology has come to understand the relevance of ultrasound and its application to the head and neck well beyond this small central organ. The time for formal curricula and courses within residency just for residents in training has arrived.

The multitude of postgraduate courses has mirrored the profusion of office-based ultrasound in clinical medicine. Its application to thyroid and parathyroid assessment is highly relevant and carries efficiencies for patients and referring physicians. Beside the reduction in size of ultrasound units and portability, they have now become affordable for purchase. The companies which manufacture these machines have realized that the market outside of radiology departments is quite substantial. In addition, the systems can be tailored to individual needs, depending on the specialty or even pooled resources of multiple clinicians. Ultrasound of the breast and head and neck can be accommodated by a single linear transducer, whereas abdominal ultrasound requires a convex probe. However, all other settings and variations can be managed through dials and changes which the sonographer does at the console.

In summary, the application of clinical ultrasound in medicine has proceeded through nearly a century of evolution along with military and industrial interests. In countries which have not been able to provide broad-reaching, sophisticated imaging technology such as CT scanning, ultrasound has been used to clinical advantage. This has occurred in spite of the fact that comparative resolution with earlier systems of even a decade ago cannot equate to what exists in today's market. The historical overview of ultrasound demonstrates that multiple individuals of diverse scientific backgrounds have collaborated in the eventual development of a remarkable product which crosses medical specialty applications. This text is designed to cover the comprehensive use of ultrasound for anatomic study and, to some degree, therapeutic management of thyroid and parathyroid disorders. It has been prepared to appeal to radiologists with a special interest in this area and clinicians who can now image this anatomic region in an outpatient, office-based setting expecting a sophisticated degree of image resolution.

References

1. Kane D. A brief history of musculoskeletal ultrasound: "From bats and ships to babies and hips". Rheumatology. 2004;43:931–3.
2. Eisenberg R. Radiology: an illustrated history. St Louis: Mosby; 1992.
3. Griffin DR, Galambos R. The sensory basis of obstacle avoidance by flying bats. J Exp Zool. 1941;86: 481–506.
4. Woo J. A short history of the developments of ultrasound in obstetrics and gynecology. http://www.ob-ultrasound.net/hydrophone.html 1999). Accessed on January 15, 2011.
5. Curie J, Curie P. Developpment par pression de l'ectricite polaire dans les cristaux hemiedres a faces inclines. CR Acad Sci (Paris). 1880;91:294.
6. Genesis Ultrasound. Breakthrough in ultrasound physics comes from Pierre Curie www.genesis-ultrasound.com/ultrasound-physics.html. Accessed on January 15, 2011.
7. Hill CR. Medical ultrasonics: an historical review. Br J Radiol. 1973;46:899–905.
8. Firestone FA. The supersonic reflectoscope, an instrument of inspecting the interior of solid parts by means of sound waves. J Acoust Soc Am. 1945;17: 287–99.
9. Dussik KT. On the possibility of using ultrasound waves as a diagnostic aid. Z Neurol Psychiatr. 1942;174:153–68.
10. Ludwig GD, Bolt RH, Hueter TF, Ballantine HT. Factors influencing the use of ultrasound as a diagnostic aid. Trans Am Neurol Assoc. 1950;51:225–8.
11. Ludwig GD, Ballantine HT. Ultrasonographic irradiation of nervous tissue. Surgical Forum, Clinical Congress of the American College of Surgeons 400, 1950.
12. Ludwig GD. The velocity of sound through tissues and the acoustic impedance of tissues. J Acoust Soc Am. 1950;22:862–6.
13. Ludwig GD, Struthers FW. Detecting gallstones with ultrasonic echoes. Electronics. 1950;23:172–8.
14. Orenstein BW. Ultrasound history. Radiol Today. 2008;9:28–30.
15. Shampo MA, Kyle RA. John Julian Wild-pioneer in ultrasonography. Mayo Clin Proc. 1997;72:234.
16. Donald I, MacVicar J. Brown TG. Investigation of abdominal masses by pulsed ultrasound Lancet. 1958;1:187–9.
17. Kurjak A. Ultrasound scanning-Prof Ian Donald (1910–1987). Eur J Obstet Gynecol Reprod Biol. 2000;90:187–9.
18. Erikson K, Fry F, Jones J. Ultrasound in Medicine-A review. IEEE Transactions on Sonics and Ultrasonics vol. SU-21 no 3, July 1974.
19. Jack B, Daniel D, Robert L. Thyroid ultrasound and ultrasound-guided FNA. 2nd ed. New York: Springer; 2008. p. 1–8.
20. Fujimoto F, Oka A, Omoto R, Hirsoe M. Ultrasonic scanning of the thyroid gland as a new diagnostic approach. Ultrasonics. 1967;5:177–80.
21. Blum M, Weiss B, Hernberg J. Evaluation of thyroid nodules by A-mode echography. Radiology. 1971;101:651–6.
22. Crocker EF, McLaughlin AF, Kossoff G, Jellins J. The gray scale echographic appearance of thyroid malignancy. J Clin Ultrasound. 1974;2:305–6.
23. Wallfish PG, Hazani E, Strawbridge HTG, Miskin M, Rosen IB. Combined ultrasound and needle aspiration cytology in the assessment and management of hypofunctioning thyroid nodule. Ann Intern Med. 1977; 87:270–4.
24. Kossoff G, Garrett W. in Behm A(quoted in Frentzel-Beyme B) Als die Bilder laufen Lenten. Ultraschall Klin Prax. 1994;8:265–87.
25. Uber das farbige licht der Doppellsterne und eininger anderer Gestirne des Himmels. Read on May 25, 1842. Abjandlungen derr Koniglich Bohmischen Gesellschaft der Wissenschaften Prague 1842 2:465–82.
26. White DN. Johann Christian Doppler and his effect- a brief history. Ultrasound Med Biol. 1982;8(6):583–91.
27. Kainberger F, Leodolter S. Christian Doppler and the influence of his work on modern medicine. Wiener Klinische Wochenschrift. 2004;116(4):107–9.
28. Lagalla R, Cariso G, Midiri M, Cardinale AE. Echo-Doppler couleur et pathologic thyroidienne. J Echography Med Ultrasons. 1992;13:44–7.
29. Cerbone G, Spiezia S, Colao A, Di Sarno A, et al. Power Doppler improves the diagnostic accuracy of color Doppler ultrasonography in cold thyroid nodules: follow-up results. Horm Res. 1999;52:19–24.
30. Staren ED, Knudson NM, Rozycki GS, Harness JK, Wherry DC, Shackford SR. An evaluation of the American College of Surgeon's ultrasound education. Am J Surg. 2006;191:489–96.
31. Mann W. Ultraschall im Kopf/Hals-Bereich. Tokyo, Berlin, Heidelberg, New York. Springer, 1984
32. Orloff L. Head and neck ultrasonography. San Diego: Plural Publishing Inc; 2008. p. 6–7.

Physics and Principles of Ultrasound

2

Robert A. Sofferman

Ultrasound has a storied history which achieved reality during World War II in finding German submarines in the protection of North Atlantic convoys. It was initially employed for its therapeutic benefits in physical therapy to produce deep heat and ablation of brain lesions for Parkinson's disease. The wave characteristics have been altered in diagnostic ultrasound to the point where energy transfer is limited, and deep tissue heat is virtually nonexistent. Ultrasound systems are comprised of a transducer, console (which contains the computer software, electrical components, Doppler technology, and storage), and the display. The physics of ultrasound waves and the means of their delivery are important to meld into this discussion. Artifacts which are demonstrated in the display of clinical ultrasound can be used to advantage in understanding what is actually portrayed.

Before delving into the applied physics of ultrasound, it is helpful to turn attention to the natural world and some of the creatures which use sound waves to remarkable advantage. As will become apparent in the formal discussion to follow, sound waves depend on a support transport medium. Liquids and animal soft tissues transmit sound waves efficiently and to nearly the same velocity since the aggregated molecules are compact and noncompressible. Bone transmits sound waves even better due to its even compact nature, but bone reflectivity obviates the practical use of ultrasound. On the other hand, air is a poor supporter of sound waves due to the compressibility of the molecules and their reduced concentration. In the ocean, dolphins and odontocetes such as toothed whales emit very-high-pitched single-frequency clicks to communicate with others of their species [1]. It is also used for echolocalization of schools of fish upon which they prey. In contrast, baleen whales which feed on plankton do not transmit in the high-frequency range but more on the order of 10–30 Hz. These sound waves travel extreme distances due to both their low frequency and the medium of transport which has important communication advantages. Above ground, elephants also transmit in this approximate low-frequency range with a volume level which may reach 117 dB [2, 3]. These transmissions can be identified as far as 10 km from the source and may also be sensed by the broad elephant's feet or the trunk which it may place along the ground to "hear" in this unique way. Once again, the sound transmission through a more solid medium is more effective than through air. Bats [2, 4] emit sounds in the ultrasound range to identify insects and obstructions, but the waves are disadvantaged by having to travel in air. As will be noted in the subsequent discussion of sound wave physics, high-frequency sound attenuates rapidly with reduction in returning wave energy. The massive

R.A. Sofferman (✉)
Division of Otolaryngology-Head and Neck Surgery, Fletcher Allen Health Care, University of Vermont School of Medicine, 111 Colchester Ave., Burlington, VT 05401, USA
e-mail: robert.sofferman@vtmednet.org

R.A. Sofferman and A.T. Ahuja (eds.), *Ultrasound of the Thyroid and Parathyroid Glands*, DOI 10.1007/978-1-4614-0974-8_2, © Springer Science+Business Media, LLC 2012

ears of the bat relative to its body are critical to reception of the returning waves. Since their emitted sounds have high frequency in an air medium, the distances the sound must travel are short to overcome these disadvantages of acoustic physics.

Physics of Ultrasound

As just illustrated, sound waves travel readily through fluid medium and very ineffectively through air. In contrast with light which can travel in a vacuum, sound requires a support medium. The sound waves travel effectively through liquids which are comprised of closely compacted molecules. In fact, water and soft tissues have approximately the same transmission velocity with the latter averaging 1,540 m/s. In addition, the attenuation or loss of sound wave amplitude occurs rapidly in an air medium. Thus, structures which are retrotracheal or retroesophageal are difficult or impossible to visualize.

The principles of ultrasound are complex, relying on sophisticated physics and mathematics. Many of these applied concepts to be described have been simplified from the comprehensive text by Kremkau [5] entitled "Diagnostic Ultrasound, Principles and Instruments." Sound is transmitted as sequential sine waves whose height represents amplitude or loudness (Fig. 2.1). A single full cycle is measured from peak to peak, and the number of these cycles per one second represents the frequency. The frequency (cps) is also described in Hertz (Hz) which by convention is in honor of the German physicist Heinrich Hertz for his work on electromagnetic transmission [6]. It is of interest that the son of Heinrich Hertz's nephew, Carl Hellmuth Hertz, is said to be credited with invention of medical ultrasound [6]. The human ear can recognize sounds as low as 20 Hz and as high as 20,000 Hz (Fig. 2.2), and ultrasound is so named because its frequency emission is in the range of more than a million cycles per second or in the megahertz (mHz) range. An ultrasound wave is transmitted to human tissues through the transducer by physical deformation of the tissue surface. This is accomplished through piezoelectric crystals which elongate and shorten in response to applied alternating electrical current (Fig. 2.3). These crystals are organized in 128 parallel channels which emit sound waves of equal frequency into the tissues (Fig. 2.4). Besides containing the vibrating crystals, the transducer at the contact interface with the skin contains a structure of matching layers which permits better energy transfer. Piezoelectric crystals employed for

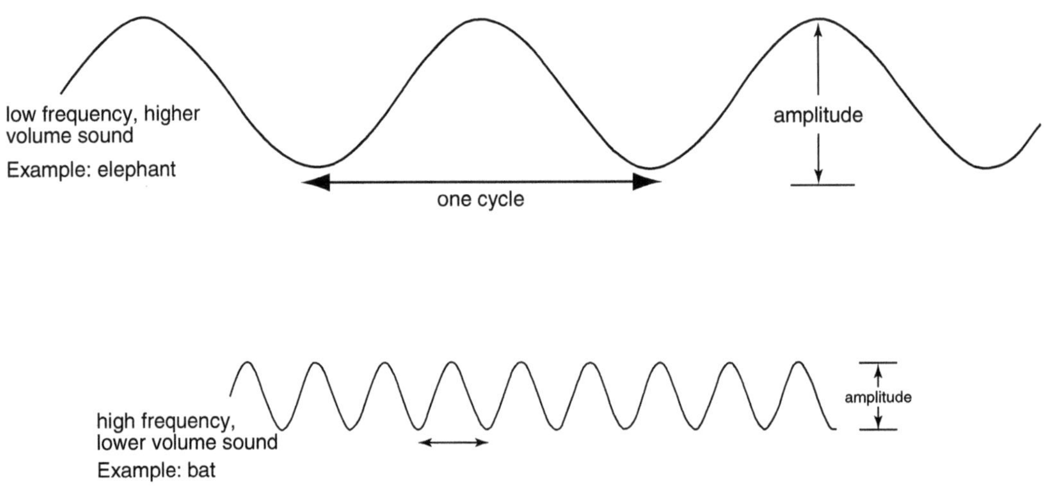

Fig. 2.1 Sound travels as linked sine waves. The frequency is determined by the number of cycles per unit of time and loudness by the amplitude. Sound travels at varying speeds through tissues depending on tissue density and properties

ultrasound are synthetic (PZT=lead zirconate titanate) as opposed to naturally existing crystals such as quartz.

As these emitted sound waves enter the skin and deeper structures, they are reflected back toward the transducer by a variety of tissue elements. Most waves either reflect at angles from these reflectors or pass through without returning directly to the transducer. Only 1% of entering sound is reflected directly back, but it is these waves which are responsible for presenting the eventual images. The tissues contain structures which are of varying density, and these adjacent contrasting elements produce an acoustical mismatch. This mismatch or interface acts as a reflector. When the tissues or fluid through which the sound waves travel is of even consistency and the reflector is broadly uniform such as the posterior wall of a cyst, a bright evident, hyperechoic signal just deep to the entire posterior wall is produced. This artifact is consistently helpful in diagnosing a cystic structure and occasionally a mass lesion such as a pleomorphic adenoma. This solid mass can be noted in the submaxillary or parotid gland, is comprised in large part by a diffuse myxoid stroma, and with ultrasound often demonstrates the same posterior enhancement identified with cysts.

Sound waves are emitted in packets of pulsed cycles and then stop for one frequency cycle to allow the same transducer to receive these reflected impulses and convert them into electrical energy. This is accomplished by the same emitting piezoelectric crystals which are set into vibration on the mechanical return. Acoustic waves progressively lose amplitude as they pass through tissues, a phenomenon known as attenuation. The extent of this attenuation depends on the tissue density and depth required for sound waves to reach the visual desired target (Fig. 2.5).

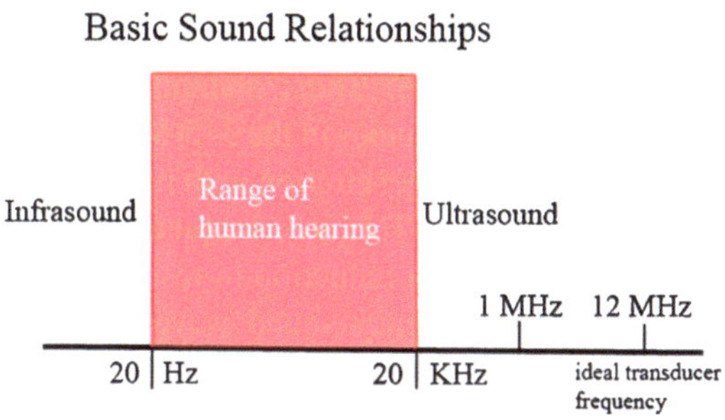

Fig. 2.2 Humans hear frequencies from 20 to 20,000 cycles/s. Ultrasound is above 20 kHz and infrasound below 20 Hz

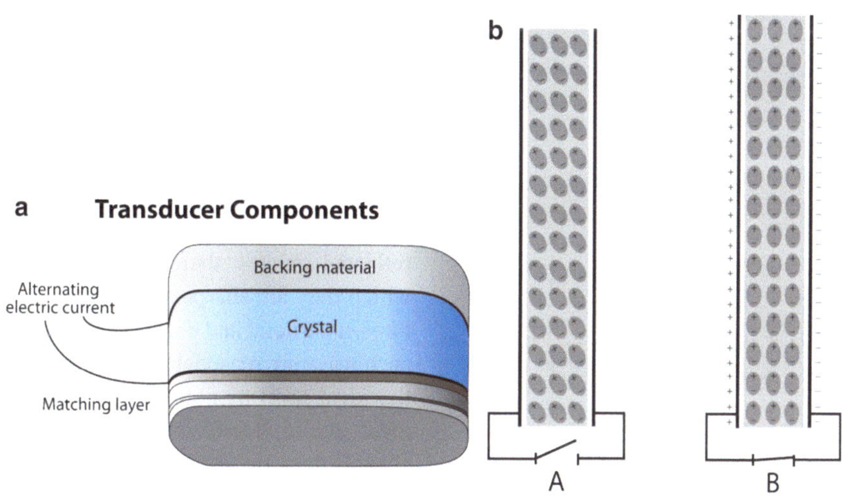

Fig. 2.3 (**a**) The transducer is comprised of piezoelectric crystals surrounded by insulating material and matching layers at the exit port which allow ideal transmission of the sound waves through the skin into the tissues. (**b**) Piezoelectric crystals elongate and shorten with realignment of the crystal dipoles in response to applied alternating current

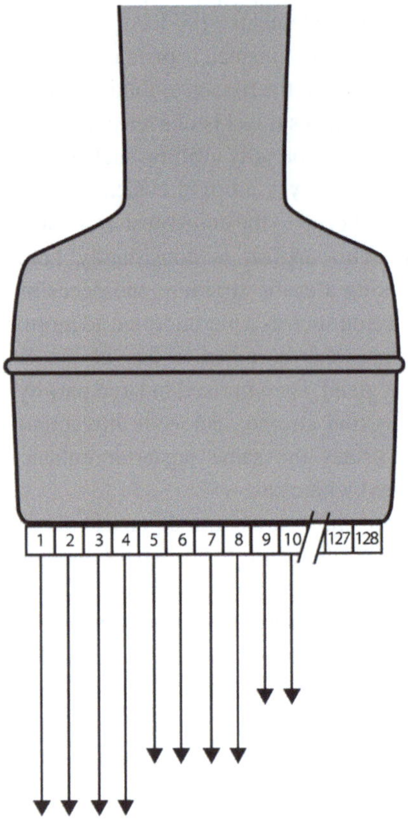

Fig. 2.4 Each crystal resides in its own sectored compartment adjacent to others which will send waves into the tissues upon command

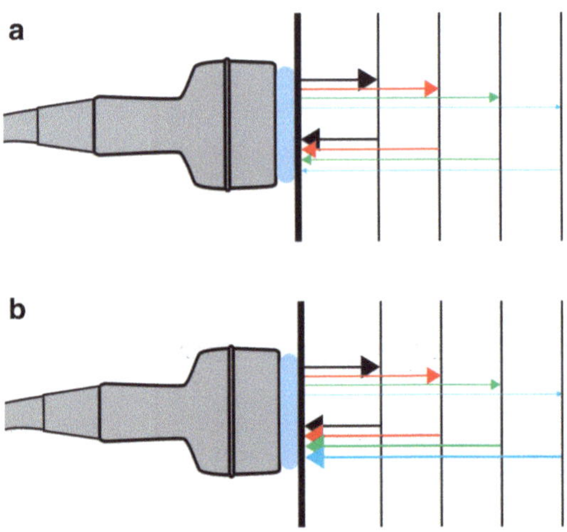

Fig. 2.5 (**a**) As ultrasound waves enter tissues, they attenuate with depth from the surface. High-frequency waves attenuate more than those of low frequency. (**b**) Time-gain compensation allows selective amplification of the weaker deep and intermediate returning echoes

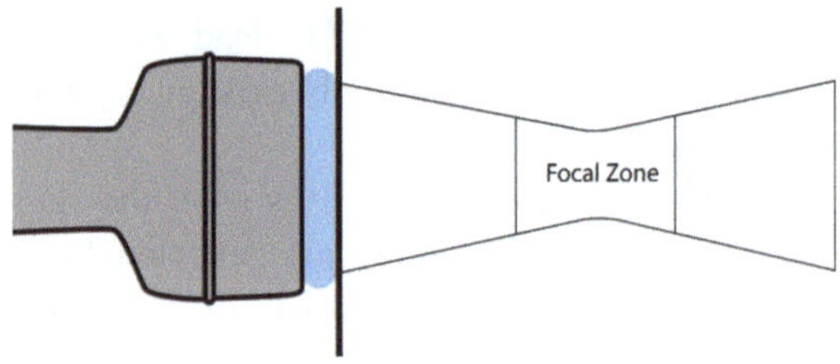

Fig. 2.6 The focused penetrating sound waves do not have a rectangular or linear pattern. The hourglass shape is typical, and the focal zone is the narrowest portion of this configuration

Another critical consideration in attenuation is the frequency of the penetrating sound waves. Low-frequency waves do not attenuate until arriving at a deeper level than those of high-frequency ultrasound. Thus, abdominal ultrasound utilizes frequencies in the 3–5-MHz range to achieve adequate penetration with retention of adequate reflection. This low frequency comes at a cost as there is a reduction in resolution. In contrast, high-frequency sound waves produce greater resolution which if possible is always desirable to achieve. Structures in the head and neck are relatively superficial in location and do not require the lower-frequency deep penetrating waves. A 10–12-MHz transducer readily demonstrates all of the relevant anatomy of the thyroid gland, parathyroid glands, and adjacent lymph nodes.

In addition to frequency, other characteristics of sound waves are highly relevant to attainment of ideal resolution. Sound waves emit and do not maintain a purely linear shape. Its physical form becomes centrally narrowed ("focal point") as it passes through tissue in the approximate shape of an hourglass (Fig. 2.6). If one examines the reflected images, there is an optimum depth at which they are sharpest in resolution. The structures superficial and deep to this narrowed area of each wave are reasonably well resolved but not to the ideal level as noted at the focal point. This ideal area or "focal zone" can be adjusted on the console to a preferred shallow or deeper depth. The image clarity at the focal zone is designated its "lateral resolution" (Fig. 2.7). The frequency of the transmitted wave determines another type of clarity-designated "axial resolution."

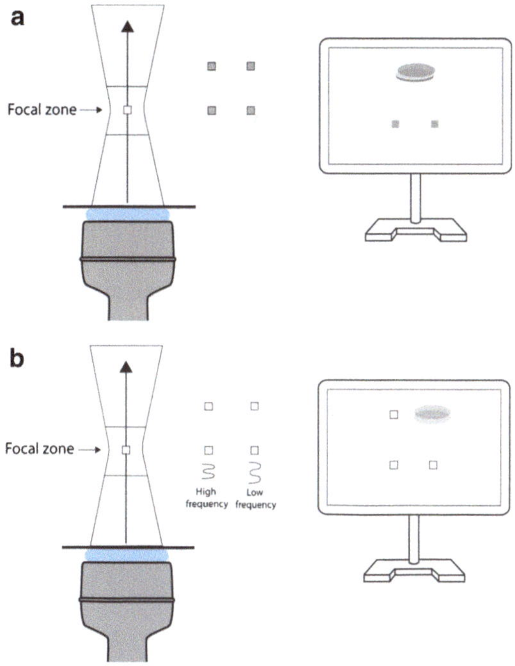

Fig. 2.7 (**a**) Lateral resolution depends more on alignment of the ideal focal zone to the region in question. Those points near or within the focal zone will be discerned as separate and better resolved. (**b**) Linear resolution depends on the frequency of the emitting ultrasound wave with higher frequencies permitting better definition of adjacent points. As well, this image demonstrates that both linear and lateral resolution work together to provide the optimum resolution

As indicated above, high-frequency sound waves produce a profile of resolution which is superior to that produced by low-frequency waves. The ability to separate adjacent points of interest into their individual components is what produces both contrast and clarity. High-frequency waves produce better ability to resolve adjacent tissue elements in the direct path of the sound wave, and this "axial resolution" in concert with a preferred level of "lateral resolution" allows the sonographer to achieve the best image quality. In summary, where depth of penetration is the most important priority such as a thick multinodular or substernal goiter, the lower-frequency waves must be utilized with some sacrifice in resolution. In most other circumstances involving the neck tissues, high-frequency waves may be selected since only a 3–4-cm tissue depth is under study.

Besides these frequency issues, other manipulations of the image can be performed from the console. The overall image brightness can be adjusted by a turn of the gain control knob, but this is not selective and affects all structures on the display. As previously described, ultrasound waves attenuate at greater depth from surface entry. The attenuation is especially problematic when higher frequencies are employed as in thyroid and parathyroid imaging. When the deeper aspects of a large goiter with 6–7 cm of A–P dimension are difficult to see, the time-gain compensation knob can be manipulated to brighten the attenuating structures. The deeper attenuated waves can be selectively amplified with time-gain compensation by increasing the gain of these waves while leaving unaltered the more superficial waves which have never lost their image brightness. Thus, the overall image has a more even distribution of brightness. There are other proprietary methods of improving image quality. SonoCT [7] changes the way sound waves are delivered from the transducer. Adjacent channels send divergent waves from a central point which then intersect with several adjacent waves which similarly have been modified. The intersections of these waves produce an image which has better contrast and sharpness. Electronic noise is an undesirable but unavoidable element in amplification systems. This noise can be reduced by band pass filtering which eliminates the frequencies above and below the ideal selected frequency. Harmonic imaging is a common refinement which manipulates both the fundamental and second harmonic frequency echo reception. The fundamental frequency is filtered while allowing passage of the second harmonic, a postprocessing method which improves image quality. Modern ultrasound units have employed several unique methods beyond the traditional elements of acoustic physics to refine image quality which were simply unimaginable less than a decade ago.

Artifacts

Artifacts are images which appear on the display and do not represent actual physical structures. These shadows or enhanced representation of tissue elements tell a story. Pure thyroid or parathyroid cysts have a thin capsule and are fluid-filled without significant solid components. Sound enters the cyst as strong signals penetrating the anterior capsule. Since the interior of the cyst is fluid which readily transmits sound without interruption, the parallel sound waves then strike the posterior capsule which through the acoustical mismatch acts as a reflector. A large proportion of these waves penetrate just beyond this capsule and concentrate as uniform returning reflecting signals. This produces a relatively broad area which is hyperechoic to adjacent tissues and the cyst itself. "Posterior enhancement" is the designated artifact invariably diagnostic of a cyst (Fig. 2.8). As described above, the unique tissue characteristics of a pleomorphic adenoma also produce posterior enhancement due to the uniform tissue matrix (Fig. 2.9). In contradistinction to this permissive transmission, coarse calcifications or close aggregates of microcalcifications block transmission of the sound waves to deeper tissue planes. This produces a dark rectangular area deep to the densely hyperechoic structure. Known as posterior shadowing artifact (Fig. 2.10), this particular image is representative of a consolidation of calcium. In contrast, microcalcifications (Fig. 2.11) generally seen in papillary carcinoma of the thyroid gland do not produce posterior shadowing artifact as a result of their small size. These microcalcifications are small points of hyperechoic signal and represent either psammoma bodies defined histologically in papillary

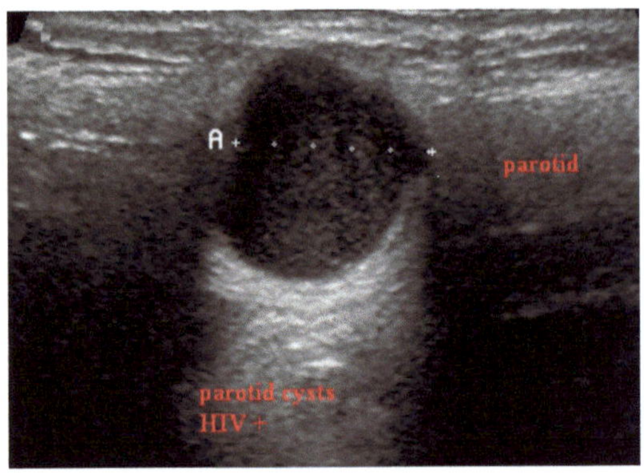

Fig. 2.8 Posterior enhancement deep to the posterior capsule of a cyst

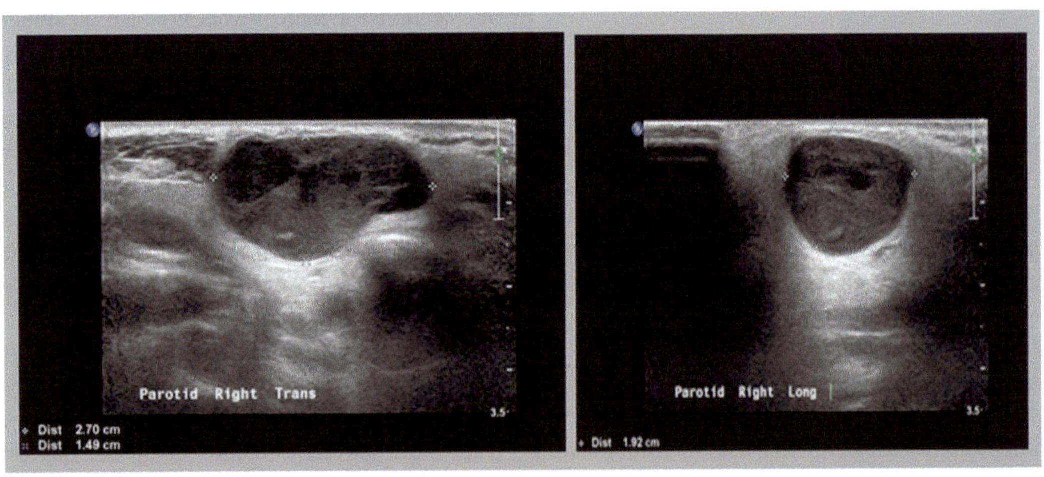

Fig. 2.9 Similar posterior enhancement deep to a pleomorphic adenoma, a testimony to the uniform character of its tissues and even transmission of sound waves with little attenuation

carcinoma or aggregates of amyloid or fibrosis noted in some medullary carcinomas. Microcalcifications may be identified in either the primary thyroid carcinoma or metastatic adenopathy (Fig. 2.12). When planning fine needle aspiration cytology, the areas selected for sampling under ultrasound guidance are often those with a large proportion of microcalcification. Other artifacts may be confused with microcalcifications. "Comet tail" artifacts (Fig. 2.13) are hyperechoic points with a tapering image of hyperlucency extending from and deep to the circular dot. The "tail" portion of this hyperechoic artifact is actually a form of reverberation. Small areas of colloid within the nodule crystallize and serve both as finite obstructions to transmission and deeper reverberation of the ultrasound waves in typical comet tails. Ahuja has studied comet tail artifacts in a large number of thyroid conditions and invariably has found that this is a marker for an underlying benign process [8]. Reverberation artifact is more of a curiosity than one which defines an important anatomic correlation. Reverberation suggests that the sound waves are reflected one or more times deeper into the tissues than the actual target but retain the same pattern and echogenicity. Some of the initial primary waves pass alongside the target but deep to it and on the return are redirected back into the tissues from the deepest aspect of the lesion. When they finally make their way back to the transducer after one or more of these delays, the signal processor incorrectly assumes and displays them as deeper structures rather than the delayed secondary echoes they really are. The anterior wall of the trachea, anterior wall of the carotid artery, biopsy needles in their long axis, and the trailing tapering region of comet tails are all examples of reverberation artifact (Fig. 2.14).

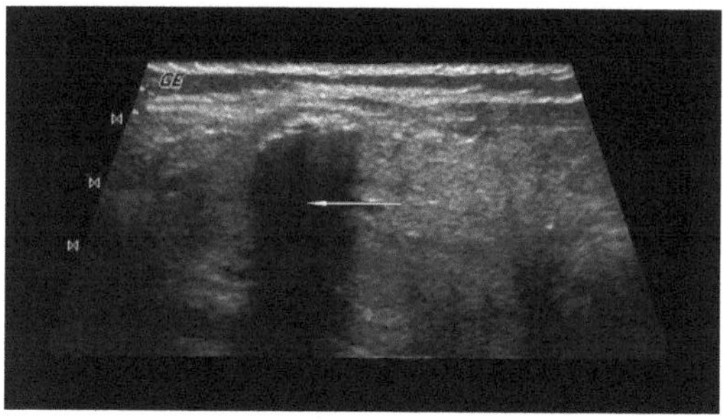

Fig. 2.10 Dense calcification prevents penetration of sound beyond the lesion resulting in posterior shadowing artifact (demonstrated by *arrow*)

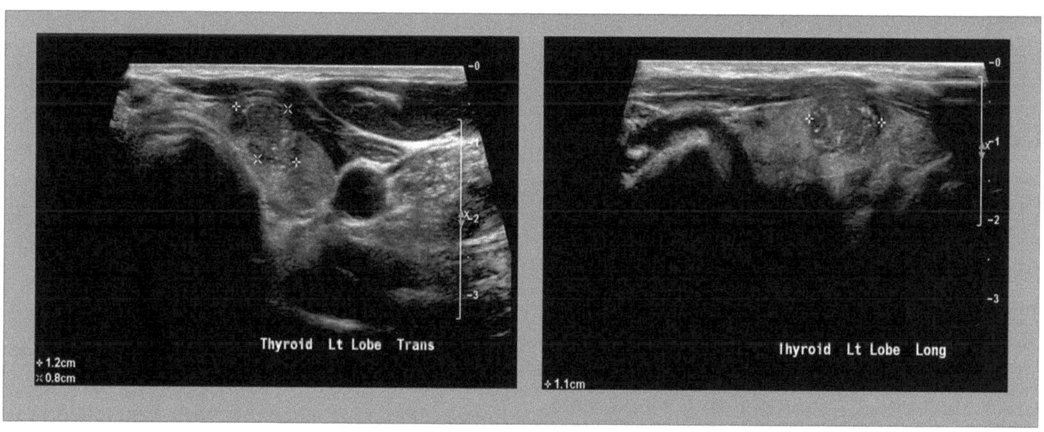

Fig. 2.11 Microcalcifications do not produce posterior shadowing artifact

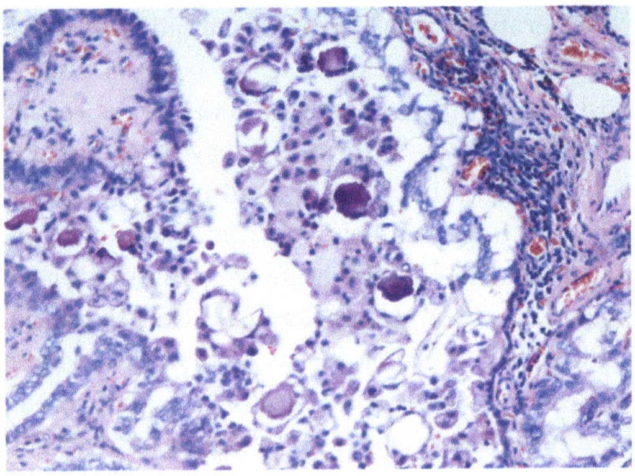

Fig. 2.12 Psammoma bodies are small, discrete calcifications commonly found in papillary carcinoma

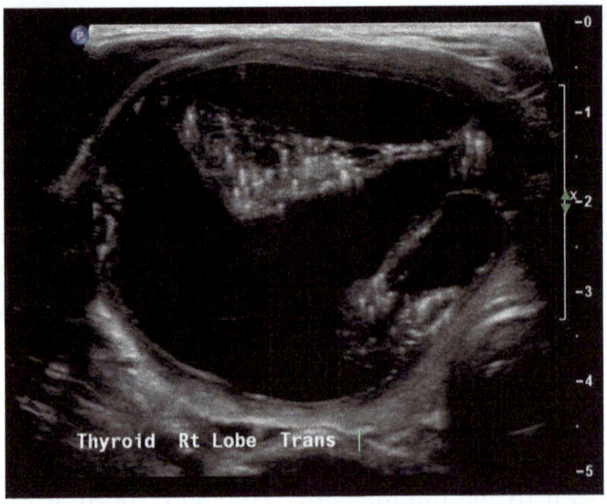

Fig. 2.13 Comet tail artifact is similar in appearance to microcalcifications, but the comet tail clearly differentiates it from the representations of psammoma bodies

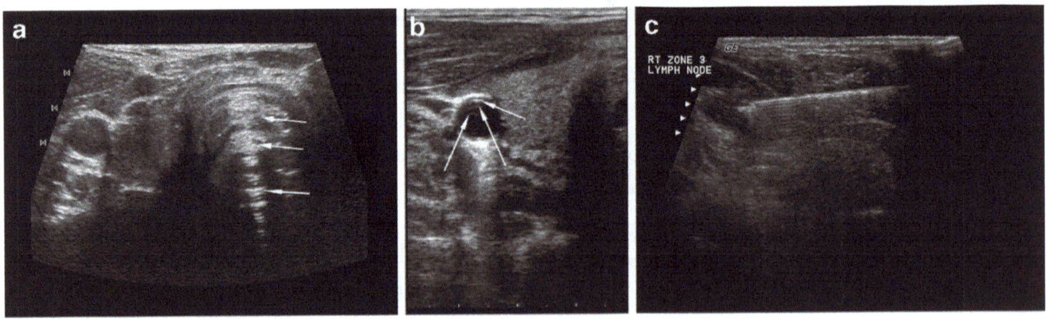

Fig. 2.14 Reverberation artifact can be seen in the following: (**a**) Anterior tracheal wall. (**b**) Anterior wall of the carotid artery. (**c**) Biopsy needles in the long axis. *Arrows* demonstrate the reverberating artifacts

Doppler

Doppler is a unique and technically different process than gray scale ultrasound. This methodology can assess the vascularity of anatomical and pathological elements. [9] The Doppler shift of sound waves occurs when waves imparted at an angle to a blood vessel penetrate the wall and strike directionally moving red blood cells. These waves are then reflected by the flowing red cells, and the reflected sound is either augmented or reduced in intensity depending on both the direction and velocity of this movement (Fig. 2.15). This velocity of red cell movement can be calculated and directional flow given a color designation, i.e., flow toward the transducer is red and away from it blue by convention. The mathematical Doppler equation can be transformed into a visual graph where systolic and diastolic velocity can be measured over a unit of time to compute actual blood flow through vessels large enough in caliber to be measured. The system then determines the exact color image and coordinates this with a matched gray scale representation of the same view. The corresponding B mode image is then alternated so rapidly with its twin Doppler representation that a moving rendition is the end product. The eye sees this as a moving color video or cine loop.

This color Doppler imaging and flow interpolation produces not only a representative image but also a quantification of the vascular activity. Although this feature is highly relevant to the study of carotid and peripheral vascular anatomy and restriction of flow, the clinician interested in Doppler application for thyroid and parathyroid work has little need of this exact realm of the technology. Power Doppler is a separate console setting which ignores these calculations and directional relationships. Power Doppler is more sensitive to low-flow states and produces a sharp image of even the smallest blood vessel. Through their sensitivity and resolution capabilities, good power Doppler systems may display a discrete blood supply through the hilum of a lymph node or vascular pattern of a hyperplastic parathyroid adenoma (Fig. 2.16). In fact, power Doppler can often be used as a differentiating tool between these two structures in the clinical setting. Color rather than power may still be used to identify a large vessel in the neck, but the quantitative issues have little clinical relevance (Fig. 2.17). Of course, one can still identify a vessel as such without any Doppler technology by observing the persistence of a rounded structure as the transducer is moved up or down over the target. The sagittal view demonstrates the vessel as well by confirming it as a long continuous structure. However, the Doppler button produces a level of efficiency in identifying a vascular structure without changing planes or leaving the area of interest. In salivary duct ectasia, where there may be confusion over whether a tubular anechoic structure is a vessel or obstructed duct, Doppler can answer this question and store the imaged result (Fig. 2.18).

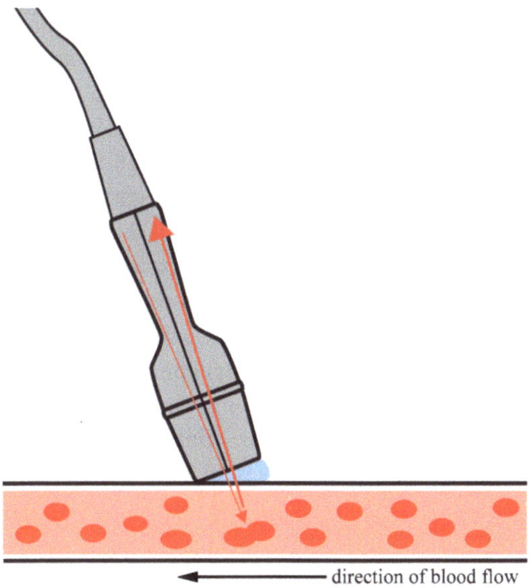

Fig. 2.15 Doppler waves reflect differentially off moving red cells. Depending on whether these cells are moving toward or away from the transducer, direction of flow and its velocity can be determined by the Doppler system

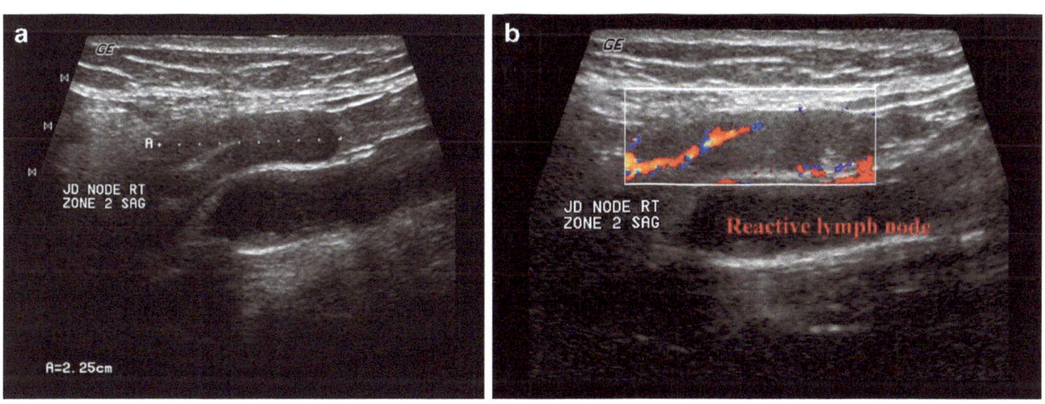

Fig. 2.16 Gray scale image of a hyperplastic lymph node with a typical "hilar line" (**a**). Power Doppler demonstrates the axial vessel penetrating the hilum of the node and representing the "hilar line" (**b**)

In summary, the modern ultrasound system is based on the physics of sound energy and transmission/reflection in tissues. It is not critical to understand in detail these principles and mathematical relationships, but a general working knowledge does provide the clinician with tools to better apply this technology to his or her clinical craft. A full understanding of artifacts with gray scale imaging is pivotal to proper ultrasound interpretation, and there are certain subtle tricks which involve manipulating the technology. As an example, there is often confusion between microcalcifications and other less important punctate hyperlucencies. It is possible to apply Doppler to these areas, turn down the color gain to a negligible degree, and demonstrate very small posterior shadowing in true microcalcifications. Another method is to eliminate harmonic imaging or SonoCT and only employ the fundamental frequency, once again to bring out the fine posterior shadowing artifact which may have been eliminated by the modern system refinements [Ahuja AT, personal communication, 2011]. In fact, there is a significant difference between reviewing the static images which someone else has obtained and the real-time study either in static or cine loop form by the treating clinician. Cine loops are the best means of reviewing an ultrasound case on referral since the study seems dynamic and as if the reviewing physician is doing the actual procedure. In the hands of the clinician, ultrasound will provide opportunities to better understand pathologic conditions and obtain more information at the time of the patient encounter than has ever before been possible.

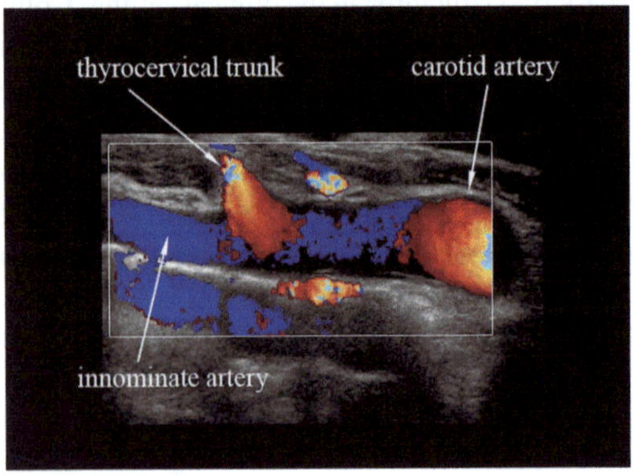

Fig. 2.17 Color Doppler demonstrates the innominate, thyrocervical trunk, and carotid artery relationships

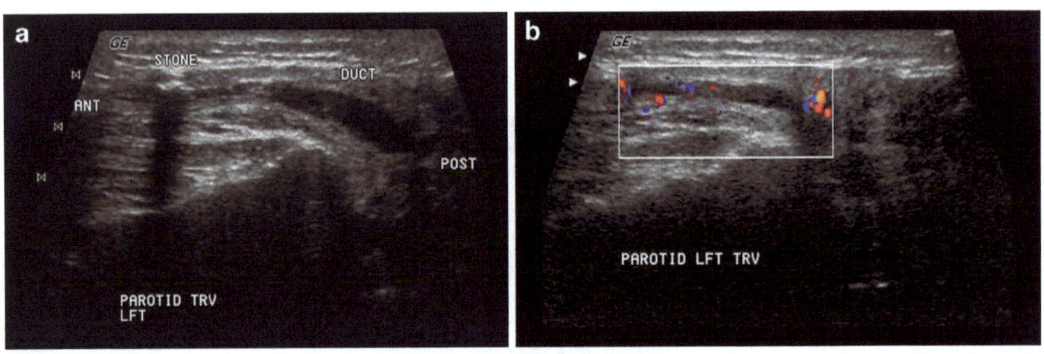

Fig. 2.18 (**a**, **b**) The use of Doppler to distinguish a vessel from duct is demonstrated in this salivary duct calculus producing obstruction and duct ectasia. The gray scale image alone cannot easily make that determination, but the addition of Doppler confirms that the widened anechoic structure is not a vessel

References

1. Au W, Popper A, Fay R. Hearing by Whales and Dolphins. Springer handbook of auditory research Vol. 12, pp. 72, 85, 89, 2000.
2. Simmons JA et al. Echolocation and hearing in the mouse-tailed bat, *Rhinopoma hardwickei*: acoustic evolution of echolocation in bats. J Comp Physiol. 1984;154:347–56.
3. Reuter T, Nummela S. Elephant hearing. J Acoustic Soc Am. 1998;104:1122–3.
4. Payne K. Silent thunder: in the presence of elephants. New York: Penguin Group; 1998. p. 121.
5. Kremkau FW. Diagnostic ultrasound. 6th ed. Philadelphia: WB Saunders; 2002. 18–37, 62–64, 71–76, 86–92, 167–194, 273–318.
6. Hertz H. Wikipedia, en.wikipedia.org. Accessed January 3, 2011.
7. Freedman MT, et al. Ultrasound images of implanted tumors in nude mice using Sono-CT correlated with MRI appearance. In: Chin-Tu Chen, Anne V. Clough (eds) Medical Imaging 2001: Physiology and Function from Multidimensional Images; 2001. pp.163–167.
8. Ahuja A, Evans R. Practical head and neck ultrasound. London: Greenwich Medical Media Ltd; 2000. p. 41.
9. Deane C. Doppler ultrasound: principles and practice. In: Nicolaides K, Rizzo G, Hecker K, and Ximines R. (eds) Doppler in Obstetrics. http://www.centrus.com/commonultrasoundcases/principlesofultrasound.html. Accessed January 15, 2011.

3 Practical Concepts of Ultrasound

Robert A. Sofferman

When to Use Ultrasound

The use of office-based ultrasound depends on the type of practice the clinician has developed. Whether performing from the perspective of otolaryngology or general surgery, the head and neck surgeon with a thorough knowledge of anatomy is ideally suited to perform thyroid ultrasound and assessment of adjacent structures. Similarly, the endocrinologist has a need to understand the conditions affecting the thyroid and parathyroid glands even though a direct surgical intervention is not part of his or her practice realm. In the past, all ultrasound images were obtained in the radiology department, and they were transferred to the clinician as a composite either in an envelope or through a digital format. The static nature of these images was a real limitation in the process and really did little to engage the clinician. In addition, the prohibitive cost of ultrasound units and their size did little to move the technology to an office base. Within the past decade, this has all undergone an accelerated transition. Ultrasound companies have understood the value in this new market and have become flexible in configuring systems to the needs of different specialties. Of course, obstetrical ultrasound has preceded these concepts and likely led the way to where we have finally arrived. In general surgery, ultrasound of the breast has been a basic technique for obtaining guided biopsies both in the clinic and operating room. Ultrasound has become a standard method of determining the presence of intraperitoneal blood after mechanical blunt or penetrating trauma usually performed in the emergency room by residents, surgeons, and emergency room physicians. In fact, the FAST examination has allowed these clinicians to quickly determine whether retroperitoneal and/or pericardial blood has also become part of the trauma equation. Vascular laboratories have developed in the surgical office setting which allows the vascular surgeon to have a firsthand understanding of applied flow dynamics. Intracavitary transducers have expanded the management of rectal and prostate cancer again for the clinician in the outpatient setting. There are many other uses of outpatient ultrasound, and these few examples are only an introduction to its application in thyroidology.

Ultrasound of the thyroid gland is its most effective imaging tool. Not only is it efficient and readily available, but the advances in resolution place it on a par with CT and MRI scans. It allows precise measurements of single or multiple thyroid nodules, definition of whether lesions are likely benign or suspect for malignancy, identification of conditions other than nodular change, and adjacent lymphadenopathy, just to illustrate a few common uses of the modality. With transportation of ultrasound to the office, endocrinologists and surgeons can measure change in size of

R.A. Sofferman (✉)
Division of Otolaryngology-Head and Neck Surgery, Fletcher Allen Health Care, University of Vermont School of Medicine, 111 Colchester Ave, Burlington, VT 05401, USA
e-mail: robert.sofferman@vtmednet.org

R.A. Sofferman and A.T. Ahuja (eds.), *Ultrasound of the Thyroid and Parathyroid Glands*, DOI 10.1007/978-1-4614-0974-8_3, © Springer Science+Business Media, LLC 2012

nodules over time. In addition to allowing the same examiner to perform measurements at each time interval, this procedure provides a significant level of efficiency for the patient. This is especially important when a patient travels long distances from a small community where high-resolution ultrasound may not be readily available. The initial office-based clinical evaluation or follow-up can be combined with this imaging opportunity to provide a cost-effective and convenient assessment.

Of course, in addition to the diagnostic side of ultrasound, the opportunity to not only perform general fine needle aspiration of a lesion but also more importantly to sample specific subareas creates a specificity which is now possible with higher-resolution imaging. Lymphadenopathy is an important adjunct to assessment of thyroid disease, especially in the realm of postthyroidectomy surveillance in papillary carcinoma. The ability to identify subtle lymph node enlargement is an important element of this surveillance, especially when there is only mild elevation in thyroglobulin or the patient has thyroglobulin antibodies. The addition of Tg washout to the basic cytologic detail comes from an ultrasound opportunity.

In consideration of hyperparathyroidism, ultrasound is a critical component of the surgical evaluation. When there is concordance with the sestamibi scans, the surgical approach may clearly change to a focused limited-access procedure. Occasionally, an enlarged parathyroid gland cannot be identified in one or more cardinal positions, but a separate suspect site within the thyroid gland or elsewhere in the neck must be clarified. With ultrasound guidance, these lesions can be sampled with PTH washout of the needle. There are circumstances when a mass in the thymus or atypical location cannot be defined as being of parathyroid origin. The use of high-resolution Power Doppler can often illustrate the vascularity which defines either hyperplastic lymph node or parathyroid adenoma.

With this brief introduction, let us travel through the basic ultrasound examination of the thyroid gland, parathyroid glands, and lymph node basins of the neck.

Gray-Scale Imaging of the Thyroid Gland

Position

Traditionally, the patient is placed in the supine position with a roll of fabric such as a sheet or compressed pillow beneath the shoulders such that the neck is in mild hyperextension. This has the effect of elevating the thyroid gland somewhat and bringing it slightly closer to the surface of the neck. However, patients do not tolerate significant extension for a prolonged period, especially the older patient who may have cervical arthritis or neck inflexibility. In the outpatient otolaryngology clinic, patients are examined sitting upright in a mobile chair which can change to a horizontal attitude. Even in the sitting position, the head rest can be retracted such that the neck extension is adequate for complete inspection of the neck and thyroid glands. During fine needle aspiration, the chair is changed to a horizontal position to reduce the likelihood of a vasovagal response. In conventional ultrasound, the examiner is at the right side of the patient and the console just above the level of the right shoulder. The patient's head is in the midline for thyroid examination, but slight rotation of the head away from the midline can be employed for inspection of lymph nodes or other lateral areas of interest. During aspiration cytology, patient and relative clinician position may vary depending on preferred techniques. In the usual aspiration, there is no change in these relative positions, and it is preferable to have an assistant on the left side of the patient to perform certain functions. If simple capillary techniques are utilized for aspiration, the needle and expelling syringe can be handed directly to the operator who is focused on the transducer and target relationships. If aspiration is preferred, an intervening length of tubing can be inserted between the aspiration needle which the operator holds and a syringe which the assistant controls. Upon request, the assistant aspirates slightly and then discontinues this as the needle is withdrawn. Additionally, the assistant can hold pressure on the entry site if bleeding or hematoma formation seems to be developing.

Hand position on the transducer is often overlooked and an important topic to address. The radiologic technologist who is performing ultrasound examinations all day long must use a technique which is comfortable and ergonomic. Similarly, the clinician should hold and apply the transducer in a way which is stable and comfortable. It is preferable to hold the transducer with the right hand as low as possible such that the fourth and fifth fingers actually rest on the patient's neck skin. With this method, there is less chance that the transducer will slip and require repositioning. Abundant gel should be used to maximize image quality and smooth slide of the transducer over the skin. Because of this, all annotations and manipulations of the dials and knobs on the console should be done with the free, non-gel-covered left hand so that the equipment can be best protected.

Thyroid Gland

The neck is examined with a high-frequency linear transducer with ideal range from 10 to 12 mHz. Certainly frequencies of 7 mHz can produce acceptable images but likely of lesser resolution. Images of the thyroid gland are performed in the transverse plane from the most superior to inferior aspect of the thyroid gland in a slow and careful manner to make certain that any pathology is not missed. In fact, occasionally nodules of thyroid origin can be identified as separate from but close to the thyroid gland in the upper mediastinum. The careful examination can identify these lesions as the lower pole of the thyroid is surveyed. After "freezing" the maximum dimension of the lobe in question, measurements are produced in the mid-transverse and mid-anteroposterior dimension and appropriately saved and annotated. The isthmus is inspected from its superior to inferior position and its AP dimension measured. The opposite lobe of the thyroid is similarly measured. Once the overall dimensions of the thyroid are established, individual lesions are examined. It is important to establish a pattern of examination which is consistent from one patient to another such that no omissions are made. Perhaps the simplest technique is to examine and characterize each lesion independently from a superior to inferior direction, taking care to record and annotate both transverse and AP dimensions of each lesion, as well as defining the lateral or medial positions. Power Doppler of each lesion is important, as nodules which demonstrate increased internal vascularity are suspicious and often the principal target of aspiration cytology. Whether to perform the Doppler after each gray-scale measurement or after the entire gland is surveyed depends on operator preference, but again standardization is a most important methodology. Once the gland is surveyed, an efficient screening examination of lymph node zones II through VI should be performed. Of course, the nature of the thyroid lesion will depend on just how much time is spent in examining the lymph node regions. A highly suspect thyroid nodule may require a more detailed and repeated examination of adjacent lymph nodes to the thyroid gland, especially zones III–VI.

Circumstances in which the lesion or structure in question is quite large can pose a problem beyond routine scanning methods. The cine loop is one means of visualizing the entirety of a large structure in transverse, sagittal, or both planes. However, this will not permit the image to be rendered static or frozen for measurement. A simple way to achieve approximate measurements is to select a recognizable element in the middle of the target, such as a cyst margin, vessel, or calcification. A measurement from the perimeter to that point can be determined and the process then repeated from that point to the opposite perimeter in a second image. These two distances can then be manually added together providing the full dimension (Fig. 3.1a). This method may be required for very large thyroid masses or the dimensions of a goiter. Another technique is somewhat analogous but allows display of both of these images as a composite for biplanar measurement. With the split- or dual-screen technique, the large lesion can be divided into approximate halves and then one half is frozen while the other remains mobile. Using simple visual estimation on the screen, the transducer is

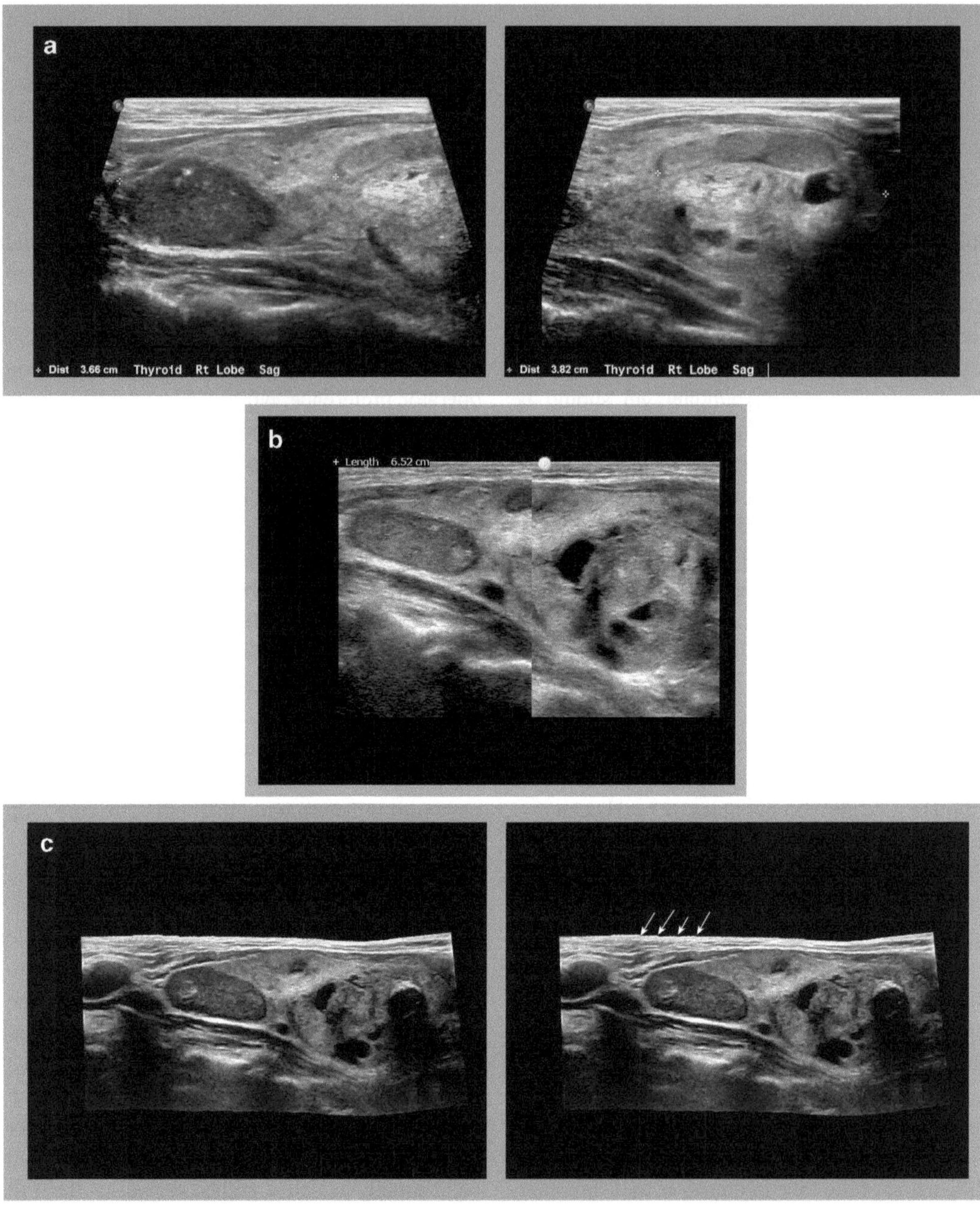

Fig. 3.1 Three methods of measuring large thyroid glands are illustrated in the same patient with a multinodular goiter. The sagittal view is utilized. (**a**) Linear measurement. The measurements are obtained in two parts to a common central point of reference. (**b**) Dual-screen merge and measurement. (**c**) Panoramic measurement. Some systems allow panoramic accrual of images. The *arrows* denote the linkage of each of multiple images. The completed product is similar to the way panoramic "stitching" photographic software programs produce a composite wider view than can be obtained with a single photograph

moved such that the mobile image appears to move toward the static half to the point where a selected same element from each half is overlapped as closely as possible. At this exact point the moving image is frozen as well, producing a composite image. From this point the completed image can be measured and stored (Fig. 3.1b). Panoramic imaging is a technique which some contemporary ultrasound systems employ to display large masses. In this method, the transducer is moved in the direction of the scan plane while the panoramic process is activated from the console. The immediate previous echo information is retained and displayed while the new images are sequentially added as the transducer moves to the next area. This method requires a slow, steady movement of the transducer along a precise path so that the new and previous images are in register. Once the end point is reached and the approximate termination element on the console activated, the entire panorama is displayed as a composite image again allowing measurement and storage (Fig. 3.1c). The image acquisition must be done as the transducer is moved along its long axis. For example, a panorama cannot be obtained by moving the transducer from the inferior to superior aspect of a transverse image with the transducer in a transverse orientation. It must be changed to a sagittal position and then moved from the inferior to superior aspect of the target. As with all scanning techniques, the operator's left index finger should rest slightly on the freeze button to appropriately end the study at the desired point.

Parathyroid Glands

The normal parathyroid glands cannot be visualized with routine ultrasound, at least not with the current technology. Ultrasound is very appropriate for the surgeon to perform since he/she has a strong vested interest in accurate preoperative localization. It is preferable to perform the ultrasound without knowledge of the sestamibi result so there is no bias and better objective comparisons can be rendered. In primary hyperparathyroidism, there is likelihood that a single adenoma will be responsible and if large enough readily identified. In fact there are many circumstances where the sestamibi scan will be negative and ultrasound will actually identify a defined adenoma. In patients with diffuse hyperplasia, the sestamibi scan will usually fail to demonstrate delayed washout of all or even some of the enlarged parathyroid glands. However, ultrasound will usually demonstrate more than one enlarged parathyroid glands which indicates the need for inspection of all parathyroids rather than a focused exploration. The cardinal positions of the parathyroid glands are examined sequentially, and those which are enlarged are hypoechoic and extrathyroidal in position. Power Doppler invariably identifies a large vessel immediately anterior to the enlarged gland which is an extension of the inferior thyroid artery. This parathyroid artery continues as its extension and enters the parathyroid adenoma as a single blunt vessel. When the expected enlarged parathyroid gland cannot be identified, careful inspection of the thyroid gland should be performed. Any mass or cystic lesion within the thyroid should be sampled with needle washout for parathyroid hormone (PTH). If there is nothing suspect for a parathyroid enlargement in or near the thyroid gland, ectopic sites should be examined. A systematic examination of the neck should proceed with review of the entire carotid sheath, paraesophagus, and upper neck to include the submandibular region to identify the enlarged gland. Once again, Doppler may be helpful in differentiating a mass of parathyroid origin from a lymph node, and any question can usually be settled with aspirate for PTH.

Lymph Nodes

For clinical purposes, the cervical region is divided into six separate regions. Zone I is essentially the submandibular triangle bounded by the anterior and posterior bellies of the digastric muscle and superiorly by the mandible. The next three zones are equally divided into thirds along the internal jugular vein. Zone II starts at the jugulodigastric region and the junction between zones II and III rather loosely defined. Zone III borders superiorly at the level of the hyoid bone and inferiorly at the level of the cricoid cartilage.

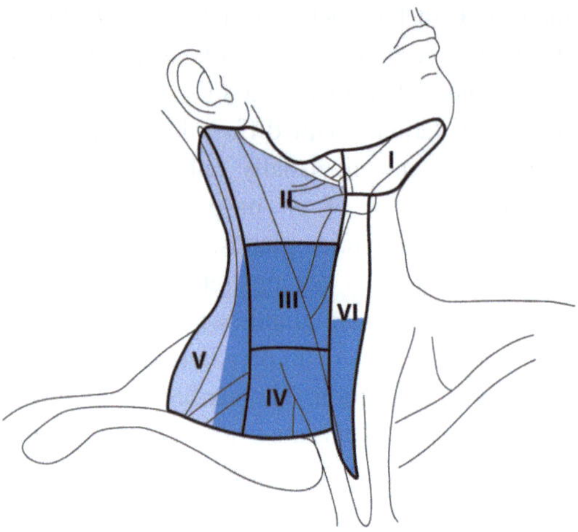

Fig. 3.2 The six primary neck zones are illustrated. Areas in *dark blue* are the most common sites and *lighter blue* the less frequent areas of metastatic papillary carcinoma

Zone IV extends from inferior zone III to the clavicle. Zone V covers the entire posterior triangle with its perimeter, the sternocleidomastoid and trapezius muscles and the clavicle inferiorly. It is actually divided into two segments, with Va craniad to the accessory nerve and Vb inferior to it. Lastly, zone VI is essentially a midline compartment bounded superiorly by the hyoid bone, inferiorly by the sternal manubrium, and laterally by the carotid arteries. Some authors indicate that there is a zone VII between the upper manubrium and innominate artery. Others consider this as part of zone VI. Metastatic lymph nodes from thyroid cancer do not generally present in zone I, and even zone II adenopathy is uncommon. Metastatic nodes from thyroid malignancy are usually found in zones III, IV, Vb, and VI (Fig. 3.2). Examination of zone VI can be problematic as the clavicle and manubrium often interfere with ideal placement of the transducer. The performance of a comprehensive survey of the entire neck for metastatic lymphadenopathy can be accomplished in many ways and depends on nothing more than a complete, careful standardized method. The authors prefer a systematic Z-shaped pattern which is simple and allows inspection of all above-mentioned zones with efficiency. The neck is examined with the transducer in the transverse position, beginning in zone I and ending at the jugulodigastric region and carotid bulb. The second limb of the "Z" follows the full course of the internal jugular vein again with transverse imaging. The transducer is positioned such that the entire anterior aspect of Zone V can be surveyed at the same time as the neck is examined to the clavicle inferiorly. The third limb of the "Z" is completed by examining the supraclavicular region posteriorly to the trapezius muscle. The posterior aspect of zone V is examined by sweeping the transducer superiorly along the anterior border of the trapezius to the mastoid tip. Lastly, zone VI is examined on either side of the midline from the hyoid to the manubrium with the transducer then angled inferiorly into the mediastinum. The examiner's eye watches for enlarged hypoechoic masses as the transducer passes through the scanning Z survey. If after the entire neck is examined in this way an area of concern has been identified, the transducer comes back to that area for a more deliberate inspection. Any suspicious node(s) is examined in both transverse and sagittal planes, and Power Doppler is applied as well. All images are properly annotated as to side and zone. If the node is obviously malignant, there is no need to perform an FNA for cytology if thyroidectomy and a neck dissection are planned. If there are any doubts, an FNA can be performed for cytology along with Tg washout.

The Ultrasound System

It is instructive to discuss the actual instrument which is responsible for performing ultrasound. Each system is comprised of a transducer, monitor or display, and console. In an effort to best explain the way these components work, the technical details are extracted and hopefully again simplified from Frederick Kremkau's text [1].

Beam Former

The pulser produces the voltage that transforms electrical into mechanical energy and generation of the desired frequency. The pulse repetition frequency (PRF) is the number of ultrasound pulses per second and averages 4–5 kHz. In order for echoes to be properly timed for reception, the emitted pulses must be received before the next pulse is transmitted. When deeper structures are imaged, the returning echoes take longer to return to the transducer. Thus, a slower PRF is required, as well as a reduced "frame rate," which is the number of images which are then generated on the display per second. Wider images and differing focuses also mandate that the PRF be reduced to avoid echo displacement.

The maximum output amplitude is approximately 100 V, and the voltage is displayed as a percentage or decibel value from 0 to 100. When amplitude is reduced, the gain dial can compensate somewhat for this. There are some variations in coded sequencing that can produce more advantageous imaging. This coded excitation produces specific pulse groupings in listening sequences, i.e., a series of three pulses followed by a missing pulse or gap, then two pulses followed by another gap, are examples of how the patterns are altered by the system automatically. Each independent delay sequence and transmission is complicated and is part of a channel comprised of the transmitting crystal, the specific amplifier, an analog-to-digital converter, and delay pattern. The typical high-resolution system has 128 of these units aligned in parallel in the transducer.

Amplifier

The amplifier exists for each channel in the beam former. The amplifiers increase the small voltages received by the transducer to larger logarithmic dimensions more suitable for additional processing. The process of amplification is linked directly to time-gain compensation. Those signals which arrive later and are of weaker amplitude are selectively amplified.

Analog-to-Digital Converters (Digitizers)

Once the echoes are amplified, they are converted to a digital form by analog-to-digital converters (ADC). Analog is the actual voltage amplitude, and its conversion to discrete numbers allows numerical coding and processing of the signals as is done with all digital electronic systems, such as CD and DVD players.

Signal Processor

Once the reception stream of echoes occurs, they are modified by the signal processor. In order for the amplified sounds to be clear without electronic noise, a band-pass filter is employed to eliminate frequencies immediately above and below the primary returning echo frequency. Another filtering modality known as harmonic imaging filters out the fundamental frequency after the sound travels through the band-pass filter and allows the second harmonic frequency to pass. This process improves image quality. The dynamic range is used to describe amplifier abilities in decibels and characterizes the ability to handle the range between the weakest and stronger returning echoes. Most amplifiers have a dynamic range of 100–160 dB. The human visual system can only appreciate a dynamic range of 20 dB. A smaller dynamic range produces an image of higher contrast. Through a process known as compression, the dynamic range can be appropriately narrowed, and this is controlled by the sonographer through the gain control knob.

The image processor converts these detected, filtered, compressed, and digitized sound echoes into images that are processed prior to storage into memory. Each emitted pulse returning to the transducer stores as information at a memory location in either a column or row depending on whether the received pulse is directly vertical or off that axis. Each scan line from one of the emitting 128 channels is received by the scan converter in a fraction of a second. When this process is duplicated multiple times per second and presented on the display, real-time sonography has occurred.

The number of pixels per unit area determines contrast resolution which is the ability of the gray-scale display to distinguish echoes of only the slightest difference in intensity. All of these aforementioned techniques prior to storage in memory are designated as preprocessing modalities. Anything done after the image is frozen and stored is referred to as postprocessing. B color is an example of postprocessing manipulation which is not ordinarily employed in ultrasound of the head and neck. Since the eye can differentiate more color tints than gray shades, a colorized display can provide improved contrast resolution.

Display

Brightness mode, also known as B mode, produces a gray-scale image on the monitor or display. This is performed with a cathode ray tube (CRT), which generates a focused beam of electrons which register a spot of light on the phosphor, fluorescent inner aspect of the tube adjacent to the display glass. These beams can move across the tube by application of electromagnetic deflection coils which surround the neck of the CRT. When the image spot reaches a margin or completed pattern, it returns to the starting point so the next image can form. These spots are activated across the monitor left to right and proceed to the next line as one would read a text in a book. The refresh rate is the number of these images per second that can be displayed. In order for the echoes to be portrayed with the proper intensity(brightness) on the CRT, a conversion back from digital to analog must be accomplished (digital-to-analog converter or DAC). The frame rate is the number of sonographic images which are stored in image memory per second, and the refresh rate is the number of times per second that a stored image is retrieved from memory and displayed. Displays must also present color information since Doppler is now most often displayed in color. The color CRTs have three cathodes and thousands of very small triple-group aggregates of color phosphor dots on the inner face of the tube. The electron beam aims at the appropriate color dot and stimulates projection of that color. These color dots are the primary colors red, green, and blue and are so close together that combinations of stimulation can produce nearly any color. A standard display (SVGA) has a pixel matrix of 1,024 × 728 and display refresh rate of 60 Hz.

The CRT displays are now replaced by flat screen LCD monitors which are lighter, do not require much power, and do not have the deep bulk of the CRT systems. LCD is an abbreviation for liquid crystal display. Liquid crystals are molecules that are somewhere between the physical characteristics of a liquid and a solid. Solids are comprised of molecules which are static and cannot move, whereas liquid molecules can both change shape and move randomly. Liquid crystals do not change their orientation but can change position. Special liquid crystals known as twisted nematics can untwist when electrical current is applied to them. In a most simplistic description, these crystals are sandwiched between two glass plates, and the rear screen is back illuminated. When an electrical current is applied to the twisted nematic, depending on the voltage, some or all of the light is transmitted as certain crystals are untwisted. The display is organized into 1,024 columns and 768 rows, and there is a specific organization to the display which allows a charge to travel down a column until it reaches a ground in one of the rows. This interaction produces a voltage emission which untwists a nematic crystal allowing specific shades of light and dark to be emitted as gray-scale projections. With color, there are subpixels with red, green, and blue filters which are activated in specific ways to produce color on the screen.

Temporal Resolution

As stated, the frame rate is the number of sonographic images which can be stored. As the transducer moves across an area of interest, the display reflects the real time changes at that rate. However, the display also depends on its refresh rate which may not be equivalent to the more rapid frame rate. It is advantageous to store at a higher frame rate, i.e., 100 Hz, to retain as much information as possible. Echo information is retrieved from memory at a lower rate, i.e., 75 Hz but can be displayed at its original frame rate through technical manipulation in the console. With cine loops, a form of movie if you will, less time between images elapses. This improved temporal resolution presents a smoother cine loop. As stated earlier, the pulse repetition frequency (PRF) must be such that deeper penetrating images have sufficient time to return before the next pulse is emitted. Thus, frame rates decrease with interest in deeper and wider structures which require more scan lines and corresponding more time to generate each frame. Frame rates may need to be controlled manually when there is interest in deeper or broader images.

Console

The console is the element which provides the operator maximum control over generated and stored images. There are variations in how each manufacturer presents these options as either knobs, sliders, or dials and precisely where these are positioned. Some systems reduce these physical elements to a greater degree but assign multiple tasks to one or more of the controls. Manufacturers try to make these activities intuitive and simple to learn, but regardless of advertised information there is always a bit of a learning curve for the sonographer when trying to adapt to a new device. In order to simplify this presentation, the principal focus will be on those elements which are useful for a clinician using ultrasound for thyroid, parathyroid, and neck imaging. Thus, details which are germane to 3D and 4D ultrasound, abdominal, and vascular studies will not be discussed.

The transducer is a critical part of the system which should be covered in brief. The footprint or size of the part that contacts the skin can vary in size depending on the manufacturer. Smaller footprints may be easier to hold and manipulate low in the neck, especially when examining for nodes in zone VI adjacent to the clavicle and sternal manubrium. The disadvantage of the small footprint is that a narrower image is produced with less anatomical area covered. The transducer is the most expensive accessory and must be properly cared for. It must be carefully replaced into its holder after each individual scan, as a fall to the floor can break delicate crystal elements and reduce resolution. In addition, the backing and cover of the transducer are very sensitive to alcohol which will eventually lead to cracking and likely void the warranty. One solution during FNA is to wrap the transducer with saran wrap after gel is applied. Thereafter generous use of alcohol to sterilize both the transducer and skin will have no adverse effects on the equipment. If the skin is appropriately wet with alcohol and gel has been appropriately applied between the saran wrap and transducer, excellent image quality can be expected. Some individuals employ a surgical glove or commercial cover, but the saran wrap is a cheaper alternative and conforms better than any other item.

The console, display, and stand are on wheels which allow easy manipulation about the examining room or transport beyond. Every console has knobs or dials which permit image modification. A keyboard for typing function allows alterations in annotation beyond any organized preset. Some annotations are created through a "touch screen"; others, through either a key stroke or full-typed notation. The most commonly manipulated buttons on the console except for the trackball and those which allow measurements are indicated in *italics* in the next few sentences in the text. Each area of interest is identified and captured with the *freeze* button, and thereafter the appropriate annotation is applied on the display screen. Every image of interest is **saved** to the hard drive. Every image is examined in three planes: transverse, anteroposterior (AP), and sagittal. The most basic manipulation is the *gain* button, which changes the brightness of the image on the display. It is simply a matter of operator preference, what appeals to his/her eye and seems to allow the best contrast appearance. The *focus button* is rotated to position one or more markers at the appropriate depth where the structure of interest resides. This optimizes specific lateral resolution. The *depth* button produces a range of interest, from the surface into the tissues. As a rule, depths of greater than 6 cm are rarely used in head and neck ultrasound. When the depth is increased, the overall image size decreases. The *time-gain compensation* (TGC) sliders are set for average imaging when they are all aligned in the middle position. It is possible to selectively brighten portions of the image rather than using the gain knob to change the entire image itself. This would brighten the deep regions but increase the more superficial and middle images to an abnormal extent. Items of interest can be measured by using cursors providing accurate, reproducible renderings. In fact, the depth of a lesion from the surface can also be determined which may be important for certain techniques such as core biopsy. Most systems used for thyroid and neck ultrasound have specific settings which optimize the image quality by establishing presets of frame rates which usually do not require alteration. Breast and soft part imaging uses the same presets.

In gray scale, vessels may appear as circular structures that could be confused with cysts, especially since there may be posterior enhancement from blood in a vessel. However, as the transducer is moved vertically maintaining its transverse orientation, the circular structure persists as such, defining this as a blood vessel. If the transducer is rotated to a sagittal position, the structure can easily be demonstrated as a long vessel if the axis of the transducer is synchronous with the vessel orientation. Of course, another technique simply involves pressing one of the Doppler buttons to display the internal color as blood flow. *Power Doppler* is preferred for most thyroid, parathyroid, and node identification applications. It demonstrates low flow in small vessels allowing interpretation of pattern rather than direction or magnitude of flow.

Other imaging qualities may be proprietary for different manufacturers. As an example, SonoCT is a setting whereby each channel emits three to nine diverging sound waves from a point along the full length of the mid-central axis of the transducer (Fig. 3.3). In an analogy to CT X-ray scanning, these multiple sound waves intersect at selected depths to produce a more refined image at the multiple points of intersection. This setting can be turned on and off from the console. One disadvantage of the use of SonoCT is the loss of posterior-shadowing artifact seen with calcifications. In cases where identification of a calculus or calcification is important, it would be best to perform at least the search for the calcification without SonoCT. Some units provide a sector type of image even though the transducer array is linear. This provides a wider field of display. Other systems allow a wider image than standard with a simple selection of "wide scan" on the console. These are but a few examples of advances in the console and system technology which optimize image quality and presentation.

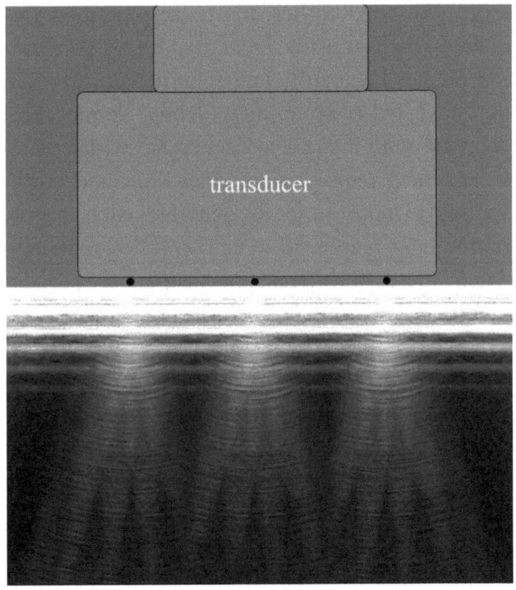

Fig. 3.3 The principle of SonoCT is demonstrated by three paper clips positioned transverse to the long axis of the transducer. The sound waves spread from a central point at the skin level and then spread to a vector pattern. Although these three beams are quite separated in distance, there is still some overlap which is much more complex in the actually SonoCT mode where channels are closely adjacent to one another. Each crystal can emit anywhere from 3 to 9 divergent beams in this mode. The larger number of beams produces a more refined image, but this is at the expense of frame rate

The Machine

Many available ultrasound machines come in different sizes, shapes, and portability (Fig. 3.4). In fact some systems are genuinely portable approaching laptop dimensions. In addition, each company has its own size and proprietary transducer system, although only linear transducers are used for B-mode ultrasound of the thyroid, parathyroid, and cervical lymph nodes (Figs. 3.5 and 3.6).

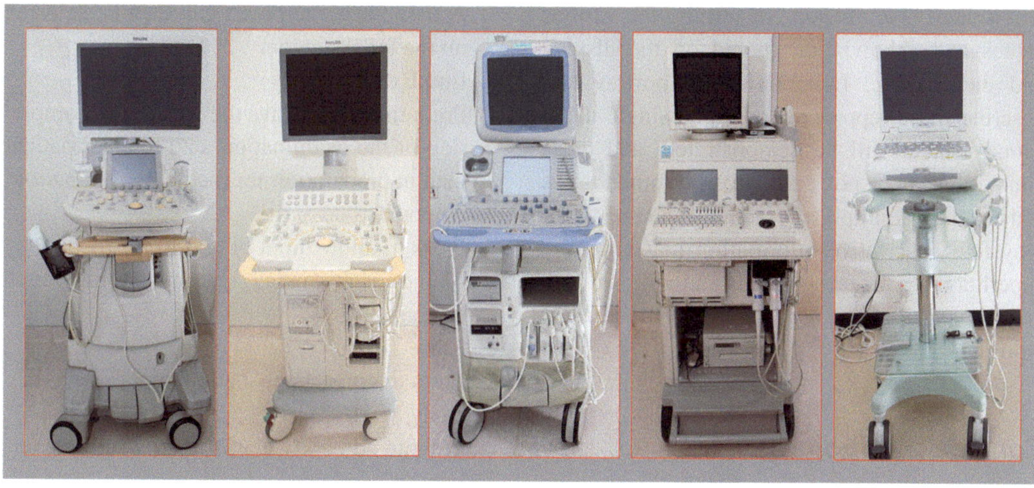

Fig. 3.4 Various ultrasound units are displayed. These are all console models, but very small portable devices have been developed. Some have all of the general capabilities of the larger standard systems

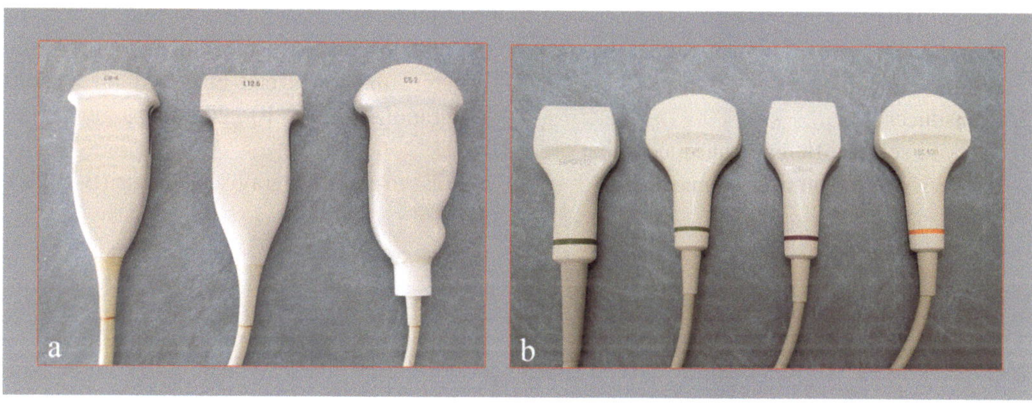

Fig. 3.5 Two sets of transducers (**a**, **b**) from separate machines are demonstrated. The linear transducer is used for neck ultrasound and is the only one with a flat footprint

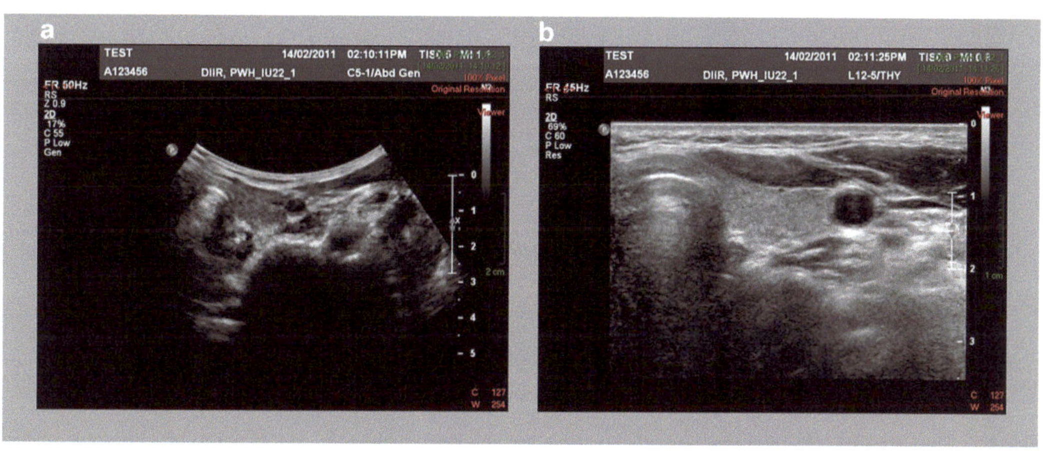

Fig. 3.6 Two thyroid scans from the same patient are obtained with a convex abdominal transducer (**a**) and a high-frequency linear transducer (**b**) to illustrate the improvement in thyroid image quality with the linear footprint

Often there is confusion concerning the various values and abbreviations noted on the display and the console. In an effort to portray and describe these representations, one single ultrasound system will be demonstrated, and these annotations may not carry over to other units. This attempt is simply a beginning, and the reader may find descriptive information that is totally superfluous to his or her needs and others which are relevant with similar function but different wording.

Console "Knobology"

The following knobs on the console are depicted in Fig. 3.7, and a brief description of individual functions is rendered in the following narrative:

1. Patient Data
   Press to enter patient information at the start of the examination.
2. Transducer
   Press to select different transducers that are connected to the ultrasound machine. A tissue-specific preset can then be selected on the touch screen.
3. End Exam
   Press to end and save the study after completion of the examination, and to clear patient data in preparation for the next examination.
4. Annotate
   Press to allow input of text to the display by typing or by using buttons on the touch screen.
5. Erase Text
   Press to erase the text annotation.
6. Body Mark
   Press to add body marks to the display.
7. Freeze
   Press to freeze/unfreeze image.
8. Print
   Press to save image onto hard disk.
9. Capture
   Press to capture a cine loop. In the setup menu, the loops can be saved for various durations, i.e., 5-, 10-, 20-s loops.
10. 2D
    Press to enter 2D gray-scale mode (B-mode).

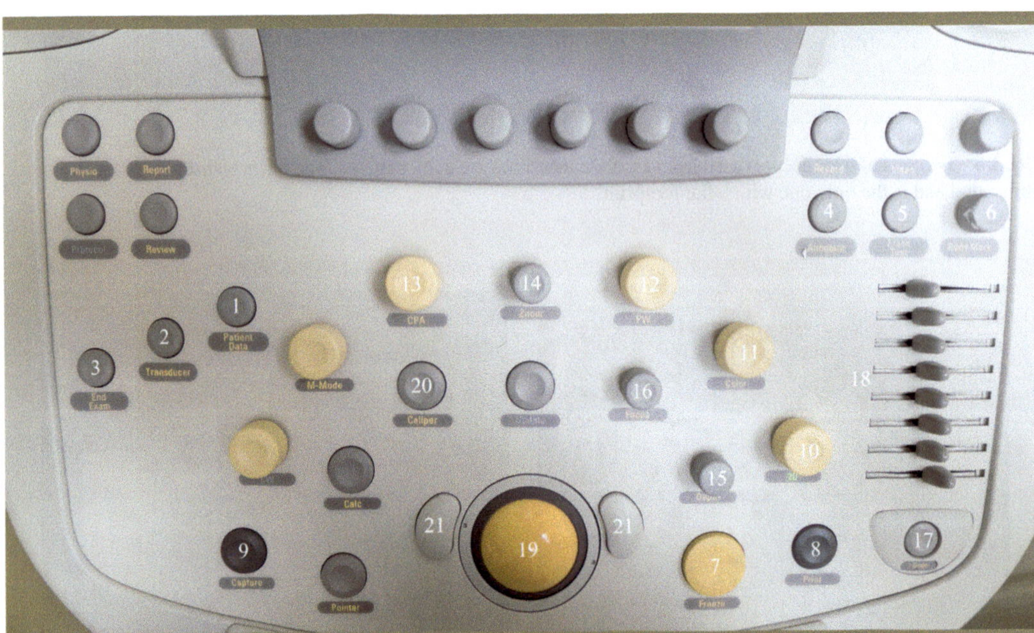

Fig. 3.7 The various knobs on a representative console are annotated and linked to the text to provide some understanding of what each one accomplishes

Rotate knob to adjust the overall gain (brightness) of the displayed image. On many consoles, pressing 2D brings the examiner back to the home display.

11. Color
    Press and rotate knob to enter color flow imaging mode and adjust color gain.
    Color flow imaging adds color-coded quantitative information concerning the relative velocity and direction of fluid motion within the gray-scale image.
12. PW
    Press and rotate knob to enter pulsed-wave Doppler mode and to adjust the Doppler gain.
    Pulsed-wave imaging maps the flow velocity and allows display of the Doppler wave spectrum. This is not generally required for thyroid assessment.
13. CPA
    Press and rotate knob to enter power imaging and adjust power gain. Power Doppler imaging maps the strength of the Doppler signal coming from the flow. The magnitude of the flow is displayed based on the number of reflectors that are moving, regardless of their velocity. The best way to use this power Doppler knob is to increase the gain until speculation occurs and then reduce its amplitude to produce the ideal pattern display.
14. Zoom
    A region of interest can be magnified for closer examination. Two types of zoom are available: Digital Zoom and HD Zoom.
    Rotate knob to adjust the digital zoom factor. Digital zoom is a postprocessing magnifying function. It has no effect on the frame rate.
    Press knob to enter HD zoom mode and select a region of interest. HD zoom concentrates the data acquisition on a specific region of interest. This results in a reduced field of view, but greater detail and higher frame rate, giving better image quality over the selected region of interest.
15. Depth
    Rotate knob to adjust the depth to visualize deeper/shallower structures. When the depth is increased, echoes from deeper in the body are captured. It takes longer for the transducer to receive all of the signal, and the time between two ultrasound beams is increased, hence resulting in a decreased frame rate.
16. Focus
    The focal zone is the depth at which the transmitted ultrasound energy is focused, and hence the lateral resolution is highest at this depth.
    This knob can be pressed or rotated to adjust the position and size of the focal zone.
    Changing the size of the focal zone affects the frame rate; the larger the focal zone, the slower the frame rate.
17. i-scan
    Press to automatically adjust the 2D gray-scale gain for different tissue attenuations.
18. Time-Gain Compensation (TGC) Curve
    The individual slide pods can be moved individually or simultaneously to adjust the uniformity of brightness throughout the image.
19. Trackball
    The trackball can be rolled to move the position of the pointer on the display monitor.
20. Caliper
    Press and use trackball to move pointer on display for distance and other 2D measurements.
21. Set buttons (each on either side of the trackball is identical to its twin)
    These have multiple functions, the most common of which is completion of the second part of a measurement before another caliper icon is activated.

Touch Screen

This particular ultrasound system has a touch screen which allows the examiner to perform manipulative functions quickly with the non-scanning hand. These touch functions are produced on a small screen between the console and the display (Fig. 3.8). The touch screen has some

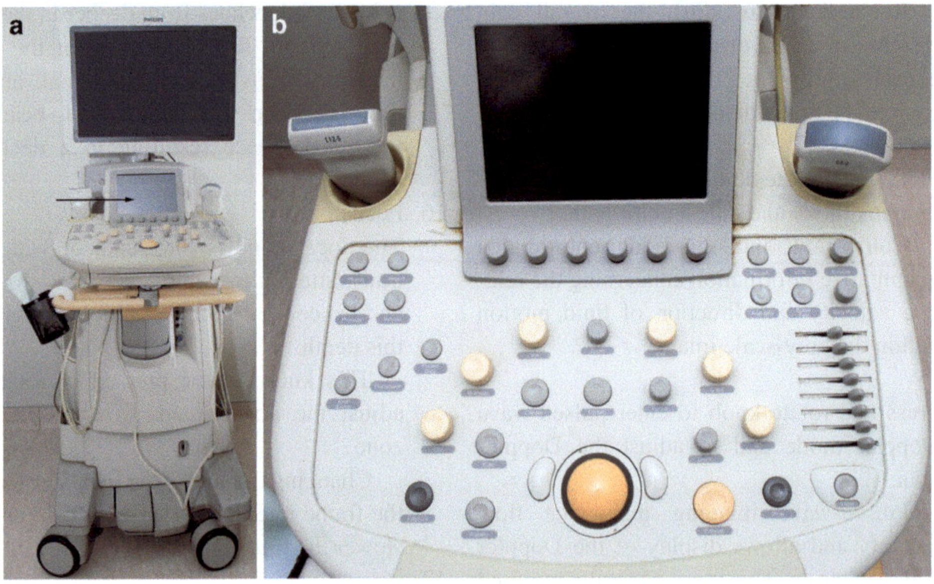

Fig. 3.8 (**a**) Views of the ultrasound machine with touch screen. (**b**) All of the console, touch screen, and display details are associated with this same unit

efficiency advantages but is similar in ways other systems manipulate the images. The ultrasound manual, whether in hard copy or online, is the best reference for understanding one's individual unit. The following narrative information correlates with Fig. 3.9:

1. Left/Right
   Touch to flip the image along the left–right axis.
2. Top/Bottom
   Touch to flip the image along the up–down axis.
3. Dual
   Touch to activate or deactivate dual mode. Two images are placed alongside each other, and the imaging settings can be maintained independently. This can be used to demonstrate a transverse and sagittal image on the same screen. It can also be used to demonstrate a gray scale and Doppler image side by side. A common use of dual screen is to merge halves of a large image into one composite.
4. Res/Spd
   Resolution/Speed provides different settings which varies the balance between image quality (resolution) and the frame rate (speed).
5. Gray Map
   Displays the echo amplitudes as a range of gray scale. Five gray maps are available numbered 1–5. A gray map of 3 is generally used for head and neck imaging.
6. Compress
   This assigns the compression curve for the image display with values ranging from 36 to 70 dB. A higher compression curve softens the image while a lower compression curve produces a high-contrast image. For head and neck imaging, this is preset to 60 dB.
7. Wide Scan
   Used during SonoCT imaging to produce a wide-screen display especially when an image is just beyond the dimensions of the transducer or cannot be entirely displayed. This is a very useful technique with large nodules or goiter.
8. SonoCT
   This setting reduces noise and improves contrast resolution. This setting is used for most imaging except when artifacts such as calcifications are present and better observed with conventional scanning.
9. X Res
   This setting enhances gray-scale imaging by reducing noise while maintaining resolution.

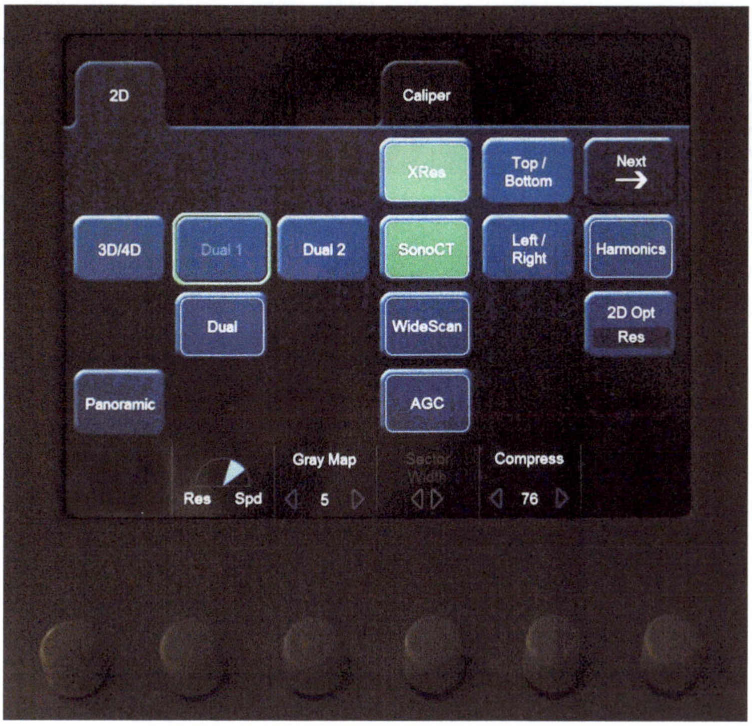

Fig. 3.9 This illuminated mid-screen portrayed from Fig. 3.8 demonstrates many of the special manipulations possible with this particular ultrasound system

With this system both X Res and SonoCT are usually activated for most scanning (green color on the touch area signifies that the function is active). X Res aligns the random pixels in an ultrasound image in real time for better delineation of borders. It also decreases noise artifact.

10. Harmonics

    This function is used to reduce image noise and reverberation and enhance borders. In this system, SonoCT obviates the need to employ harmonics.

11. 2D opt

    Optimizes imaging for resolution (Res), penetration (Pen), or general (Gen), which is a balance of resolution and penetration. For most images, Gen is used to give a balanced image but it may be helpful in special situations to trial the other 2 settings.

The display often demonstrates a lot of confusing information much of which is irrelevant to the practical use of the system with appropriate predetermined customized or factory preset settings. The following information correlates with Figs. 3.9 and 3.10 and is presented in an elementary manner to assist the reader who wishes to have a more comprehensive understanding of that which is displayed.

Monitor Display

The elements in parentheses are taken from the monitor display of an actual patient study and are included to illustrate how these values are presented (Fig. 3.10).

1. Frame rate (FR 45 Hz)

   Displays the frame rate of the scan.
2. Resolution/Speed (S1)

   This indicates the chosen setting for the image quality (resolution) versus the frame rate (speed).
3. Overall gain (68%)

   This indicates the overall gain of the B-mode image.

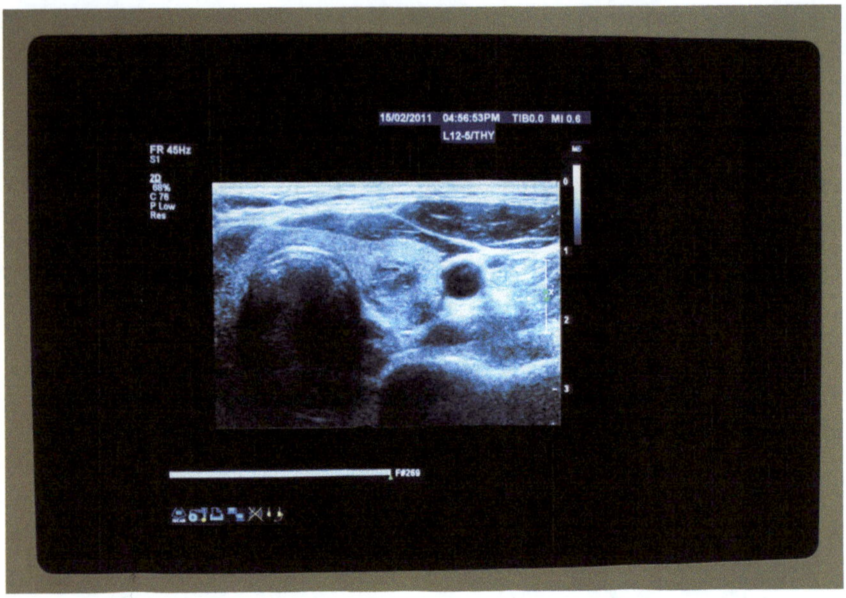

Fig. 3.10 Displays demonstrate the variety of numerical data which correlate with the ultrasound examination

4. Compression (C76)
   Displays the compression value.
5. Persistence (P low)
   Persistence determines the frame averaging for image display. Higher persistence values give a smoother appearance with less noise. A lower persistence is useful for imaging fast-moving structures. This is usually set to medium or low for imaging the head and neck.
6. Penetration/Resolution (Res)
   This shows one of three settings: resolution (Res), penetration (Pen), or general (Gen), which is a balance of resolution and penetration. Most often the Gen setting is adequate.
7. and 8. Transducer and presets (L12-5/thy)
   Indicates the selected transducer and presets which are designated for different anatomical regions and body build. One's own preferred presets can be established and stored in the menu.
9. and 10. MI and TI (T1B0.0 and MI 0.6)
   These are values which depict safety levels with diagnostic ultrasound machines. These do not affect the resolution or any desired manipulation of the image.

The output power changes the amount of ultrasound acoustic power that is produced by the transducer (measured in Watts per square centimeter). Increasing the output power increases the thermal and mechanical indices.

Mechanical index (MI) – Mechanical bioeffects are threshold phenomena that occur when a certain level of output is exceeded. However, the threshold level varies with the type of tissue. The higher the MI value, the greater the likelihood of mechanical bioeffects occurring. There is no specific MI value that means that a mechanical effect is actually occurring. The MI should only be used as a guide for implementing the ALARA principle, and generally the MI should not be greater than 0.5.

Thermal index (TI) – The TI informs the user of the potential for temperature rise in body tissue. It is an estimate of temperature increase with specific properties. The actual amount of any temperature rise is influenced by tissue type, vascularity, mode of operation, and others. The TI should be used as a guide for implementing the ALARA principle, and generally the TI should not exceed 1.0.

11. Gray-scale or color bar (M5 and gray-scale bar)
    Displays the gray scale or color in a graphic bar depending on mode of imaging.
12. Depth scale (3.5 cm)
    The depth scale is shown in centimeters to the right of the image.
13. Focus (green arrows depict the focal point along the white bar just to the left of the depth scale)
    Indicates the selected focal depth and range.

Output

The hard drive on all ultrasound systems has a finite limitation in its storage capacity. Thus, it is critical to develop a strategy to store the images on some form of electronic media. Perhaps the most basic is an output to a CD or DVD burner, and most contemporary systems provide this capability. A USB 2.0 port can usually permit output to any other device such as an external hard drive. With this storage capability, cine loops are preserved for playback.

It is also useful to link the system to a printing device where static images can be printed as either a single image or along with other related images as a group. The advantage of a group format of 4 images is that for thyroid both lobes can be visualized in transverse and sagittal views along with assigned measurements. The disadvantage is the reduction in size of each specific image. This method allows storage of the images in the clinical paper record. With the transition to electronic medical records, the images can be configured into a composite which includes the dictated description.

Perhaps the most widely used option, especially in radiology departments, is the PACS (picture archiving and communication system). This allows images to be stored and retrieved at will wherever there is a work station connected to the system. The output from the ultrasound unit into PACS is altered into a standardized format known as DICOM (Digital Imaging and Communications in Medicine). Examination of DICOM images requires some form of software conversion with an associated viewer. Alternatively, there are software programs which allow manipulation of the images (i.e., erasure of the patient name and a lot of distracting numerical data) in either static or cine loop format so that the images can be displayed in PowerPoint presentations or publication without revealing confidential patient information.

Lastly the benefits of storage of cine loops should be profiled. Many PACS systems do not store cine loops since they are so storage intensive, although some institutions have augmented their ability to save larger amounts of imaging information and can take the loops. When a clinician wishes to review an ultrasound examination, the cine loop is much easier to interpret especially if he or she had not performed the initial examination. It is an ideal format for teaching as it allows real-time demonstration of adjacent relationships. These points suggest that some personal form of storage of images and especially cine loops should be considered. Even a simple printout of 1–4 of the most salient images has some practical value. For example, the surgeon who performs the ultrasound in the clinic and at some future point in time will be doing the actual procedure may want to have the printed image in the operating room for reference. The printed image is an excellent way to store interesting cases where the catalog information is present in the formal annotation and the diagnosis or interesting features can be handwritten on the back as a means of future reference. Finally, some patients may want a copy of the ultrasound study and it is quite simple to produce this copy with the press of a button.

In summary, this chapter has attempted to illustrate practical ultrasound in as comprehensive a manner as possible. It is not necessary to understand or manipulate every option on the console or those which are presented on the display. There are a few important functions which the experienced sonographer will become intimately familiar with and will employ with every study. Others will be required only on occasion and may demand reference to the manual to refresh that function's proper use. In addition, there are several manipulations which overlap and produce the same net result. The only means of understanding these variables is to experiment with the machine and determine how it can best serve the examiner in the simplest and most efficient manner.

Reference

1. Kremkau FW. Diagnostic ultrasound. 6th ed. Philadelphia, PA: WB Saunders; 2002. p. 10.

Section II

Thyroid and Parathyroid Glands

Sonography of the Normal Thyroid

4

Hok Yuen Yuen, Cina Shin-Loong Tong, and
Anil T. Ahuja

Introduction

Patients with thyroid disease may present with local signs such as a palpable diffuse (goiter) or focal (nodular) enlargement of the gland and/or with systemic symptoms due to endocrine disturbance resulting in altered metabolism (hyperthyroidism or hypothyroidism). While physiological derangement is well assessed by clinical examination and laboratory biochemical tests, the evaluation of the structural anomaly relies heavily on modern ultrasound imaging which provides high-resolution anatomical details of any morphological alteration.

The major indications for sonography of the thyroid gland include:

1. Confirm that a clinically palpable mass or nodule indeed arises from the thyroid and try to determine its nature.
2. Guide fine needle aspiration cytology (FNAC) or biopsy.
3. Follow up patients postoperatively for excluding local or regional disease.
4. Screen patients with increased risk of developing thyroid malignancies, such as patients with Hashimoto's thyroiditis who have increased risk of thyroid lymphoma [1, 2], and those who may have been exposed to previous radiation, particularly children [3–5].
5. Distinguish simple goiter from multinodular goiter or other thyroid disease.
6. Evaluate a nonpalpable thyroid lesion seen on other imaging modalities such as a cold nodule on a thyroid scan, a hypermetabolic nodule on an FDG-PET scan, and incidental nodules seen on CT, MRI, and Doppler of neck vessels.
7. Provide complementary assessment in patients with deranged thyroid function tests.

Scanning Technique

Position the patient comfortably in the supine position with the neck slightly extended/hyperextended by placing a pillow under the shoulders. This may not be possible in the elderly and in children. In such instances, the examination is best performed by positioning the patient in a supine position. In addition, children/infants may be calmed by placing them comfortably in their parents' arms. In a situation that the patient cannot lie supine, a diagnostic examination can be carried out with the patient sitting up. The patient should be instructed to refrain from swallowing and maintain normal, shallow breathing during the scan. No specific preparation is required prior to the scan. One must remember that lying supine

H.Y. Yuen (✉) • A.T. Ahuja
Department of Imaging and Interventional Radiology, The Chinese University of Hong Kong, Prince of Wales Hospital, Shatin (NT), Hong Kong (SAR), China
e-mail: drhyyuen@gmail.com

C.S.-L. Tong
Department of Imaging & Interventional Radiology, Prince of Wales Hospital, The Chinese University of Hong Kong, Shatin, NT, Hong Kong

R.A. Sofferman and A.T. Ahuja (eds.), *Ultrasound of the Thyroid and Parathyroid Glands*,
DOI 10.1007/978-1-4614-0974-8_4, © Springer Science+Business Media, LLC 2012

with the neck extended/hyperextended is uncomfortable for patients. Therefore, all examinations must be efficiently performed to reduce scanning time and patient discomfort. Some patients may feel dizzy as they get off the couch at the end of the examination, particularly the elderly. Therefore, make sure the patients are well supported and cared for.

Higher ultrasound frequencies have shorter wavelengths and higher spatial resolution but limited penetration due to increased absorption. Ideally, a high-frequency transducer (7–12 MHz) should be used for scanning the thyroid to obtain the benefit of better spatial resolution, since penetration is not a major issue due to the superficial location of the thyroid. However, in cases such as large masses, deep seated tumors, lesions with retrosternal or retroclavicular extension, obese patients with short necks, and patients who cannot extend their neck adequately, a lower-frequency transducer may also be used in order to identify the relevant pathology and to obtain more complete anatomical information. In such cases, the use of a standoff gel may help to improve the quality of the examination. A linear transducer with vector format is usually preferred, but a curved linear array probe may be used for obtaining a larger field of view (FOV) in scanning large glands. Hyperextension of the neck may occasionally be required for full sonographic assessment of the bases of the lobes very low in the neck at the cervicothoracic junction. Hyperextension of the neck elevates the lower lobes into the neck, improving their visualization. Most modern equipments now routinely use harmonic imaging, crossbeam/multidirectional imaging, etc., to improve the quality of the image. However, with their use, the fine shadowing from the punctate calcification is often difficult to see. Such shadowing is best seen/evaluated using the basic/fundamental gray scale.

The entire thyroid gland should be scanned in both the transverse and longitudinal planes. Transverse scan is useful to locate thyroid nodules; to determine their relationship to the trachea, carotid sheath, and any associated nodes; and to evaluate their internal architecture and extrathyroid extension. Longitudinal scan evaluates internal architecture, vascularity on Doppler, and extrathyroid extension. The longitudinal scan is particularly useful in identifying the "pseudo-mass" of hypertrophic tongue of thyroid tissue which on the transverse scan may mimic a "separated" portion of the gland, a discrete nodule, or even a parathyroid lesion (Figs. 4.1 and 4.2). Such pseudo-mass is more common at the lower pole of the thyroid especially in a rounded, hypertrophied gland as in Graves' disease or thyroiditis. Doppler study should be performed when appropriate for assessment of glandular or tumor vascularity and flow pattern.

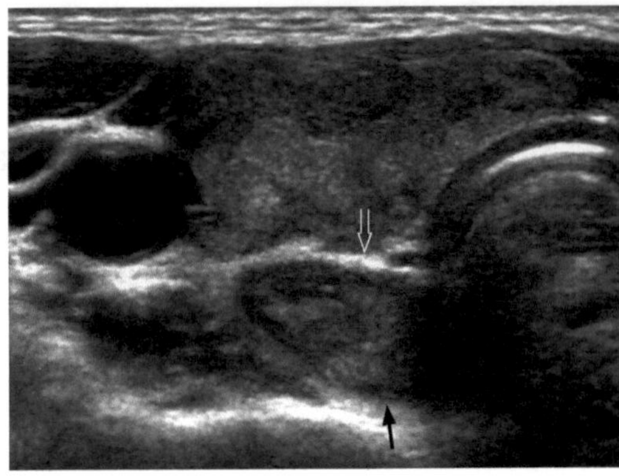

Fig. 4.1 Transverse gray scale ultrasound shows the "pseudo-mass" of hypertrophic tongue of thyroid tissue (*black arrow*) which mimics a "separated" portion of the gland, a discrete nodule, or a parathyroid lesion. Note the apparent echogenic capsule (*open arrow*) separating the "pseudo-mass" from the parent gland

The adjacent structures in the neck including the trachea, esophagus, strap muscles, carotid arteries, internal jugular veins, and the cervical lymph nodes must also be carefully examined in every case to complete a full examination of the thyroid.

Normal Anatomy and Sonography of Thyroid

Embryologically, the thyroid is derived from the first and second pharyngeal pouches (medial anlage) as proliferations of endodermal epithelial cells on the median surface of the developing pharyngeal floor known as the foramen cecum.

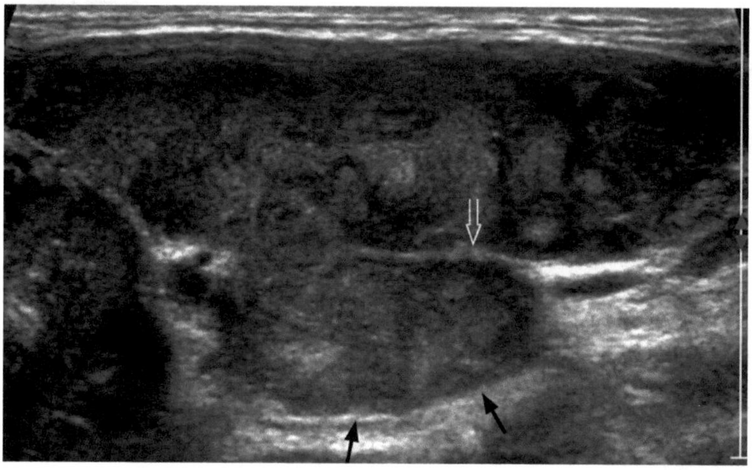

Fig. 4.2 Longitudinal gray scale ultrasound (same patient as in Fig. 4.1) confirms that the "pseudo-mass" (*black arrows*) is in fact due to a hypertrophic tongue of thyroid tissue protruding from the parent gland (*open arrow*)

The bilobed thyroid gland then descends anterior to the pharyngeal gut along the thyroglossal duct with further inferior migration anterior to the hyoid bone and laryngeal cartilages. As such, developmental anomaly such as thyroglossal duct cyst (due to failure of involution of a portion of the thyroglossal duct), remnant of thyroid tissue (due to sequestration of thyroid tissue along the thyroglossal duct), and ectopic thyroid gland (due to incomplete descent of the thyroid into the lower neck) may be found anywhere along this path of descent (Figs. 4.3–4.5). The most common location for ectopic thyroid in the neck is just deep to the foramen cecum in the posterior tongue base known as the lingual thyroid (Figs. 4.6–4.12).

The thyroid is an "H"- or "U"-shaped endocrine gland located in the visceral space of the infrahyoid neck, usually extending from the level of C5 to T1 (Fig. 4.13). It is composed of two pear-shaped lateral lobes with a narrow upper pole and a broader lower pole and connected in the midline by a narrow isthmus anterior to the second, third, and fourth tracheal rings (Figs. 4.14–4.16). Each lateral lobe appears triangular on a transverse scan.

Anterolaterally, the thyroid is covered by the sternocleidomastoid muscle, the strap muscles (sternohyoid and sternothyroid), and the superior belly of the omohyoid muscle (Figs. 4.17–4.20). Posterolaterally, the thyroid is in close proximity to the carotid sheath (containing the common carotid artery [CCA], internal jugular vein [IJV], and the vagus nerve [CN X]) (Fig. 4.21) and the scalenus anterior muscle. The thyroid isthmus is covered anteriorly by the strap muscles, the anterior jugular vein, fascia, and skin.

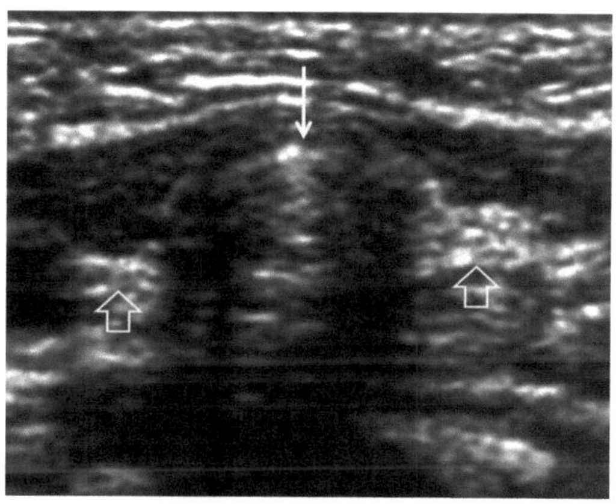

Fig. 4.3 Transverse gray scale ultrasound shows an empty thyroid bed (*open arrows*) in a patient with ectopic thyroid gland. Note the trachea (*white arrow*)

The larynx and trachea are located medial to the thyroid. The dense shadowing from the

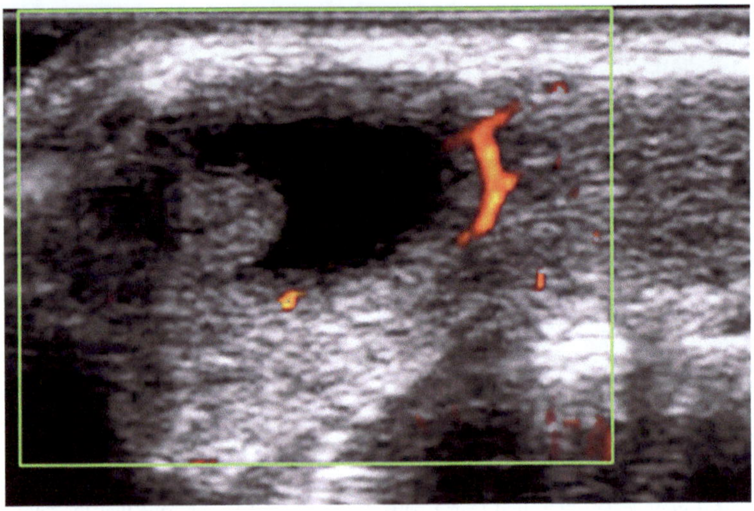

Fig. 4.4 Longitudinal power Doppler ultrasound (same patient as in Fig. 4.3) demonstrates the ectopic thyroid tissue with cystic nodule in the infrahyoid neck

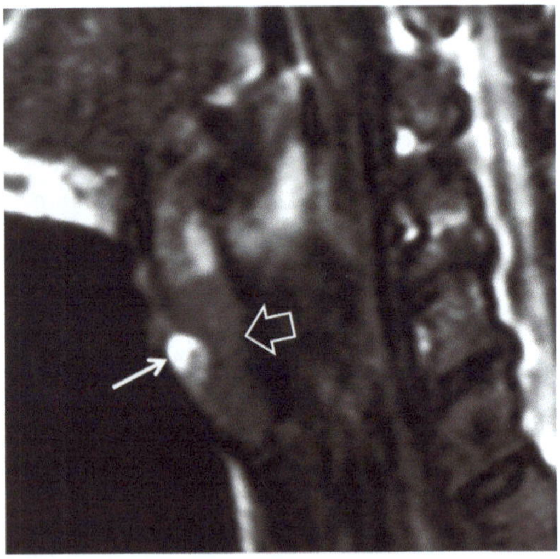

Fig. 4.5 Sagittal T2-weighted MRI shows the ectopic thyroid tissue in the midline infrahyoid neck (*open arrow*). Note the cystic nodule (*white arrow*) seen on ultrasound

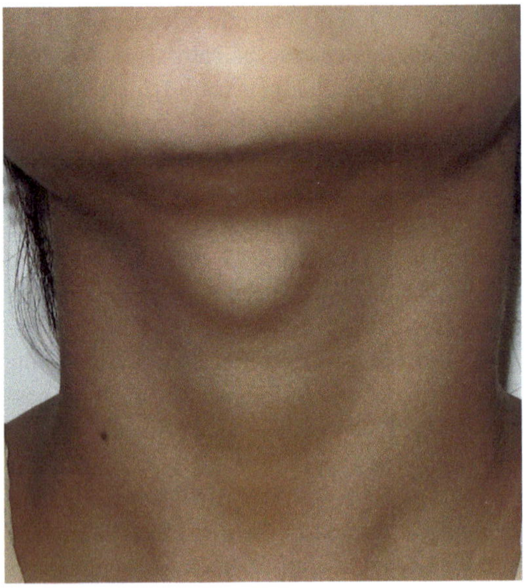

Fig. 4.6 Clinical photograph of a patient with an ectopic thyroid gland presenting as a midline anterior neck mass. Courtesy of Dr. Sanjay Vaid

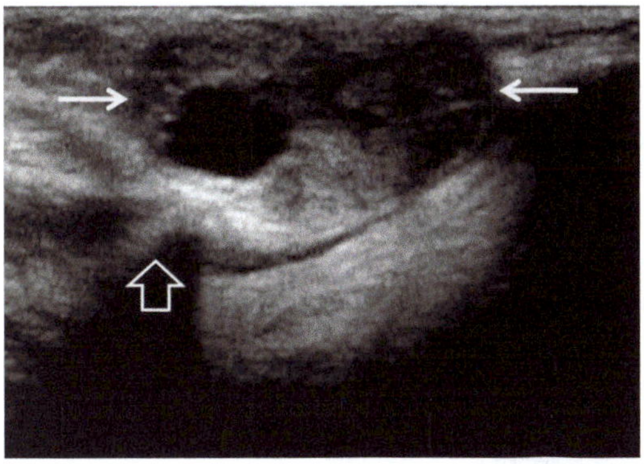

Fig. 4.7 Longitudinal gray scale ultrasound (same patient as in Fig. 4.6) demonstrates the ectopic thyroid tissue (*white arrows*) at the infrahyoid neck. Note the relationship to the hyoid bone (*open arrow*). Courtesy of Dr. Sanjay Vaid

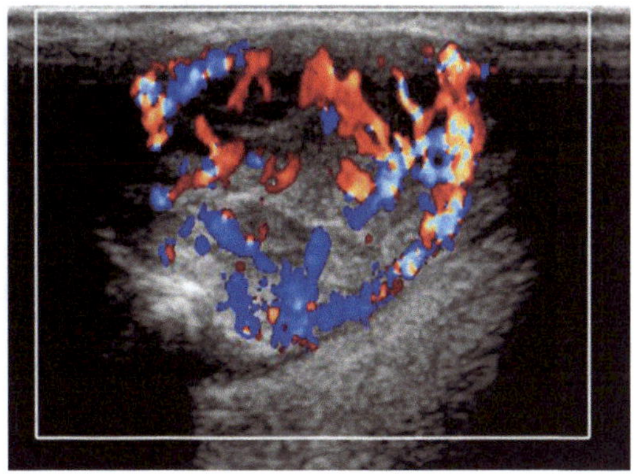

Fig. 4.8 Corresponding color Doppler ultrasound (same patient as in Figs. 4.6 and 4.7) shows prominent parenchymal vascularity in the ectopic thyroid tissue. Courtesy of Dr. Sanjay Vaid

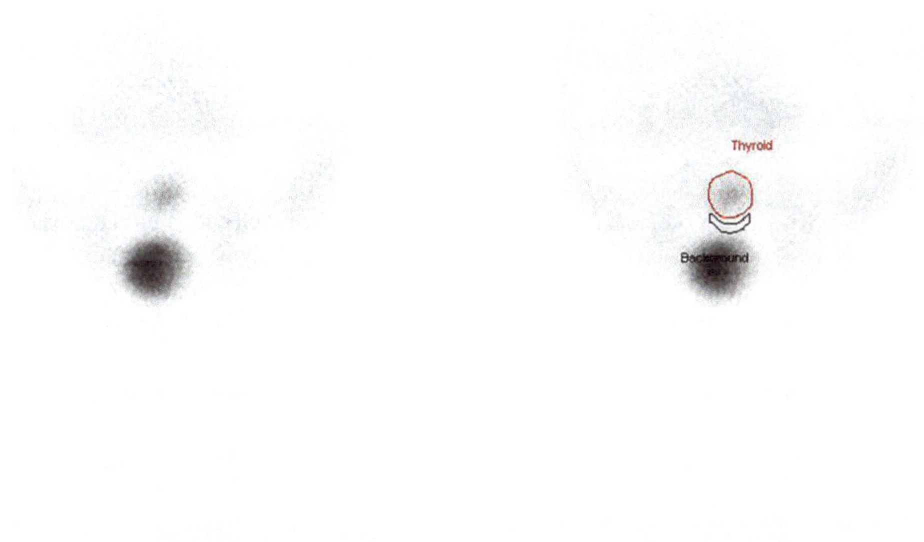

Fig. 4.9 Radionuclide scan (same patient as in Figs. 4.6–4.8) shows two foci of iodine avid ectopic thyroid tissue in the midline. The lower focus corresponds to the infrahyoid ectopic thyroid tissue seen on ultrasound. The upper focus is likely in the region of the foramen cecum at the posterior tongue base. Courtesy of Dr. Sanjay Vaid

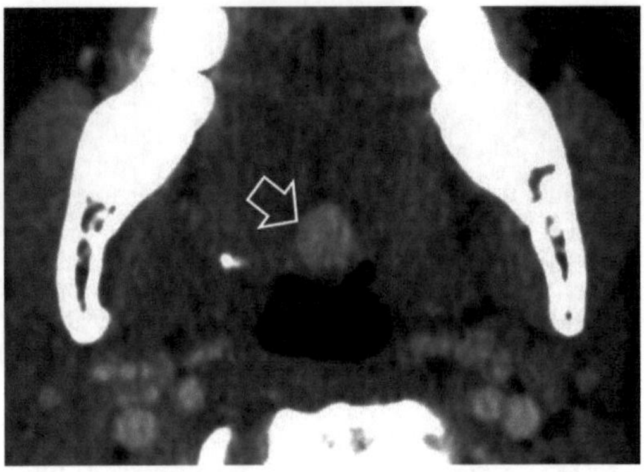

Fig. 4.10 Contrast-enhanced axial CT (same patient as in Figs. 4.6–4.9) confirms the presence of ectopic thyroid tissue in the region of the foramen cecum (open arrow). Courtesy of Dr. Sanjay Vaid

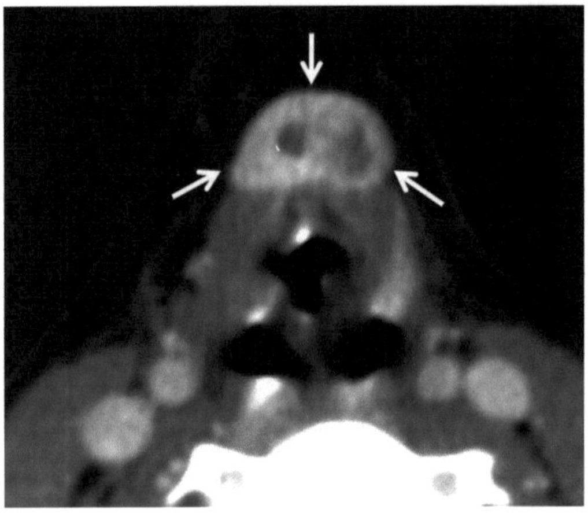

Fig. 4.11 Contrast-enhanced axial CT (same patient as in Figs. 4.6–4.10) at the level of the piriform fossa demonstrates ectopic thyroid tissue in the infrahyoid neck (*white arrows*). Courtesy of Dr. Sanjay Vaid

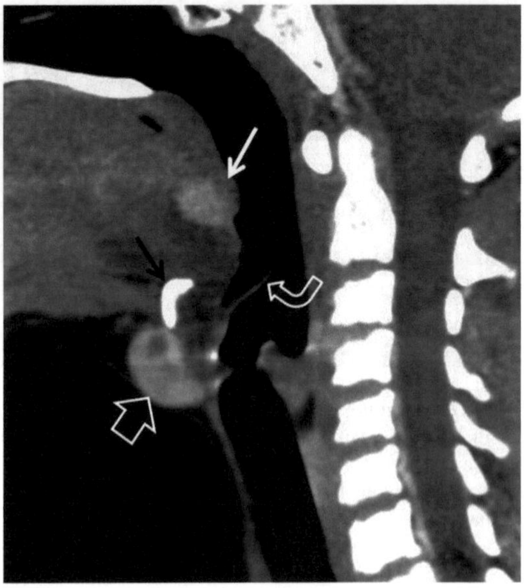

Fig. 4.12 Contrast-enhanced sagittal CT (same study as in Figs. 4.10–4.11) demonstrates the two foci of ectopic thyroid tissues at the foramen cecum (*white arrow*) and the infrahyoid neck (*open arrow*), respectively. Note the hyoid bone (*black arrow*) and the epiglottis (*curved open arrow*).Courtesy of Dr. Sanjay Vaid

tracheal/laryngeal cartilage obscures the trachea and larynx, making their examination suboptimal on an ultrasound examination (compare to CT and MRI). Posteriorly, the esophagus is usually located slightly to the left and can be identified as a "bull's eye" (the echogenic center is due to air and fluid within the lumen, and the hypoechoic rim represents the esophageal musculature), and should not be mistaken for a mass lesion, lymph node, or parathyroid lesion (Figs. 4.17 and 4.22). The location of the esophagus varies with rotation of the neck. When the head is turned toward the left, the esophagus may be seen on the right, posterior to the right lobe of thyroid. With the head turned to the right, the esophagus is seen on the left.

In about 10–30% of people, there is a third lobe (the pyramidal lobe) arising from the isthmus which projects superiorly along the midline or slightly to the left, anterior to thyroid cartilage, toward the hyoid bone (Figs. 4.23–4.26). This pyramidal lobe is only rarely visualized on ultrasound due to its small anteroposterior diameter and is more commonly detected in the young as it becomes progressively atrophic in adulthood. There is often mild asymmetry of the thyroid, and the right lobe tends to be slightly larger than the left lobe. The two lobes are also often not at the same level in the neck, and in such cases, the location of the parathyroid glands/lesions is also altered.

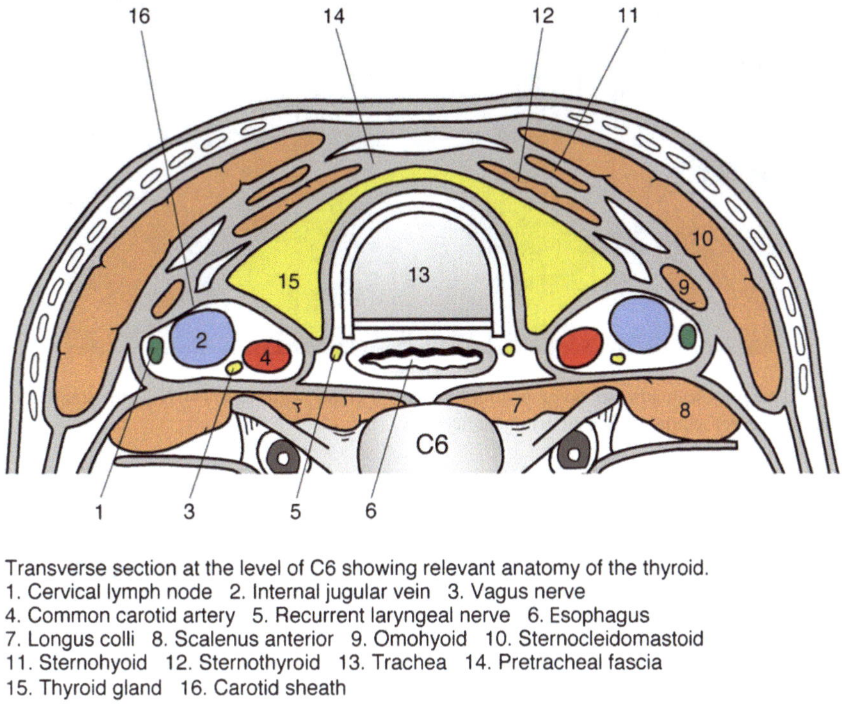

Fig. 4.13 Schematic diagram, transverse section at the level of C6 showing the relevant anatomy of the thyroid

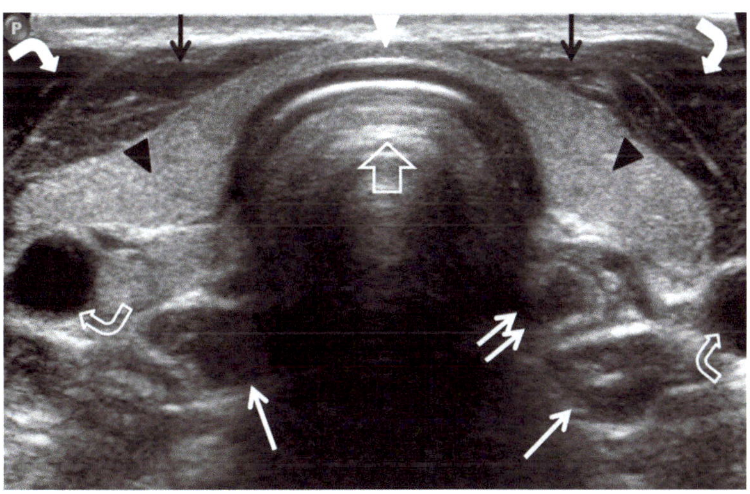

Fig. 4.14 Transverse gray scale ultrasound of the normal thyroid gland. Note the isthmus (*white arrowhead*), right and left lobes (*black arrowheads*), strap muscles (*black arrows*), sternocleidomastoid muscles (*curved solid arrows*), esophagus (*double white arrows*), longus coli muscles (*white arrows*), and the common carotid arteries (*curved open arrows*). The normal thyroid parenchymal echoes are fine, homogeneous, and hyperechoic

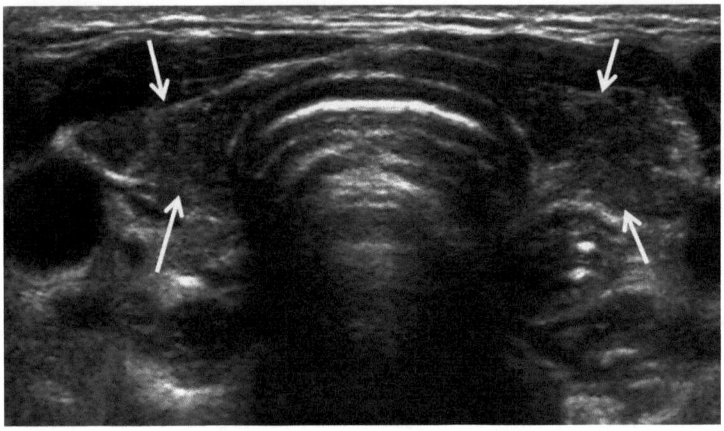

Fig. 4.15 Transverse gray scale ultrasound of an atrophic thyroid gland (*white arrows*). Note the small size of the gland with heterogeneous decreased parenchymal echogenicity

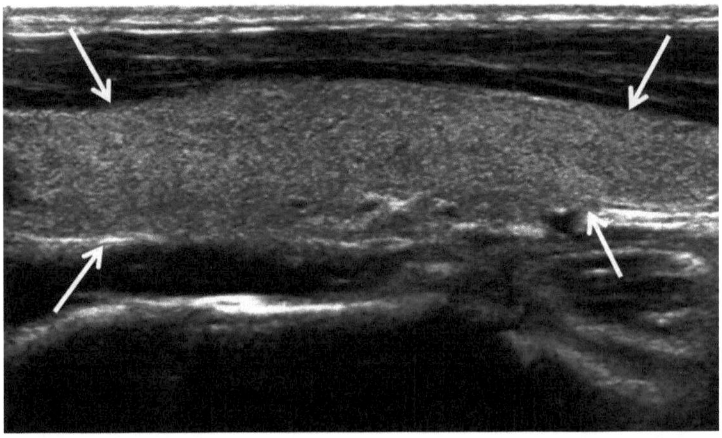

Fig. 4.16 Longitudinal gray scale ultrasound of the normal thyroid gland (*white arrows*). Note the normal homogeneous, fine, hyperechogenicity of the thyroid parenchyma

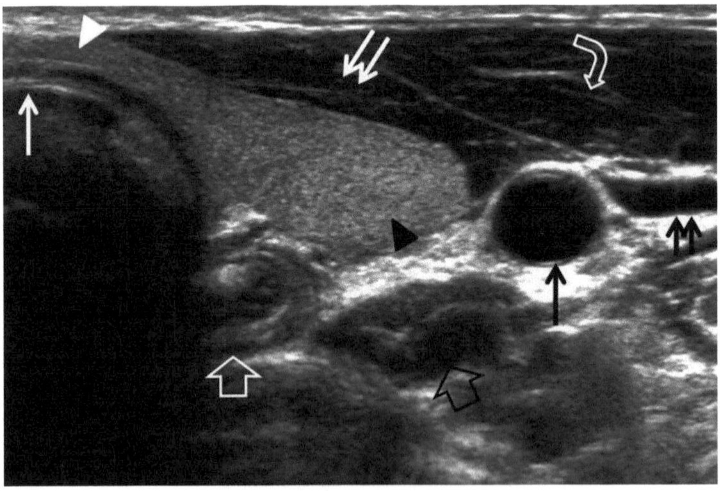

Fig. 4.17 Transverse gray scale ultrasound of the left lobe of thyroid. Note the isthmus (*white arrowhead*), trachea (*white arrow*), left lobe (*black arrowhead*), esophagus (*white open arrow*), left longus coli muscle (*black open arrow*), left common carotid artery (*black arrow*), left internal jugular vein (*double black arrows*), left strap muscles (*double white arrows*), and sternocleidomastoid muscle (*white curved open arrow*)

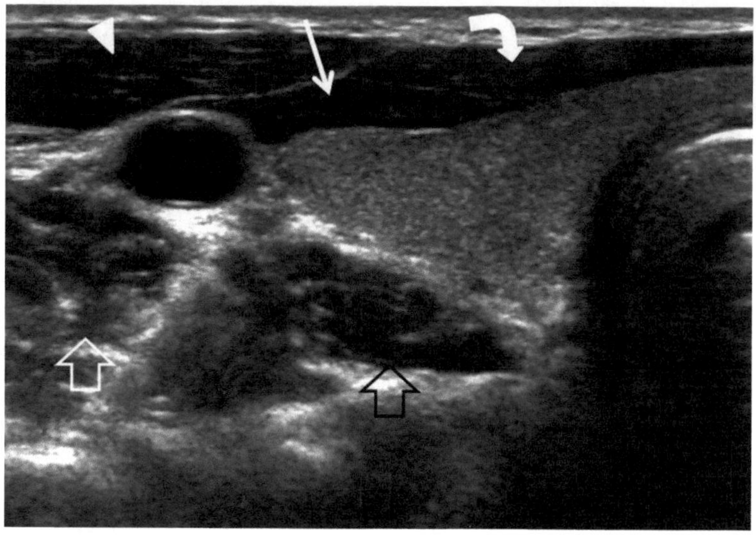

Fig. 4.18 Transverse gray scale ultrasound of the mid-portion of the right lobe of thyroid. Note the right sternohyoid muscle (*curved white arrow*), sternothyroid muscle (*white arrow*), sternocleidomastoid muscle (*white arrowhead*), longus coli muscle (*black open arrow*), and scalenus anterior muscle (*white open arrow*)

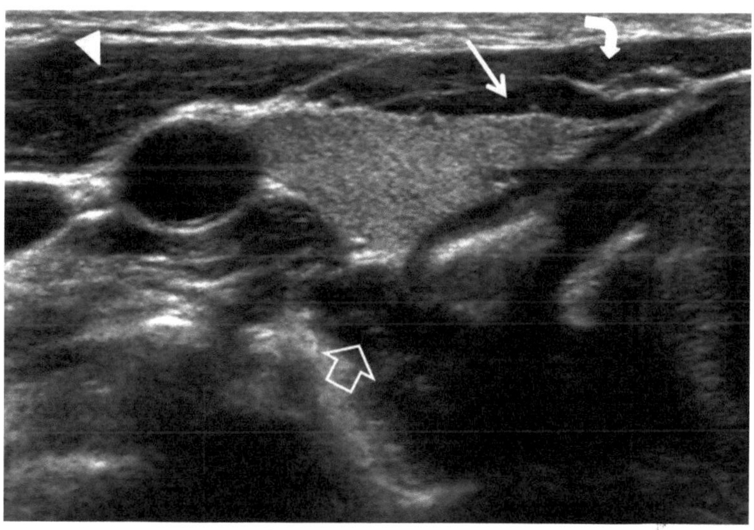

Fig. 4.19 Transverse gray scale ultrasound of the lower pole of the right lobe of thyroid. Note the right sternohyoid muscle (*curved white arrow*), sternothyroid muscle (*white arrow*), sternocleidomastoid muscle (*white arrowhead*), and longus coli muscle (*white open arrow*)

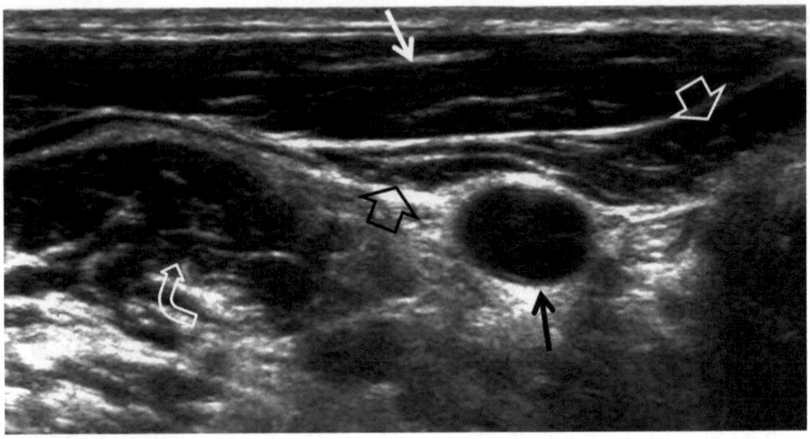

Fig. 4.20 Transverse gray scale ultrasound of the right lower neck. Note the right sternocleidomastoid muscle (*white arrow*), strap muscles (*white open arrow*), omohyoid muscle (*black open arrow*), common carotid artery (*black arrow*), and scalenus anterior muscle (*curved open arrow*)

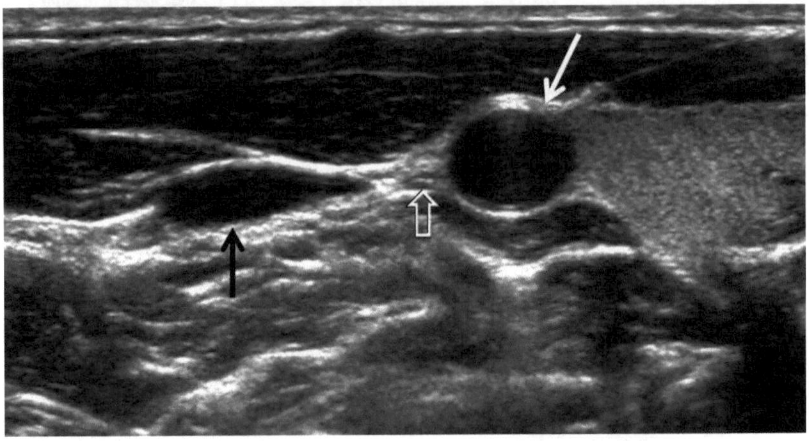

Fig. 4.21 Transverse gray scale ultrasound of the right carotid space. Note the vagus nerve (*open arrow*) posterior to and between the common carotid artery (*white arrow*) and internal jugular vein (*black arrow*). On transverse scans, the vagus nerve is seen as a small echogenic structure with central hyperechogenicity

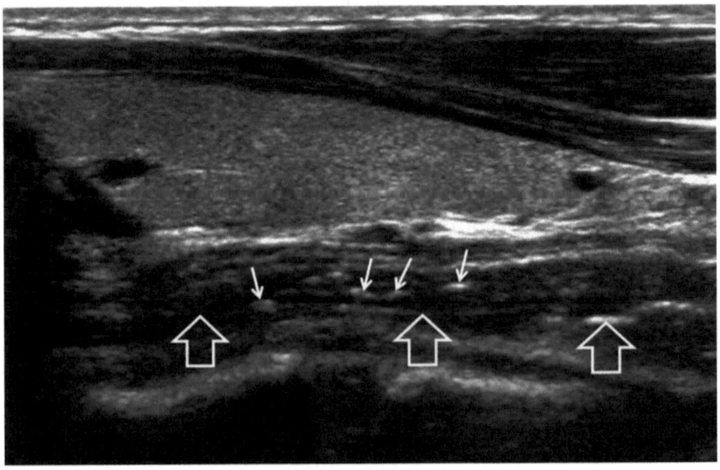

Fig. 4.22 Longitudinal gray scale ultrasound shows the esophagus (*open arrows*) just posterior to the left lobe of thyroid. Note the echogenic foci (*arrows*) which represent air within the lumen and the hypoechoic peripheral rim representing the esophageal musculature

The tracheoesophageal grooves on both sides lie posteromedial to the thyroid and contain the paratracheal lymph nodes, recurrent laryngeal nerve, and the parathyroid glands. The recurrent laryngeal nerve runs anterior to the longus colli muscle and is very often difficult to see. It may be visualized as a thin, linear, hypoechoic structure with echogenic edges formed by the thyroid capsule and muscle.

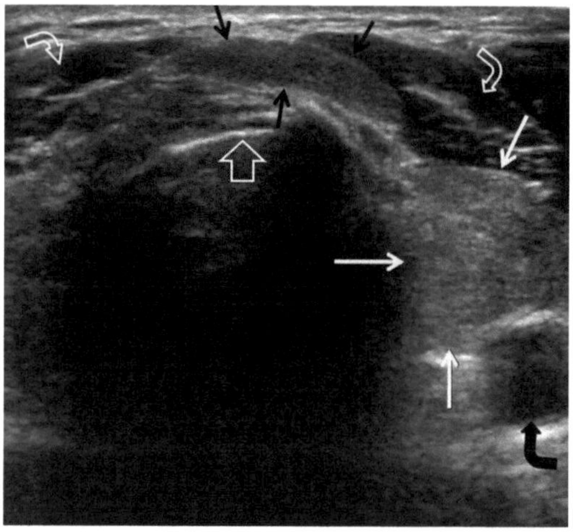

Fig. 4.23 Transverse gray scale ultrasound shows the pyramidal lobe (*black arrows*) of thyroid projecting superiorly from the isthmus (*not shown*) and slightly to the left. Note the thyroid cartilage (*open arrow*), strap muscles (*curved open arrows*), left lobe of thyroid (*white arrows*), and left common carotid artery (*curved black arrow*)

On gray scale ultrasound, the normal thyroid parenchymal echoes are fine, homogeneous, and hyperechoic (bright) compared to the adjacent muscles (Figs. 4.14–4.16). The thyroid gland is completely invested by a sheath derived from the pretracheal layer of the deep fascia attaching the gland to the larynx and trachea. The thyroid capsule appears echogenic on ultrasound and aids in distinguishing thyroid nodules from adjacent extrathyroid lesions.

The thyroid vessels are best seen at the poles of the thyroid. The thyroid is supplied by the superior and inferior thyroid arteries. The superior thyroid artery is the first branch of the external carotid artery, and its proximal course is immediately anterior to the superior laryngeal nerve. It runs superficially over the anterior border of the upper pole to send a branch deep into the gland (Fig. 4.27) and divides into an anterior branch curving toward the isthmus to anastomose with the contralateral artery and a posterior branch running down the back of the lobe to anastomose with an ascending branch of the inferior thyroid artery. A separate branch from the left superior thyroid artery may supply the pyramidal lobe.

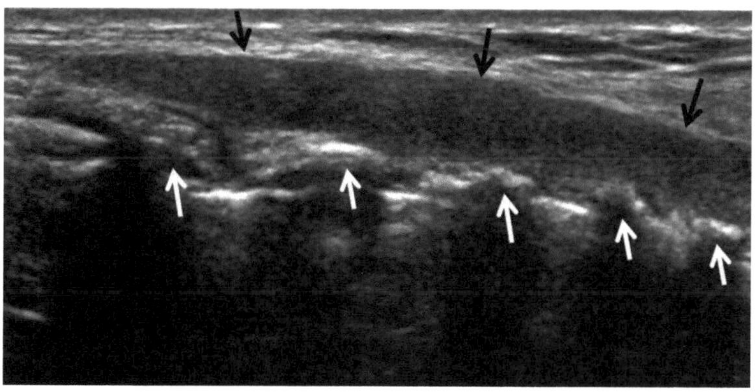

Fig. 4.24 Longitudinal gray scale ultrasound shows the pyramidal lobe of thyroid (*black arrows*) anterior to the tracheal rings (*white arrows*)

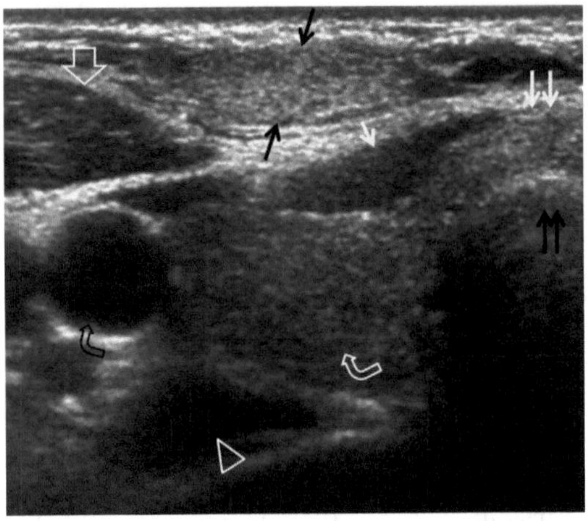

Fig. 4.25 Transverse gray scale ultrasound shows the pyramidal lobe (*black arrows*) of thyroid. Note the isthmus (*double white arrows*), trachea (*double black arrows*), right lobe of thyroid (*white curved open arrow*), right strap muscles (*white arrow*), longus coli muscle (*white arrowhead*), sternocleidomastoid muscle (*white open arrow*), and common carotid artery (*black curved open arrow*)

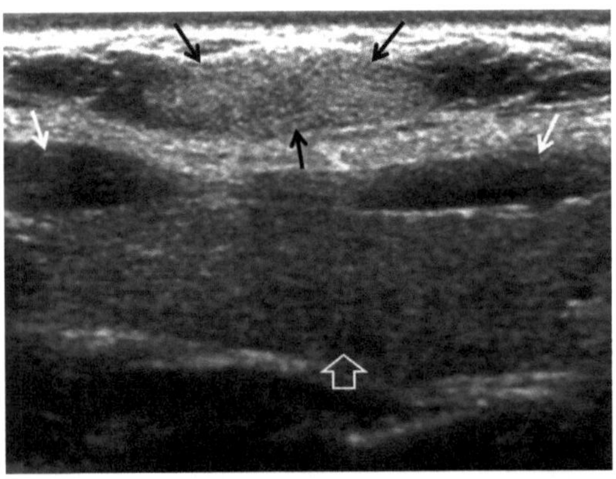

Fig. 4.26 Longitudinal gray scale ultrasound (same patient as in Fig. 4.25) shows the pyramidal lobe (*black arrows*) of thyroid. Note the right lobe of thyroid (*white open arrow*) and right strap muscles (*white arrows*)

The inferior thyroid artery arises from the thyrocervical trunk, a branch of the subclavian artery. It enters the tracheoesophageal groove posterior to the carotid space and is closely associated with the recurrent laryngeal nerve. Behind the lower pole, it divides into four or five branches which pierce the fascia separately to penetrate the posterior aspect of the lower pole (Fig. 4.28). Occasionally (3%), there is a thyroidea ima artery arising from the brachiocephalic trunk, right common carotid artery, or directly from the aortic arch, and it enters the inferior border of the isthmus.

During thyroid surgery, the inferior thyroid artery serves as a useful anatomical landmark to aid in the identification and preservation of the recurrent laryngeal nerve and the parathyroid glands. Its identification helps to avoid the potential complications of nerve injury causing cord palsy and inadvertent removal, damage, or devascularization of the parathyroid glands resulting in hypoparathyroidism and hypocalcaemia [6–8].

Normal Doppler parameter values in the thyroid arteries in healthy individuals have been described [9]. The median and mean references for the systolic peak velocity (SPV), resistive index (RI), and pulsatility index (PI) are 24.80 cm/s and 25.85 cm/s, 0.60 and 0.62, and 0.98 and 1.04, respectively, for superior thyroid arteries; these reference values for the inferior thyroid arteries are 20.92 cm/s and 21.50 cm/s, 0.57 and 0.57, and 0.84 and 0.88, respectively. Women tend to have greater SPV values. The SPV is higher in the superior thyroid artery than in the inferior thyroid artery, presumably because the superior thyroid artery is supplied by the external carotid artery, larger than the thyrocervical trunk, which is a vessel afferent to the inferior thyroid artery. In addition to the use of Doppler vascularity in the differential diagnosis of diffuse and neoplastic diseases, vascular change of parenchymal color flow pattern and decreased maximum systolic velocity of the inferior thyroid artery after thyroid hormone replacement may be used as an adjunct in determining the effects of medical treatment in hypothyroidism (in addition to hormonal evaluation [10]).

There are three pairs of veins arising from venous plexus on the surface of the thyroid gland. The venous return from the upper pole follows the superior thyroid artery. The superior thyroid vein drains either into the internal jugular vein or into the facial vein in approximately equal

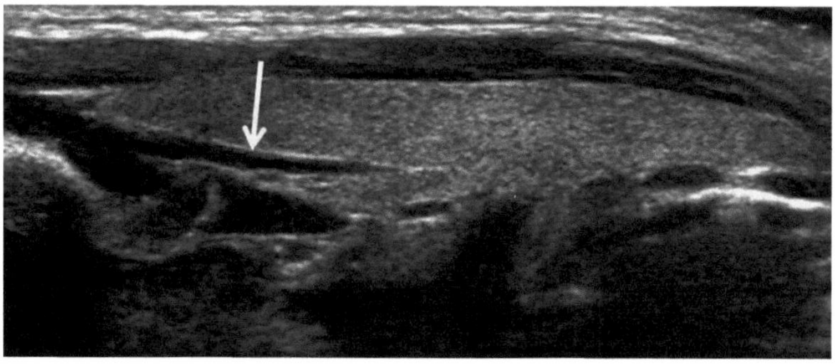

Fig. 4.27 Longitudinal gray scale ultrasound shows the superior thyroid artery (*white arrow*) entering the upper pole of thyroid

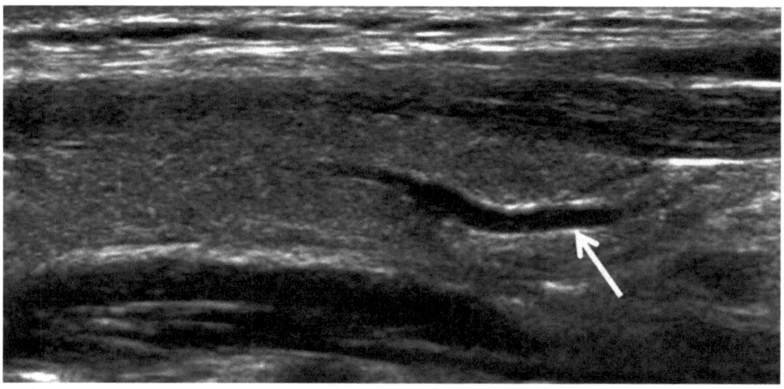

Fig. 4.28 Longitudinal gray scale ultrasound shows the inferior thyroid artery (*white arrow*) entering the lower pole of thyroid

proportions. The middle thyroid vein drains into the internal jugular vein. From the isthmus and the lower poles, the inferior thyroid veins form a plexus which drains into the brachiocephalic veins, mostly into the left one.

The lymphatic vessels from the thyroid form a subcapsular network and lateral and medial collecting trunks, with extensive and multidirectional lymphatic drainage. These drain laterally into the internal jugular chain (levels 2–4) and spinal accessory chain (level 5) and medially to the prelaryngeal, pretracheal (Delphian), and paratracheal nodes along the recurrent laryngeal nerve, the latter also into the mediastinum. In addition to lymphatic spread of cancer to neck nodes, this extensive lymphatic network is responsible for the intrathyroid lymphatic spread of malignancy leading to multiple foci of cancer within the thyroid, particularly in the case of papillary thyroid cancer.

In cases of thyroid malignancy, extrathyroid spread may occur with local infiltration of the adjacent structures including the trachea, esophagus, strap muscles, and recurrent laryngeal nerve. These structures must be scrutinized for integrity, and normally, the fascial planes between the thyroid and the adjacent structures should be maintained. The lymph nodes most commonly involved by metastatic deposits from primary thyroid malignancy are the pretracheal and paratracheal nodes (Fig. 4.29) and the deep cervical nodes along the internal jugular vein, and these areas should be carefully examined. Shadowing from the trachea obscures the paratracheal nodes,

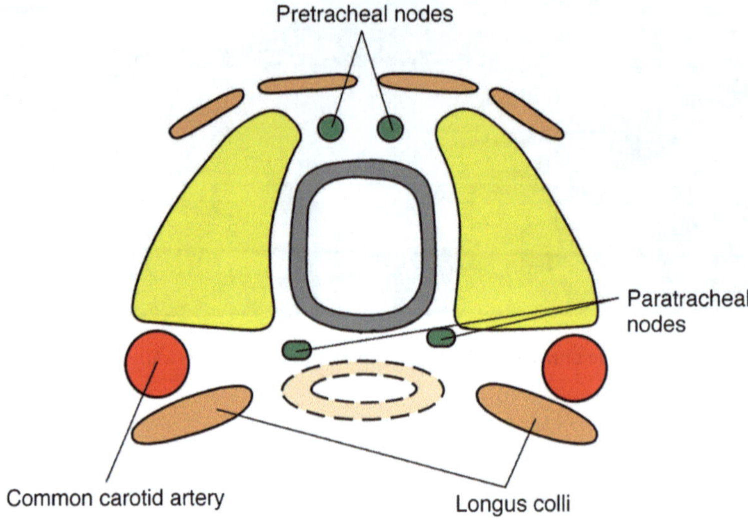

Fig. 4.29 Schematic transverse section at the level of the thyroid gland shows the relationship of the pretracheal and paratracheal lymph nodes to the adjacent structures

and their visualization on ultrasound is often suboptimal, particularly when the involved nodes are small.

Although thyroid and parathyroid conditions usually do not involve submental, submandibular, and parotid areas, they are included in the following discussion for the sake of completion. In addition, incidental thyroglossal duct cysts and sublingual/ectopic thyroid may be seen at the floor of the mouth, and large second branchial cleft cysts may displace the submandibular gland and appear inseparable from the apex of the parotid gland. Therefore, in addition to ultrasound of the thyroid gland, we routinely examine the following areas with their key structures:

Submental region (Figs. 4.30 and 4.31): platysma, anterior belly of digastric, mylohyoid, genioglossus and geniohyoid muscles, sublingual glands, and lingual artery. It should be noted that the posterior border of the mylohyoid muscle is free, allowing communication between the sublingual and submandibular spaces.

Submandibular region (Fig. 4.32): submandibular gland, lymph nodes, mylohyoid muscle and hyoglossus muscles, anterior and posterior bellies of digastric muscles, and facial vein and anterior division of retromandibular vein.

Parotid region (Figs. 4.33 and 4.34): parotid gland (superficial lobe), intraparotid duct, retromandibular vein, external carotid artery, intra/periparotid lymph nodes, and masseter and buccinator muscles.

Cervical region: upper/mid/lower cervical/internal jugular nodes, jugulodigastric node (Fig. 4.35), common carotid artery, internal jugular vein, omohyoid muscle, esophagus, vagus nerve, and subclavian artery.

Posterior triangle (Figs. 4.36–4.40): cranial nerve XI, accessory nodal chain, and brachial plexus trunks/divisions.

Supraclavicular fossa (Fig. 4.41): trapezius, sternocleidomastoid, omohyoid, brachial plexus trunks/divisions, and transverse cervical chain of nodes. The transverse cervical chain of nodes links the spinal accessory nodal chain laterally with the jugular chain medially.

Midline: hyoid bone, strap muscles, tracheal rings, and larynx.

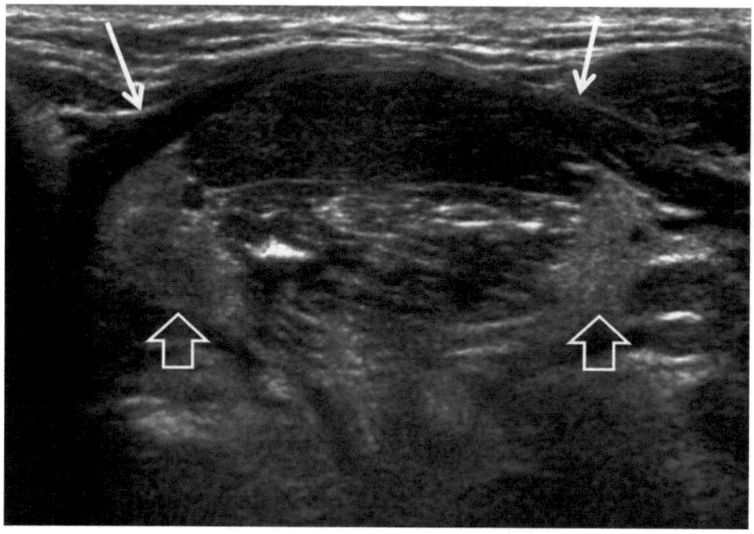

Fig. 4.30 Transverse/coronal gray scale ultrasound of the submental region. Note the mylohyoid muscles (*white arrows*) and the sublingual glands (*white open arrows*)

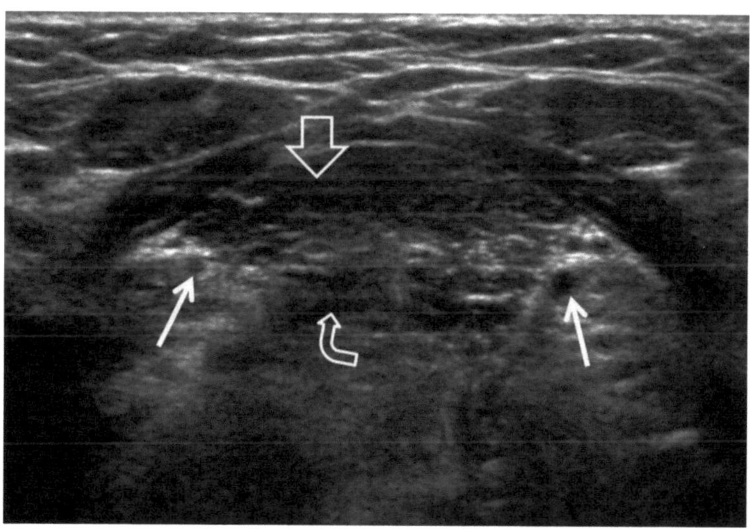

Fig. 4.31 Transverse/coronal gray scale ultrasound of the submental region. Note the branch of lingual arteries (*white arrows*), geniohyoid muscle (*white open arrow*), and genioglossus muscle (*curved white open arrow*)

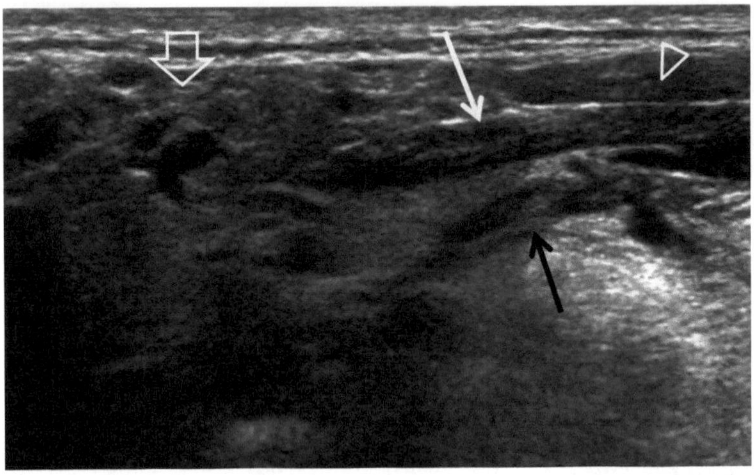

Fig. 4.32 Oblique coronal gray scale ultrasound of the submandibular region. Note the submandibular gland (*white open arrow*), the anterior belly of the digastric muscle (*white arrowhead*), the mylohyoid muscle (*white arrow*), and the hyoglossus muscle (*black arrow*)

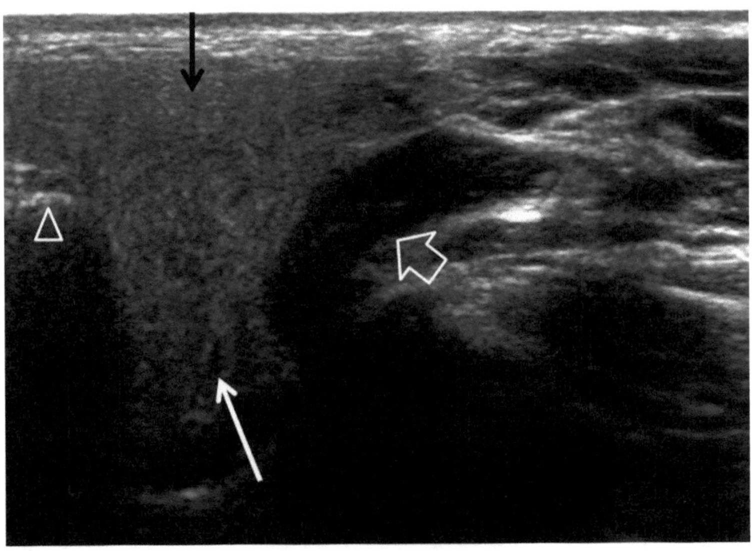

Fig. 4.33 Transverse gray scale ultrasound of the left parotid region. Note the superficial (*black arrow*) and part of deep (*white arrow*) lobes of the parotid gland, the ramus of mandible (*white arrowhead*), and the posterior belly of digastric muscle (*white open arrow*)

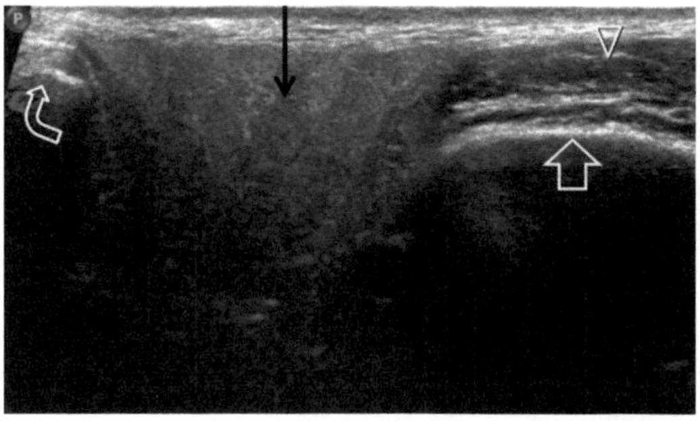

Fig. 4.34 Transverse gray scale ultrasound of the right parotid region. Note the superficial (*black arrow*) lobe of the parotid gland, the ramus of mandible (*white open arrow*), the tip of mastoid process (*white curved open arrow*), and the masseter muscle (*white arrowhead*)

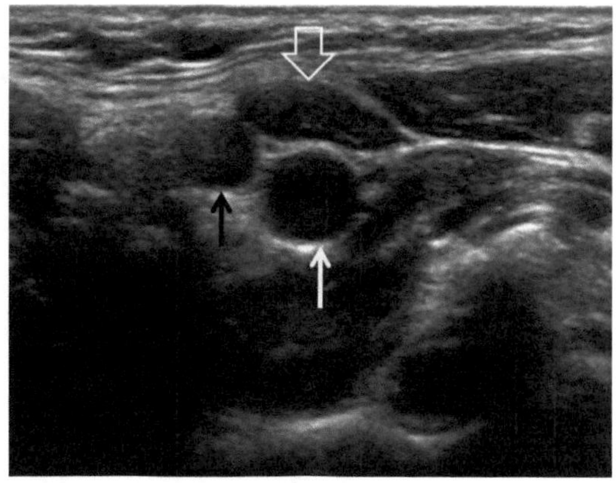

Fig. 4.35 Transverse gray scale ultrasound of the right upper cervical region. Note the jugulodigastric lymph node (*white open arrow*) and its relation to the external (*black arrow*) and internal (*white*) carotid arteries

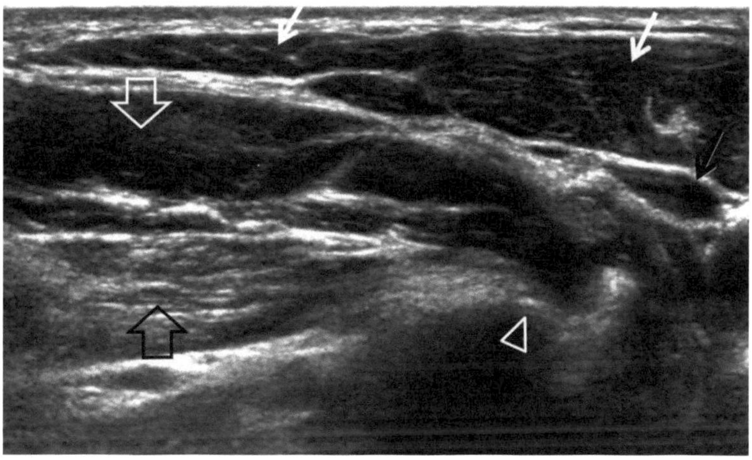

Fig. 4.36 Transverse gray scale ultrasound of the posterior triangle. Note the internal jugular vein (*black arrow*), sternocleidomastoid muscle (*white arrows*), levator scapulae muscle (*white open arrow*), semispinalis capitis muscle (*black open arrow*), and vertebral transverse process (*white arrowhead*)

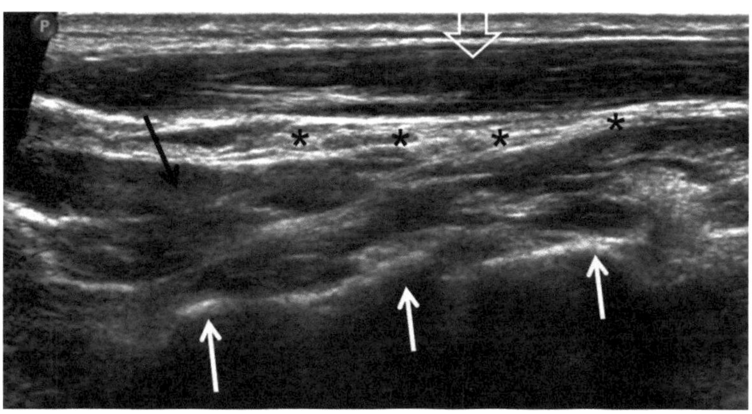

Fig. 4.37 Longitudinal gray scale ultrasound of the posterior triangle. Note the sternocleidomastoid muscle (*white open arrow*), levator scapulae muscle (*black arrow*), and the vertebral transverse processes (*white arrows*). The accessory chain of nodes lies in the thin echogenic fat tissue (*asterisk*) along with the spinal accessory nerve (XI), preaxillary brachial plexus, and dorsal scapular nerve

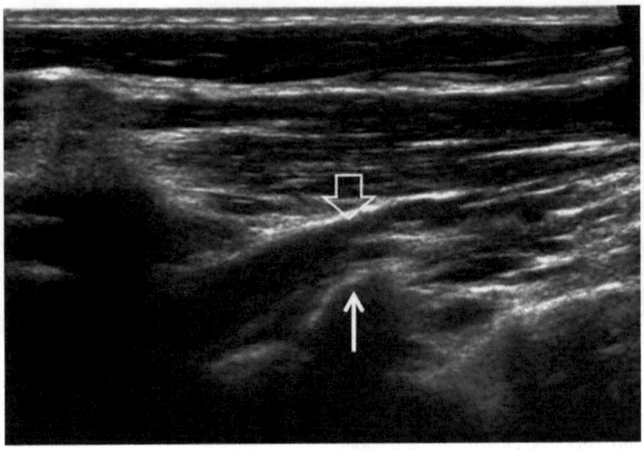

Fig. 4.38 Longitudinal gray scale ultrasound of the posterior triangle shows the upper brachial plexus trunk exiting the spine (*white open arrow*) and the vertebral transverse process (*white arrow*)

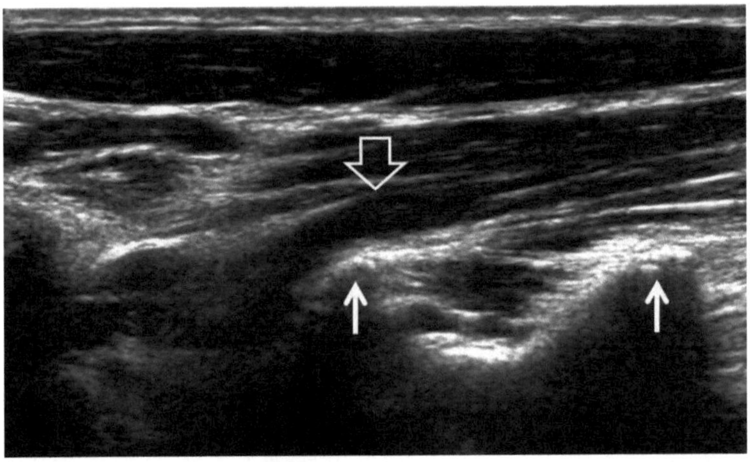

Fig. 4.39 Longitudinal gray scale ultrasound of the posterior triangle shows the mid brachial plexus trunk (*white open arrow*) exiting the spine and the vertebral transverse processes (*white arrows*)

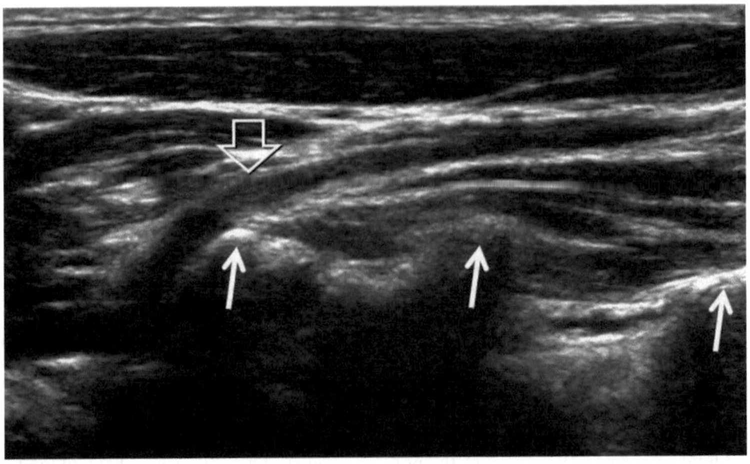

Fig. 4.40 Longitudinal gray scale ultrasound of the posterior triangle shows the lower brachial plexus trunk (*white open arrow*) exiting the spine and the vertebral transverse processes (*white arrows*)

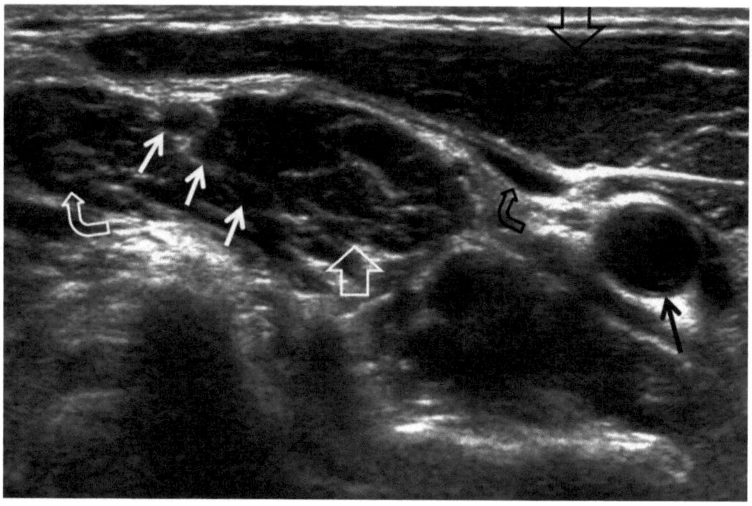

Fig. 4.41 Transverse gray scale ultrasound of the supraclavicular region. Note the brachial plexus elements (*white arrows*), the scalenus anterior muscle (*white open arrow*), the scalenus medius muscle (*white curved open arrow*), the sternocleidomastoid muscle (*black open arrow*), the internal jugular vein (*black curved open arrow*), and the common carotid artery (*black arrow*)

Thyroid Physiology and Thyroid Function Tests

An understanding of the thyroid physiology and basic thyroid function tests (TFTs) may aid in the interpretation of thyroid imaging.

Thyrotropin-releasing hormone (TRH) is secreted by the hypothalamus and acts to stimulate the production of thyroid-stimulating hormone (TSH) by the anterior pituitary gland. Thyroid-stimulating hormone stimulates the production and release of thyroxine (T4) and triiodothyronine (T3) from the thyroid under the control of a negative feedback mechanism. The thyroid produces predominantly T4 which is fivefold less active than T3, and 85% of T3 is formed from the peripheral conversion of T4. Most T3 and T4 in plasma are protein-bound, mainly to thyroxine-binding globulin (TBG), but it is the unbound portion which is the active part. T3 and T4 increase cell metabolism and are vital for growth and mental development.

Measurement of free T4 and T3 levels, which are unaffected by thyroxine-binding globulin, is clinically more useful than total T4 and T3 levels.

↑TSH, ↓ T4 - Hypothyroidism
↑TSH, = T4 - Treated or subclinical hypothyroidism
↑TSH, ↑ T4 - TSH secreting tumor or thyroid hormone resistance
↓TSH, ↑ T4 or T3 - hyperthyroidism
↓TSH, = T4 and T3 - subclinical hyperthyroidism
↓TSH, ↓ T4 and T3 - sick euthyroid or pituitary disease

Normal TSH, abnormal T4 – consider changes in thyroxine-binding globulin, assay interference, amiodarone, or pituitary TSH tumor

Thyroid autoantibodies: Antithyroid peroxidase (TPO) antibodies or antithyroglobulin antibodies may be increased in autoimmune thyroid disease such as Hashimoto's or Graves' disease. A positive status in Graves' disease indicates an increased risk of subsequently developing hypothyroidism.

TSH receptor antibody: may be increased in Graves' disease.

Serum thyroglobulin: used in monitoring the treatment of differentiated carcinoma. It should be undetectable in patients whose thyroid has been ablated and are on a suppressive dose of thyroxine. Detectable thyroglobulin is suggestive of tumor recurrence or metastatic disease.

References

1. Moshynska OV, Saxena A. Clonal relationship between Hashimoto thyroiditis and thyroid lymphoma. J Clin Pathol. 2008;61:438–44.
2. Holm LE, Blomgren H, Lowhagen T. Cancer risks in patients with chronic lymphocytic thyroiditis. N Engl J Med. 1985;312:601–4.
3. Ron E, Lubin JH, Shore RE, et al. Thyroid cancer after exposure to external radiation: a pooled analysis of seven studies. Radiat Res. 1995;141:259.
4. Sarne DH, Schneider AB. Evaluation and management of patients exposed to childhood head and neck irradiation. Endocrinologist. 1995;5:304.
5. Nagataki S, Hirayu H, Izumi M, et al. High prevalence of thyroid nodule in area of radioactive fallout. Lancet. 1989;2:385.
6. Xu W, Iv Z, Wang H. Relationship between RLN and inferior thyroid artery. Otolaryngol Head Neck Surg. 2010;143(2 Suppl):199–200.
7. Yalcxin B. Anatomic configuration of the recurrent laryngeal nerve and inferior thyroid artery. Surgery. 2006;139(2):181–7. Erratum: Surgery 2008;143(3):453.
8. Kapre N. Preservation of the parathyroids in thyroid surgery. Ear Nose Throat J. 2009;2-1. www.waent.org.
9. Macedo TAA, Chammas MC, Jorge PT, Pereira De Souza L, Farage L, Pegoraro BL, et al. Reference values for Doppler ultrasound parameters of the thyroid in a healthy iodine-non-deficient population. Br J Radiol. 2007;80(956):625–30.
10. Turgut AT, Cakal E, Kosar U, Kosar P, Demirbas B, Aral Y. Maximum systolic velocity of inferior thyroid artery and thyroideal color Doppler flow pattern in hypothyroid subjects before and after treatment. J Med Ultrasound. 2009;17(1):44–51.

Further Reading

Ahuja AT. The thyroid and parathyroids. In: Practical head & neck ultrasound. London: Greenwich Medical Media; 2001. p. 37–43.

Ahuja AT, et al. Diagnostic imaging: ultrasound. 1st ed. Salt Lake City: Amisys; 2007. 11-2-5.

Ahuja AT, et al. Diagnostic and Surgical imaging anatomy: ultrasound. 1st ed. Salt Lake City: Amisys; 2007. II-52-57.

Evans RM. Anatomy and technique. In: Practical head & neck ultrasound. London: Greenwich Medical Media; 2001. p. 1–16.

Fultz PJ, Crowley JC. Thyroid, parathyroid, and neck lymph nodes. In: Ultrasound secrets. Hanley & Belfus; 2004. p. 261–262.

Longmore M, Wilkinson I, Turmezei T, Cheung CK. Oxford handbook of clinical medicine. Oxford University Press; 2007. p. 200.

McMinn RMH. Last's anatomy, regional and applied. 9th ed. Churchill Livingstone; 1994. p. 430–432.

Strachan MWJ, Walker BR. Endocrine disease. In: Davidson's principles and practice of medicine. 20th ed. Churchill Livingstone; 2006. p. 760–761.

Strang J. Basic ultrasound technology. In: Ultrasound Secrets. Hanley & Belfus; 2004. p. 1.

Yuen HY, Ahuja AT, King AD, Wong KT. Sonography of the thyroid gland. ASUM Bull. 2003 May;6:6–17.

Benign Thyroid Conditions

5

Ka Tak Wong, and Anil T. Ahuja

Introduction

The thyroid gland is a crucial endocrine organ and its primary endocrine function is to synthesize thyroid hormone. The secretion of thyroid hormone is mediated by thyrotropin-stimulating hormone (TSH) secreted by the anterior pituitary gland. Disturbances of the normal glandular function of the thyroid gland may result in hyperthyroidism/thyrotoxicosis or hypothyroidism. Patients with thyroid disorders may also present with diffuse enlargement (goiter), focal nodular enlargement (thyroid nodule), or compressive symptoms (dysphagia, respiratory distress). A careful clinical history and meticulous physical examination usually suggest a reasonable clinical diagnosis or a short list of differential diagnoses. Laboratory investigations including thyroid function tests allow accurate estimation of the thyroid hormonal status. Patients with high TSH levels are at an increased risk of malignancy [1]. Imaging also plays an integral role in the assessment of thyroid disorders and helps guide patient management.

The normal thyroid anatomy and common thyroid malignancies have been extensively discussed in other parts of the book. This chapter will focus on ultrasound of benign thyroid disorders, including multinodular thyroid, autoimmune thyroid disease/thyroiditis, and congenital anomalies.

Imaging Modalities

Ultrasound is an ideal imaging modality for assessment of the thyroid gland [2]. It is readily available, relatively inexpensive, and does not involve ionizing radiation. The superficial location of the gland readily lends itself to sonographic evaluation using high-resolution transducer (with its excellent spatial and contrast resolution). In addition, ultrasound is easily combined with FNAC which increases its diagnostic accuracy.

The role of ultrasound in benign thyroid disease includes:

- Characterization of thyroid nodule: Vast majority of thyroid nodules are benign. Ultrasound helps confirm benignity of most thyroid nodules and helps to reassure patients and guide subsequent management. In addition, ultrasound also helps to identify the small number of malignant nodules for better preoperative counseling of patients and timely management.
- Initial workup in patients with clinical and biochemical evidence of primary thyroid

K.T. Wong (✉)
Department of Imaging and Interventional Radiology, Prince of Wales Hospital, The Chinese University of Hong Kong, 30-32 Ngan Shing Street, Shatin, NT, Hong Kong SAR, The People's Republic of China
e-mail: wongkatakjeffrey@hotmail.com

A.T. Ahuja
Department of Imaging and Interventional Radiology, The Chinese University of Hong Kong, Prince of Wales Hospital, Shatin (NT), Hong Kong (SAR), China

R.A. Sofferman and A.T. Ahuja (eds.), *Ultrasound of the Thyroid and Parathyroid Glands*,
DOI 10.1007/978-1-4614-0974-8_5, © Springer Science+Business Media, LLC 2012

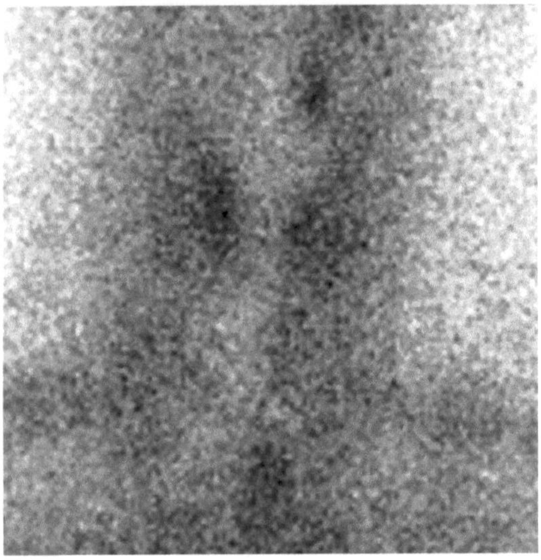

Fig. 5.1 Planar image of Tc-99m TcO4 thyroid scan shows an ill-defined thyroid in a patient with clinically painful thyroiditis. The severely inflamed thyroid with parenchymal destruction releases stored thyroxine causing hyperthyroidism. Findings are consistent with De Quervain's thyroiditis. Courtesy: Dr. Wang Ki, Prince of Wales Hospital, Hong Kong

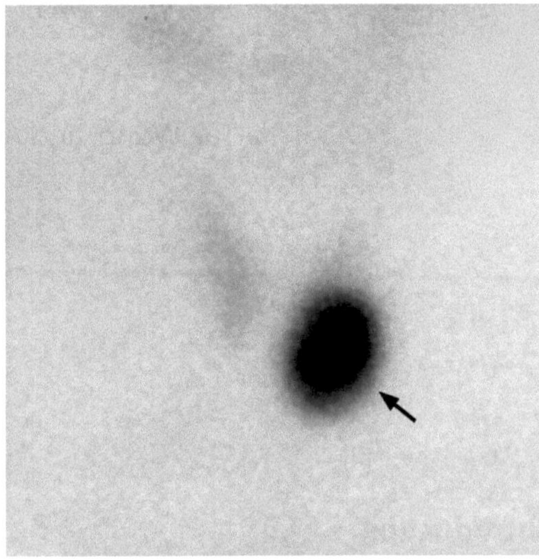

Fig. 5.2 Pinhole image of Tc-99m TcO4 thyroid scan shows a solitary hyperfunctioning nodule (hot nodule, *arrow*) in the lower pole of left thyroid, with markedly suppressed background and thyroid activity. Findings are consistent with toxic nodular goiter. Courtesy: Dr. Wang Ki, Prince of Wales Hospital, Hong Kong

dysfunction (hyperthyroidism and hypothyroidism).

- Provide imaging guidance for FNA or biopsy.
- Follow-up of benign thyroid disease and surveillance to detect any associated malignancy and sequelae/complications.

Thyroid scintigraphy using technetium (Tc-99m) pertechnetate is the principal nuclear medicine investigation in thyroid disease. The more common clinical use of thyroid scintigraphy in benign thyroid disease includes [3]:

- Differential diagnosis of hyperthyroidism: A very low thyroid uptake suggests destructive ("subacute") thyroiditis (Fig. 5.1), a self-limiting disorder, whereas a normal or increased uptake ("superscan") is consistent with toxic nodular goiter (Fig. 5.2) and Graves' disease (Fig. 5.3). Scintigraphic characteristics also help to differentiate between nodular goiter (Fig. 5.4) and Graves' disease.

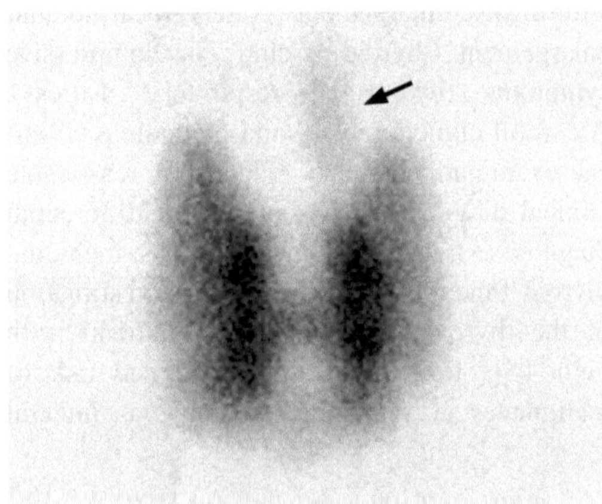

Fig. 5.3 Pinhole image of Tc-99m TcO4 thyroid scan shows a mildly hypertrophic thyroid with enlarged pyramidal lobe (*arrow*). The thyroid is hyperfunctioning with suppressed background and salivary gland activity. Findings are consistent with Graves' disease (clinically hyperthyroid and positive antithyroglobulin and antimicrosomal antibodies). Courtesy: Dr. Wang Ki, Prince of Wales Hospital, Hong Kong

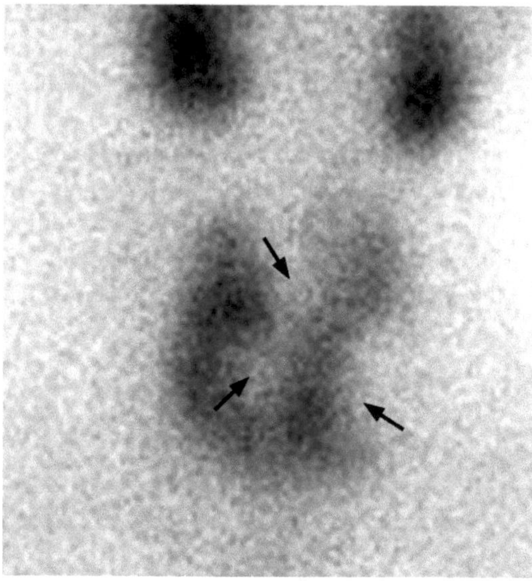

Fig. 5.4 Planar image of Tc-99m TcO4 thyroid scan shows multiple hypofunctioning nodules (*arrows*) in both lobes of thyroid. Overall uptake of thyroid is slightly diminished, while the submandibular glands and background activities are normal. Findings are consistent with nontoxic multinodular goiter. Courtesy: Dr. Wang Ki, Prince of Wales Hospital, Hong Kong

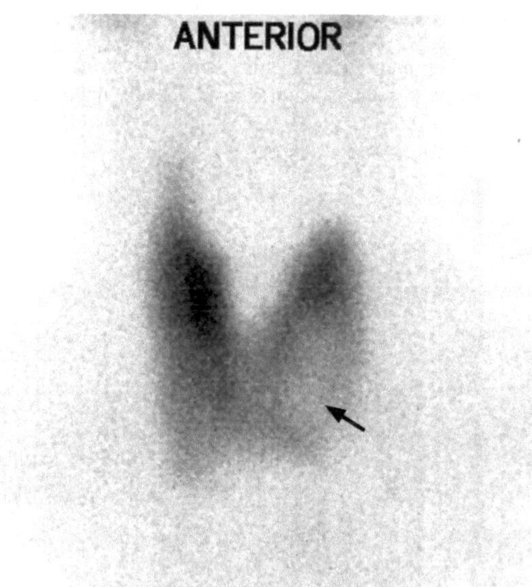

Fig. 5.5 Planar image of Tc-99m TcO4 thyroid scan shows a hypofunctioning (cold nodule, *arrow*) in the lower pole of left thyroid for in a patient with clinically palpable goiter. FNAC showed benign hyperplasia, consistent with nontoxic nodular goiter. Courtesy: Dr. Wang Ki, Prince of Wales Hospital, Hong Kong

- Functional assessment of thyroid nodules prior to FNAC: Scintigraphy helps to determine the necessity of FNAC. "Hot" nodules are generally benign and do not require FNAC, whereas "cold" nodules (Fig. 5.5) may be malignant and warrant a lower threshold for needle sampling.
- Differential diagnosis of congenital hypothyroidism: Scintigraphy combined with ultrasound helps to identify thyroid agenesis, dyshormonogenesis, and incomplete thyroid descent.

Multinodular Thyroid

2–6% of the population have multinodular thyroid with a clinically palpable mass [4]. The vast majority of these thyroid nodules are benign hyperplastic nodules. Compared with the very high prevalence of nodular thyroid disease, thyroid cancer is not common [5]. Patients with multinodular thyroid are frequently asymptomatic, but may present with an anterior neck lump or swelling. Occasionally, patients present acutely with compressive symptoms or with a rapidly enlarging neck mass, most commonly caused by hemorrhage into an underlying hyperplastic thyroid nodule.

Thyroid ultrasound has been widely used to differentiate benign from malignant nodules and to guide fine needle aspiration cytology (FNAC) [5, 6]. However, the accuracy and predictive values of sonographic criteria are variable and no single ultrasound feature has both high sensitivity and positive predictive value for prediction of benignity or malignancy. The Society of Radiologists in Ultrasound consensus panel acknowledged that "although there are certain trends in the ultrasound distinction of benign and malignant thyroid nodules, there is also overlap in their appearances. Because of the inconsistent predictive value of ultrasound features, most agree that FNA and cytopathologic evaluation of a thyroid nodule are usually required before a patient undergoes surgical resection for a possible thyroid malignancy" [5].

Ultrasound Features of Multinodular Thyroid [2]

- *Number*: Presence of multiple oval- to round-shaped nodules (Figs. 5.6 and 5.7) in both lobes of thyroid gland particularly in the inferior poles.
- *Solid/cystic*: Predominantly solid (<50% cystic component) in the majority (87%) of benign nodules [7]. 13% of benign nodules are predominantly cystic in composition (>50% cystic component) with multiple internal septa (Figs. 5.8 and 5.9). A purely cystic nodule, although rare (<2% of all nodules), is highly unlikely to be malignant [8]. Spongiform appearance, defined as aggregation of multiple microcystic components in more than 50% of the volume of the nodule (Figs. 5.10 and 5.11),

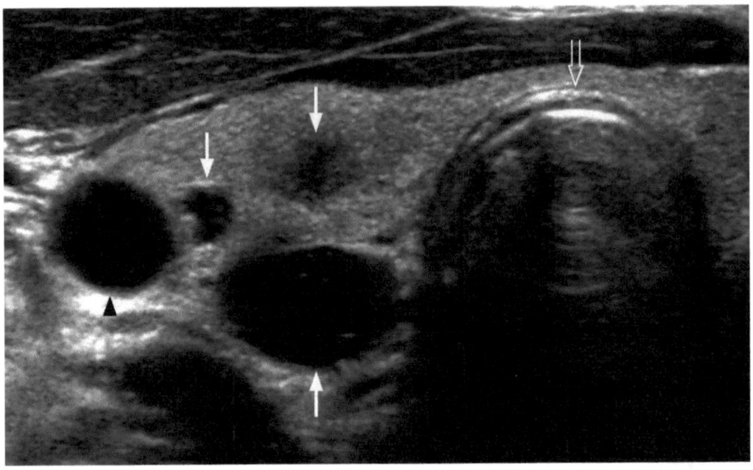

Fig. 5.6 Transverse gray scale thyroid ultrasound shows multiple, heterogeneous nodules in the right lobe of the thyroid (*arrows*). Note some nodules show cystic component (with comet-tail artifacts) and others are isoechoic solid component with cystic elements. None of the nodules show obvious features suspicious for malignancy. Note *open arrow* shows trachea and *arrowheads* mark the common carotid artery (CCA)

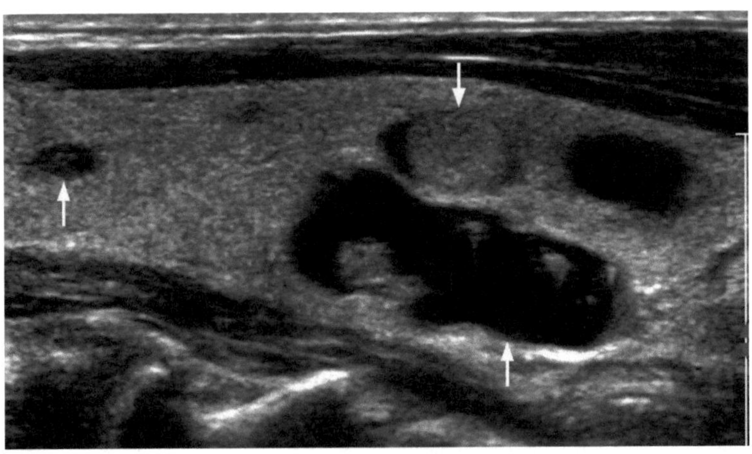

Fig. 5.7 Longitudinal gray scale thyroid ultrasound of the same patient demonstrated in Fig. 5.6 shows multiple, heterogeneous nodules in the right lobe of the thyroid (*arrows*)

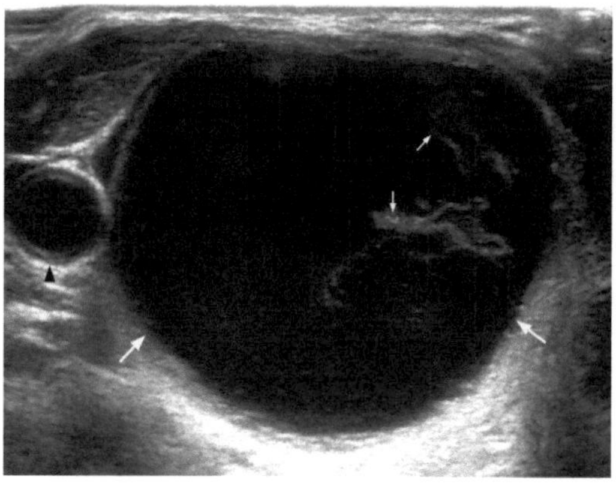

Fig. 5.8 Transverse gray scale ultrasound shows a large, cystic thyroid nodule (*large arrows*) with fine internal debris and septa (*small arrows*). The ultrasound appearances are of a hemorrhagic thyroid nodule. Although benign looking on ultrasound, an FNAC may be indicated to aspirate the contents (invariably altered blood) to reduce the size of the nodule for cosmetic reasons. *Arrowhead*=CCA

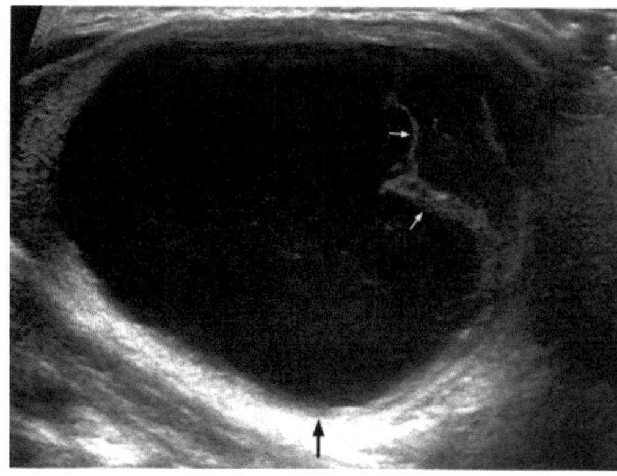

Fig. 5.9 Longitudinal gray scale ultrasound of the same patient demonstrated in Fig. 5.8 shows a large, cystic thyroid nodule (*large arrows*) with fine internal debris and septa (*small arrows*)

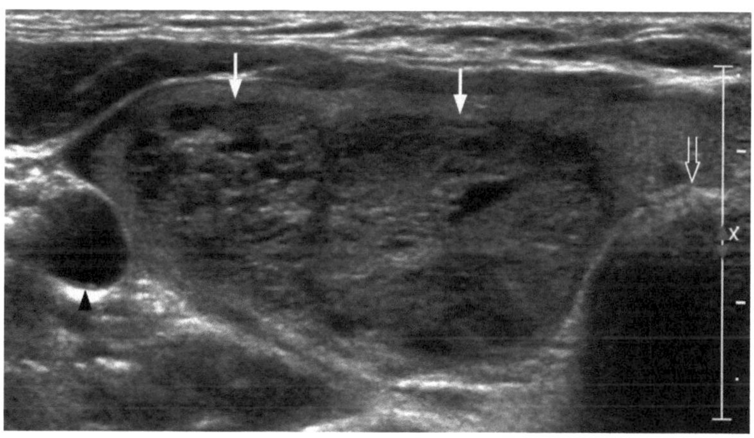

Fig. 5.10 Transverse gray scale ultrasound shows a typical, spongiform appearance of the thyroid nodule (*arrows*). Such nodules are invariably benign and may not require confirmatory FNAC. *Open arrow*= trachea, *arrowhead*=CCA

is 99.7% specific for benign hyperplastic nodule with a negative predictive value for malignancy of 98.5% [7, 9, 10].

- *Echogenicity*: Isoechogenicity (Fig. 5.12) of the solid component, present in 57% of hyperplastic nodules, is a good indicator of benignity. However, hypoechogenicity (often seen in malignant thyroid nodules) is also seen in 34% of benign hyperplastic nodules. Some large cystic nodules may demonstrate the presence of isoechoic, avascular "mural nodule" (Figs. 5.13 and 5.14). These represent intranodular clots following intranodular hemorrhage and feel soft on FNAC.
- *Edge/margins*: Well-defined, smooth margin in 76%.
- *Calcification*: Present in 15–25% and may be curvilinear/annular or dysmorphic in appearance,

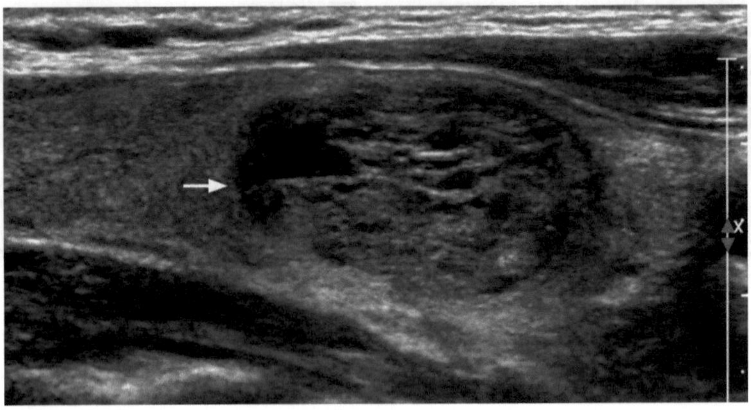

Fig. 5.11 Longitudinal gray scale ultrasound of the same patient demonstrated in Fig. 5.10 shows a typical, spongiform appearance of the thyroid nodule (*arrow*)

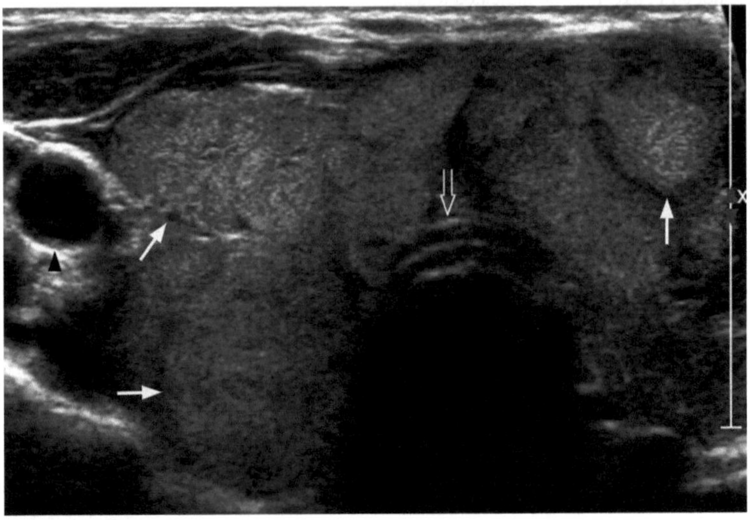

Fig. 5.12 Transverse gray scale ultrasound showing multiple, well-defined, solid, homogeneous, isoechoic nodules (*arrows*) in a patient with multinodular goiter. None of the nodules show any suspicious-appearing features such as hypoechogenicity, punctate calcification, and taller than wide appearance. *Open arrow*=trachea, *arrowhead*=CCA

dense, and with posterior acoustic shadowing (Figs. 5.15–5.17).

- *Comet-tail sign*: Indicating the presence of colloid within a nodule, is often seen in multinodular thyroid. On ultrasound, these are seen as multiple, tiny, nonshadowing echogenic foci with posterior comet-tail artifacts (Fig. 5.7) [11].
- *Doppler*: Predominantly peripheral pattern of vascular flow on power Doppler examination is suggestive of benign hyperplastic nodule rather than a malignant nodule (Figs. 5.18 and 5.19) [12–15].

What is the Role of Ultrasound in Multinodular Thyroid?

The diagnosis of multinodular thyroid is readily established clinically, by surgeons/endocrinologists/clinicians. Therefore, what role if any does ultrasound have in such patients? It was previously

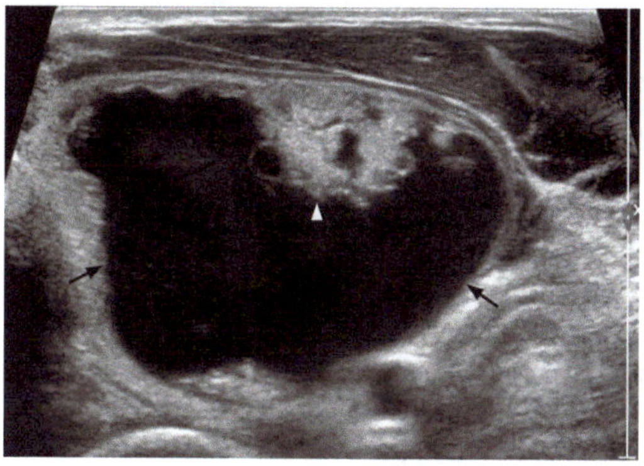

Fig. 5.13 Transverse gray scale ultrasound show a large predominantly cystic nodule (*arrows*) with a focal, "solid" component (*arrowheads*). This is a fairly common appearance of a hemorrhagic component within a thyroid nodule and the avascular solid component represents blood clot

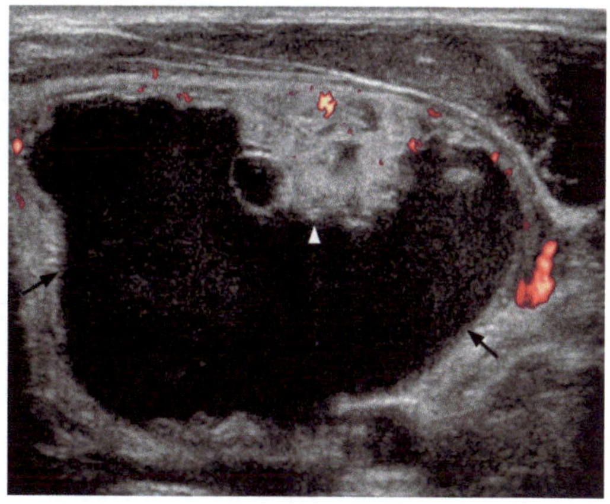

Fig. 5.14 Transverse gray scale and Doppler ultrasound of the same nodule demonstrated in Fig. 5.13. *Arrows* designate the cystic area and the focal "solid" component is indicated by the *arrowhead*. Note that no significant vascularity is seen within the solid component

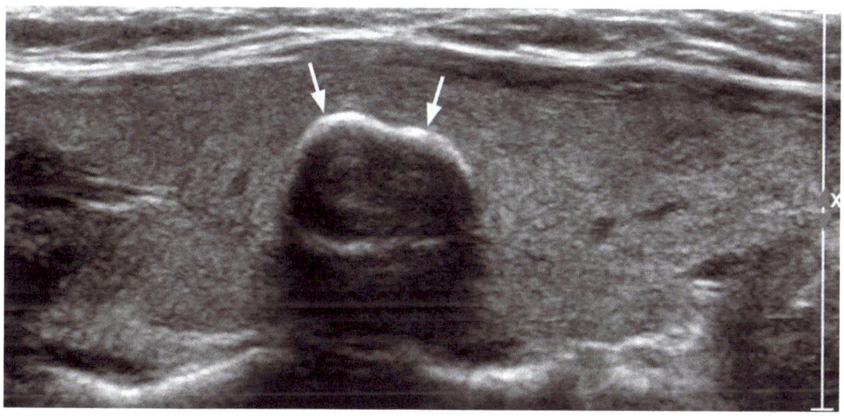

Fig. 5.15 Longitudinal gray scale ultrasound shows an area of dense, solid, shadowing dysmorphic calcification (*arrows*) seen in MNG

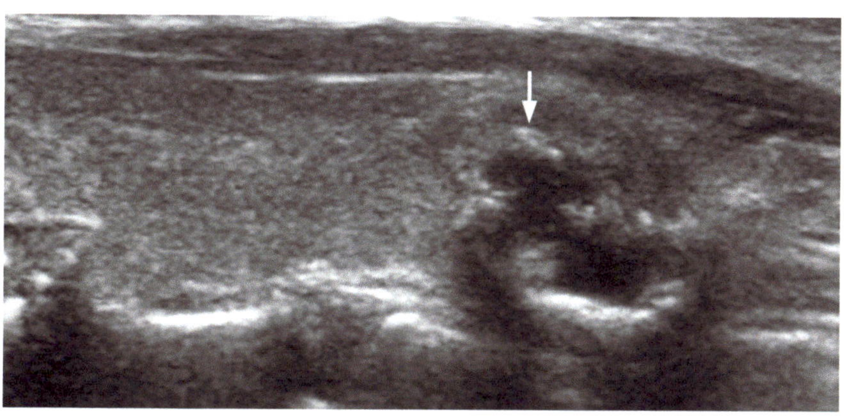

Fig. 5.16 Longitudinal gray scale ultrasound shows an additional region of dysmorphic calcification (*arrow*) in MNG

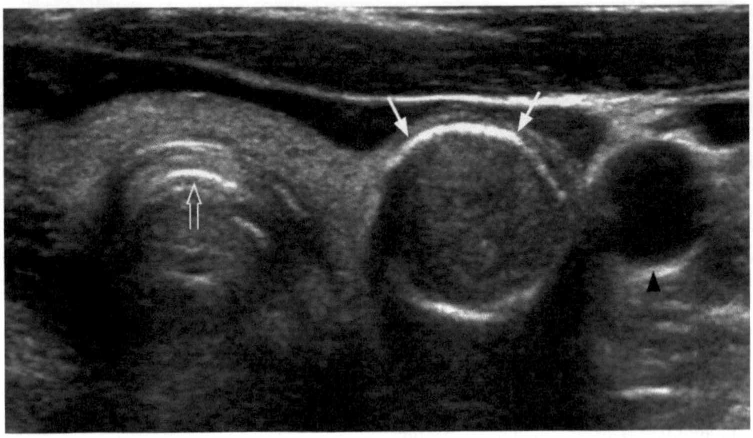

Fig. 5.17 Transverse gray scale ultrasound shows dense, curvilinear shadowing calcification (*arrows*) in the thyroid. *Open arrow*=trachea, *arrowhead*=CCA

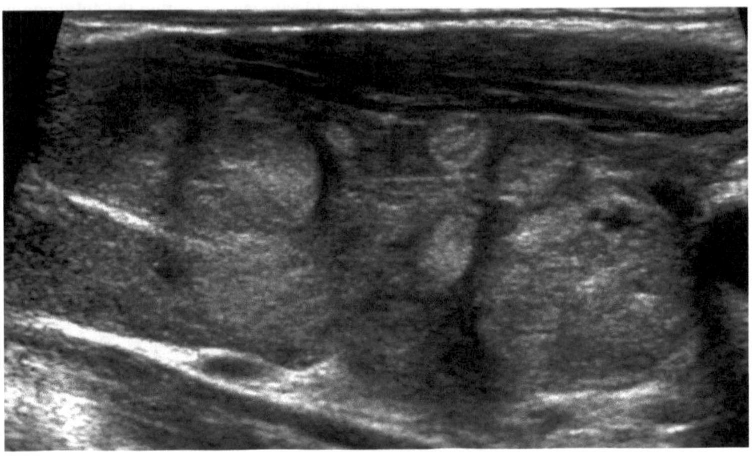

Fig. 5.18 Longitudinal gray scale shows multiple, solid, isoechoic, noncalcified nodules

believed multinodularity conferred benignity on thyroid nodules and any further imaging may not be necessary. However, it is now well documented that patients with multiple nodules have the same risk of malignancy as those with solitary nodules [6, 8, 12]. It is reported that 33% of malignant disease is found in solitary nodules and 22% in MNGs [16]. Also, with modern high-resolution transducers, it is quite unusual to sonographically encounter a solitary nodule. Therefore, ultrasound is crucial in detecting the presence of a thyroid malignancy against the background of multinodularity.

The common cancers seen in multinodular thyroid include differentiated thyroid cancers (papillary and follicular cancers) and anaplastic carcinoma, papillary carcinoma being the most common. In a previous study, 52% of papillary carcinomas were found in solitary nodules and 48% in MNGs [17].

The roles of ultrasound in patients with multinodular thyroid are:

- Identify the presence of thyroid malignancy against the background of multinodularity (Figs. 5.20–5.22) and guide a confirmatory

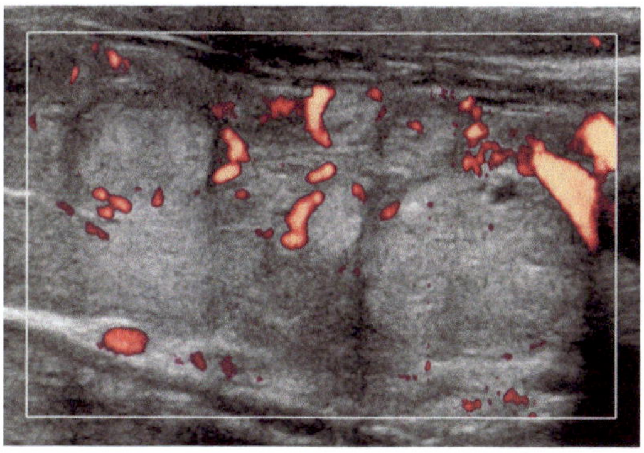

Fig. 5.19 Longitudinal gray scale and Doppler ultrasound shows multiple, solid, isoechoic, noncalcified nodules with a predominantly benign-looking perinodular vascularity

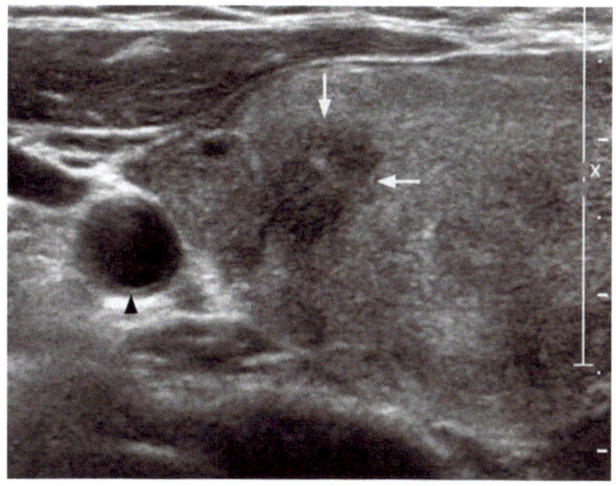

Fig. 5.20 Transverse gray scale ultrasound demonstrates a solid, ill-defined, hypoechoic nodule (*arrows*), confirmed as a papillary carcinoma with FNAC. *Arrowheads*=CCA. The diagnosis of MNG is invariably suggested by a clinician. The main role of ultrasound is to detect the presence of any malignancy against this background of MNG

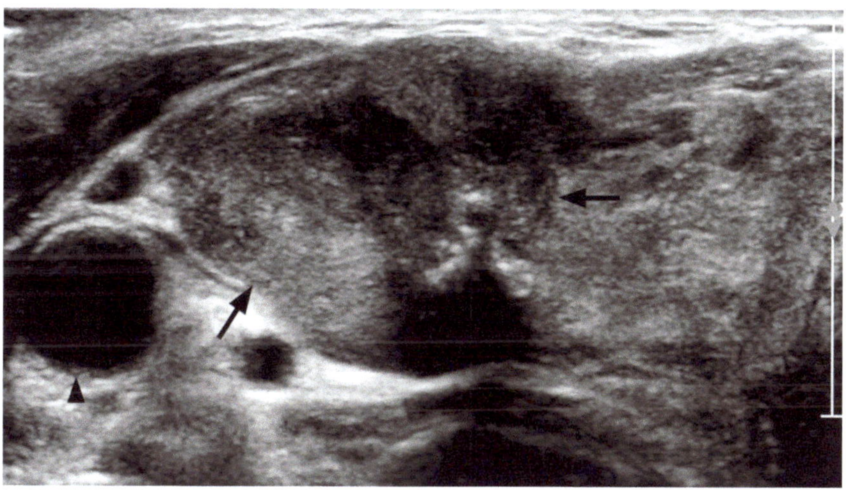

Fig. 5.21 Transverse gray scale ultrasound demonstrates a solid, ill-defined, hypoechoic nodule (*black arrow*) with punctate calcification confirmed on FNAC as papillary carcinoma. This nodule exists in a background of MNG. *Black arrowhead*=CCA

FNAC/biopsy [16]. Ultrasound-guided FNAC increases the accuracy of FNAC from 85% to 95% and reduces the inadequate rate from 15% to 3% [18, 19].

- Evaluate the neck for the presence of associated metastatic nodes, if any.

In addition, ultrasound is useful in:

- Follow-up of patients who are otherwise asymptomatic but apprehensive about their thyroid nodule
- Guide FNAC/biopsy of nodules that show a rapid, substantial growth on serial examination

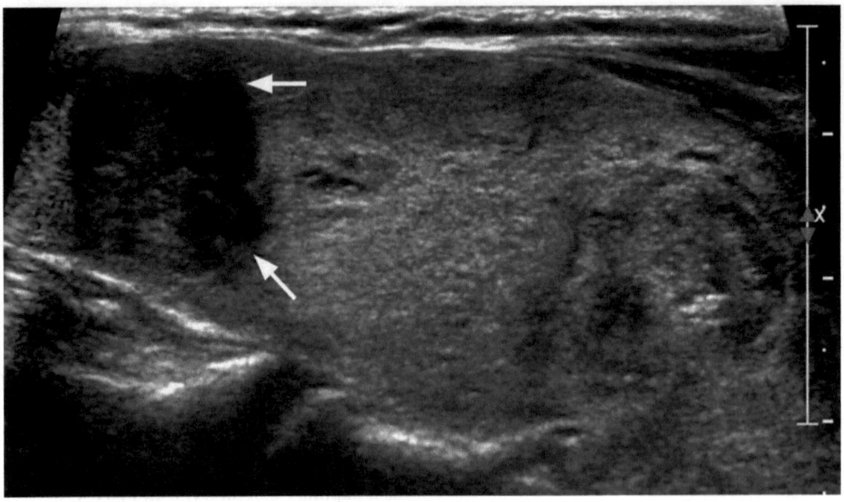

Fig. 5.22 Longitudinal gray scale ultrasound demonstrates a hypoechoic nodule (*arrows*) against a background of MNG. It is "taller-than-wide" and has been proven to be a papillary carcinoma with FNAC

Limitations of ultrasound in multinodular goiter:

- In large multinodular goiters, ultrasound may be unable to identify the presence of tiny foci of malignancy (solitary or multiple). In patients with MNG with a dominant nodule, ultrasound may be unable to detect the suspected thyroid malignancy if the thyroid volume is high. When the thyroid volume is less than 38 mL, the detection of suspicious nodules with ultrasound is increased [20].
- Ultrasound cannot evaluate the entire extent of large goiters, particularly its mediastinal extension.
- Ultrasound cannot accurately evaluate the presence or extent/severity of airway compression.

In the Presence of Multiple Discrete Thyroid Nodules on Ultrasound, is FNAC Necessary, and Which Nodule Should Be FNAed?

In a multinodular thyroid, it is obvious that not every nodule can be FNAed. It is therefore essential to pick the nodule against the background multinodularity that requires further evaluation by FNAC. The established consensus is that the choice of nodule for FNAC is based primarily on ultrasound characteristics of the nodule rather than nodule size (i.e., dominant) [5, 21].

Any nodule with suspicious feature (presence of punctuate calcification, markedly hypoechoic, solid, ill-defined margins, abnormal vascularity, taller than wide) should be selected for FNA rather than a dominant nodule with no/little suspicious features.

Although the natural history for both benign and malignant nodules is growth over time [22], it is generally agreed that rapid growth of a nodule indicates an increase risk for malignancy [23, 24]. Therefore, FNAC is recommended for nodules demonstrating substantial growth on serial ultrasound.

Is FNAC Required if None of the Nodules Show Any Sonographic Suspicion of Malignancy?

In the absence of any sonographically suspicious nodule, a dominant nodule with nonsuspicious features may be FNAed [25] to allay the concerns of apprehensive patients. In our practice, in addition, large, predominantly cystic nodule may be FNAed to aspirate the fluid and reduce the size of the nodule for cosmetic purposes/provide symptomatic relief. However, following FNAC of a predominantly cystic nodule, one must note that the residual post-FNAC nodule may mimic a malignant nodule with a taller than wide shape, hypoechogenicity and ill-defined/crenated margins [26] (Figs. 5.23–5.27). Therefore, when follow-up examinations are performed for benign nodules, one must clearly inquire for a history of previous FNAC and the approximate site of the FNAC in order not to mistake a post-FNAC nodule with a malignant nodule.

In some centers, if all nodules in multinodular thyroid appear sonographically nonsuspicious, FNAC may not be performed, and a follow-up examination is suggested to monitor change in size and appearance.

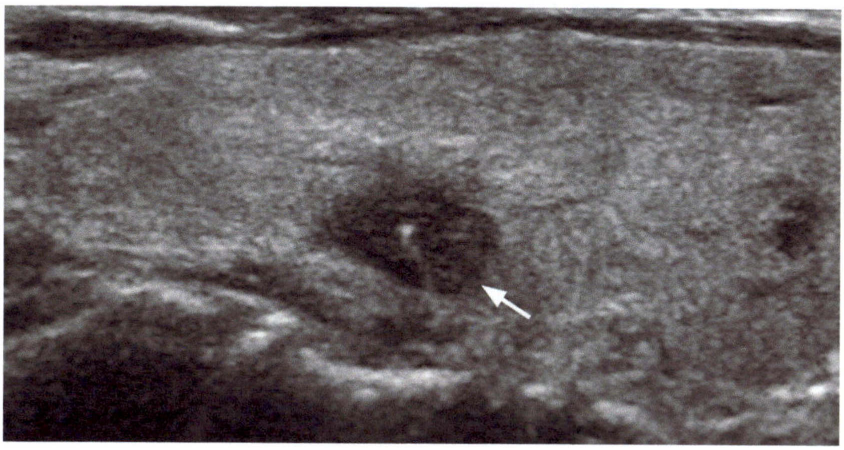

Fig. 5.23 Longitudinal gray scale of a postaspirated collapsed benign thyroid nodule (*arrow*). This nodule was predominantly cystic in nature prior to FNAC. Note the hypoechogenicity, ill-defined margins simulating a malignant thyroid nodule.

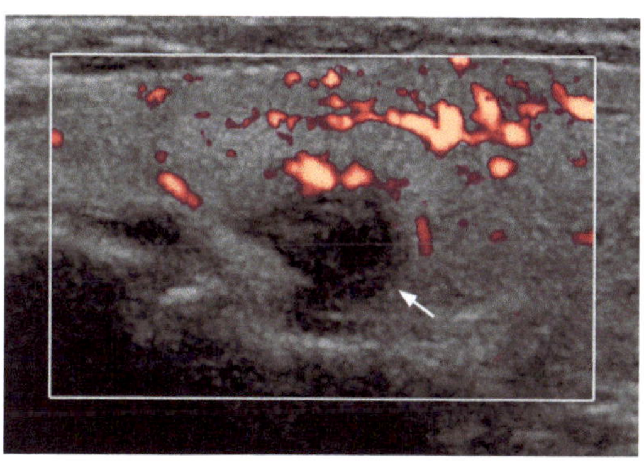

Fig. 5.24 Longitudinal gray scale and Doppler ultrasound of a postaspirated collapsed benign thyroid nodule (*arrow*). This nodule was predominantly cystic in nature prior to FNAC. Note the hypoechogenicity, ill-defined margins simulating a malignant thyroid nodule. The complete absence of vascularity and a history of previous FNAC will help in its evaluation

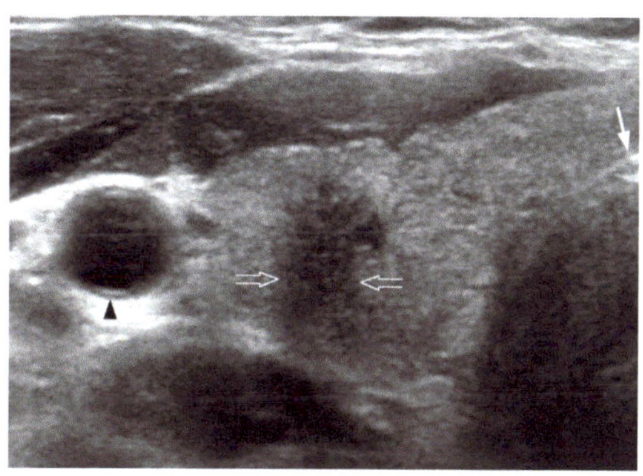

Fig. 5.25 Transverse image of a postaspirated benign thyroid nodule (*open arrow*). Note its hypoechogenicity, ill-defined margins, taller than wide nature simulating a malignant thyroid nodule. *Arrow*=trachea, *arrowhead*=CCA

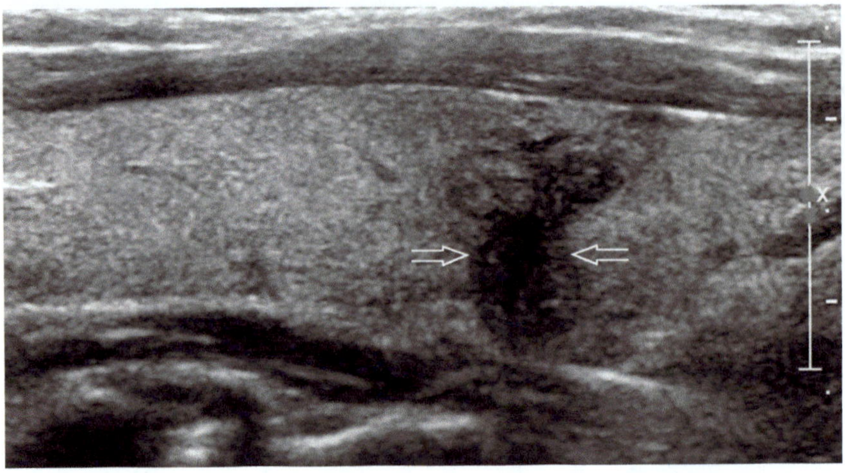

Fig. 5.26 Longitudinal gray scale image of a postaspirated benign thyroid nodule (*open arrow*). Note its hypoechogenicity, ill-defined margins, taller than wide nature simulating a malignant thyroid nodule. *Arrow*=trachea, *arrowhead*=CCA

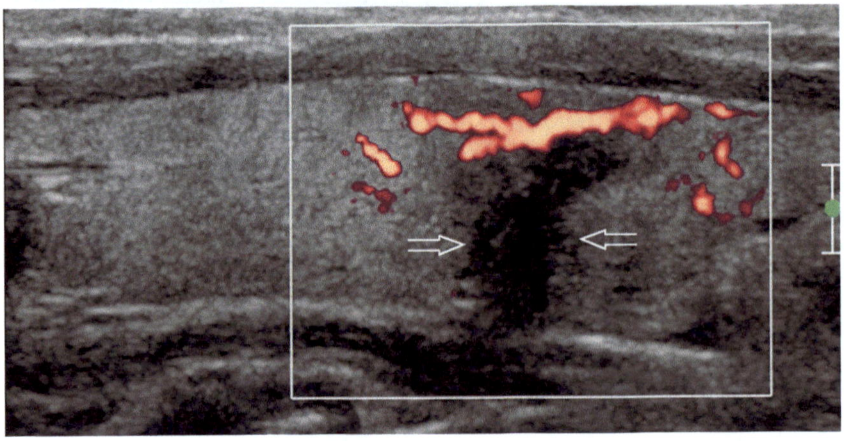

Fig. 5.27 Longitudinal gray scale and Doppler image of a postaspirated benign thyroid nodule (*open arrow*) in patient demonstrated in Fig. 5.26

What is the Suggested Frequency of Follow-Up?

In patients who have had a previous FNAC suggesting benign disease, a follow-up is routinely suggested and effective as the false-negative rate of FNAC is quite low [27, 28]. In a patient, the probability of benignity correctly identified by FNAC is 90%, and this increases to 98% if a subsequent second FNAC is also benign [29]. The false-negative rate of FNAC also drops from 5.2% to 1.2% when a diagnostic second FNAC is performed [30].

Against this background of information, some of the follow-up recommendations are:

- All benign thyroid nodules be followed with serial ultrasound 6–18 months after the initial FNAC. If nodule size is stable (i.e., no more than a 50% change in volume or <20% increase in at least two nodule dimensions in solid nodules or in the solid portion of mixed cystic-solid nodules), the interval before the next follow-up clinical examination or ultrasound may be longer, e.g., 3–5 years [25]. If growth is detected, an ultrasound-guided FNAC is indicated [25].
- After the first thyroid ultrasound and FNA, follow-up ultrasound should be repeated in 6 months and once a year thereafter, if there are no changes [31].

- The British Thyroid Association recommends a repeat FNAC 3–6 months after the initial diagnosis of benign disease [32].

In other patients, although there is no consensus [in the statement issued by the Society of Radiologists in Ultrasound [5]], some of the recommendations for follow-up are:

- The frequency of routine ongoing follow-up depends on the size of the nodule and rapidity of appearance, ultrasound appearances, and history and clinical assessment. Larger nodules that have appeared suddenly need to be followed more frequently than an incidental 6-mm nodule detected on ultrasound [33].
- The American Association of Clinical Endocrinologists recommended that thyroid incidentalomas should be followed by ultrasound in 6–12 months and regularly thereafter [34].

Autoimmune Thyroiditis

There are two major forms of autoimmune thyroiditis (AITD) and these include chronic autoimmune thyroiditis (CAITD) and Graves' disease [35, 36]. CAITD has two forms, atrophic form referred to atrophic thyroiditis and a goitrous form called Hashimoto's thyroiditis [37]. The other forms of CAITD include postpartum thyroiditis and silent thyroiditis [36]. These are usually self-limiting, and when the inflammatory process happens in the absence of pregnancy, it is termed painless thyroiditis.

The Need for Imaging in AITD?

In most instances, the diagnosis of AITD is made by the clinician based on clinical signs and symptoms of thyroid disease and laboratory investigations which include measurement of thyroid hormone level, thyrotropin (TSH), and thyroid antibodies. However, as discussed by Pedersen et al. [37], in some patients the symptoms may be absent and nonspecific. In the elderly, the symptoms may overlap with other chronic medical diseases, and the laboratory data may be inconclusive or not requested [38, 39].

Imaging may help to differentiate: (1) AITD from non-AITD conditions such as De Quervain's thyroiditis; (2) differentiate between forms of AITD i.e., Graves' disease from Hashimoto's thyroiditis; (3) follow-up of patients with AITD: (a) focal lymphocytic thyroiditis [40] and (b) evaluate response to treatment as the degree of hypoechogenicity correlates with levels of circulating antibodies [41] and persistence of hypoechogenicity and elevated thyroid antibody levels correlate with higher chance of relapse following cessation of medication [42].

Which is the Ideal Initial Imaging Modality?

In patients with AITD, particularly Graves' disease, scintigraphy is suggested by many guidelines [43–45] and still considered an essential step in the diagnosis of Graves' disease [46]. However, ultrasound is now being increasingly performed, and considered a good alternative to scintigraphy [47–50] if not the gold standard in the evaluation of hyperthyroid patients [42].

Cappelli et al. [46] found that in patients with Graves' disease, there was no difference in terms of diagnosis between scintigraphy and ultrasound, and ultrasound was significantly better than scintigraphy in detection of nodules ≥10 mm. The inability of scintigraphy to reliably visualize nodules <10 mm is well established [3].

As established by Cappelli et al. [46], ultrasound (+color Doppler) should be performed in all hyperthyroid patients and scintigraphy limited to uncommon cases when clinical features, laboratory data, and ultrasound are not diagnostic.

Sonographic Appearances in AITD

Echogenicity

Decrease in thyroid echogenicity is a strong predictor of AITD [37], and the relationship between low echogenicity and AITD has been known for decades [39, 51]. This reduction in echogenicity occurs early in the disease process, often before overt thyroid failure [37]. The degree of hypoechogenicity significantly correlates with levels of circulating thyroid antibodies [41], and there is a linear relationship between positive/abnormal laboratory tests and the reduction in thyroid echogenicity [37]. Thyroid echogenicity depends on cellularity, and vascularization, reduced colloid content, lymphocytic infiltration, and hypervascularization all contribute to the hypoechogenicity in AITD [41, 52–56].

Diffuse lymphocytic infiltration accounts for decreased echogenicity in Hashimoto's and postpartum thyroiditis. In Graves' disease, the hypoechogenicity may be due to reduced colloid content, increased cellularity and reduction of cell-colloid interface, and increased blood flow [52].

Doppler

The marked increase in intrathyroid vascularity seen on Doppler in patients with Graves' disease has also been known for years [54]. This pulsatile hypervascularity was termed as "thyroid inferno" seen diffusely in both systole and diastole. Such increase in vascularity is not seen in patients with toxic multinodular goiter and Hashimoto's thyroiditis [57]. The reduction in such vascularity in patients responding to medical treatment is also reported [54].

In addition to the thyroid blood flow, others have studied the peak systolic velocity (PSV) in patients with AITD [58]. Patients with Graves' disease showed a proportional increase in thyroid blood flow and PSV (normal PSV = 17.7 ± 3 cm/s). This is again useful in differentiating Graves' disease from Hashimoto's thyroiditis where the vascularity in the thyroid gland may range from hypovascular to hypervascular [59].

Doppler also helps to differentiate between Type 1 and Type 2 amiodarone–induced thyrotoxicosis [60, 61]. Type 1 amiodarone-induced thyrotoxicosis resembles Graves' disease and responds to treatment with thionomides and perchlorate. It shows normal vascularity or diffuse glandular hypervascularity. Type 2 amiodarone-induced thyrotoxicosis resembles painless thyroiditis and may respond to glucocorticoid therapy rather than thionomides or perchlorate. The thyroid gland may be hypovascular on Doppler.

Lymph Nodes

The presence of enlarged lymph nodes is another feature of autoimmune thyroiditis and may sometimes be the first clue to the presence of disease. The lymph nodes are frequently multiple, may be along the cervical chains and/or pretracheal in location [62]. Their overall appearances are reactive in nature, i.e., oval, hypoechoic, noncalcified, presence of echogenic hilum with hilar vascularity, and nonnecrotic.

Graves' Disease

Graves' disease is an autoimmune disorder characterized by hyperthyroidism due to circulating thyroid-stimulating hormone (TSH) receptor autoantibodies (TRAb) with thyroid-stimulating activity [63]. It is the commonest cause of primary hyperthyroidism, with an estimated prevalence in iodine-sufficient areas of 20/1,000 females and 2.3/1,000 males [64]. It is most common in females between 20 and 50 years of age. The diagnosis of Graves' disease is based on clinical (diffuse goiter with clinical symptoms and signs of hyperthyroidism) and laboratory evidence (high serum thyroid hormone, undetectable serum TSH concentrations associated with circulating thyroglobulin and thyroperoxidase antibodies).

Ultrasound is not routinely required in management of patient's with Graves' disease. It may be necessary in patients:

- Who does not respond to routine medical treatment
- For thyroid volume estimation in patients who choose to undergo radioactive iodine treatment
- To rule out other causes of thyroiditis, if indicated

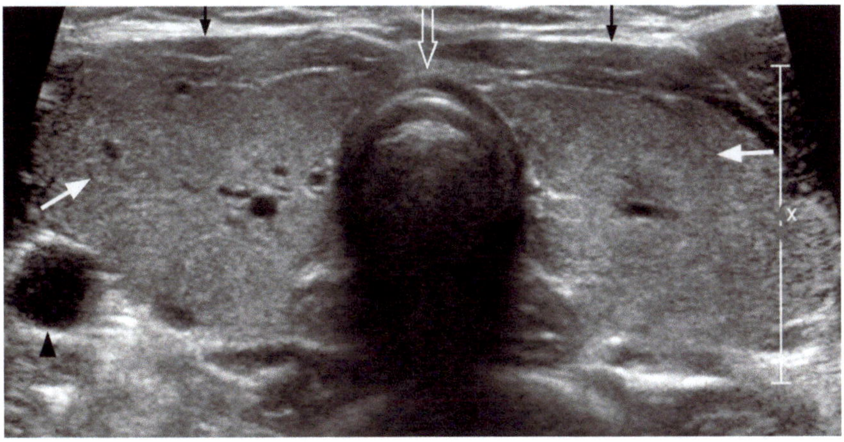

Fig. 5.28 Transverse gray scale ultrasound of the thyroid shows a slight decrease in thyroid echogenicity (*large arrows*), but not as hypoechoic as the strap muscles anteriorly (*small arrows*). The parenchymal hypoechogenicity is the clue toward the diagnosis of autoimmune thyroiditis, Graves' disease in this case. *Open arrow*=trachea, *arrowhead*=CCA

Ultrasound Features of Graves' Disease [47]

- Diffuse glandular enlargement, ± rounded contour, increase in volume up to 90 mL.
- Diffuse low echogenicity of the glandular parenchyma in ~70% [42, 65] due to reduced colloid content with increased cellularity and reduction of the cell-colloid interface and/or to the increased blood flow [52]. The degree of hypoechogenicity (as compared to the adjacent strap muscle) may range from slightly hypoechoic to markedly hypoechoic (Figs. 5.28–5.36). The presence of hypoechogenicity is associated with a higher frequency of TRAb positivity and its persistence on cessation of treatment with relapse of hyperthyroidism [65].
- Marked diffuse hypervascularity ("thyroid inferno") in the glandular parenchyma and around periphery of parenchyma on power Doppler ultrasound (Figs. 5.29, 5.30, 5.35 and 5.36) [48, 54, 58]. The degree of increased vascularity appears to be less marked in patients well controlled by medical therapy. The peak flow velocity in the inferior thyroid artery may be increased up to 120 cm/s. The increased vascularity is a reflection of the inflammatory process and does not correlate with thyroid function.

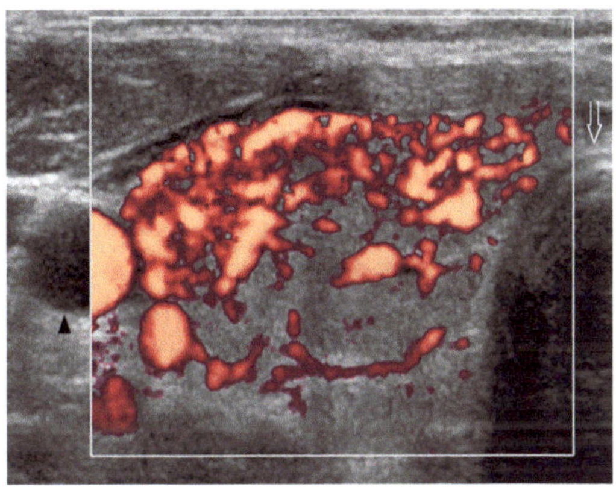

Fig. 5.29 Corresponding Doppler ultrasound (same patient as Fig. 5.28) shows marked increase in thyroid parenchymal vascularity in right lobe of the thyroid, consistent with Graves' disease. *Open arrow*=trachea, *arrowhead*=CCA

On scintigraphy, the thyroid gland is diffusely enlarged with diffuse intense homogeneous tracer uptake (Fig. 5.3). This is in contrary to findings in acute phase of thyroiditis (inhomogeneous reduced tracer uptake), toxic multinodular thyroid (patchy heterogeneous areas of increased and decreased tracer uptake in enlarged gland), and toxic adenoma (focal uptake in single nodule).

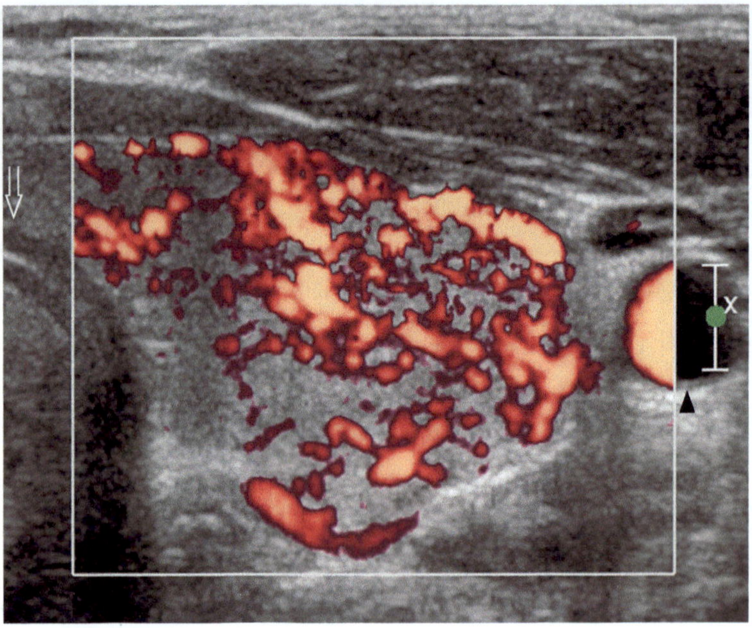

Fig. 5.30 Corresponding Doppler ultrasound (same patient as Fig. 5.28) shows marked increase in thyroid parenchymal vascularity in left lobe of the thyroid, consistent with Graves' disease. *Open arrow*=trachea, *arrowhead*=CCA

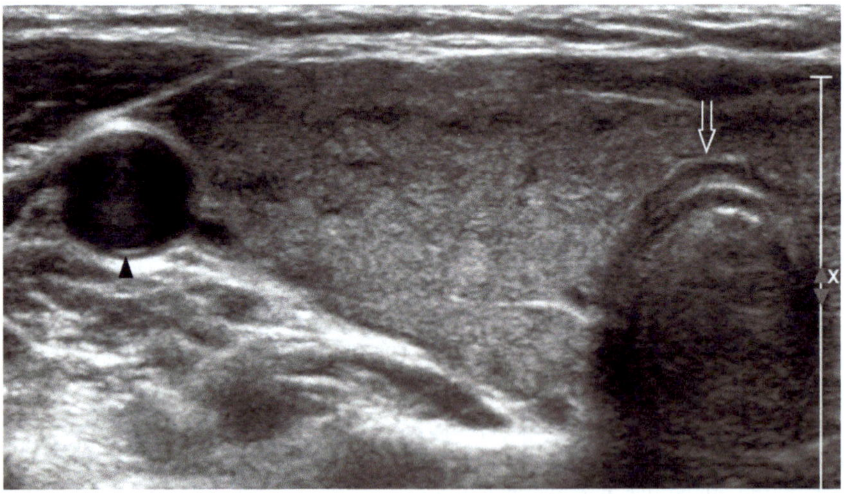

Fig. 5.31 Transverse gray scale ultrasound of the right lobe of the thyroid gland showing diffuse, parenchymal hypoechogenicity. Note areas of the gland are as hypoechoic as the strap muscles anteriorly. The ultrasound appearances are consistent with AITD, in this case Graves' disease. *Open arrow*=trachea, *arrowhead*=CCA

Hashimoto's Thyroiditis

Hashimoto's thyroiditis (chronic lymphocytic thyroiditis) is the commonest cause of acquired hypothyroidism. It is an autoimmune disorder; pathologically, the thyroid gland is enlarged and demonstrates lymphocytic and plasma cell infiltration, colloid-depleted follicles with atrophy, and interlobular fibrosis [66]. Clinically, patients usually present with goiter and symptoms of hypothyroidism. It is more common in females with a peak incidence between 40 and 60 years of

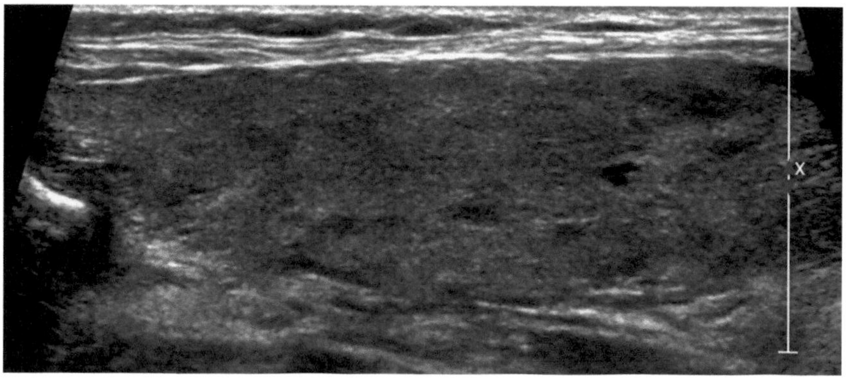

Fig. 5.32 Longitudinal gray scale ultrasound of the right lobe of the thyroid gland in the same patient as Fig. 5.31 shows diffuse, parenchymal hypoechogenicity

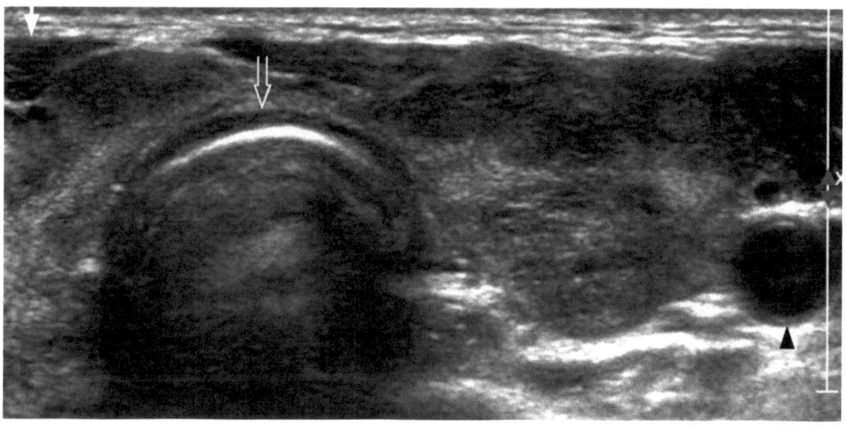

Fig. 5.33 Transverse gray scale ultrasound of the left lobe of the thyroid showing diffuse, marked parenchymal hypoechogenicity. Note areas of the gland are more hypoechoic compared to the strap muscles anteriorly (*arrow*). The ultrasound appearances are consistent with AITD, Graves' disease. *Open arrow* = trachea, *arrowhead* = CCA

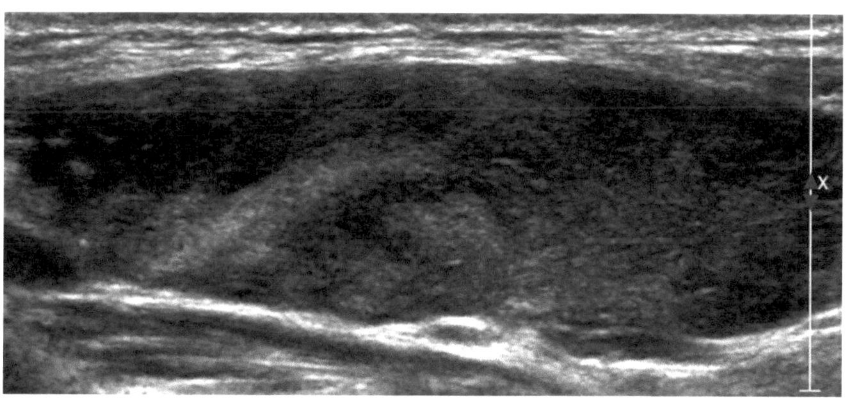

Fig. 5.34 Longitudinal gray scale ultrasound of the left lobe of the thyroid as in the same patient demonstrated in Fig. 5.33 showing diffuse, marked parenchymal hypoechogenicity. The ultrasound appearance is consistent with AITD, Graves' disease

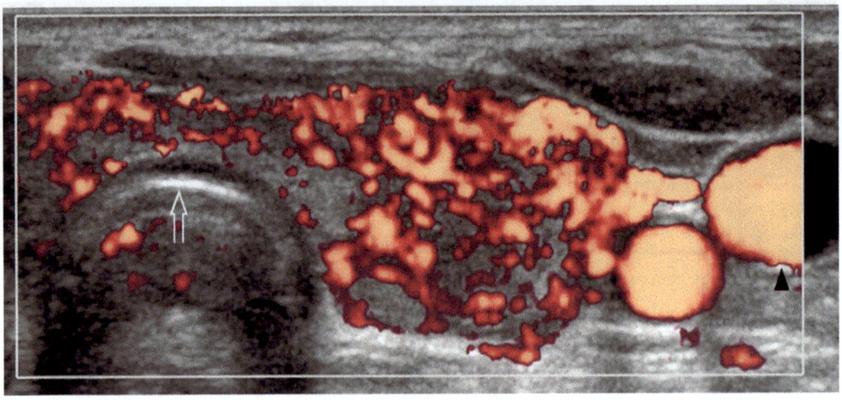

Fig. 5.35 Corresponding Doppler ultrasound (same patient as in Figs. 5.33 and 5.34) shows marked increase in thyroid parenchymal vascularity (even with increase PRF and wall filter, in this case) consistent with Graves' disease. *Open arrow* = trachea, *arrowhead* = IJV

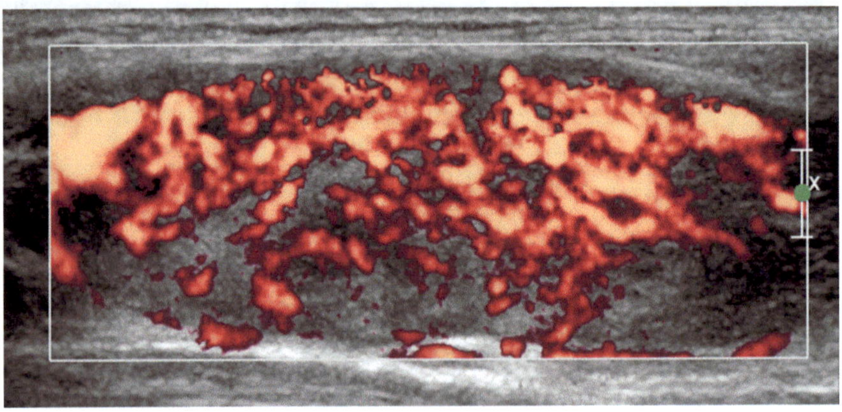

Fig. 5.36 Corresponding Doppler ultrasound (same patient as in Figs. 5.33 and 5.35), left lobe, longitudinal view

age. The diagnosis is primarily based on positive serology for thyroid autoantibodies (such as antimicrosomal antibodies, antithyroglobulin, thyroid peroxidase) in symptomatic cases. However, the diagnosis may be missed when thyroid autoantibodies are negative. Ultrasound has been shown to be of value in the diagnosis of Hashimoto's thyroiditis and other autoimmune thyroid diseases with typical ultrasound appearances [67–69].

Ultrasound Features of Hashimoto's Thyroiditis [2]

The ultrasound appearances vary in different phases of the disease. The hypoechogenicity may vary from being slightly hypoechoic to markedly hypoechoic (echogenicity less than adjacent muscle) [37].

Focal Nodular/Lymphocytic Thyroiditis/ Pseudotumor (Figs. 5.37–5.40)

- Discrete nodules against an altered or normal thyroid parenchymal echopattern [70, 71].
- ≈5% of all biopsied nodules [39].
- Lower incidence of hypothyroidism (10%) among patients with only nodular thyroiditis compared to 43% in patients with nodular thyroiditis and diffuse Hashimoto's thyroiditis [72].
- Nodular Hashimoto's thyroiditis occurs in almost equal frequency against a background of diffuse Hashimoto's thyroiditis and in otherwise normal thyroid parenchyma [72].

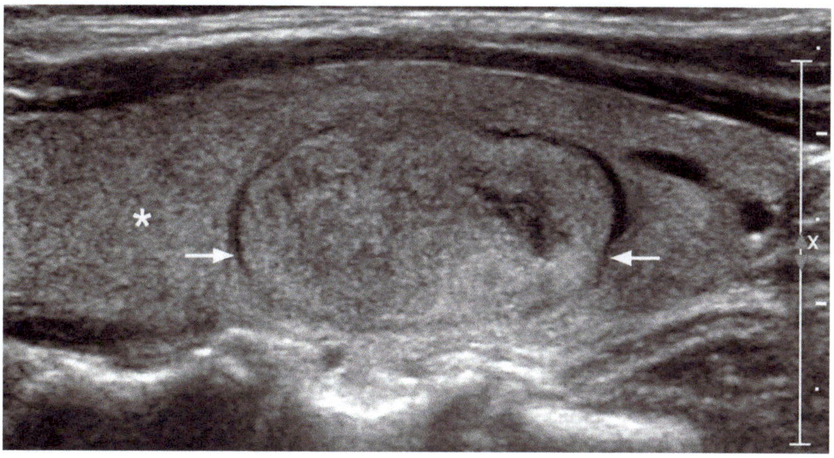

Fig. 5.37 Longitudinal gray scale showing a well-defined/haloed, noncalcified, predominantly solid, and isoechoic thyroid nodule (*arrows*) with a small cystic portion. FNAC revealed it to be focal nodular Hashimoto's thyroiditis. Note the relatively normal looking background thyroid parenchymal echoes (*asterisk*)

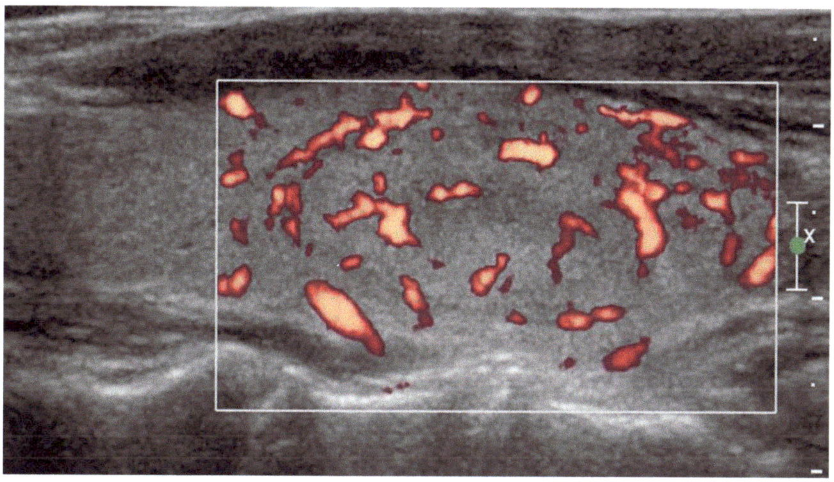

Fig. 5.38 Longitudinal gray scale and Doppler of same thyroid nodule demonstrated in Fig. 5.37

- In nodular Hashimoto's thyroiditis along with diffuse Hashimoto's thyroiditis, the "nodule" is solitary, solid, noncalcified, hyperechoic, and haloed. However, without diffuse Hashimoto's thyroiditis, the "nodule" may have cystic change and eggshell calcification [72].
- Vascularity in nodular Hashimoto's thyroiditis is variable and showed appearances simulating both benign and malignant thyroid nodules [72].

Diffuse Thyroiditis (Figs. 5.41–5.51)

- Diffuse hypoechoic enlargement of the thyroid gland ± lobulated outlines.
- Patchy ill-defined hypoechoic areas separated by echogenic fibrous septa [73] (Figs. 5.43–5.48).
- Multiple small (≈2–6 mm) nodules with a micronodular pattern involving the whole gland (Figs. 5.49–5.51). The nodules are hypoechoic and represent lymphocyte infiltration and their

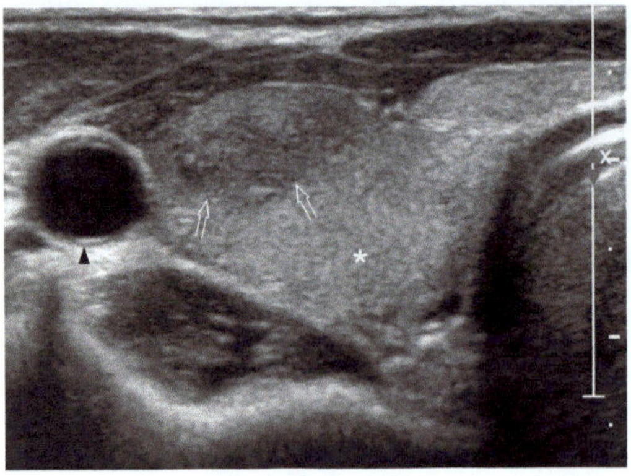

Fig. 5.39 Transverse gray scale showing a relatively isoechoic thyroid nodule (*open arrow*) in the right lobe anteriorly. Note the small bulge in thyroid contour indicating the presence of the nodule. FNAC confirmed focal nodular Hashimoto's thyroiditis. Note the relatively normal thyroid parenchymal echoes (*asterisk*). *Arrow*=trachea, *arrowhead*=CCA

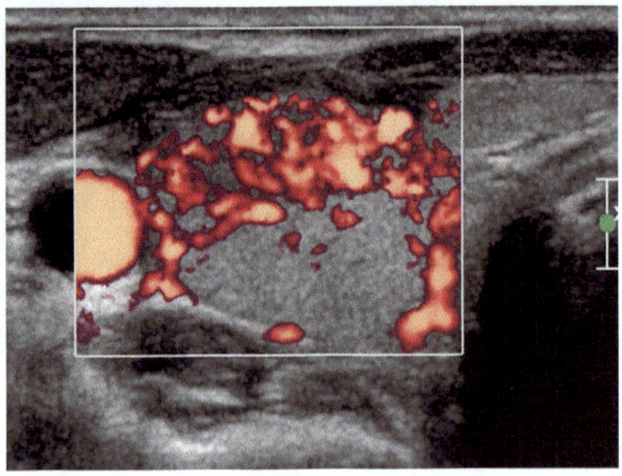

Fig. 5.40 Transverse Doppler image of same thyroid nodule designated in Fig. 5.39 demonstrates its hypervascularity

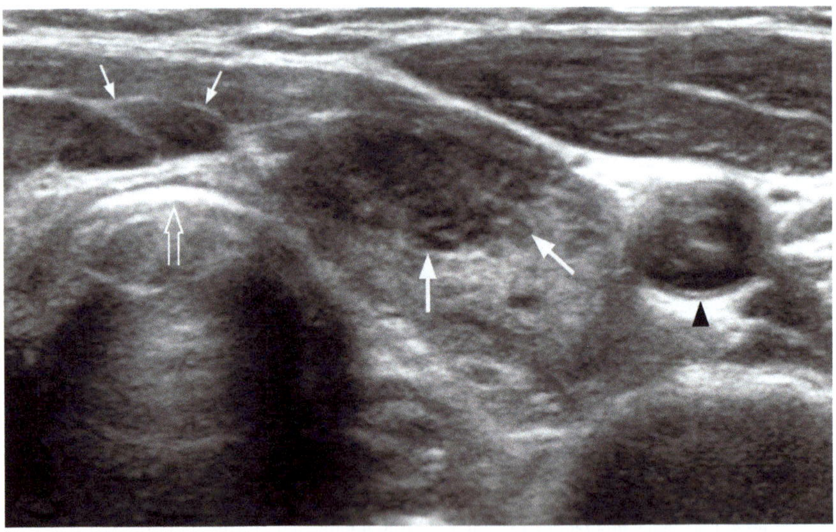

Fig. 5.41 Transverse gray scale ultrasound of the thyroid gland in a patient with Hashimoto's thyroiditis. Note the focal ill-defined, solid, hypoechoic area (*large arrows*) seen in the thyroid parenchyma, a reflection of lymphoid infiltration. Also note the enlarged reactive looking pretracheal lymph node (*small arrows*), a frequent finding in patients with thyroiditis. *Open arrow*=trachea, *arrowhead*=CCA

bright rims are due to the fibrous septa seen within the gland [74].

- The vascularity within the gland may be variable from the gland being hypovascular to diffuse hypervascularity [70], and the flow velocities are normal. This hypervascularity in Hashimoto's thyroiditis is due to the hypertrophic action of TSH [75]. When the TSH levels return to normal, the hypervascularity decreases [75].

End/Late Stage

- Small atrophic glandular parenchyma (Figs. 5.52–5.54)
- More often hypovascular on power Doppler

Apart from the ultrasound findings on the thyroid gland, the presence of enlarged pretracheal/paratracheal lymph nodes, and less commonly nodes in lateral compartment, is not uncommon [62]. They typically resemble reactive lymph nodes with elliptical shape and preserved echogenic hilum. Nodes exhibiting suspicious features may warrant FNA under ultrasound guidance.

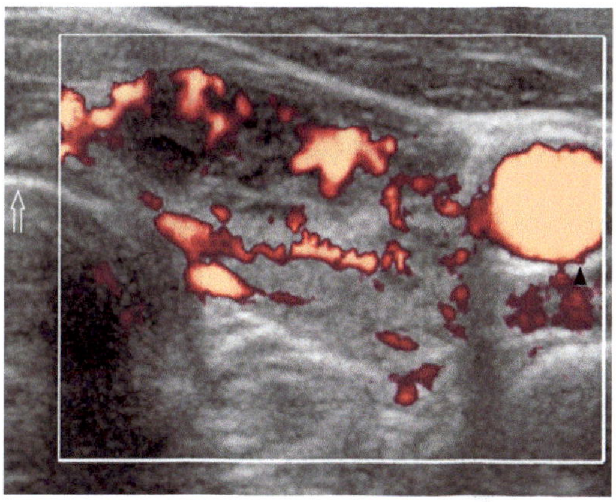

Fig. 5.42 Transverse Doppler ultrasound of the thyroid gland in the same patient with Hashimoto's thyroiditis demonstrated in Fig. 5.41. *Open arrow*=trachea, *arrowhead*=CCA

In addition, thyroid non-Hodgkin lymphoma and antecedent Hashimoto's thyroiditis are strongly associated [76, 77]. There have also been recent reports indicating a higher risk of papillary carcinoma in patients with Hashimoto's thyroiditis [78–80] (Fig. 5.55). The reported incidence of 16% [81] is higher than the 9–13% incidence of cancer in the general population of patients with thyroid nodules [5]. Therefore, in a patient with Hashimoto's thyroiditis, the development of thyroid nodule or recent increase in size should be viewed with a high degree of suspicion and followed by thyroid nodule/pseudonodule/lymph node FNAC. The sonographic features (gray scale and Doppler) of benign and malignant nodules in Hashimoto's thyroiditis are generally similar to the ultrasound appearance of benign and malignant thyroid nodules in the general population. Therefore, the nodule chosen for FNAC/biopsy in Hashimoto's thyroiditis follows the same established criteria for nodules seen in the general population. However, presence of calcification (of any pattern) in nodules associated with Hashimoto's thyroiditis should raise

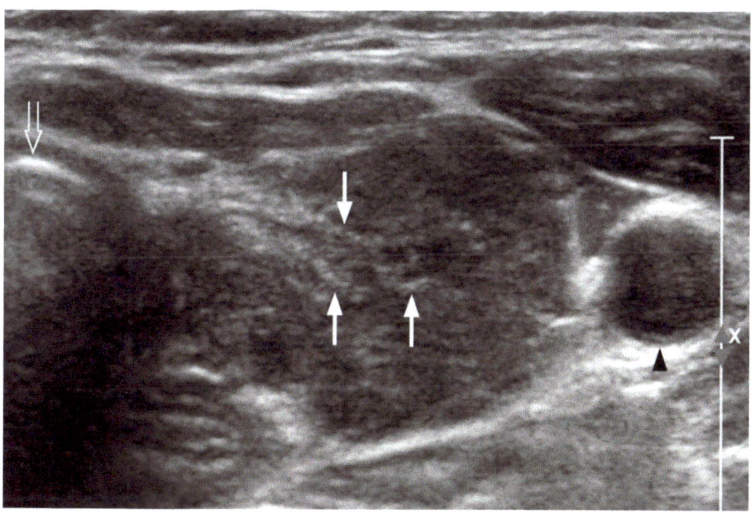

Fig. 5.43 Gray scale transverse ultrasound of the left lobe of the thyroid in a patient with Hashimoto's thyroiditis shows a mildly enlarged gland with rounded contours and diffuse marked parenchymal hypoechogenicity. Note the bright streaks (*arrows*) within the gland corresponding to intraglandular fibrosis in Hashimoto's thyroiditis. *Open arrow*=trachea, *arrowhead*=CCA

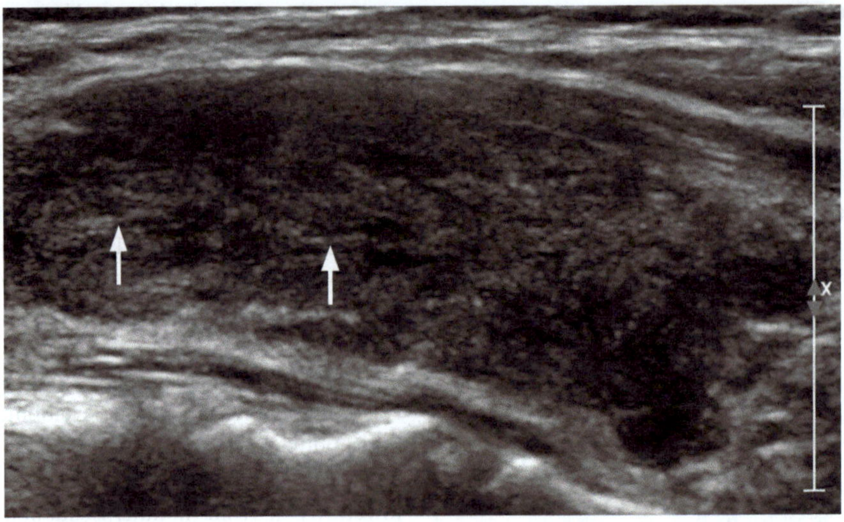

Fig. 5.44 Gray scale longitudinal ultrasound of the left lobe of the thyroid in a patient with Hashimoto's thyroiditis shows a mildly enlarged gland with rounded contours and diffuse marked parenchymal hypoechogenicity. Note the bright streaks (*arrows*) within the gland corresponding to intraglandular fibrosis in Hashimoto's thyroiditis

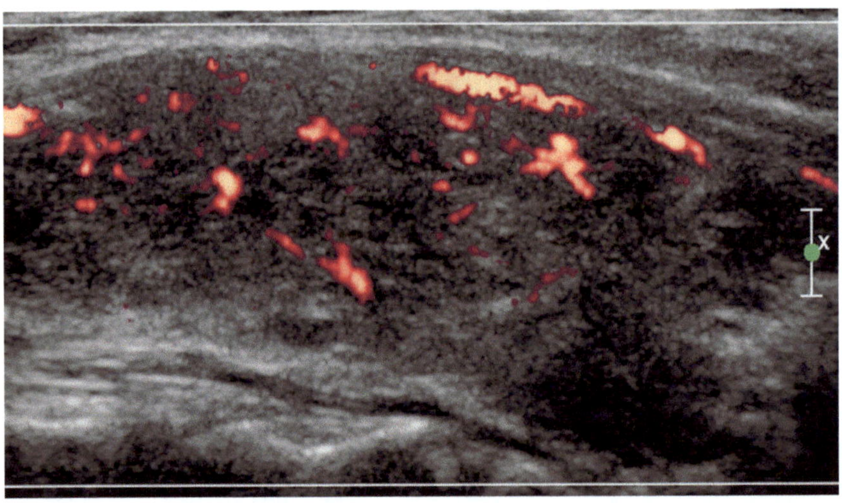

Fig. 5.45 Doppler longitudinal ultrasound of the left lobe of the thyroid in the patient with Hashimoto's thyroiditis demonstrated in Fig. 5.44

the suspicion of malignancy. In a recent report, calcification of any kind in nodules associated with Hashimoto's thyroiditis had a 50% risk of being malignant compared to 4.7% in noncalcified nodules [81].

On scintigraphy, the appearance of Hashimoto's thyroiditis also depends on the stage of the disease [82]. In early stage, due to presence of TSH stimulation in response to thyroid glandular inflammation, there is diffuse increased tracer uptake in the whole gland. Thyroid follicles demonstrate a variable response to the chronic TSH stimulation, leading to patchy proliferation of these follicles, resulting in patchy areas of increased activity (follicles that respond to TSH) and of decreased activity (those that do not respond). In late stage, when more thyroid parenchyma is replaced by fibrous tissue, the

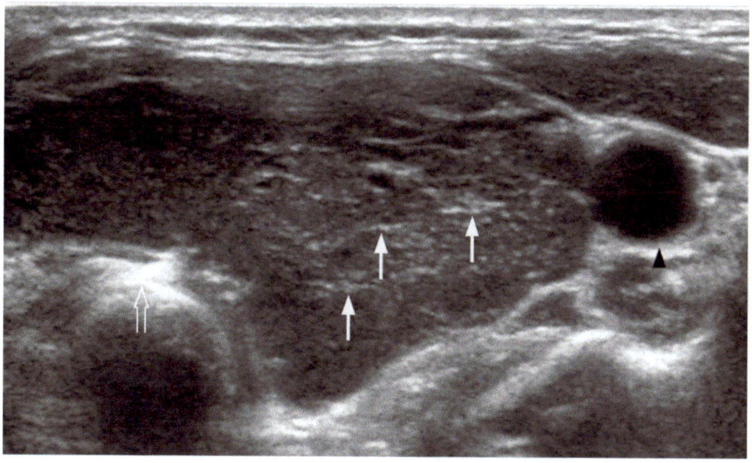

Fig. 5.46 Transverse gray scale ultrasound in a hypothyroid patient with Hashimoto's thyroiditis. Note the diffuse parenchymal hypoechogenicity and evidence of fibrosis within the gland (*arrows*). *Open arrow* = trachea, *arrowhead* = CCA

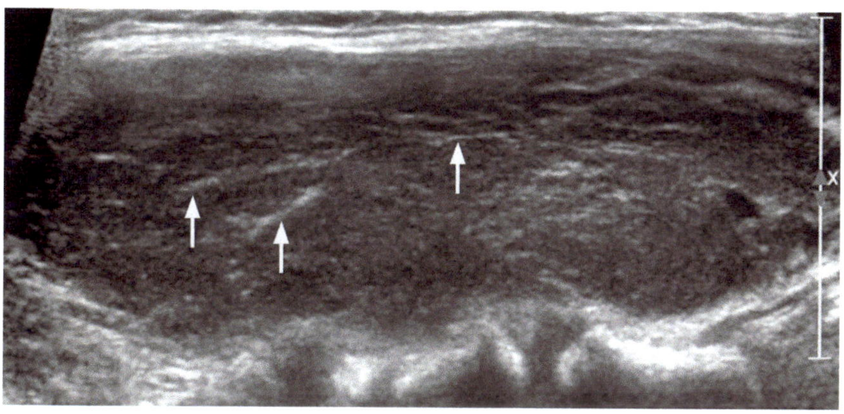

Fig. 5.47 Longitudinal gray scale ultrasound in a hypothyroid patient with Hashimoto's thyroiditis. Note the diffuse parenchymal hypoechogenicity and evidence of fibrosis within the gland (*arrows*)

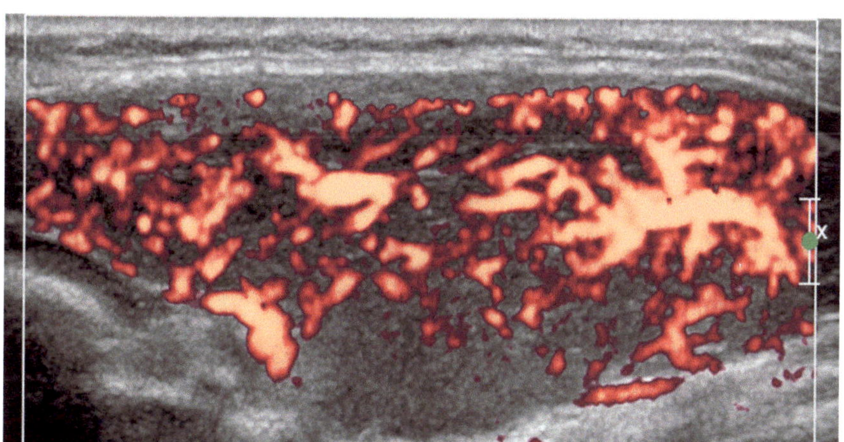

Fig. 5.48 Corresponding Doppler ultrasound (same patient as in Figs. 5.46 and 5.47) shows marked thyroid parenchymal vascularity. Such hypervascularity in a hypothyroid patient with Hashimoto's thyroiditis is due to the hypertrophic action of TSH. The hypervascularity decreases when the TSH normalizes

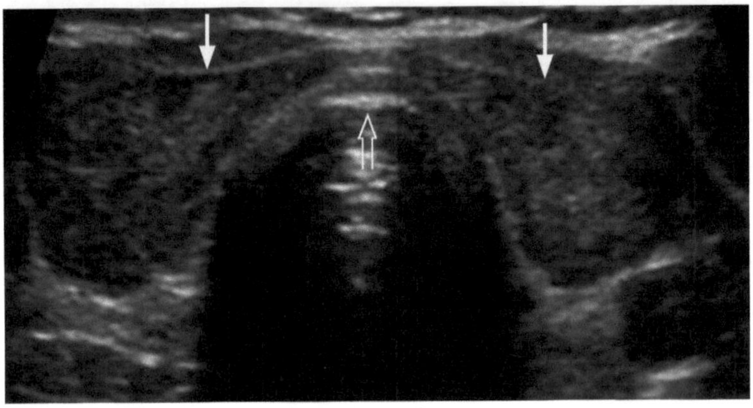

Fig. 5.49 Transverse gray scale ultrasound of the thyroid in a patient with Hashimoto's thyroiditis. Note the diffuse hypoechoic "ghostlike" thyroid parenchymal echoes (*arrows*), a feature of Hashimoto's thyroiditis. *Open arrow*=trachea

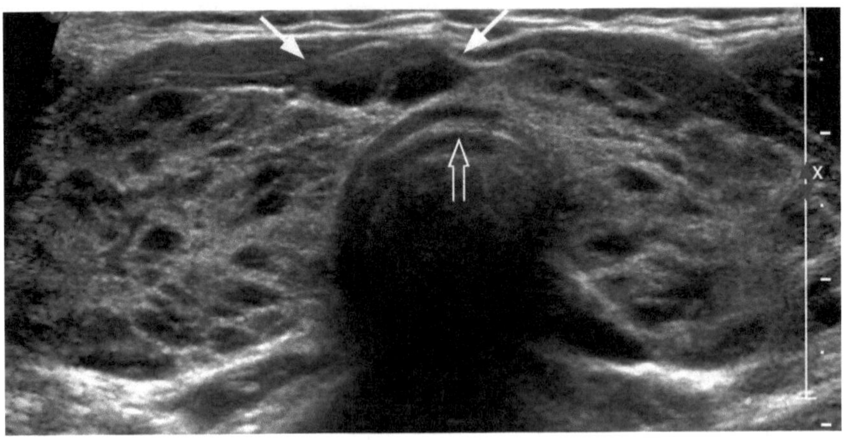

Fig. 5.50 Transverse gray scale ultrasound of the thyroid in a patient with Hashimoto's thyroiditis. Note the diffuse heterogeneous pattern with focal hypoechoic areas giving the gland a "leopard skin"/"Swiss cheese" appearance. The focal hypoechoic areas represent lymphocytic infiltration. Also note the enlarged, reactive pretracheal lymph node (*arrow*), a common association with thyroiditis. *Open arrow*=trachea

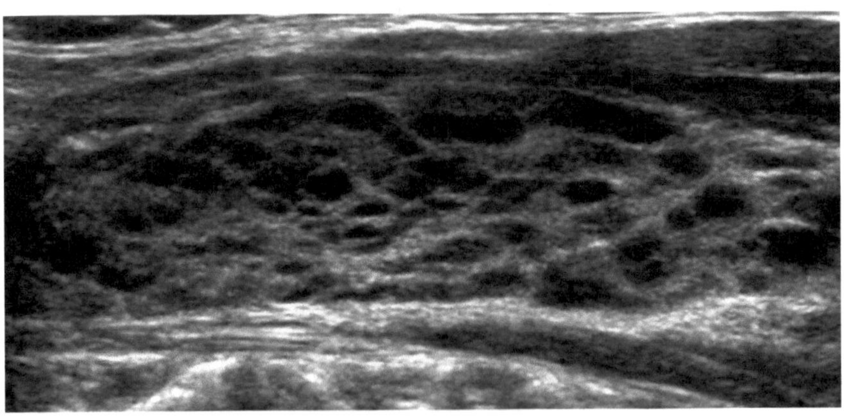

Fig. 5.51 Longitudinal gray scale ultrasound of the thyroid in the patient with Hashimoto's thyroiditis demonstrated in Fig. 5.50

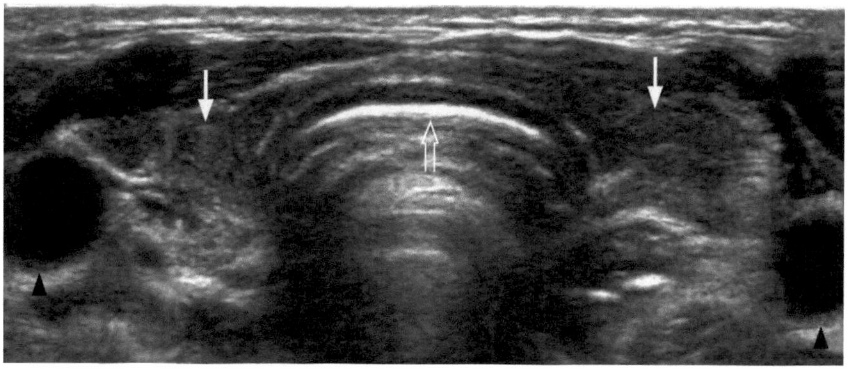

Fig. 5.52 Transverse gray scale ultrasound in a patient with Hashimoto's thyroiditis shows a diffuse reduction in thyroid (*arrow*) size/volume and a hypoechoic parenchymal echopattern. *Open arrow*=trachea, *arrowhead*=CCA

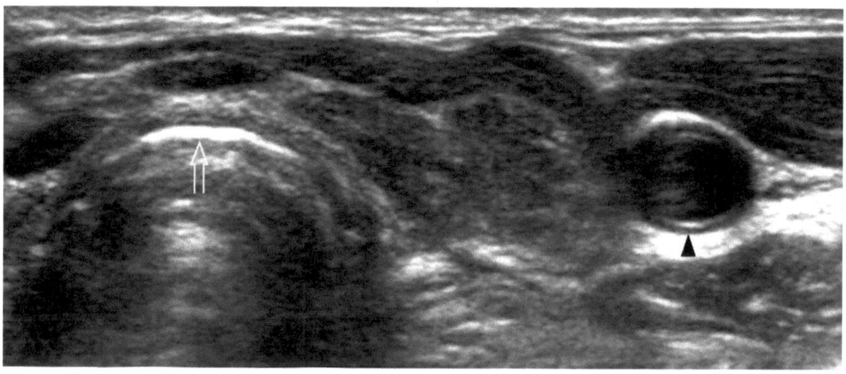

Fig. 5.53 Transverse gray scale ultrasound of the left lobe of the thyroid, in a patient with atrophic Hashimoto's thyroiditis. Note the reduction in thyroid size/volume, and hypoechogenicity. *Open arrow*=trachea, *arrowhead*=CCA

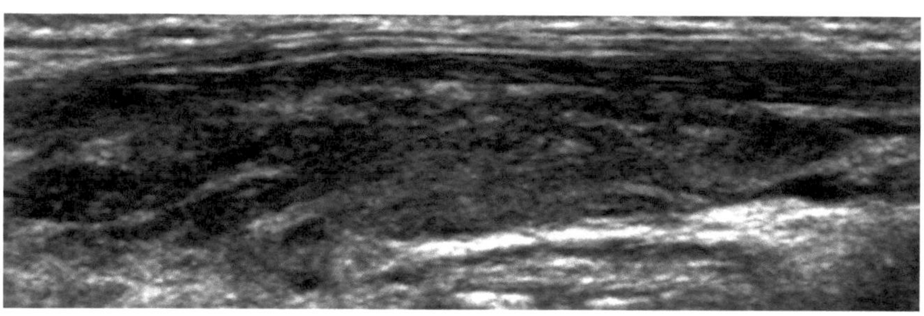

Fig. 5.54 Longitudinal gray scale ultrasound of the left lobe of the thyroid, in the patient with atrophic Hashimoto's thyroiditis as demonstrated in Fig. 5.53

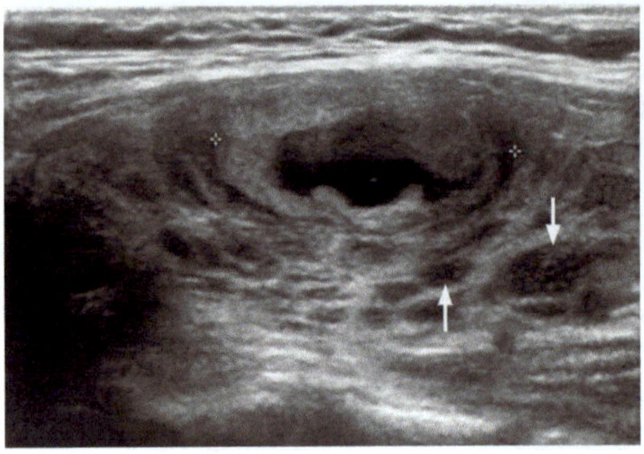

Fig. 5.55 Longitudinal gray scale ultrasound in a patient with known Hashimoto's thyroiditis. Note the background parenchymal echoes are hypoechoic, heterogeneous with multiple small hypoechoic foci [lymphocytic infiltration (*arrows*)]. Against this background is a well-defined nodule (calipers) with a thick solid rim and cystic centre. FNAC revealed this to be a papillary carcinoma against a background of Hashimoto's thyroiditis, a known association

gland fails to respond to TSH stimulation, giving rise to clinical hypothyroidism and nonuniform decreased tracer uptake in varying degree throughout the thyroid gland.

De Quervain's Thyroiditis

De Quervain's thyroiditis, also known as subacute granulomatous thyroiditis, is a self-limiting inflammatory condition that usually occurs following an upper respiratory tract viral infection. Patients typically present with neck pain, thyroid tenderness, odynophagia, and systemic symptoms of inflammatory disease [83]. There may be a palpable thyroid nodule or diffuse goiter. In acute stage, the patient may be thyrotoxic, followed by progress to a hypothyroid state in 2–4 months and euthyroid 6 months from the onset of symptoms.

Ultrasound Features of De Quervain's Thyroiditis [2]

Acute Phase (Figs. 5.56–5.58)

- Focal, ill-defined, hypoechoic nodule in subcapsular location.
- Transducer pressure elicits pain.

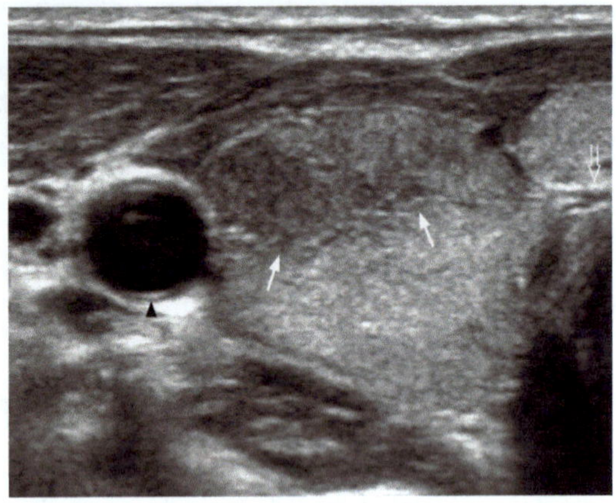

Fig. 5.56 Transverse gray scale ultrasound in a patient with De Quervain's thyroiditis shows a focal, ill-defined, hypoechoic area (*arrow*) merging imperceptibly with normal thyroid parenchyma. The area was tender on transducer pressure and an FNAC confirmed De Quervain's thyroiditis. *Open arrow*=trachea, *arrowhead*=CCA

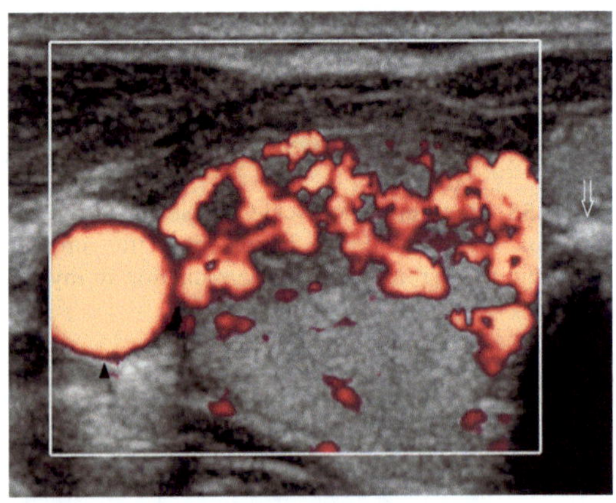

Fig. 5.57 Transverse power Doppler ultrasound of the right lobe with De Quervain's thyroiditis corresponds to the focal, hypoechoic area demonstrated in the same patient in Fig. 5.56

- Adjacent thyroid glandular parenchyma may appear heterogeneously hypoechoic/normal in echopattern.
- Inflammatory nodes in its vicinity.
- Hypovascularity/avascularity of the nodule on power Doppler ultrasound.

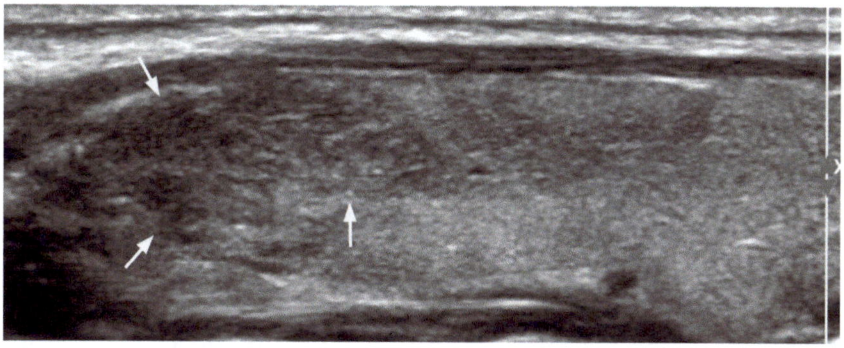

Fig. 5.58 Longitudinal gray scale ultrasound in the patient with De Quervain's thyroiditits demonstrated in Figs. 5.56, 5.57 shows the same ill-defined focal hypoechoic area (*arrows*) which merges with the adjacent normal parenchyma

Subacute Phase (Figs. 5.59–5.64)

- Glandular enlargement of the entire lobe or whole gland.
- Diffuse hypoechoic echopattern.
- Residual localized tenderness on transducer pressure.
- Adjacent inflammatory nodes.
- Hypovascular parenchyma.

After several months, when the thyroid function is normalized, the ultrasound appearance of the thyroid gland usually returns to normal. However, cases of residual nodule/pseudonodule formation or glandular atrophy do occur.

The sonographic appearances in acute phase of De Quervain's thyroiditis may mimic a thyroid nodule. The involvement is focal, hypoechoic, subcapsular in location, ± vascularity, and simulates a hypoechoic thyroid nodule. This may raise the concern of a malignant thyroid nodule (particularly the hypoechogenicity and the presence of lymphadenopathy) and the need for a FNAC.

However, the presence of clinical inflammatory signs and symptoms and thyroid tenderness should guide the sonologist toward the diagnosis. A follow-up ultrasound a week to 10 days later shows the progression of the inflammatory process to the other parts of the gland thus obviating the need of a FNAC.

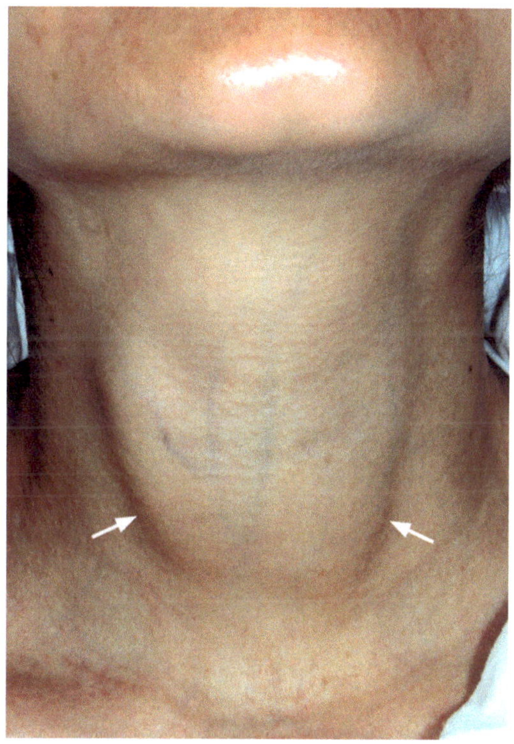

Fig. 5.59 Clinical photograph in a patient with De Quervain's thyroiditis showing diffuse enlargement of the thyroid gland (*arrows*). The patient had fever and the gland was tender on palpation and transducer pressure

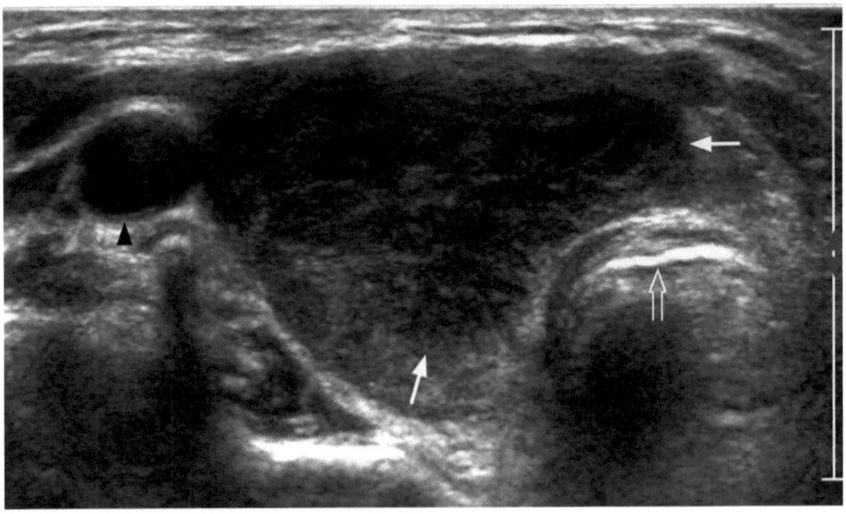

Fig. 5.60 Transverse gray scale ultrasound of the thyroid shows ill-defined, patchy, hypoechoic areas (*arrows*) in both lobes of the thyroid gland. Note they are nonhaloed/marginated with adjacent areas of normal echogenicity. The thyroid gland was tender on transducer pressure and the sonographic appearances are consistent with De Quervain's thyroiditis. *Open arrow*=trachea, *arrowhead*=CCA

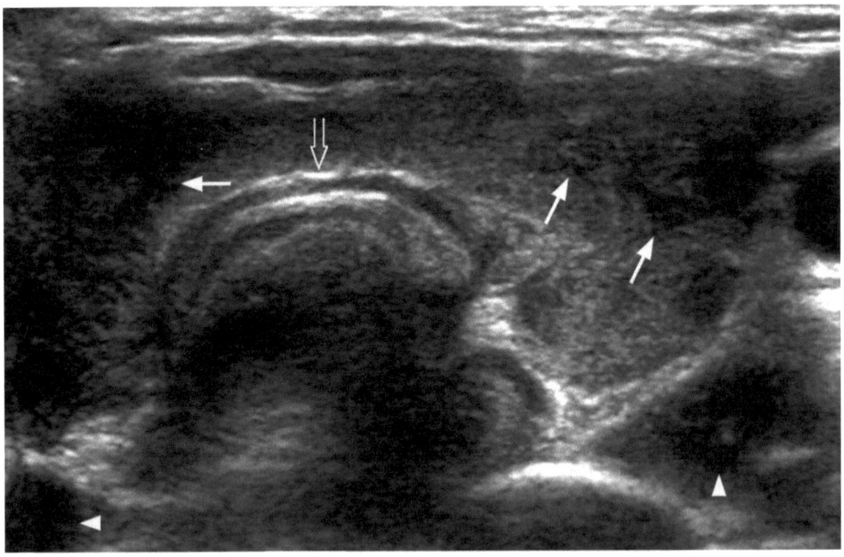

Fig. 5.61 Transverse gray scale ultrasound of the left lobe of the thyroid gland in the same patient demonstrated in Fig 5.60. Note the same ill-defined hypoechoic areas designated by the white arrows. Open arrow=trachea, arrowhead=CCA.

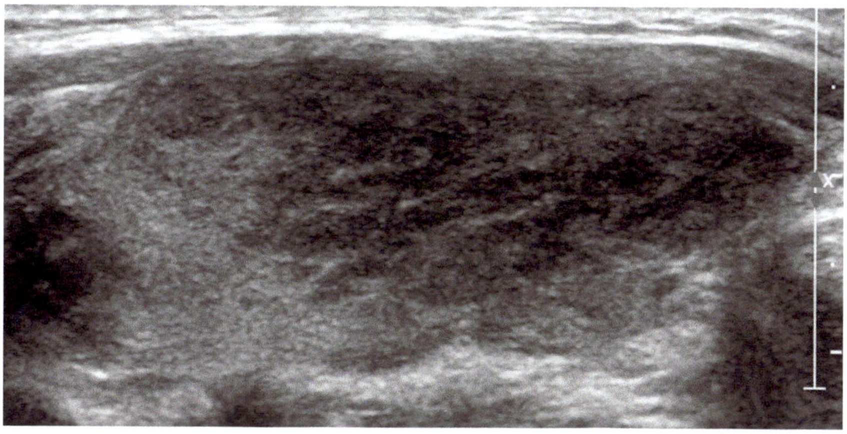

Fig. 5.62 Longitudinal/oblique gray scale ultrasound in a patient with De Quervain's thyroiditis (same patient as in Figs. 5.60 and 5.61)

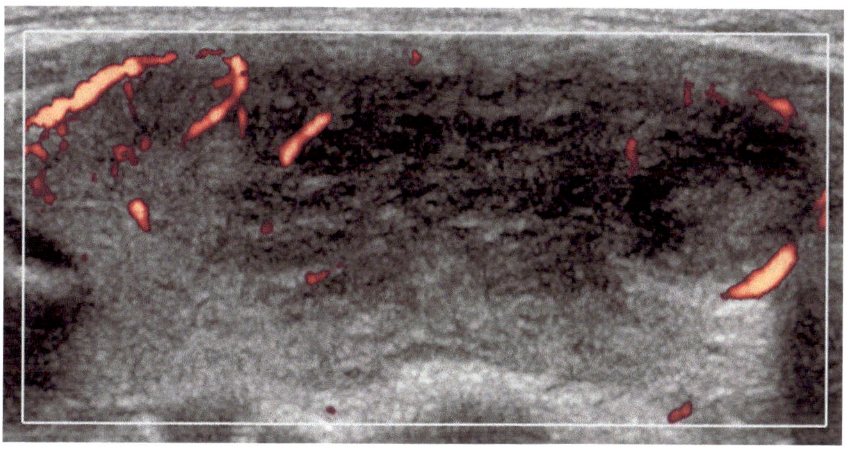

Fig. 5.63 Longitudinal/oblique gray scale and Doppler ultrasound in a patient with De Quervain's thyroiditis (same patient as in Figs. 5.60 and 5.61)

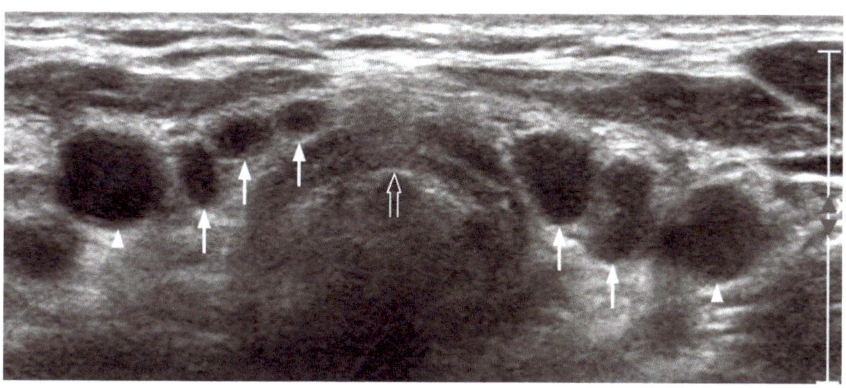

Fig. 5.64 Transverse gray scale ultrasound in a patient with De Quervain's thyroiditis (same patient as in Figs. 5.60–5.63) showing multiple, solid, round, hypoechoic enlarged inflammatory pre-/paratracheal lymph nodes (*arrows*). *Open arrow* = trachea, *arrowhead* = CCA

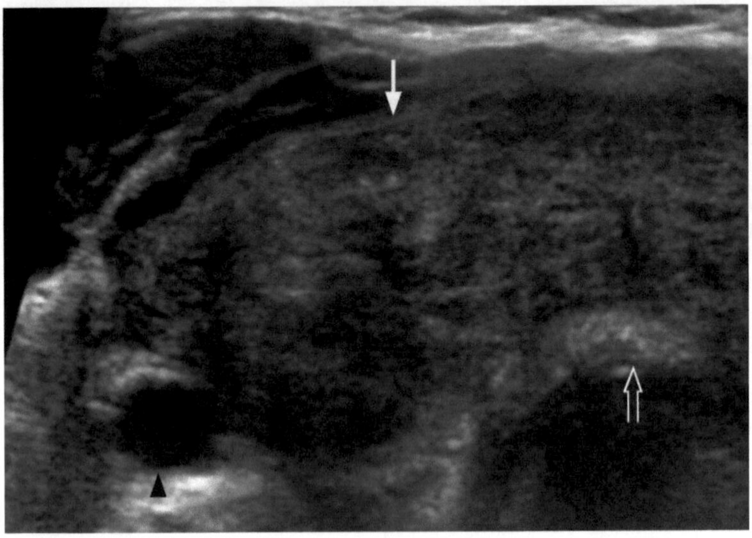

Fig. 5.65 Transverse gray scale ultrasound in a patient with Riedel's thyroiditis showing a diffuse, hypoechoic, heterogeneous echopattern (*arrow*) of the right lobe and thyroid isthmus. The thyroid was hard and difficult to penetrate on a core biopsy. Note the marked fibrosis seen on the biopsy specimen (Fig 5.66) *Open arrow*=trachea, *arrowhead*=CCA

Silent Thyroiditis and Postpartum Thyroiditis

Silent thyroiditis, also known as painless thyroiditis, is a clinical syndrome that manifests as transient hyperthyroidism followed by transient hypothyroidism. It is an autoimmune disease that is characterized by elevated levels of thyroid peroxidase antibodies and thyroglobulin antibodies [83]. Pathologically, there is lymphocytic infiltration of thyroid follicles resulting in follicular cell damage with release of excess thyroxine into the circulation, resulting in transient thyrotoxicosis. This is followed, usually after 1–4 weeks, by transient hypothyroidism before the thyroid function becomes normalized. On ultrasound, the gland appears mildly enlarged with heterogeneous hypoechoic echopattern and shares similar ultrasound features with other autoimmune thyroid diseases. Thyroid scintigraphy reveals marked decrease in thyroid uptake [82], which helps to distinguish silent thyroiditis from Graves' disease.

Postpartum thyroiditis is a subtype of silent thyroiditis that appears during the first postpartum year. It occurs in up to 5% of postpartum women and has a high recurrence rate in subsequent pregnancy [84]. Thyrotoxicosis usually occurs 2–6 months after delivery and lasts for 2–6 weeks, followed by a period of hypothyroidism that usually lasts 2–6 weeks. Approximately 20–25% of patients develop permanent hypothyroidism [85]. Ultrasound shows glandular enlargement with diffuse hypoechogenicity of the parenchyma which may persist in patients with biochemical hypothyroidism [86]. Thyroid scintigraphic appearance resembles silent thyroiditis with markedly decreased tracer uptake [82].

Riedel's Thyroiditis (Figs. 5.65 and 5.66)

Riedel's thyroiditis is a rare form of chronic thyroiditis, characterized by a fibroinflammatory process that partially destroys the thyroid and often involves surrounding tissues [87]. Clinically, it may be indistinguishable from thyroid malignancy due to firm to hard consistency of the thyroid gland due to extensive fibrosing inflammatory

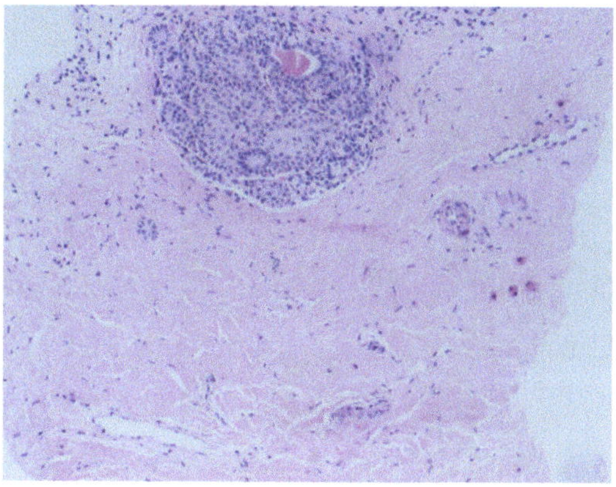

Fig. 5.66 The patient with Riedel's thyroiditis demonstrated in Fig. 5.65 underwent core biopsy. The specimen demonstrates marked fibrosis with islands of normal thyroid follicles

process and extension to perithyroidal soft tissues. Diffuse hypoechogenicity is the most common ultrasound finding based on limited case series [88]. Riedel's thyroiditis may be associated with mediastinal or retroperitoneal fibrosis as well as sclerosing cholangitis.

Infection

Acute infectious thyroiditis is a rare condition of the thyroid gland as the thyroid gland itself is relatively resistant to infection because of its thick fibrous capsule, vascularity, high iodine content, and extensive lymphatics.

Acute suppurative thyroiditis is the commonest form of infection affecting the thyroid gland and perithyroidal soft tissue [89]. It is mostly seen in children with congenital conditions connecting the thyroid directly to the oropharynx such as a piriform sinus fistula or thyroglossal duct remnant. Rarer forms of infection, including tuberculous abscess [90] and septic emboli derived from infective endocarditis [91], have also been reported.

Acute Suppurative Thyroiditis

It is the most common form of acute infection of the thyroid gland. Gram-positive bacteria (staphylococci and streptococci) are the common causative microorganisms. It predominantly affects children/adolescent and has a left-sided predominance. Typically, the affected child presents acutely with pain, fever, and painful swelling of thyroid gland. There is usually history of multiple similar episodes in the past requiring incision and drainage indicating the recurrent nature of the disease.

Ultrasound Features of Acute Suppurative Thyroiditis [2, 92]

- The inflammatory/infective changes first occur in perithyroid soft tissues producing hypoechoic soft tissue thickening due to edema and inflammation.
- Obliteration/blurring of fascial planes between thyroid gland and adjacent soft tissue.
- Intra- and extrathyroidal abscess formation: ill-defined, hypoechoic, heterogeneous mass with internal debris, thick wall, and ± internal gas (Figs. 5.67–5.70).
- Presence of inflammatory lymph nodes in adjacent jugular chain and central compartment.

The role of ultrasound is to confirm the diagnosis, assess extent of infection (e.g., extrathyroidal ± thyroid involvement), detect abscess formation supplemented by image-guided aspiration, and monitor response to antibiotic treatment. Further imaging is essential to demonstrate the piriform sinus fistula and may include barium swallow (Fig. 5.71) [93], CT (Fig. 5.72) [94], or MRI [95].

Radiation-Induced Thyroiditis

Thyroiditis Induced by External-Beam Radiotherapy (Figs. 5.73–5.79)

External-beam radiotherapy induces a variety of thyroid abnormalities and these include: primary hypothyroidism (3–92%), Graves' disease (0.1–2%), silent thyroiditis (0.6–3%), Hashimoto's thyroiditis (0.7–48%), Graves' ophthalmopathy (0.2–1.3%), benign adenoma (0.6–3%), and

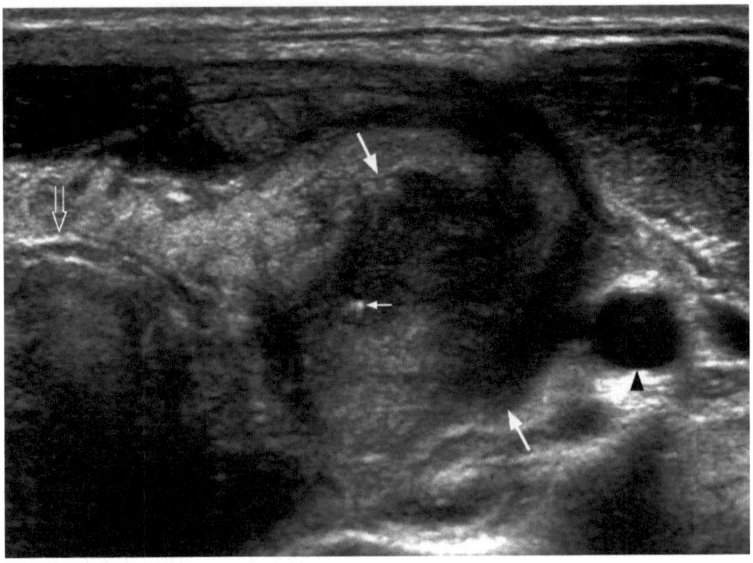

Fig. 5.67 Transverse gray scale ultrasound in a patient with acute suppurative thyroiditis. Note the presence of an ill-defined, necrotic/cystic, hypoechoic area/abscess (*large arrows*) with internal debris and gas (*small arrows*). This patient had a history of multiple left-sided neck infections requiring incision and drainage. *Open arrow*=trachea, *arrowhead*=CCA

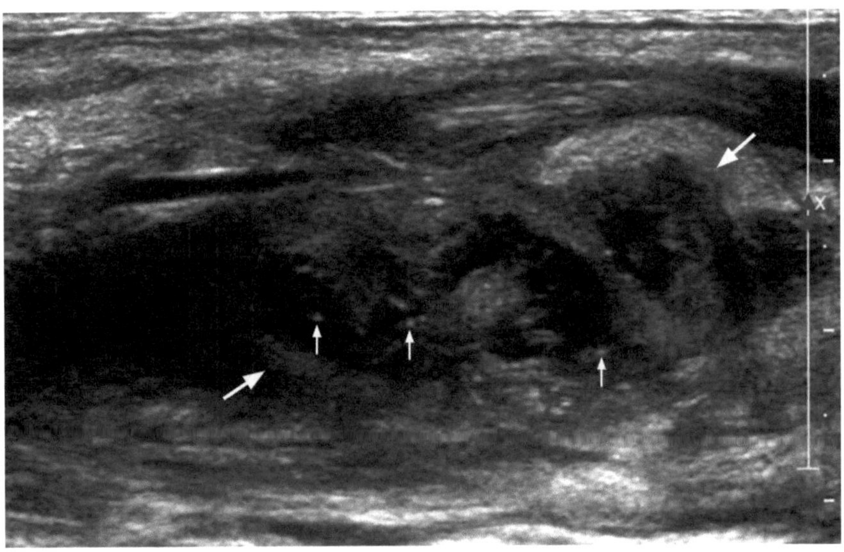

Fig. 5.68 Longitudinal gray scale ultrasound in the same patient in Fig 5.67 with acute suppurative thyroiditis. Note the presence of an ill-defined, necrotic/cystic, hypoechoic area/abscess (*large arrows*) with internal debris and gas (*small arrows*). This patient had a history of multiple left-sided neck infections requiring incision and drainage. *Open arrow*=trachea, *arrowhead*=CCA

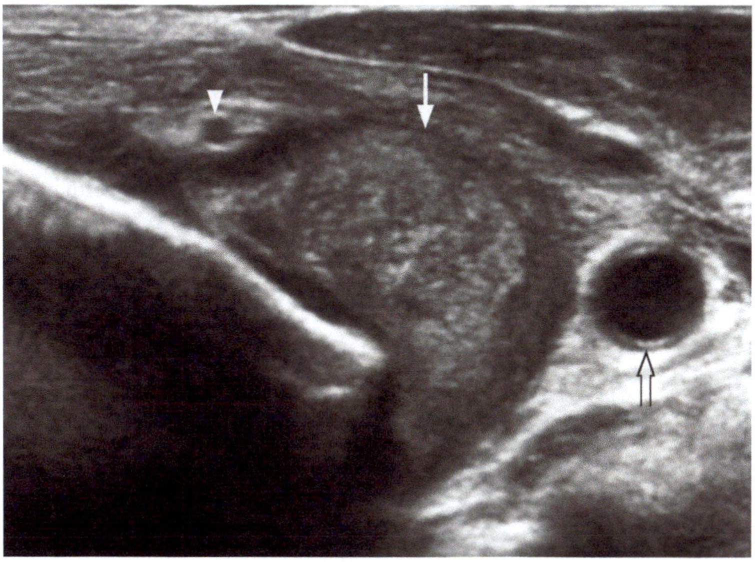

Fig. 5.69 Transverse gray scale ultrasound in a patient with fever, raised WCC, and a tender left-sided mass. Note the heterogeneous "mass" (*arrow*) anterior to the thyroid cartilage and medial to the left CCA (*open arrow*). It was soft on aspiration, and the location, appearance, and clinical signs are suggestive of acute suppurative thyroiditis. Note the associated pyriform sinus fistula (*arrowhead*) clearly demonstrated on the ultrasound.

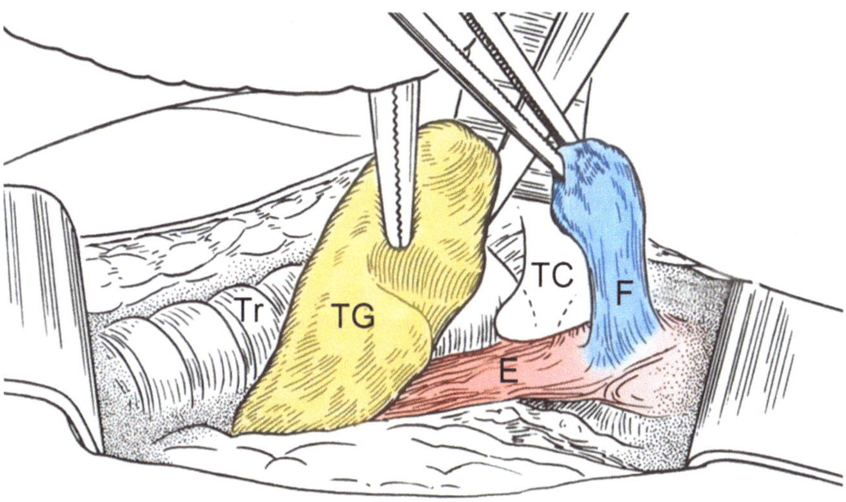

Fig. 5.70 The relationships between 4th branchial pouch fistula (F), thyroid cartilage (TC), thyroid gland (TG), trachea (Tr), and esophagus (E) are artistic renditions from the patient in Fig. 5.69

thyroid cancer (0.35%) [96–99]. Thyroid storm after IMRT has also been reported [100]. The radiation-related thyrotoxicosis is usually transient, whereas the hypothyroidism is usually permanent [101]. External-beam radiation releases excessive thyroid hormones during treatment and suppresses TSH through the negative feedback mechanism [99]. Thyroid damage is initially seen within the first 6 months [102], and the peak incidence of hypothyroidism is seen 2–3 years after treatment with half of the cases occurring within the first 5 years following radiotherapy [96, 98, 103]. A shorter latency period is seen in patients who have received higher doses of radiation treatment [103]. Autoimmune-induced reaction, thyroid parenchymal cellular damage, and vascular damage are listed as the supposed causes of radiation-induced damage [96].

Thyroiditis induced by radioactive iodine treatment: The induced thyrotoxicosis is transient; however, the hypothyroidism induced by such treatment is often permanent [101].

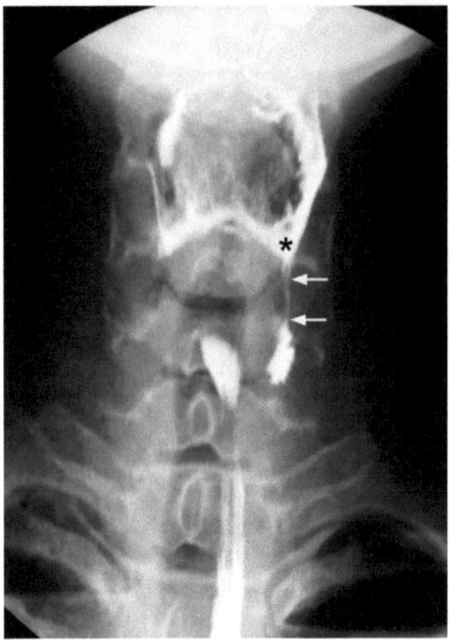

Fig. 5.71 Barium swallow in a patient with acute suppurative thyroiditis showing the presence of a fistula (*arrows*) arising from the left pyriform sinus (*asterisk*). The fistula usually tracks through the perithyroid tissue and the left thyroid gland (95%) and is the cause of the recurrent thyroid infection

Congenital Anomalies

The thyroid gland develops in the first trimester of pregnancy, beginning around the fifth week of gestation and is completed by the 10th week [104]. It develops from median and paired lateral anlages which fuse at midline by the tenth week giving the bilobed appearance of the thyroid gland. During fetal development, the thyroid gland descends from the foramen cecum down to the lower anterior neck via the thyroglossal duct, which subsequently degenerates and atrophies. Abnormal development or aberrant caudal descent of the thyroid gland results in a variety of congenital anomalies.

Dysgenesis of the thyroid gland accounts for 80–90% of congenital primary hypothyroidism [105]. Approximately two-thirds of these patients have thyroid ectopia and one-third with thyroid agenesis. The roles of ultrasound and thyroid scintigraphy are to identify presence of functional ectopic thyroid tissue, most commonly at the

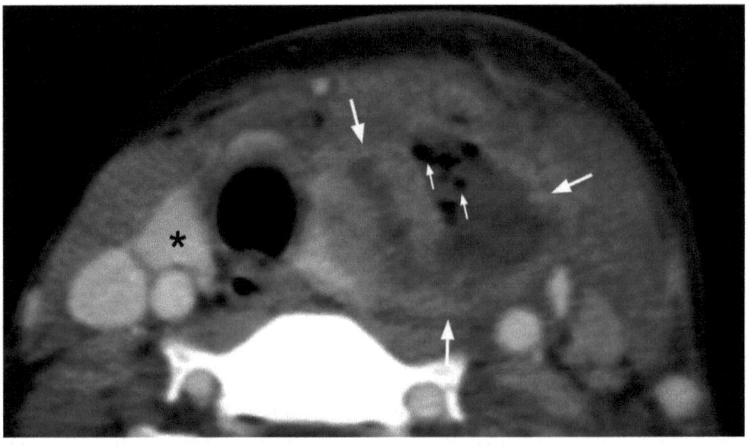

Fig. 5.72 Axial CECT (another patient) shows a left acute suppurative thyroiditis (*large arrows*) with focal areas of gas within (*small arrows*). Note normal contralateral thyroid gland (*asterisk*)

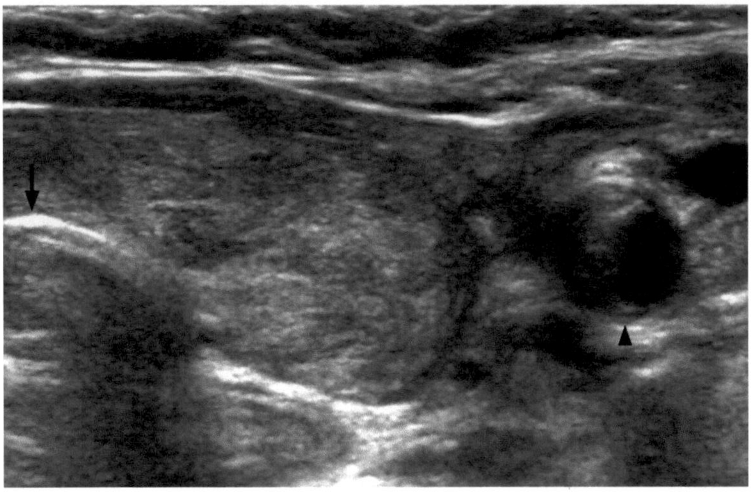

Fig. 5.73 Transverse gray scale ultrasound of the thyroid in a patient who received external-beam RT for a head and neck carcinoma. Note the heterogeneous, hypoechoic parenchymal thyroid echopattern. The U/S appearances are of an RT-induced thyroiditis. *Arrow* = trachea, *arrowhead* = CCA

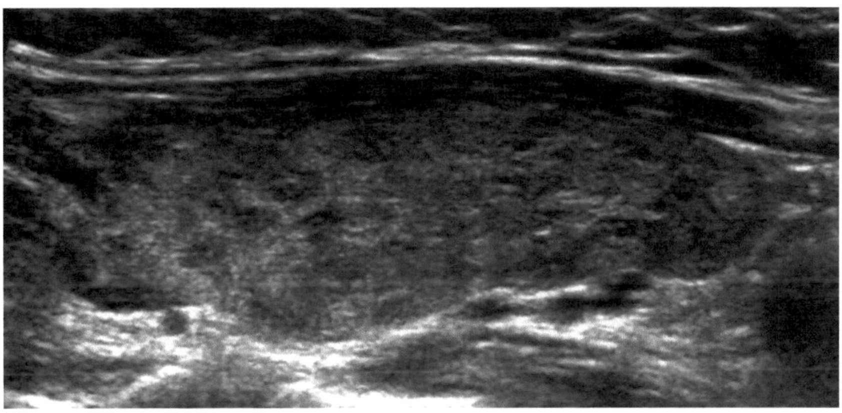

Fig. 5.74 Longitudinal gray scale ultrasound of the patient who received external-beam RT for head and neck carcinoma demonstrated in Fig. 5.73

tongue base, and detection/presence of normal/hypofunctioning thyroid tissue in the anterior neck [106].

Aberrant descent of the thyroid gland may give rise to ectopic thyroid and thyroglossal duct cyst/fistula. Ectopic thyroid can occur anywhere along the line of embryonic descent of the thyroid gland. Lingual thyroid gland at the base of the tongue is the commonest type of functioning ectopic thyroid tissue (Figs. 5.80–5.84). Ectopic thyroid has also rarely been found in the submandibular and lateral neck regions [107, 108] and may be misinterpreted as metastatic disease. Thyroid scintigraphy helps to confirm presence of functioning ectopic thyroid tissue (Fig. 5.85). Thyroglossal duct cyst/fistula is described in another chapter in this book discussing miscellaneous neck lesions.

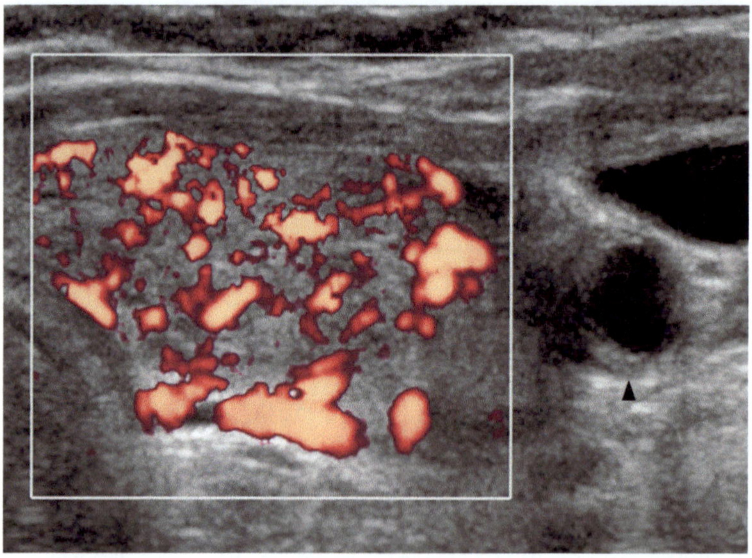

Fig. 5.75 Transverse Doppler Ultrasound of the thyroid in the patient who received external-beam RT for a head and neck carcinoma as demonstrated in Fig. 5.73. *Arrowhead* = CCA

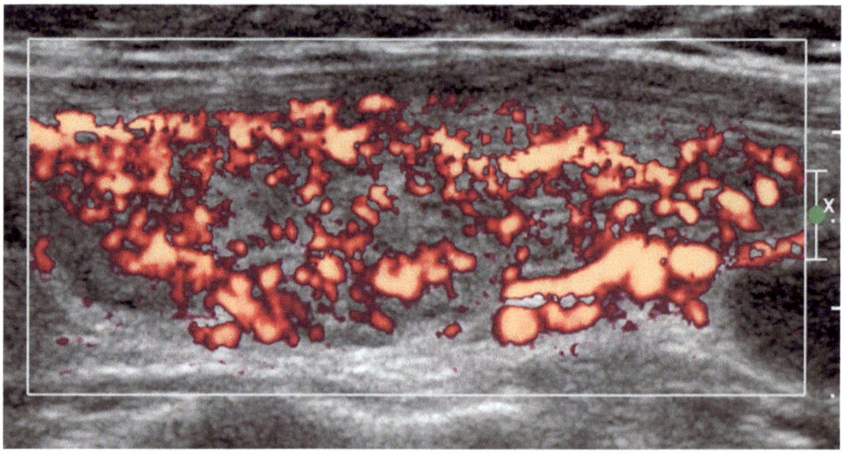

Fig. 5.76 Longitudinal Doppler Ultrasound of the thyroid in the patient who received external-beam RT for a head and neck carcinoma which corresponds to the longitudinal gray scale image in Fig. 5.74, note the heterogeneous, hypoechoic parenchymal thyroid echopattern with marked increase in vascularity. The U/S appearances are of an RT-induced thyroiditis.

Postoperative Thyroid Hypertrophy

Patients who have had surgery for previous benign thyroid disease may present for routine follow-up examination or with palpable thyroid mass/enlarging thyroid.

In patients who have had previous surgery for benign multinodular goiter, the residual thyroid may show evidence of multinodular change [2]. The nodules usually have the appearance of benign hyperplastic nodules, and the role of ultrasound is to determine the presence of any suspi-

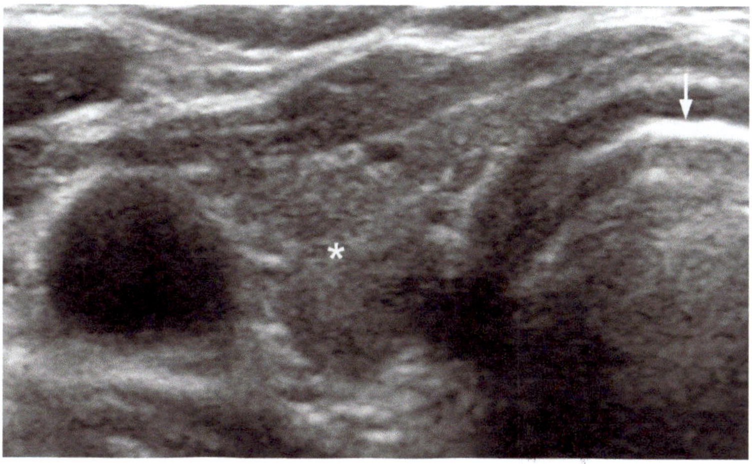

Fig. 5.77 Transverse gray scale image of right lobe of post-RT atrophic thyroid (*asterisk*). Note the small volume gland which is hypovascular on Doppler. Note the thick carotid walls (*arrowhead*), also a post-RT feature. *Arrow* = trachea

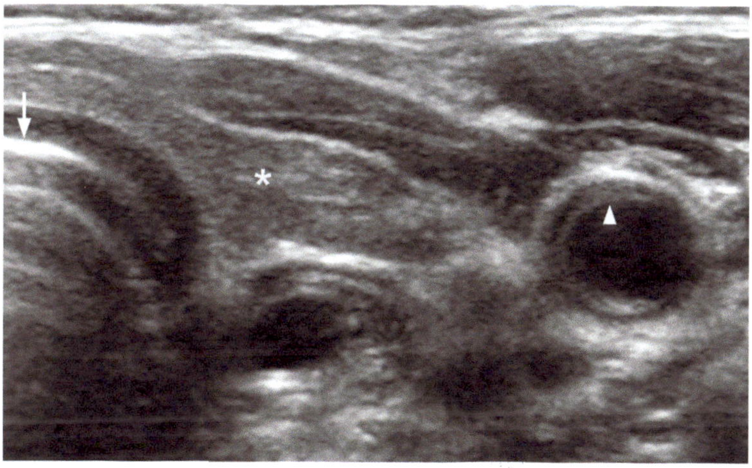

Fig. 5.78 Transverse gray scale image of left lobe of post-RT atrophic thyroid (*asterisk*). Note the small volume gland. Note the thick carotid walls (*arrowhead*), also a post-RT feature. *Arrow* = trachea

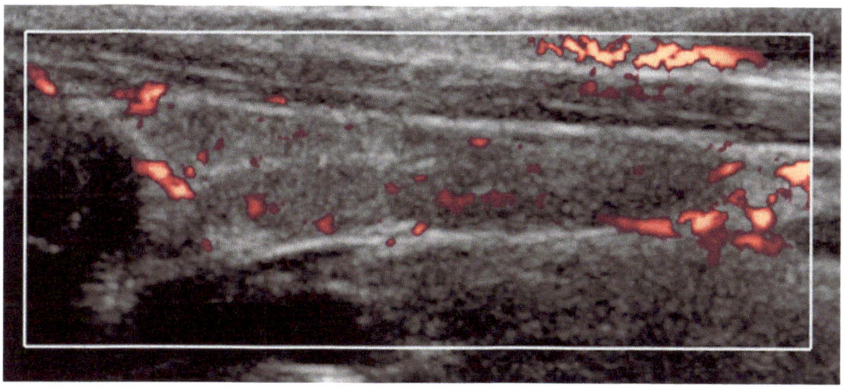

Fig. 5.79 Doppler image of post-RT atrophic thyroid. Note the small volume gland which is hypovascular on Doppler.

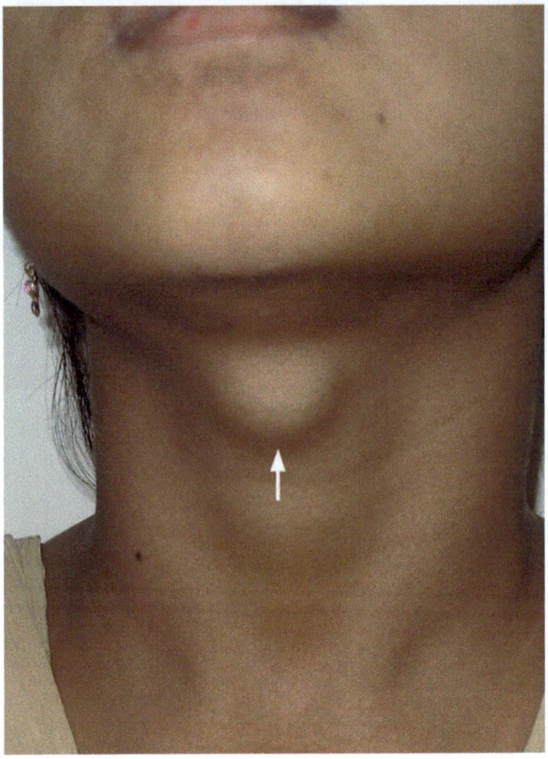

Fig. 5.80 Clinical photograph of a young patient with a focal, well-defined, clinically obvious midline neck mass (*arrow*). Courtesy: Dr. Sanjay Vaid, Pune

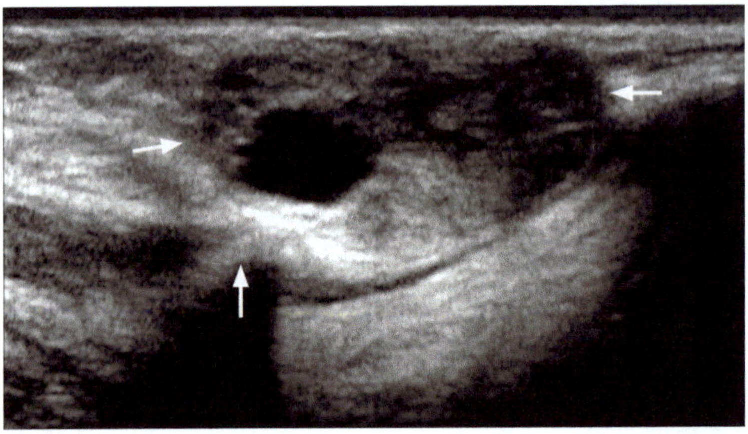

Fig. 5.81 Longitudinal gray scale ultrasound of the clinically obvious neck mass shows it to be at the level of the hyoid bone (*horizontal arrows*). Note the nodule is heterogeneous on gray scale (*vertical arrow*). The thyroid bed did not show the presence of normal thyroid tissue. The appearances suggest the "nodule" to be ectopic thyroid tissue. Courtesy: Dr. Sanjay Vaid, Pune

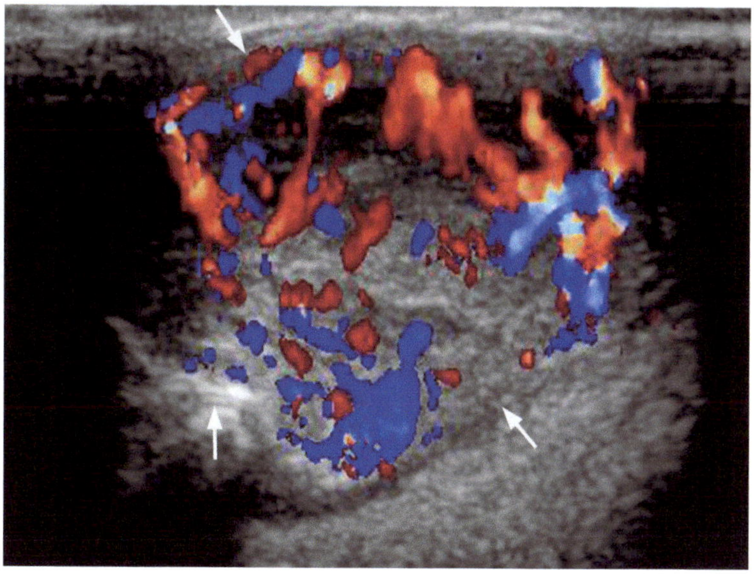

Fig. 5.82 Longitudinal color Doppler ultrasound of the clinically obvious neck mass shows it to be at the level of the hyoid bone (*vertical arrow*). Note the nodule is hypervascular on Doppler (*Oblique arrow* designates margin of nodule). The thyroid bed did not show the presence of normal thyroid tissue. The appearances suggest the "nodule" to be ectopic thyroid tissue. Courtesy: Dr. Sanjay Vaid, Pune

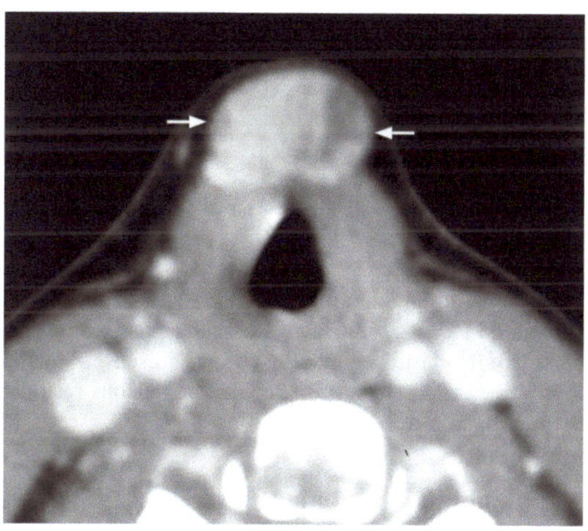

Fig. 5.83 Axial CECT shows the ectopic thyroid tissue at the level of the hyoid bone (*arrows*), which was also visualized on ultrasound. Courtesy: Dr. Sanjay Vaid, Pune

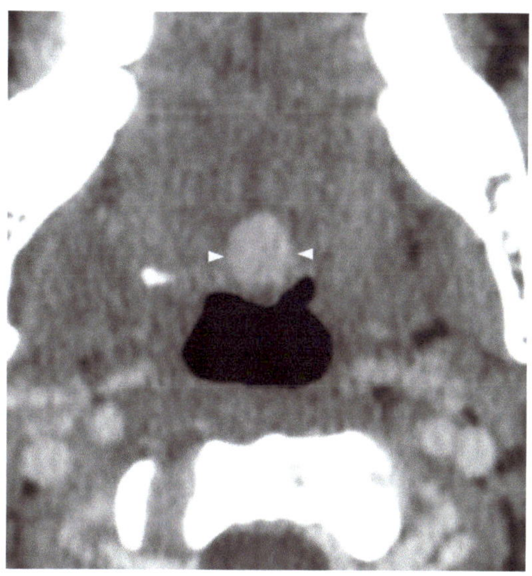

Fig. 5.84 Axial CECT shows the ectopic thyroid tissue at the floor of mouth (*arrowheads*), which was also visualized on ultrasound. Courtesy: Dr. Sanjay Vaid, Pune

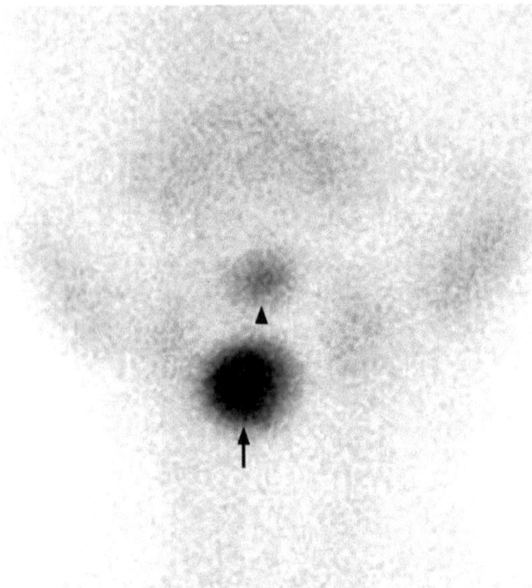

Fig. 5.85 A scintigram confirms two foci of ectopic thyroid tissue (*arrow and arrowhead*), seen on ultrasound and CT.Courtesy: Dr. Sanjay Vaid, Pune

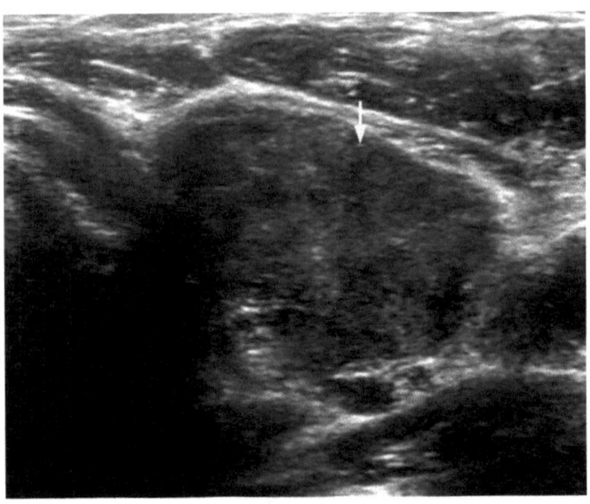

Fig. 5.86 Transverse left gray scale ultrasound in the same patient in Fig 5.85 with a previous history of subtotal thyroidectomy in Graves' disease. In the thyroid bed is the hypertrophied, heterogeneous residual thyroid gland (*arrow*)

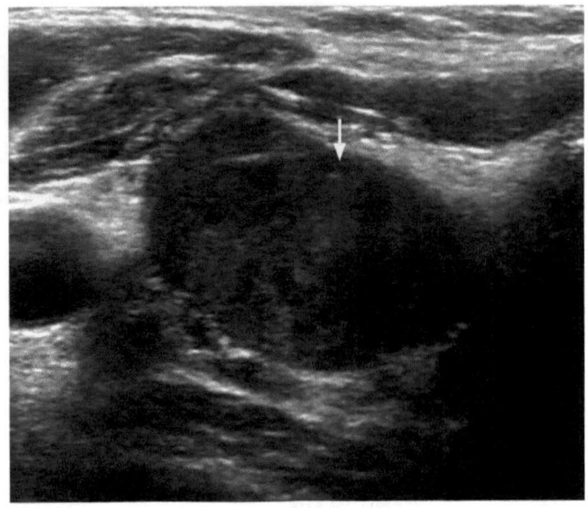

Fig. 5.87 Transverse right gray scale ultrasound in the patient with a previous history of subtotal thyroidectomy for Graves' disease demonstrated in Figs. 5.85 and 5.86. In the thyroid bed is the hypertrophied, heterogeneous residual thyroid gland (*arrow*)

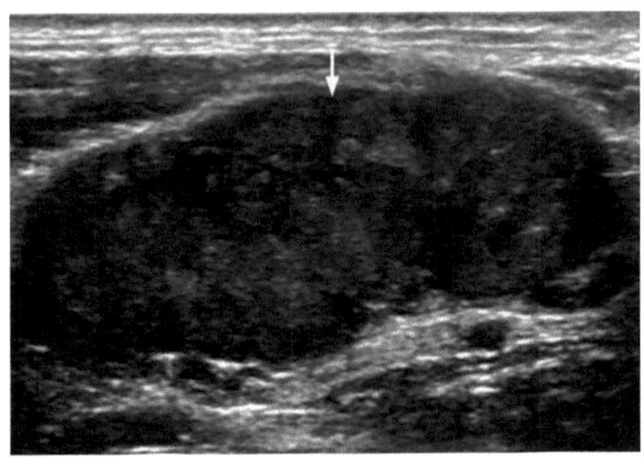

Fig. 5.88 Longitudinal gray scale ultrasound in the patient in Figs 5.85, 5.86, and 5.87 with a previous history of subtotal thyroidectomy for Graves' disease. In the thyroid bed is the hypertrophied, heterogeneous residual thyroid gland (arrow)

cious/malignant thyroid nodule, ± associated lymphadenopathy.

In patients who have had previous surgery for Graves' disease, the residual thyroid tissue [in patients with subtotal thyroidectomy (Figs. 5.86–5.89)] and any lateral aberrant thyroid [in patients with total thyroidectomy (Figs. 5.90–5.95)] may show postoperative hypertrophy. These patients often present with palpable "nodules" ± recurrent symptoms of thyrotoxicosis. The hypertrophied thyroid "nodules"/glands may be palpable and are usually round, hypoechoic with a heterogeneous parenchymal echopattern, vascular on Doppler [2], and intensely enhancing on contrast-enhanced CT. These must not be mistaken for abnormal nodes.

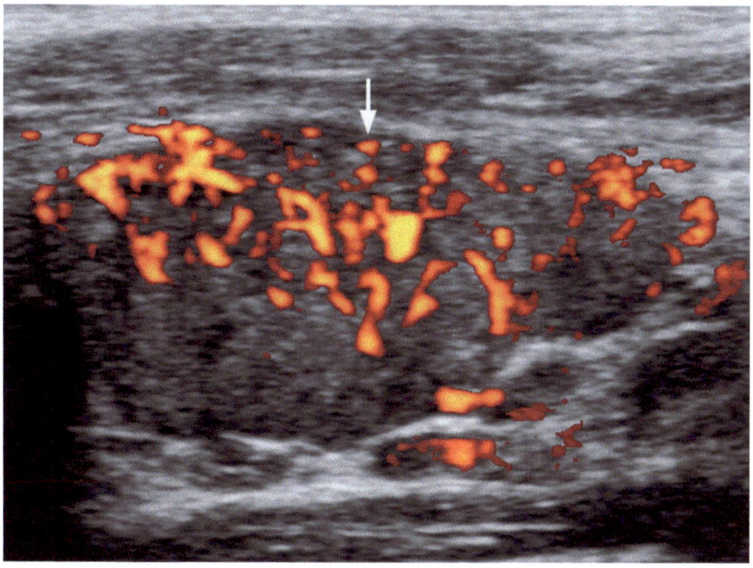

Fig. 5.89 Doppler longitudinal ultrasound in a patient with the previous history of subtotal thyroidectomy for Graves' disease as demonstrated in Fig. 5.88. In the thyroid bed is the hypertrophied, heterogeneous residual thyroid gland (*arrow*) with increased vascularity

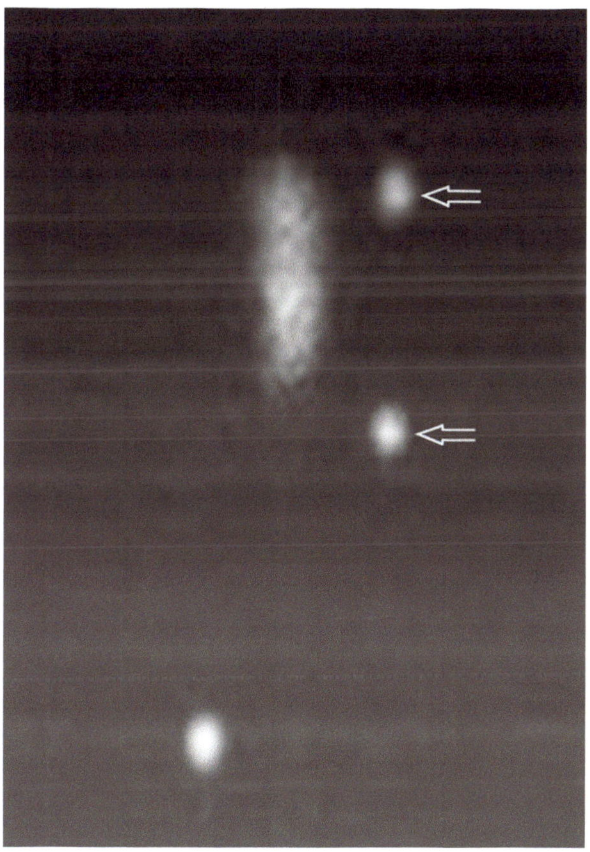

Fig. 5.90 Scintigram of a lateral aberrant thyroid in a patient with previous history of thyroidectomy for Graves' disease. Note the two foci of uptake on the scintigram (*open arrows*) which correspond to the hypertrophied, heterogeneous, hypoechoic "nodules" on ultrasound and intensely enhancing on CECT. These were confirmed as lateral aberrant thyroid tissue at surgery and histology

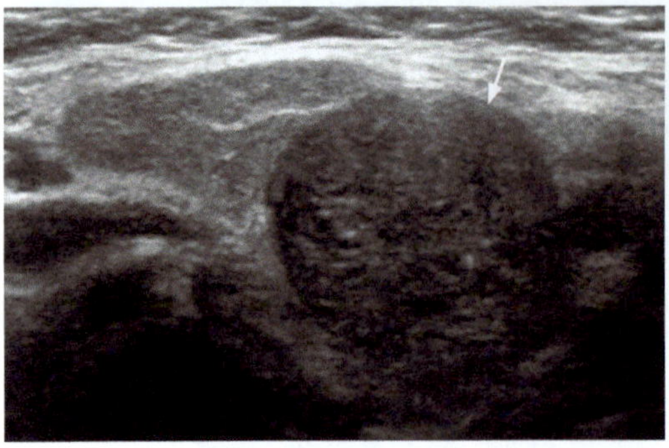

Fig. 5.91 Transverse gray scale ultrasound of discrete superior left neck nodule, Zone IIa adjacent to the submandibular gland. This is one of two confirmed lateral aberrant thyroid tissue nodules confirmed at surgery and histology

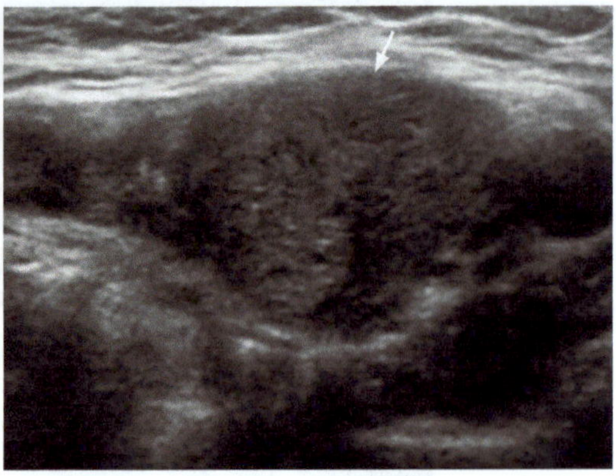

Fig. 5.92 Transverse gray scale ultrasound image of discrete left inferior zone III nodule adjacent but separate from the mass demonstrated in Fig. 5.91 in the patient with prior total thyroidectomy for Graves disease

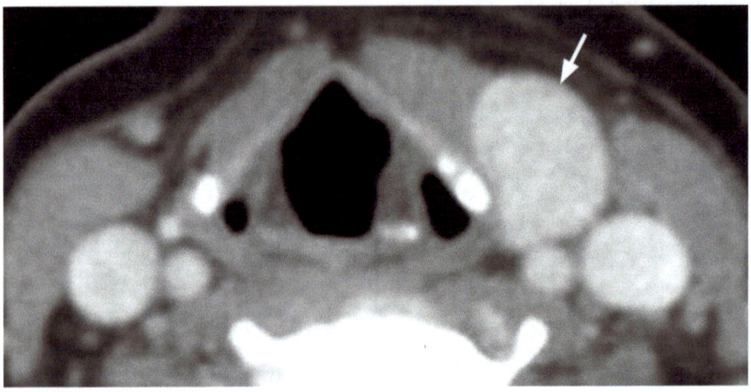

Fig. 5.93 Contrast-enhanced axial CT in the patient with prior thyroidectomy for Graves disease and recurrent hypertrophied lateral aberrant rest. This left sided mass corresponds to the nodule in zone III on ultrasound in Fig. 5.92

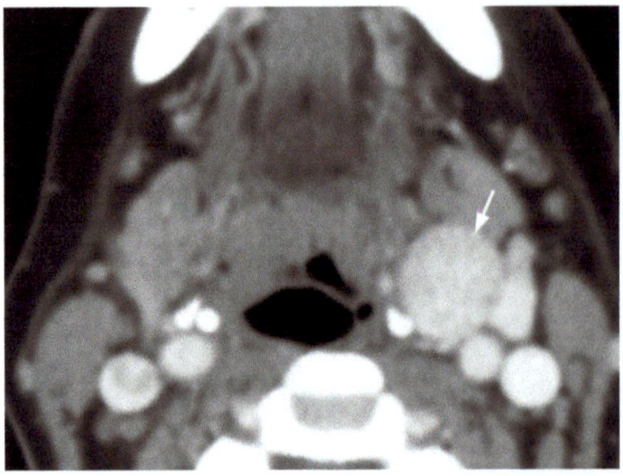

Fig. 5.94 Contrast enhanced axial CT scan demonstrating left neck mass in zone IIa corresponding to the ultrasound image demonstrated in Fig. 5.91. This is one of the two confirmed hypertrophied lateral thyroid rests in this patient with recurrent Graves disease

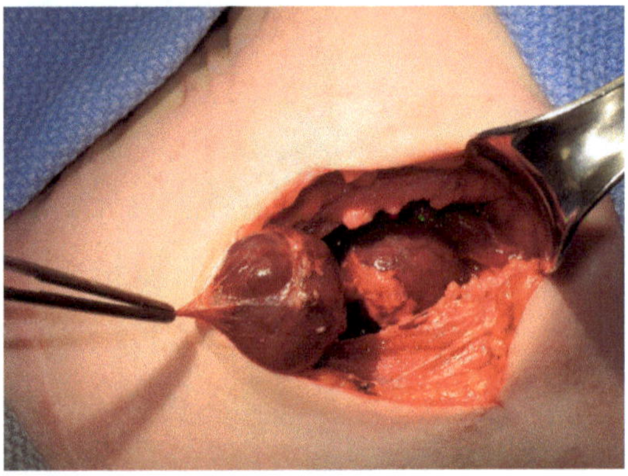

Fig. 5.95 Demonstration of the two lateral aberrent thyroid rests corresponding to the ultrasound and CT images noted in Figs. 5.91–5.94

Conclusion

Benign thyroid disease is commonly encountered in routine clinical practice, and imaging, particularly ultrasound, plays an important role in the diagnostic workup and subsequent follow-up of these patients. Every practicing sonologist should be familiar with the common use of ultrasound/thyroid scintigraphy and typical imaging features of these common benign thyroid diseases.

References

1. Boelaert K, Horacek J, Holder RL, Watkinson JC, Sheppard MC, Franklyn JA. Serum thyrotropin concentration as a novel predictor of malignancy in thyroid nodules investigated by fine-needle aspiration. J Clin Endocrinol Metab. 2006;91:4295–301.
2. Ahuja AT. The thyroid and parathyroids. In: Ahuja AT, Evans RM, editors. Practical head and neck ultrasound. London: Greenwich Medical Media Limited; 2000. p. 35–64.
3. Sarkar SD. Benign thyroid disease: what is the role of nuclear medicine? Semin Nucl Med. 2006;36:185–93.
4. LiVolsi VA. Pathology of thyroid disease. In: Flak SA, editor. Thyroid disease: endocrinology, surgery, nuclear medicine and radiotherapy. Philadelphia: Lippincott-Raven; 1997. p. 75–8.
5. Frates MC, Benson CB, Charboneau JW, et al. Management of thyroid nodules detected at US: Society of Radiologists in Ultrasound consensus conference statement. Radiology. 2005;237: 794–800.
6. Marqusee E, Benson CB, Frates MC, et al. Usefulness of ultrasonography in the management of nodular thyroid disease. Ann Intern Med. 2000;133:696–700.
7. Moon WJ, Jung SL, Lee JH, et al. Thyroid Study Group, Korean Society of Neuro- and Head and Neck Radiology. Benign and malignant thyroid nodules: US differentiation – multicenter retrospective study. Radiology. 2008;247:762–70.
8. Frates MC, Benson CB, Doubilet PM, et al. Prevalence and distribution of carcinoma in patients with solitary and multiple thyroid nodules on sonography. J Clin Endocrinol Metab. 2006;91:3411–7.
9. Moon WJ, Kwag HJ, Na DG. Are there any specific ultrasound findings of nodular hyperplasia ("leave me alone" lesion) to differentiate it from follicular adenoma? Acta Radiol. 2009;50:383–8.
10. Bonavita JA, Mayo J, Babb J, et al. Pattern recognition of benign nodules at ultrasound of the thyroid: which nodules can be left alone? AJR Am J Roentgenol. 2009;193:207–13.
11. Ahuja A, Chick W, King W, Metreweli C. Clinical significance of the comet tail artifact in thyroid ultrasound. J Clin Ultrasound. 1996;24:129–33.
12. Papini E, Guglielmi R, Bianchini A, et al. Risk of malignancy in nonpalpable thyroid nodules: predictive value of ultrasound and color-Doppler features. J Clin Endocrinol Metab. 2002;87:1941–6.
13. Rago T, Vitti P, Chiorator L, Mazzeo S, et al. Role conventional ultrasonography and colour flow Doppler sonography in predicting malignancy in 'cold' thyroid nodules. Eur J Endocrinol. 1998;138:41–6.
14. Bakhshaee M, Davoudi Y, Mehrabi M, et al. Vascular pattern and spectral parameters of power Doppler ultrasound as predictors of malignancy risk in thyroid nodules. Laryngoscope. 2008;118:2182–6.
15. Giammanco M, Di Gesù G, Massenti MF, Di Trapani B, Vetri G. Role of color flow Doppler sonography in pre-operative diagnostics of the thyroid pathology. Minerva Endocrinol. 2002;27:1–10.
16. Deandrea M, Mormile A, Veglio M, et al. Fine-needle aspiration biopsy of the thyroid: comparison between thyroid palpation and ultrasonography. Endocr Pract. 2002;8:282–6.
17. Jun P, Chow LC, Jeffrey RB. The sonographic features of papillary thyroid carcinomas: pictorial essay. Ultrasound Q. 2005;21:39–45.
18. Koike E, Yamashita H, Noguchi S, et al. Effect of combining ultrasonography and ultrasound-guided fine-needle aspiration biopsy findings for the diagnosis of thyroid nodules. Eur J Surg. 2001;167:656–61.
19. Baskin HJ. Ultrasound-guided fine-needle aspiration biopsy of thyroid nodules and multinodular goiters. Endocr Pract. 2004;10:242–5.
20. Erbil Y, Barbaros U, Salmaslioglu A, et al. Effect of thyroid gland volume in preoperative detection of suspected malignant thyroid nodules in a multinodular goiter. Arch Surg. 2008;143:558–63.
21. Kim EK, Park CS, Chung WY, Oh KK, Kim DI, Lee JT, et al. New sonographic criteria for recommending fine-needle aspiration biopsy of nonpalpable solid nodules of the thyroid. AJR Am J Roentgenol. 2002;178:687–91.
22. Quadbeck B, Pruellage J, Roggenbuck U, et al. Long-term follow-up of thyroid nodule growth. Exp Clin Endocrinol Diabetes. 2002;110:348–54.
23. Alexander EK, Hurwitz S, Heering JP, et al. Natural history of benign solid and cystic thyroid nodules. Ann Intern Med. 2003;138:315–8.
24. Grant CS, Hay ID, Gough IR, McCarthy PM, Goellner JR. Long-term follow up of patients with benign thyroid fine-needle aspiration cytologic diagnoses. Surgery. 1989;106:980–5.
25. American Thyroid Association (ATA) Guidelines Taskforce on Thyroid Nodules and Differentiated Thyroid Cancer, Cooper DS, Doherty GM, Haugen BR, et al. Revised American Thyroid Association management guidelines for patients with thyroid nodules and differentiated thyroid cancer. Thyroid. 2009;19:1167–214.

26. Koo JH, Shin JH, Han BK, Ko EY, Kang SS. Cystic thyroid nodules after aspiration mimicking malignancy: sonographic characteristics. J Ultrasound Med. 2010;29:1415–21.
27. Mazzaferri EL. Management of a solitary thyroid nodule. N Engl J Med. 1993;328:553–9.
28. de los Santos ET, Keyhani-Rofagha S, Cunningham JJ, Mazzaferri EL. Cystic thyroid nodules. The dilemma of malignant lesions. Arch Intern Med. 1990;150:1422–7.
29. Oertel YC, Miyahara-Felipe L, Mendoza MG, Yu K. Value of repeated fine needle aspirations of the thyroid: an analysis of over ten thousand FNAs. Thyroid. 2007;17:1061–6.
30. Hall TL, Layfield LJ, Philippe A, Rosenthal DL. Sources of diagnostic error in fine needle aspiration of the thyroid. Cancer. 1989;63:718–25.
31. Hegedüs L. Clinical practice. The thyroid nodule. N Engl J Med. 2004;351:1764–71.
32. British Thyroid Association, Royal College of Physicians. British Thyroid Association guidelines for the management of thyroid cancer. 2nd ed. www.british-thyroid-association.org/Guidelines/ (2007). Accessed 18 Apr 2011.
33. Drucker DJ. MyThyroid.com. http://mythyroid.com/index.html (2010). Accessed 15 Dec 2010.
34. Gharib H, Papini E, Valcavi R, et al. AACE/AME Task Force on Thyroid Nodules. American Association of Clinical Endocrinologists and Associazione Medici Endocrinologi medical guidelines for clinical practice for the diagnosis and management of thyroid nodules. Endocr Pract. 2006;12:63–102.
35. Utiger RD. The pathogenesis of autoimmune thyroid disease. N Engl J Med. 1991;325:278–9.
36. Dayan CM, Daniels GH. Chronic autoimmune thyroiditis. N Engl J Med. 1996;335:99–107.
37. Pedersen OM, Aardal NP, Larssen TB, et al. The value of ultrasonography in predicting autoimmune thyroid disease. Thyroid. 2000;10:251–9.
38. Samuels MH. Subclinical thyroid disease in the elderly. Thyroid. 1998;8:803–13.
39. Gutekunst R, Hafermann W, Mansky T, Scriba PC. Ultrasonography related to clinical and laboratory findings in lymphocytic thyroiditis. Acta Endocrinol (Copenh). 1989;121:129–35.
40. Moon HJ, Kim EK, Kim MJ, Kwak JY. Lymphocytic thyroiditis on fine-needle aspiration biopsy of focal thyroid nodules: approach to management. AJR Am J Roentgenol. 2009;193:W345–9.
41. Marcocci C, Vitti P, Cetani F, Catalano F, Concetti R, Pinchera A. Thyroid ultrasonography helps to identify patients with diffuse lymphocytic thyroiditis who are prone to develop hypothyroidism. J Clin Endocrinol Metab. 1991;72:209–13.
42. Schiemann U, Gellner R, Riemann B, et al. Standardized grey scale ultrasonography in Graves' disease: correlation to autoimmune activity. Eur J Endocrinol. 1999;141:332–6.
43. Meller J, Becker W. The continuing importance of thyroid scintigraphy in the era of high-resolution ultrasound. Eur J Nucl Med Mol Imaging. 2002;29 Suppl 2:S425–38.
44. Baskin HJ, Cobin RH, Duick DS, et al. American Association of Clinical Endocrinologists. American Association of Clinical Endocrinologists medical guidelines for clinical practice for the evaluation and treatment of hyperthyroidism and hypothyroidism. Endocr Pract. 2002;8:457–69.
45. Ross DS. Diagnosis of hyperthyroidism. UpToDate.com. http://www.uptodate.com/contents/diagnosis-of-hyperthyroidism (2008). Accessed 18 Apr 2011.
46. Cappelli C, Pirola I, De Martino E, et al. The role of imaging in Graves' disease: a cost-effectiveness analysis. Eur J Radiol. 2008;65:99–103.
47. Vitti P. Grey scale thyroid ultrasonography in the evaluation of patients with Graves' disease. Eur J Endocrinol. 2000;142:22–4.
48. Arslan H, Unal O, Algün E, Harman M, Sakarya ME. Power Doppler sonography in the diagnosis of Graves' disease. Eur J Ultrasound. 2000;11:117–22.
49. Kurita S, Sakurai M, Kita Y, et al. Measurement of thyroid blood flow area is useful for diagnosing the cause of thyrotoxicosis. Thyroid. 2005;15:1249–52.
50. Saleh A, Cohnen M, Fürst G, Godehardt E, Mödder U, Feldkamp J. Differential diagnosis of hyperthyroidism: Doppler sonographic quantification of thyroid blood flow distinguishes between Graves' disease and diffuse toxic goiter. Exp Clin Endocrinol Diabetes. 2002;110:32–6.
51. Espinasse P. Thyroid echography in chronic autoimmune lymphocytic thyroiditis. J Radiol. 1983;64:537–44.
52. Müller HW, Schröder S, Schneider C, Seifert G. Sonographic tissue characterisation in thyroid gland diagnosis. A correlation between sonography and histology. Klin Wochenschr. 1985;63:706–10.
53. Li Volsi VA. Surgical pathology of the thyroid. Philadelphia: B. Saunders; 1990. p. 83–5.
54. Ralls PW, Mayekawa DS, Lee KP, et al. Color-flow Doppler sonography in Graves disease: "thyroid inferno". AJR Am J Roentgenol. 1988;150:781–4.
55. Swaenepoel L, Demeester-Mirkine N, Sacre R, Jonckheer MH, van Geertruyden J. Ultrasound examination of the thyroid. Rofo. 1982;137:12–7.
56. Zingrillo M, D'Aloiso L, Ghiggi MR, et al. Thyroid hypoechogenicity after methimazole withdrawal in Graves' disease: a useful index for predicting recurrence? Clin Endocrinol (Oxf). 1996;45:201–6.
57. Woeber KA. Graves disease: general considerations. In: Ingbar SH, Braverman LE, editors. The thyroid: a fundamental and clinical text. 5th ed. Philadelphia: Lippincott; 1986. p. 982–5.
58. Vitti P, Rago T, Mazzeo S, et al. Thyroid blood flow evaluation by color-flow Doppler sonography distinguishes Graves' disease from Hashimoto's thyroiditis. J Endocrinol Invest. 1995;18:857–61.

59. Schiefer R, Dean DS. Thyroiditis. In: Baskin HJ, Duick DS, Levine RA, editors. Thyroid ultrasound and ultrasound-guided FNA. 2nd ed. New York: Springer; 2008. p. 63–5.
60. Macedo TA, Chammas MC, Jorge PT, et al. Differentiation between the two types of amiodarone-associated thyrotoxicosis using duplex and amplitude Doppler sonography. Acta Radiol. 2007; 48:412–21.
61. Bogazzi F, Bartalena L, Brogioni S, et al. Color flow Doppler sonography rapidly differentiates type I and type II amiodarone-induced thyrotoxicosis. Thyroid. 1997;7:541–5.
62. Serres-Créixams X, Castells-Fusté I, Pruna-Comella X, Yetano-Laguna V, Garriga-Farriol V, Gallardo-Agromayor E. Paratracheal lymph nodes: a new sonographic finding in autoimmune thyroiditis. J Clin Ultrasound. 2008;36:418–21.
63. Zakarija M, McKenzie JM. The spectrum and significance of autoantibodies reacting with the thyrotropin receptor. Endocrinol Metab Clin North Am. 1987;16:343–63.
64. Vanderpump MP, Tunbridge WM, French JM, et al. The incidence of thyroid disorders in the community: a twenty-year follow-up of the Whickham Survey. Clin Endocrinol (Oxf). 1995;43:55–68.
65. Vitti P, Rago T, Mancusi F, et al. Thyroid hypoechogenic pattern at ultrasonography as a tool for predicting recurrence of hyperthyroidism after medical treatment in patients with Graves' disease. Acta Endocrinol (Copenh). 1992;126:128–31.
66. LiVolsi VA. The pathology of autoimmune thyroid disease: a review. Thyroid. 1994;4:333–9.
67. Rago T, Chiovato L, Grasso L, Pinchera A, Vitti P. Thyroid ultrasonography as a tool for detecting thyroid autoimmune diseases and predicting thyroid dysfunction in apparently healthy subjects. J Endocrinol Invest. 2001;24:763–9.
68. Hayashi N, Tamaki N, Konishi J, et al. Sonography of Hashimoto's thyroiditis. J Clin Ultrasound. 1986;14:123–6.
69. Sostre S, Reyes MM. Sonographic diagnosis and grading of Hashimoto's thyroiditis. J Endocrinol Invest. 1991;14:115–21.
70. Kerr L. High-resolution thyroid ultrasound: the value of color Doppler. Ultrasound Q. 1994;12:21–44.
71. Chonkich GD, Petti Jr GH, Goral W. Total thyroidectomy in the treatment of thyroid disease. Laryngoscope. 1987;97:897–900.
72. Anderson L, Middleton WD, Teefey SA, et al. Hashimoto thyroiditis: part 1, sonographic analysis of the nodular form of Hashimoto thyroiditis. AJR Am J Roentgenol. 2010;195:208–15.
73. Solbiati L, Livraghi T, Ballarati E, Ierace T, Crespi L. Thyroid gland. In: Solbiati L, Rizzatto G, editors. Ultrasound of superficial structures. London: Churchill Livingstone; 1995. p. 49–85.
74. Yeh HC, Futterweit W, Gilbert P. Micronodulation: ultrasonographic sign of Hashimoto thyroiditis. J Ultrasound Med. 1996;15:813–9.
75. Lagalla R, Caruso G, Benza I, Novara V, Calliada F. Echo-color Doppler in the study of hypothyroidism in the adult. Radiol Med. 1993;86:281–3.
76. Thomas Jr CG, Rutledge RG. Surgical intervention in chronic (Hashimoto's) thyroiditis. Ann Surg. 1981;193:769–76.
77. Takashima S, Ikezoe J, Morimoto S, et al. Primary thyroid lymphoma: evaluation with CT. Radiology. 1988;168:765–8.
78. Cipolla C, Sandonato L, Graceffa G, et al. Hashimoto thyroiditis coexistent with papillary thyroid carcinoma. Am Surg. 2005;71:874–8.
79. Pisanu A, Piu S, Cois A, Uccheddu A. Coexisting Hashimoto's thyroiditis with differentiated thyroid cancer and benign thyroid diseases: indications for thyroidectomy. Chir Ital. 2003;55:365–72.
80. Ott RA, McCall AR, McHenry C, et al. The incidence of thyroid carcinoma in Hashimoto's thyroiditis. Am Surg. 1987;53:442–5.
81. Anderson L, Middleton WD, Teefey SA, et al. Hashimoto thyroiditis: part 2, sonographic analysis of benign and malignant nodules in patients with diffuse Hashimoto thyroiditis. AJR Am J Roentgenol. 2010;195:216–22.
82. Intenzo CM, Capuzzi DM, Jabbour S, Kim SM, dePapp AE. Scintigraphic features of autoimmune thyroiditis. Radiographics. 2001;21:957–64.
83. Lazarus JH. Silent thyroiditis and subacute thyroiditis. In: Braverman LE, Utiger RD, editors. The thyroid. Philadelphia: Lippincott-Raven; 1996. p. 578–85.
84. Stagnaro-Green A. Recognizing, understanding, and treating postpartum thyroiditis. Endocrinol Metab Clin North Am. 2000;29:417–30.
85. Roti E, Uberti E. Post-partum thyroiditis – a clinical update. Eur J Endocrinol. 2002;146:275–9.
86. Shahbazian HB, Sarvghadi F, Azizi F. Ultrasonographic characteristics and follow-up in postpartum thyroiditis. J Endocrinol Invest. 2005;28: 410–2.
87. Papi G, LiVolsi VA. Current concepts on Riedel thyroiditis. Am J Clin Pathol. 2004;121(Suppl): S50–63.
88. Pérez Fontán FJ, Cordido Carballido F, Pombo Felipe F, Mosquera Oses J, Villalba Martin C. Riedel thyroiditis: US, CT, and MR evaluation. J Comput Assist Tomogr. 1993;17:324–5.
89. Chi H, Lee YJ, Chiu NC, et al. Acute suppurative thyroiditis in children. Pediatr Infect Dis J. 2002;21: 384–7.
90. Kang M, Ojili V, Khandelwal N, Bhansali A. Tuberculous abscess of the thyroid gland: a report of two cases. J Clin Ultrasound. 2006;34:254–7.
91. Cabizuca CA, Bulzico DA, de Almeida MH, Conceição FL, Vaisman M. Acute thyroiditis due to septic emboli derived from infective endocarditis. Postgrad Med J. 2008;84:445–6.
92. Chang YW, Hong HS, Choi DL. Sonography of the pediatric thyroid: a pictorial essay. J Clin Ultrasound. 2009;37:149–57.

93. Ahuja AT, Griffiths JF, Roebuck DJ, et al. The role of ultrasound and oesophagography in the management of acute suppurative thyroiditis in children associated with congenital pyriform fossa sinus. Clin Radiol. 1998;53:209–11.
94. Bar-Ziv J, Slasky BS, Sichel JY, Lieberman A, Katz R. Branchial pouch sinus tract from the piriform fossa causing acute suppurative thyroiditis, neck abscess, or both: CT appearance and the use of air as a contrast agent. AJR Am J Roentgenol. 1996;167:1569–72.
95. Wang HK, Tiu CM, Chou YH, Chang CY. Imaging studies of pyriform sinus fistula. Pediatr Radiol. 2003;33:328–33.
96. Hancock SL, Cox RS, McDougall IR. Thyroid diseases after treatment of Hodgkin's disease. N Engl J Med. 1991;325:599–605.
97. Hancock SL, McDougall IR, Constine LS. Thyroid abnormalities after therapeutic external radiation. Int J Radiat Oncol Biol Phys. 1995;31:1165–70.
98. Jereczek-Fossa BA, Alterio D, Jassem J, Gibelli B, Tradati N, Orecchia R. Radiotherapy-induced thyroid disorders. Cancer Treat Rev. 2004;30:369–84.
99. Nishiyama K, Kozuka T, Higashihara T, Miyauchi K, Okagawa K. Acute radiation thyroiditis. Int J Radiat Oncol Biol Phys. 1996;36:1221–4.
100. Diaz R, Blakey MD, Murphy PB, Cryar AK, Cmelak AJ. Thyroid storm after intensity-modulated radiation therapy: a case report and discussion. Oncologist. 2009;14:233–9.
101. American Thyroid Association. Thyroiditis. http://www.thyroid.org/patients/patient_brochures/thyroiditis.html. Accessed 5 Jan 2011.
102. Nishiyama K, Tanaka E, Tarui Y, Miyauchi K, Okagawa K. A prospective analysis of subacute thyroid dysfunction after neck irradiation. Int J Radiat Oncol Biol Phys. 1996;34:439–44.
103. Constine LS, Donaldson SS, McDougall IR, Cox RS, Link MP, Kaplan HS. Thyroid dysfunction after radiotherapy in children with Hodgkin's disease. Cancer. 1984;53:878–83.
104. Moore KL, Persaud TVN. Chapter 10: the pharyngeal apparatus. In: Moore KL, Persaud TVN, editors. The developing human: clinically oriented embryology. 7th ed. Philadelphia: Saunders; 2003. p. 215–7.
105. LaFranchi S. Congenital hypothyroidism: etiologies, diagnosis, and management. Thyroid. 1999;9:735–40.
106. Babcock DS. Thyroid disease in the pediatric patient: emphasizing imaging with sonography. Pediatr Radiol. 2006;36:299–308.
107. Hammond RJ, Meakin K, Davies JE. Case report: lateral thyroid ectopia – CT and MRI findings. Br J Radiol. 1996;69:1178–80.
108. Morgan NJ, Emberton P, Barton RP. The importance of thyroid scanning in neck lumps – a case report of ectopic tissue in the right submandibular region. J Laryngol Otol. 1995;109:674–6.

Malignant Thyroid Conditions

6

Ka Tak Wong, Yolanda Y.P. Lee, and Anil T. Ahuja

Introduction

Thyroid nodules are a common clinical dilemma; however, the vast majority are benign. The clinical importance of thyroid nodules rests with the need to detect thyroid cancer, which occurs in 5–10%. The risk depends on factors including age, gender, history of radiation exposure and family history [1, 2].

The main aim in the management of a thyroid nodule is to identify the small group of patients with a malignancy who warrant timely definitive treatment while avoiding unnecessary investigations and treatment in the majority of patients with benign nodules. Imaging plays an important role in providing an accurate preoperative diagnosis, and in patients with proven thyroid malignancy, it provides essential information such as local tumor extent and presence of regional and distant metastases. In addition, in patients with a high risk of tumor recurrence, imaging is an indispensible tool in the post-treatment surveillance (local, regional, and distant).

K.T. Wong (✉)
Department of Imaging and Interventional Radiology, Prince of Wales Hospital, The Chinese University of Hong Kong, 30-32 Ngan Shing Street, Shatin, NT, Hong Kong SAR, People's Republic of China
e-mail: wongkatakjeffrey@hotmail.com

Yolanda Y.P. Lee
Department of Imaging & Interventional Radiology, Prince of Wales Hospital, The Chinese University of Hong Kong, Shatin, NT, Hong Kong

A.T. Ahuja
Department of Imaging and Interventional Radiology, The Chinese University of Hong Kong, Prince of Wales Hospital, Shatin (NT), Hong Kong (SAR), China

Clinical Presentation of Thyroid Cancer

Thyroid carcinoma commonly presents as a thyroid nodule, noticed either by the patient or the clinician. Other less common clinical symptoms and signs include cervical lymphadenopathy, recent onset of hoarseness (due to vocal cord palsy), dysphagia and upper airway obstruction. Small asymptomatic thyroid cancer is most often detected incidentally on routine imaging of the neck (ultrasound, CT, MRI and PET–CT) for other indications.

Clinical features that raise the suspicion of thyroid malignancy include history of childhood head and neck irradiation, total body irradiation for bone marrow transplantation [3], history of thyroid cancer or thyroid cancer syndrome (e.g., Cowden's syndrome, familial polyposis, Carney complex, multiple endocrine neoplasia (MEN) 2, and Werner's syndrome) in a first-degree relative, exposure to ionizing radiation from fallout in childhood or adolescence [4] and rapid development of hoarseness.

Pertinent physical signs suggesting probable malignancy include hard consistency of the thyroid nodule with an irregular edge, fixation of nodule to adjacent structures (such as skin, strap muscles and cervical portion of trachea), vocal

R.A. Sofferman and A.T. Ahuja (eds.), *Ultrasound of the Thyroid and Parathyroid Glands*,
DOI 10.1007/978-1-4614-0974-8_6, © Springer Science+Business Media, LLC 2012

cord palsy and ipsilateral enlarged cervical lymph nodes. However, at presentation most patients have no overt signs of thyroid cancer. Therefore, imaging is usually indicated to evaluate a thyroid nodule and regional nodal status.

Management Protocol of Thyroid Nodule

The American Thyroid Association (ATA) published management guidelines in 2009 for patients with thyroid nodules and differentiated thyroid cancer [5].

It is suggested that with the discovery of a thyroid nodule larger than 1–1.5 cm, a serum thyrotropin (TSH) level should be obtained as part of the initial evaluation.

If the serum TSH is subnormal, a radionuclide thyroid scan should be performed using either technetium ^{99m}Tc pertechnetate or ^{123}I.

Diagnostic thyroid ultrasound (± FNAC) should be performed in all patients with a suspected thyroid nodule with normal or high TSH level (associated with increased risk of malignancy in a thyroid nodule [6]) or a thyroid nodule found incidentally on computed tomography (CT), magnetic resonance imaging (MRI) or thyroidal uptake on ^{18}FDG-PET scan.

Routine measurement of serum thyroglobulin and calcitonin level is not recommended.

Fine Needle Aspiration

FNA is inexpensive, widely available, easy to perform, accurate (>90%) [7], cost-effective method for evaluating thyroid nodules [5] and commonly regarded a part of the initial investigation. Acute complications are rare, and there is no reported case of cutaneous implantation of malignancy following FNA of a thyroid lesion [7]. However, its success depends on the skill of the person doing the procedure and the experience of the cytopathologist. FNA has an overall false negative rate of between 0.5% and 11.8% (pooled rate of 2.4%) and a false positive rate ranging from 0% to 7.1% (pooled rate of 1.2%) [8, 9]. The false negative rates can be reduced by better sampling techniques, meticulous follow-up and serial FNA examinations [7]. While the nondiagnostic rate of FNA may vary among different centers depending on the level of local expertise, 15% nondiagnosis is the maximum acceptable limit recommended by the Papanicolaou Society Guidelines [10].

The role of ultrasound-guided FNA has been a source of controversy in literature, and therefore, its use may vary among different centers. In general, an ultrasound-guided FNAC is recommended for [11–14]:

- Impalpable or poorly palpable nodules.
- Nodules with a higher likelihood of either a nondiagnostic cytology (>25–50% cystic component) or sampling error (difficult to palpate or posteriorly located nodules).
- Nondiagnostic or failed previous conventional FNA.

A false negative rate of up to 2% may occur with ultrasound-guided FNA which may be higher for nodules with suspicious ultrasound features [15]. It is therefore suggested that a repeat FNAC should be performed, for thyroid nodules that have suspicious US features, even if the initial cytologic results indicate that it is a benign lesion [15].

If the diagnostic ultrasound confirms the presence of a predominantly solid nodule corresponding to what is palpated, the FNA may be performed via palpation or US guidance.

Thyroid Imaging

Radionuclide Imaging

The use of radionuclide imaging in the work up of a thyroid nodule and management of thyroid malignancy depends on the availability of dedicated scanning equipment and appropriate radiopharmaceuticals, ^{99m}Tc pertechnetate or ^{123}I/^{131}I are the more commonly used ones.

It is recommended in a patient with a thyroid nodule and subnormal TSH level to document whether the nodule is hyperfunctioning (tracer uptake > surrounding thyroid tissue: hot), isofunctioning (tracer uptake = surrounding thyroid tissue:

warm), or nonfunctioning (tracer uptake < surrounding thyroid tissue: cold) [5]. Hyperfunctioning nodules rarely harbor malignancy; if one is found that corresponds to the nodule in question, cytologic evaluation may not be required.

For well-differentiated thyroid cancer treated with total thyroidectomy and radioiodine ablation, radioiodine whole-body scan (WBS) is recommended for high-risk patients or those with elevated TSH-stimulated thyroglobulin level [16–18].

Positron Emission Tomography

^{18}FDG-PET has been utilized in the differentiation of benign from malignant nodules [19–22]. Although it appears to have a high sensitivity for malignant nodules, its specificity is low [23]. The currently adopted clinical uses of ^{18}FDG-PET in thyroid cancers include [5]:

- Localization of thyroid cancer in thyroglobulin-positive, radioactive iodine (RAI) scan-negative patients.
- Selection tool to identify patients unlikely to respond to additional RAI therapy.
- Initial staging and follow-up of high-risk patients with poorly differentiated thyroid cancer unlikely to concentrate RAI, in which the tumor may be missed on RAI scan.
- Initial staging and follow-up of invasive or metastatic Hurthle cell carcinoma.
- Prognostic tool for identifying patients with distant metastases.
- Measurement of post-treatment response following external beam irradiation, surgical resection, embolization or systemic therapy.

In general, low-risk patients are unlikely to require ^{18}FDG-PET as part of initial staging or follow-up.

CT and MRI

CT and MRI have only limited role in the investigation of a thyroid nodule. In locally invasive thyroid malignancy (such as anaplastic carcinoma), they help to evaluate the extrathyroid spread of tumor to the larynx, trachea and adjacent major vessels (Fig. 6.1) [7, 24] and provide evidence of regional or distant metastases.

The CT and MR appearances of malignant lesions are generally nonspecific with the exception of cystic papillary carcinoma. Cystic thyroid lesions (e.g. simple serous cysts) display low

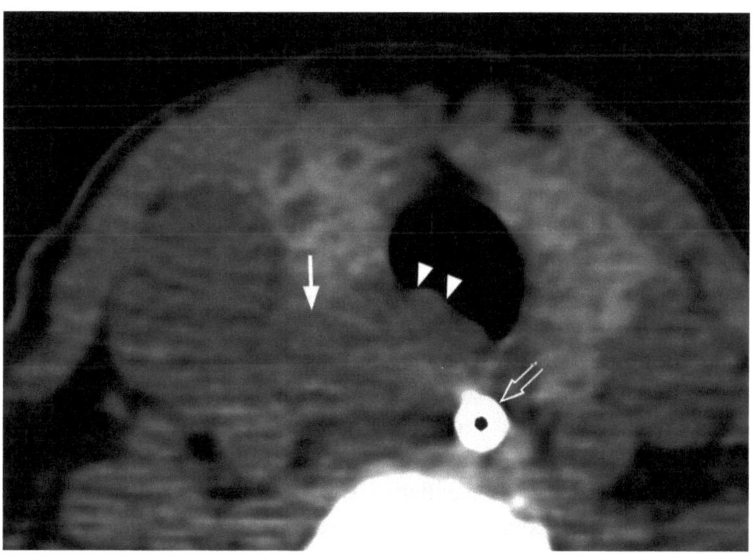

Fig. 6.1 Axial noncontrast CT of the neck at the level of thyroid gland shows a large soft tissue mass in the right lobe of thyroid gland (*arrow*) infiltrating the trachea (*arrowheads*) and cervical portion of esophagus [nasogastric tube (*open arrow*) in situ]

attenuation on CT and appear hypointense on T1-weighted and hyperintense on T2-weighted MR sequences. Due to the presence of thyroglobulin within a cystic papillary carcinoma, these tumors appear isointense (to muscle) on CT and show hyperintense signal on both T1-weighted and T2-weighted sequences on MRI [25]. Similar features are seen in cystic nodal metastases from papillary carcinoma.

Thyroid Ultrasound

Advances in ultrasound technology and transducer development have now made it possible for most modern equipment to have a lateral resolution of 2–3 mm. This makes it possible to clearly evaluate the thyroid parenchyma and detect small nodules.

The robust nature of equipment, its versatility, and reduced costs have made ultrasound a popular office-based imaging technique across multiple specialties, including head and neck. Although this improves clinical practice (as ultrasound is far more sensitive than palpation), it brings with it a unique set of problems as ultrasound now detects many small lesions/incidentalomas which would otherwise have gone undetected.

Consider these incidentalomas in the context of thyroid ultrasound. Using palpation, 4–7% of US population has a thyroid nodule compared to 50–60% detected at autopsy and 67% discovered using high-resolution ultrasound [26]. The increasing use of ultrasound has led to a 2.4-fold increase in the incidence of thyroid nodule. Adding to this pool are the incidental thyroid nodules detected using CT, MRI [27] and PET–CT done for indications unrelated to thyroid disease. This has led to an obvious increase in fine needle aspiration biopsies (FNABs), considered to be threefold in the decade 1995–2005 [28]. Despite this early detection of thyroid nodules/cancer, the incidence of thyroid cancer deaths has remained stable for the last 40 years. This is because the commonest thyroid cancer detected is papillary thyroid cancer which has a very good prognosis with a 30-year survival rate of 95% [29]. It therefore appears that the early detection of this common thyroid cancer has made no significant difference, and some suggest that occult papillary thyroid cancer may be a normal finding. Using 2–3-mm fine sections (similar to the ultrasound resolution), at autopsy papillary carcinoma was present in 36% of normal people [30].

Now, consider the following guideline issued by the American Thyroid Association [5] which suggests all thyroid nodules incidentally detected by US, CT, MRI, PET–CT (the risk of malignancy in FDG +ve nodules is about 33%, and these cancers may be aggressive [31]) should undergo further evaluation, which in many cases would involve a FNAB. The above guideline is based on the fact that the incidence of thyroid cancer in incidentally identified or nonpalpable thyroid nodules is the same as that in patients with palpable nodules [32–34]. The costs of investigation, treatment (if any), and follow-up surveillance (maybe a large number of cases) of these incidentally detected thyroid nodules will have a significant impact on the health services. This raises an ethical, financial, and philosophical dilemma which the health services will have to address and is beyond the scope of this chapter/book. This issue of increasing detection and investigation of incidentally detected thyroid nodule is eloquently discussed in an editorial entitled "Thyroid Nodules: Is It time to turn Off the Ultrasound Machines" by John Cronan [35]. Statistics quoted in this editorial have been used in the preceding paragraphs to put the clinical dilemma of a ubiquitous thyroid nodule into perspective.

The major role of ultrasound in thyroid malignancy includes [36]

- Detection, delineation and characterization of thyroid cancer.
- Detection of cervical nodal metastases.
- Follow-up of patients with benign disease.
- Follow-up of patients after thyroidectomy for early detection of local or regional nodal recurrence.
- Imaging guidance for fine needle/core biopsy.

The following paragraphs will discuss the sonographic features of a thyroid nodule, their role in distinguishing a benign from malignant nodule, and the sonographic features that may help to identify which nodule to FNA.

The sonographic evaluation of a thyroid nodule includes:

Gray-scale ultrasound – which evaluates size, shape, internal echogenicity/architecture, margins/halo, and presence or absence of cystic change and calcification.

Doppler ultrasound – assesses the presence and distribution of vessels within the thyroid nodule and intranodular intravascular resistance/flow velocity (which we do not perform at our institution, as in our experience we find it of very limited value in routine clinical practice).

Elasticity imaging (EI) – evaluates the firmness of a thyroid nodule in relation to adjacent tissues. This is discussed in detail in a separate chapter in the book.

In addition, a complete sonographic examination of the thyroid must include ultrasound assessment of nodal disease in the neck, presence/absence of extrathyroid/extracapsular spread (to adjacent soft tissues, trachea, esophagus, and muscle) and tumor thrombosis/involvement of carotid artery and internal jugular vein.

One must bear in mind that no single sonographic feature has a high accuracy, and in routine clinical practice, a combination of features (gray scale, Doppler, EI) will help in distinguishing benign from malignant disease.

Gray-scale features such as hypoechogenicity, taller than wide, irregular margin, absence of halo, microcalcification and solid nature of a nodule are useful in identifying malignancy [32, 37–44]. A combination of these features is better at predicting malignancy compared to any single feature [32, 39–44].

The role of nodule vascularity in predicting malignancy continues to be debated with some authors suggesting its useful role [32, 37, 41, 45–50], while others doubt its use in routine practice [27, 44, 51–56]. Those doubting its use report that a combination of four gray-scale features alone (taller-than-wide sign, microcalcification, marked hypoechogenicity, noncircumscribed) is better than vascularity + gray-scale features or vascularity alone [56].

Features and combination of features which have a more reasonable predictive value for malignancy:

- Presence of punctate microcalcifications and solid nature shows the highest accuracy (77%), specificity (96%), positive predictive value (75%) but a low sensitivity (30%) [57].
- Absent halo and the presence of punctate microcalcifications has a specificity of 93% and sensitivity of 27% [44].
- A combination of an absent halo, increased intranodular flow, and presence of punctate microcalcifications has a specificity of 97% and sensitivity of 16% [44].
- Taller-than-wide nodule with at least two additional sonographic features (microcalcification, hypoechogenicity and blurred margins) is the best compromise between missing a malignancy and cost benefit [58].
- Hypoechoic nodule with coarse or microcalcification, solid mass with refractive edges, central vascularity, peripheral vascularity, isoechoic nodule ± halo [59, 60].

Sonographic appearances which may be highly predictive of a benign nodule:

- A pure cystic nodule, although rare (<2% of all nodules), is highly unlikely to be malignant [61].
- A spongiform appearance, defined as an aggregation of multiple microcystic components in more than 50% of the nodule volume, is 99.7% specific for benign thyroid nodule with a negative predictive value for malignancy of 98.5% [43, 60, 62].
- The presence of a comet-tail sign in a thyroid nodule indicates a benign colloid nodule [63].
- Colloid cyst, large cystic nodule, spongiform/puff pastry appearance, hyperechoic nodule [59, 60].

These combinations continue to be refined, and the Thyroid Imaging Reporting and Data System (TIRADS) (similar to Breast Imaging Reporting and Data System, BIRADS) has been suggested to improve patient management and cost-effectiveness and avoid unnecessary FNABs [64]. We believe that every sonologist will build their own body of knowledge and identify/apply the combination of features they find useful in distinguishing benign from malignant disease. This is possible because many of the nodules will undergo FNAB, and sonographic combinations in correlation with FNAB will form the basis for such knowledge/experience acquisition.

The following paragraphs discuss each sonographic feature in greater detail.

Size of Nodule

- *Measurement method* should be standardized to minimize interobserver variability. Nodules should be measured with the calipers placed outside of any visible halo. The maximum diameter of the nodule should be measured [27].
- *Nodule size* is not predictive of malignancy; the likelihood of cancer in a thyroid nodule has been shown to be the same regardless of the size measured at US [32, 34, 39, 65]. The incidence of malignancy identified in nonpalpable nodules is the same as in patients with palpable thyroid nodule [26].
- ATA Management Guidelines 2009 suggest that only thyroid nodules (irrespective of palpable or nonpalpable) >1 cm should be evaluated as they have a greater potential to be clinically significant [5]. In addition, uncertainties exist as to whether or not diagnosis of smaller cancer improves life expectancy, as well as concern that inclusion of smaller nodules would lead to an excessive number of biopsies.
- *Nodule growth* itself is not pathognomonic of malignancy. While benign nodules may decrease in size, they often increase in size, albeit slowly [66]. The rate of thyroid nodule growth cannot distinguish between benign and malignant nodules [67]. However, nodule growth is an indication for repeat FNAC/biopsy [5]. There is no consensus on the definition of nodule growth; some groups suggest a 15% increase in nodule volume, while others recommend measuring a change in the mean nodule diameter [66, 68]. ATA recommends a reasonable definition of growth as a 20% increase in nodule diameter with a minimum increase in two or more dimensions of at least 2 mm [5]. However, others suggest that the presence or absence of growth is not a reliable indicator of the nature of a thyroid nodule [5, 69–74].
- The diagnostic accuracy of ultrasound is different for nodules smaller than 10 mm (i.e. small nodule) and those larger than 10 mm (i.e. large nodule). The US features suggestive of malignancy show a higher specificity and a lower sensitivity for large nodules than for small nodules [43]. For small nodules, the US feature of hypoechogenicity including marked hypoechogenicity showed a comparatively high sensitivity (90.9%) but a low specificity (37.4%). Malignant nodules with diameter of 10 mm or smaller showed microcalcifications less frequently than did nodules with a larger diameter (36.6% vs. 51.4%) [43]. The diagnostic value of microcalcification for cancer detection was higher for large nodule (51.4% sensitivity and 91.6% specificity) than for small nodule (36.6% sensitivity and 87.9% specificity) [43].
- Size cannot be used as a cutoff for risk of extracapsular spread or metastatic growth [32, 34, 75–80] as the prevalence of extracapsular spread, multifocality and metastatic growth is similar in nodules <10 mm and >10 mm [32].
- *Do ultrasound features of malignancy vary between small nodules ≤15 mm (SN) and large nodules ≥15 mm [81]?*
  (a) Features of malignancy irrespective of SN or LN: hypoechogenicity, presence of microcalcification, and shape (taller than wide).

  The *most sensitive* feature being hypoechogenicity, however, the specificity was low particularly in SN [81].

  The *most specific* feature was the presence of microcalcification [27, 32, 34, 39, 40, 43]. However, malignant nodules <10 mm showed microcalcification less often than larger nodules, and the overall sensitivity was low [56, 81].

  In predicting malignancy, shape of the lesion is more useful in SN compared to LN [78, 81].

(b) In selection of nodules for FNAB:
  - Some reports suggest the sonographic features associated with malignancy are similar in SN and LN [58].
  - Others indicate that the usefulness of sonographic features suggesting malignancy is lower in patients with LN compared to SN [78, 82], and the only reliable indicator was hypoechogenicity.
  - And some report the sonographic features suggestive of malignancy (taller than wide, hypoechogenicity, presence of microcalcification, spiculated margins) showed lower sensitivity and higher specificity for nodules >10 mm [43, 56].

- *Should small nodules be FNAed or followed up*?

  It is generally believed that follow-up is better than FNAB of small nodules (≤5 mm), as FNAB of such small nodules frequently lead to inadequate specimens and have a high false positive rate [83]. The reason for follow-up of such nodules is for early detection of small invasive cancers and evaluation of extracapsular spread and presence of any malignant lymphadenopathy [84, 85].

Calcification

- Calcification may be present in up to 30% of thyroid nodules and can be divided into different categories.
- Microcalcification is defined as tiny (<2 mm diameter) punctate echogenic foci with or without posterior acoustic shadowing (Fig. 6.2). Macrocalcification is defined as calcification >2 mm in diameter [69]. It is hypothesized that microcalcifications are the imaging equivalent of aggregates of psammoma bodies (infarcted papillae attracting calcium which is deposited on dying cells) characteristic of papillary carcinoma.
- The presence of microcalcifications is one of the most specific features of malignancy, with a specificity of 85.8–95% and a positive predictive value of 41.8%–94.2% [27, 32, 39, 51, 86]. The presence of microcalcifications in a predominantly solid nodule increases cancer risk threefold compared to a predominantly solid nodule without any calcification [27]. However, presence of microcalcification may not be a reliable predictor of malignancy in nodules <10 mm [56].

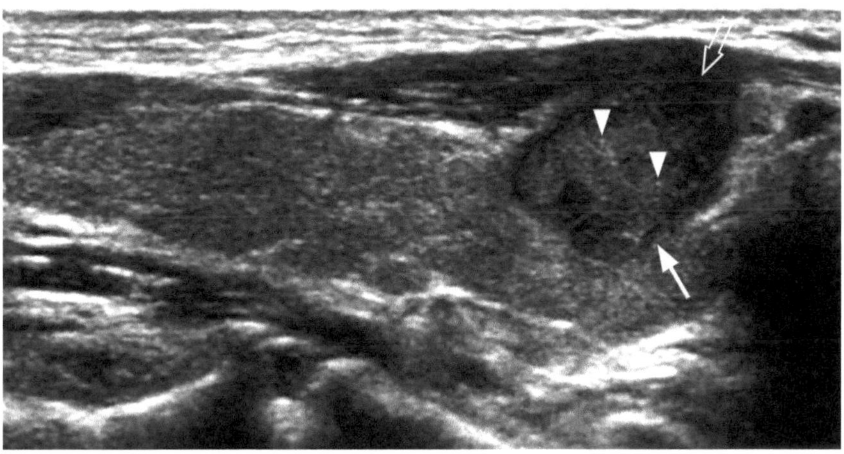

Fig. 6.2 Longitudinal gray-scale ultrasound of the thyroid gland shows a solid hypoechoic nodule (*arrow*) in the lower pole with foci of microcalcifications (*arrowheads*). Note the small size (<1 mm) and absence of posterior acoustic shadowing. Also note the anterior margins of the nodule are inseparable from the overlying strap muscle (*open arrow*) indicating extracapsular involvement

a

b

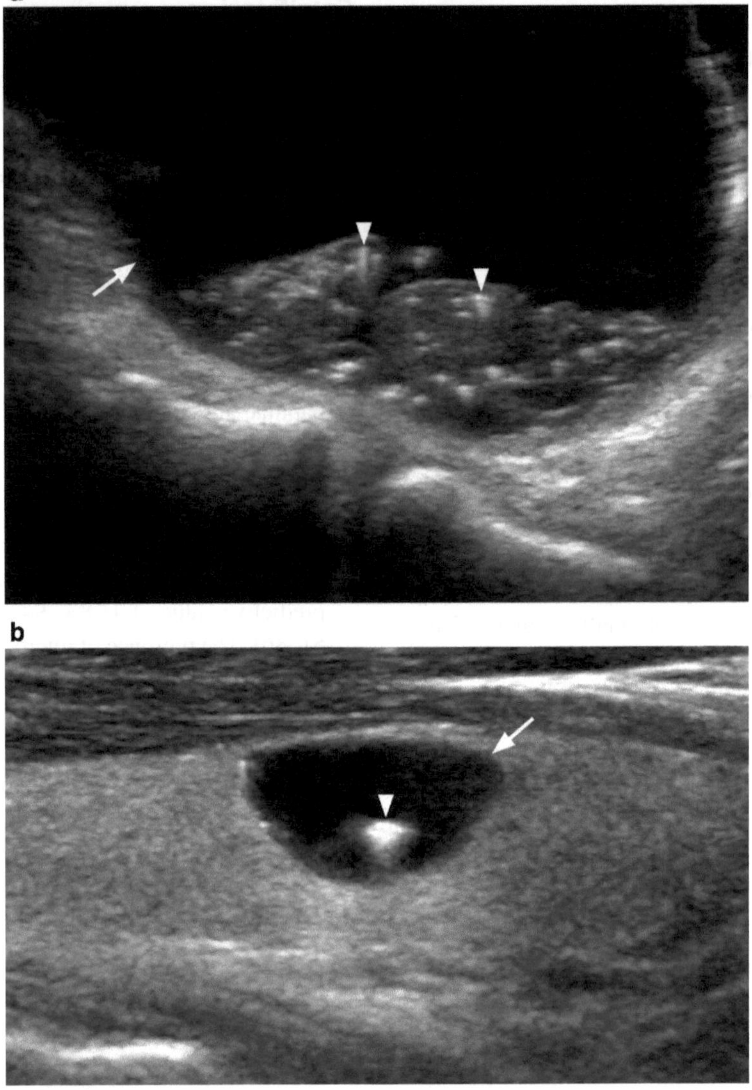

Fig. 6.3 (**a**) Longitudinal gray-scale ultrasound of a predominantly cystic thyroid nodule (*arrow*) containing echogenic foci with "comet-tail" artifacts (*arrowheads*) indicating presence of colloid within a benign colloid cyst. (**b**) Gray-scale sonogram showing a solitary comet-tail artifact (*arrowhead*) often referred to as "cat's eye" artifact within a cystic colloid nodule (*arrow*)

- The absence of fine posterior acoustic shadowing may make it difficult to reliably differentiate microcalcification from a comet-tail artifact (Fig. 6.3) (which suggests benignity). In order to better evaluate these echogenic foci:
  - Increase the scanning frequency as this facilitates the detection of fine posterior acoustic shadowing (increasing frequency increases sound attenuation and may better delineate the fine shadowing).
  - Newer equipment with multidirectional scanning and image "softening" software may make it difficult to see the microcalcification as discrete foci. Scanning in the fundamental mode (or in the Doppler mode with the color gain turned low) better delineates the fine shadowing (Fig. 6.4).

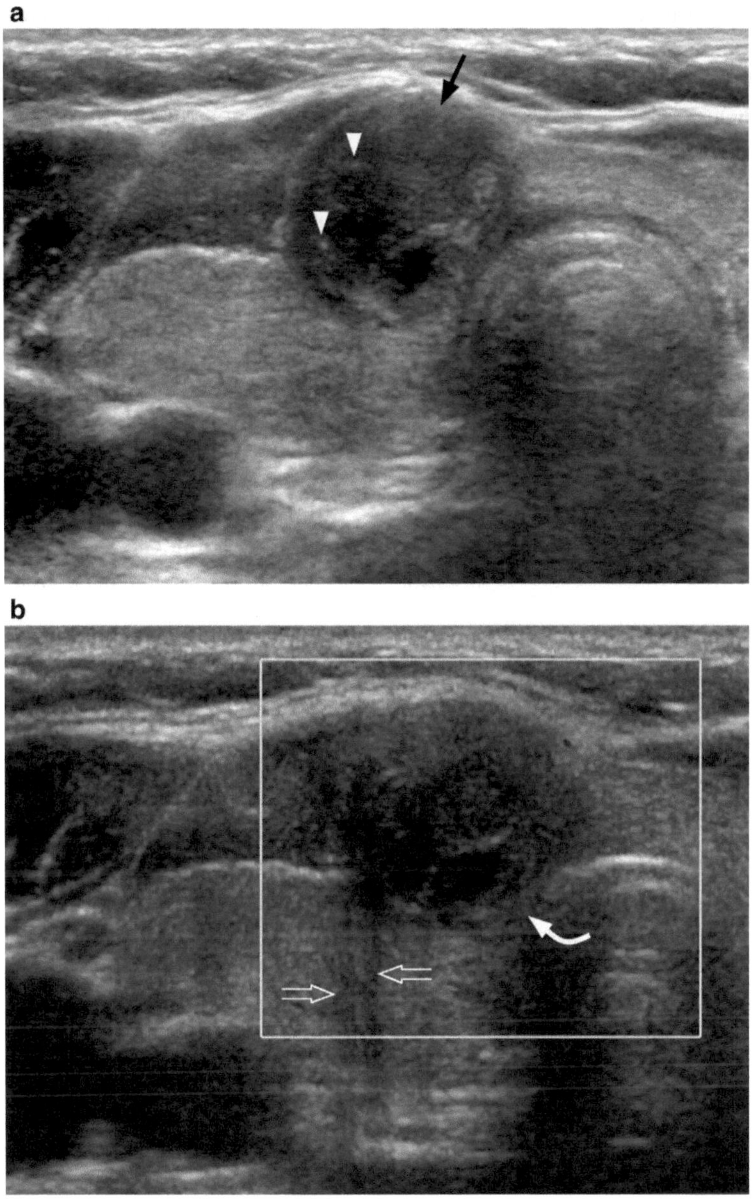

Fig. 6.4 (**a**) Transverse gray-scale sonogram of a confirmed papillary carcinoma (*arrow*). Note that it shows faint echogenic foci (*arrowheads*) within but no obvious posterior acoustic shadowing. (**b**) Corresponding power Doppler sonogram with the power gain turned down (resulting in gray-scale ultrasound in the fundamental mode) shows multiple linear posterior acoustic shadows (*open arrows*) arising from the nodule. Tracing back on real-time ultrasound shows these shadows originated from echogenic foci/microcalcification within the nodule. Also note the tumor is inseparable from the trachea (*curved arrow*)

- A twinkling artifact behind an echogenic focus is another clue to the presence of microcalcification [45].
- Coarse or dense calcification is larger than 2 mm, cast posterior acoustic shadowing (Fig. 6.5), and can be found in both benign and malignant nodules. These dystrophic calcifications are present in areas of fibrosis and tissue degeneration and necrosis. Coarse calcifications are often seen with benign nodules and indicate long-standing disease [87–89]. Coarse calcifications, either associated with microcalcifications or appearing in the center of a hypoechoic nodule, may be worrisome for malignancy [61, 90]. The presence of coarse calcifications in a predominantly solid nodule increases cancer risk twofold compared to a predominantly solid nodule without any calcification [27].

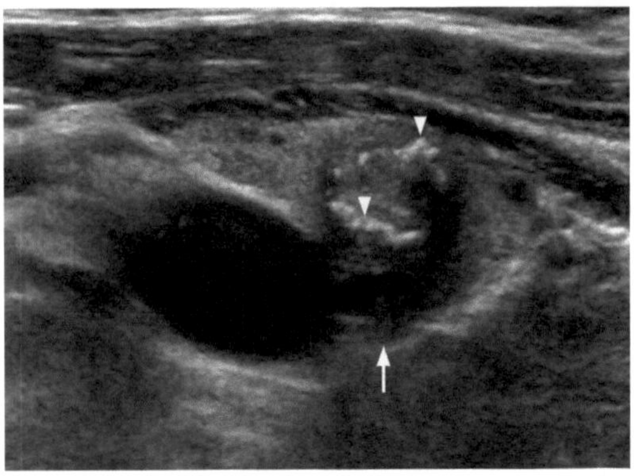

Fig. 6.5 Longitudinal gray-scale ultrasound of the thyroid gland shows a mixed cystic/solid nodule (*arrow*) with coarse calcification (*arrowheads*) casting a posterior acoustic shadow. The sonographic appearances are suggestive of a benign nodule

- Peripheral or "eggshell" calcification (Fig. 6.6), once thought to indicate benign nodule, may be found in malignant nodule [90, 91]. It is reported to have an 18.5% prevalence in malignant thyroid nodules [91]. It is particularly worrisome if the rim calcification is interrupted, indicating probable malignant tumor invasion [92]. However, the relationship of rim calcification with malignancy has yet to be definitively established, and its presence shows no statistical significance in differentiating a benign from a malignant nodule [27, 56].

Solid/Cystic Consistency

- A pure cystic nodule, although rare (<2% of all nodules), is highly unlikely to be malignant [62]. Pure cystic nodules harbor low risk of cancer compared to 30% risk of malignancy in complex cystic nodules [62].

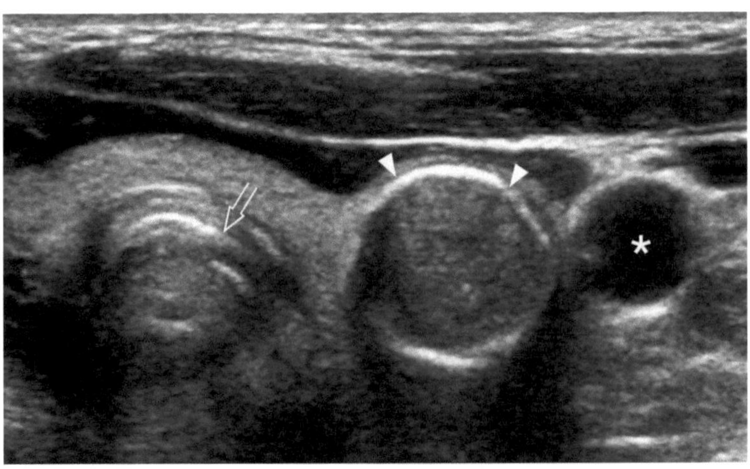

Fig. 6.6 Transverse gray-scale ultrasound of the thyroid gland shows a dense thin, complete rim calcification (*arrowheads*). *Asterisk* – left common carotid artery; *Open arrow* – trachea. The role of rim/annular calcification in suggesting malignancy is not well established and remains controversial

- The vast majority of "cystic" nodules seen in routine clinical practice are complex cystic nodules and represent colloid nodules and hyperplastic nodules as a congenital thyroid cyst is very rare. The presence of multiple or solitary ("cat's eye" artifact) comet-tail artifacts within a cystic nodule (Fig. 6.3) suggests a colloid nodule and requires no further investigation [63]. In a complex nodule that is predominantly cystic (i.e., >50% nodule volume is cystic) but has an associated solid component, the intranodular fluid represents degeneration and possible hemorrhage. The "solid" component within such a nodule is often a "blood clot" due to previous intranodular hemorrhage. On Doppler, such a solid component is invariably avascular and soft (often mobile) on FNAB (Fig. 6.7).
- A spongiform appearance (Fig. 6.8), defined as an aggregation of multiple microcystic components in more than 50% of the nodule volume, is 99.7% specific for a benign nodule [43, 60, 62]. Such an appearance is similar to the honeycomb pattern or puff pastry appearance [60]. It is believed that such a spongiform appearance may represent an earlier step of cystic degeneration of a nodular hyperplasia [62].
- A cystic component occurs in 13–26% of all thyroid malignancies [47, 93], but a predominant cystic malignancy is uncommon. A careful US assessment of the solid component often reveals suspicious features, including

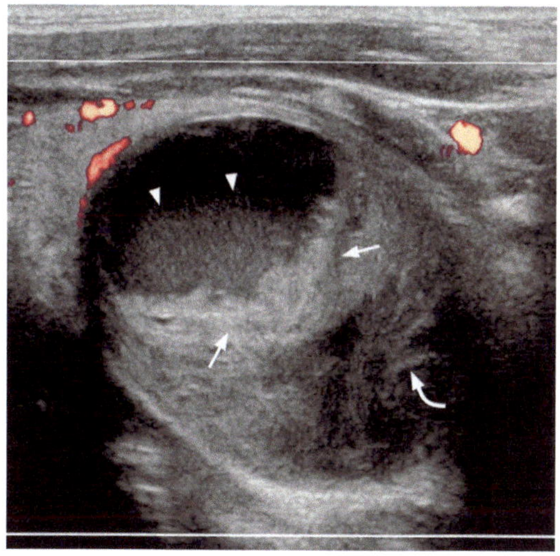

Fig. 6.7 Longitudinal power Doppler ultrasound shows a complex nodule with cystic elements containing debris (*arrowheads*), solid septa (*arrows*), and cystic septated portion (*curved arrow*). Note the absence of vascularity within the septa. The sonographic appearances are of a nodule with hemorrhage within. Aspiration of the cystic part usually yields altered blood

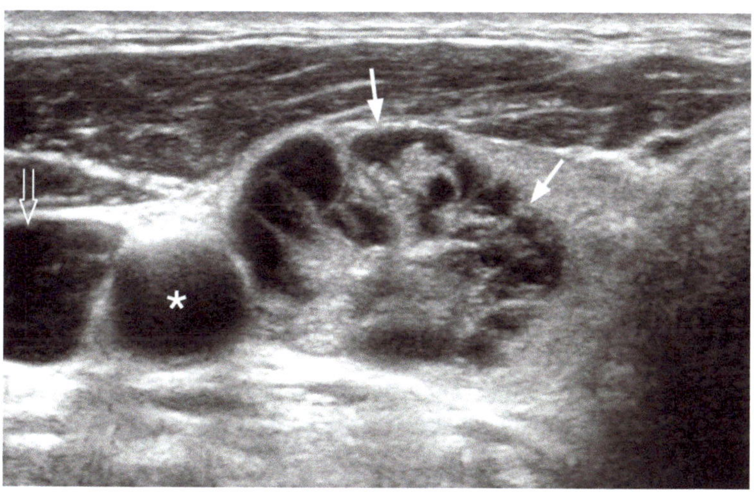

Fig. 6.8 Transverse gray-scale ultrasound of the thyroid gland shows a well-defined, heterogeneous, predominantly cystic nodule (*arrows*) with a "spongiform" appearance. *Asterisk* – right common carotid artery; *open arrow* – right internal jugular vein

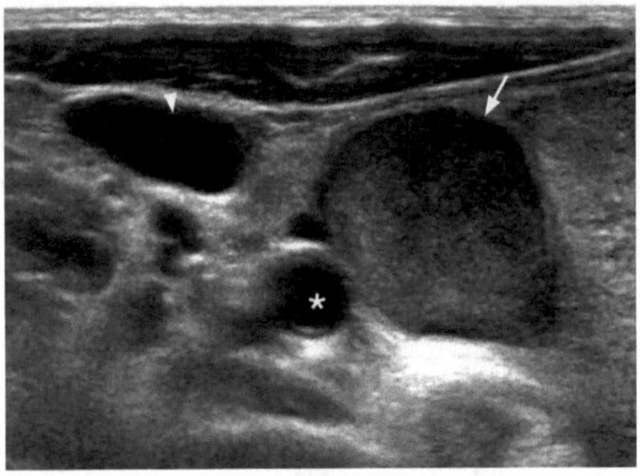

Fig. 6.9 Transverse gray-scale ultrasound of a malignant solid, hypoechoic thyroid nodule (*arrow*). *Asterisk* – right common carotid artery; arrowhead – right internal jugular vein

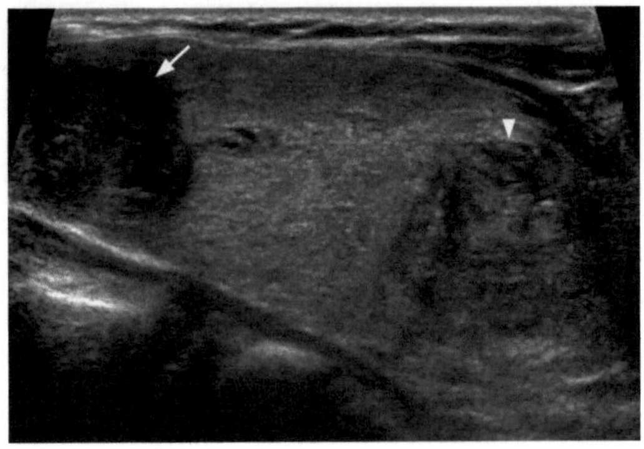

Fig. 6.10 Longitudinal gray-scale ultrasound of the thyroid gland shows a malignant nodule (*arrow*) in the upper pole of left lobe against a background of multinodular change (*arrowhead*). Most cancers detected by ultrasound are seen against a background of multinodularity, and nodule selection for FNA should be based on sonographic appearances of each nodule. With high-resolution ultrasound, it is quite unusual to see a truly solitary nodule

vascularity, solid excrescences protruding into the cyst, microcalcifications and ± associated malignant nodes.

- Predominant solid (Fig. 6.9) nature of a thyroid nodule is reported to have high sensitivity (69–75%) in predicting malignancy [27, 37, 40]. However, it has a fairly low positive predictive value in that a solid nodule has only a 15.6–27% chance of being malignant. In addition, 60–83% of benign nodules (which are far more common) are predominantly solid [51, 94]. Therefore, predominant solid nature of the nodule alone is not a useful predictor for malignancy.

Multiplicity of Nodules

- With the increasing use of high-end ultrasound equipment and improving transducer technology, it is quite common to detect the presence of multiple small (3–5 mm) nodules, bilaterally and in the lower poles of the thyroid gland. In our experience, it is unusual to see a solitary thyroid nodule on ultrasound, and most cancers detected by ultrasound are against this background of "multinodularity" (Fig. 6.10).
- Patients with multiple thyroid nodules have the same risk of malignancy as those with solitary nodules [32, 61, 95].
- The overall incidence of cancer in patients with thyroid nodules selected for FNAB is 9.2–13%, irrespective of the number of nodules detected by ultrasound [32, 34, 96, 97]. In patients with multiple thyroid nodules, the cancer rate/nodule decreases. However, the overall cancer rate/patient, 10–13%, is the same as in a patient with solitary nodule [34, 97].
  While the thyroid cancers found in patients with multiple nodules are often in the dominant or largest nodule, in approximately one-third of cases, the cancer is in a nondominant nodule [62]. Sonographic characteristics rather than size should therefore be used to prioritize nodules for FNA based on their individual risk of cancer.

Halo/Margin

- When evaluating the edges of a thyroid nodule, one assesses two aspects:
  Halo: is a thin, 1-mm, sonolucent rim that surrounds the thyroid nodule (Fig. 6.11). Benign hyperplastic nodules are slow growing and lack a true capsule. A halo around such a nodule represents compressed perinodular thy-

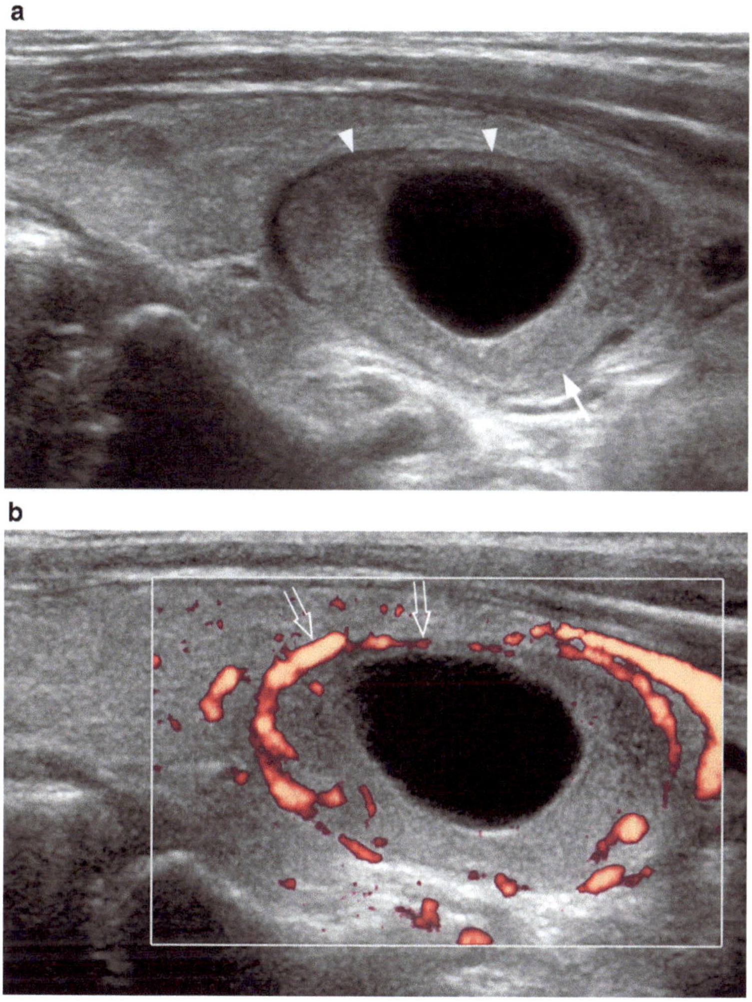

Fig. 6.11 (**a**) Longitudinal gray-scale ultrasound of the thyroid gland shows a nodule with solid and cystic elements (*arrow*) and a thin hypoechoic halo (*arrowheads*). (**b**) The hypoechoic halo is vascular (*open arrows*) on power Doppler examination and represents compressed thyroid parenchyma. The presence of thin vascular hypoechoic halo is suggestive of benignity

roid tissue and its vascularity which is often demonstrated on Doppler (50% of all benign nodules), but such vascularity is less common in invasive cancers.

A thick avascular halo (Figs. 6.12 and 6.13), which represents a fibrous capsule around a neoplastic mass (follicular or Hurthle cell), is more concerning [46]. The presence or absence of a halo is not a good indicator of the nature of the thyroid nodule as it is absent in about half of benign nodules [93, 98] and 10–24% of all papillary carcinomas may have a complete/incomplete halo around it [47, 93, 99, 100].

Margins: the margins of a thyroid nodule were previously described as well defined or ill defined (considered ill defined when more than 50% of its border is not clearly demarcated [101]). Ill-defined margins are thought to represent malignancy (specificity 15–59% [32, 94]). However, with the use of modern high-resolution transducers, the margins are now reclassified [56]:

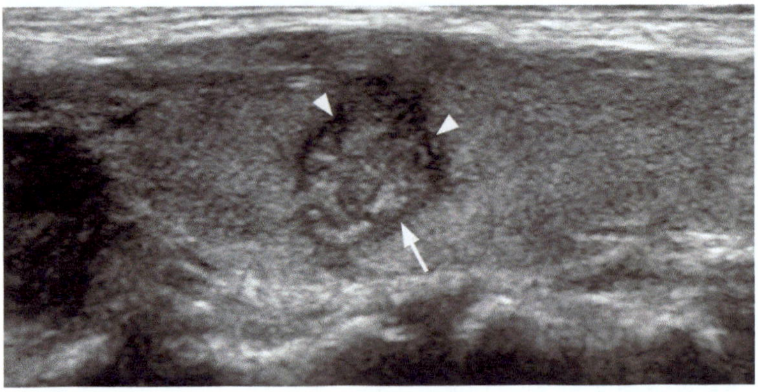

Fig. 6.12 Longitudinal gray-scale ultrasound of the thyroid gland shows a small ill-defined, solid, hypoechoic nodule (*arrow*) with a thick hypoechoic halo (*arrowheads*). Note the fine echogenic foci within and the ill-defined margins. Pathology – papillary carcinoma

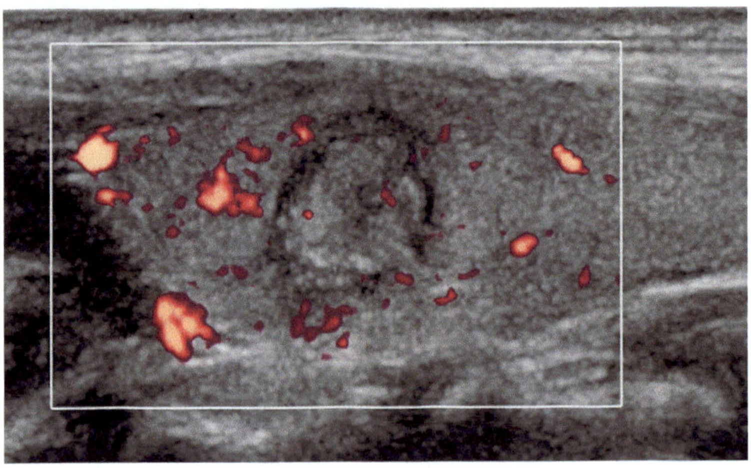

Fig. 6.13 Longitudinal power Doppler ultrasound shows a heterogeneous nodule with a thick halo which shows no obvious vascularity. Such an "avascular" halo is suspicious for a malignant nodule and represents the true capsule of the lesion. The vascular haloes seen in benign hyperplastic nodules represent compressed vessels/thyroid tissue, and such nodules do not have a true capsule around them

- Well-defined, smooth: suggestive of benignity (Fig. 6.14)
- Spiculated, sharply demarcated: indicative of malignancy (Fig. 6.15)
- Ill-defined (where the edge of the lesion cannot be demarcated from adjacent thyroid parenchyma): seen in both benign and malignant lesions

Shape

- A taller-than-wide shape (Fig. 6.16) is reported to be very specific (93% specificity [39]) in differentiating malignant thyroid nodule from its benign counterpart [39, 43, 73].
- The anteroposterior-to-transverse diameter (A/T) ratio ≥1 has been reported to have high

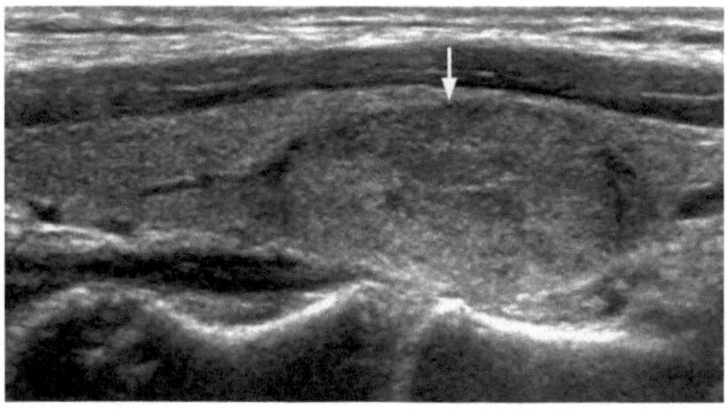

Fig. 6.14 Longitudinal gray-scale ultrasound of the thyroid gland shows a solid, isoechoic nodule (*arrow*) with well-defined margins and a thin hypoechoic halo. The sonographic appearances are more in favor of a benign nodule

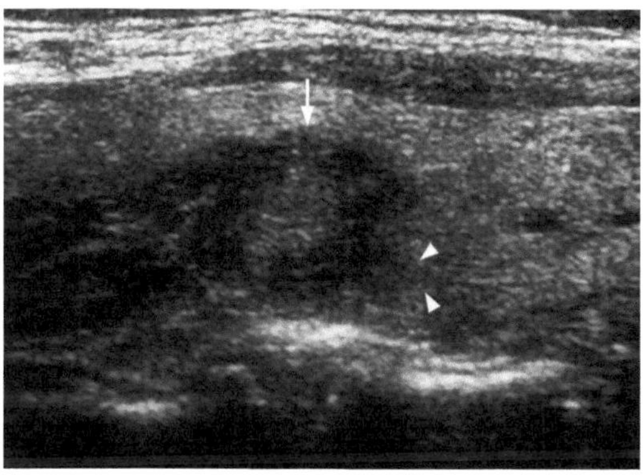

Fig. 6.15 Longitudinal gray-scale ultrasound of a malignant thyroid nodule (*arrow*) in the thyroid gland. Note its hypoechogenicity, solid nature, and spiculated margins (*arrowheads*) with the adjacent glandular parenchyma

sensitivity (84%) and specificity (82%) for detection of thyroid cancer [102].

- It is postulated that the growth behavior of thyroid malignancy is similar to that of breast cancer with growth across normal tissue planes, while benign nodules grow parallel to normal tissue planes [103]. The mechanism for the taller-than-wide sign is minimal/no compression of the nodule by the ultrasound transducer which occurs more commonly in malignant than benign thyroid nodules [104].

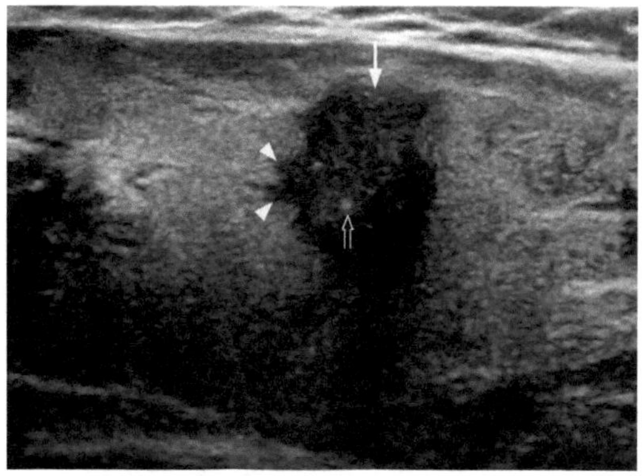

Fig. 6.16 Longitudinal gray-scale ultrasound of the thyroid gland shows a markedly hypoechoic nodule (*arrow*) which is taller than wide. Note the presence of spiculated margin (*arrowheads*) and presence of microcalcifications (*open arrow*). It demonstrates most of the sonographic features associated with malignancy

Echogenicity

- Echogenicity of a thyroid nodule is assessed in respect to the thyroid parenchyma and strap muscles and is classified as markedly hypoechoic (hypoechoic to adjacent strap muscle), hypoechoic (hypoechoic to thyroid parenchyma), isoechoic (isoechoic to thyroid parenchyma), or hyperechoic (relatively echogenic than thyroid parenchyma) (Fig. 6.17) [43].
- Hypoechogenicity in a thyroid nodule is thought to represent its microfollicular structure on histology, whereas iso/hyperechoic nodules have a macrofollicular structure [105].
- When the echogenicity of a mixed (solid and cystic) thyroid nodule is assessed, one evaluates the echogenicity of the solid component relative to thyroid parenchyma and strap muscles.
- As the echogenicity of a thyroid nodule increases, the risk of malignancy decreases and hypoechoic nodules have a higher tendency of being malignant compared to iso/hyperechoic nodules.
- Though most malignant nodules are hypoechoic, nearly 50% of benign nodules

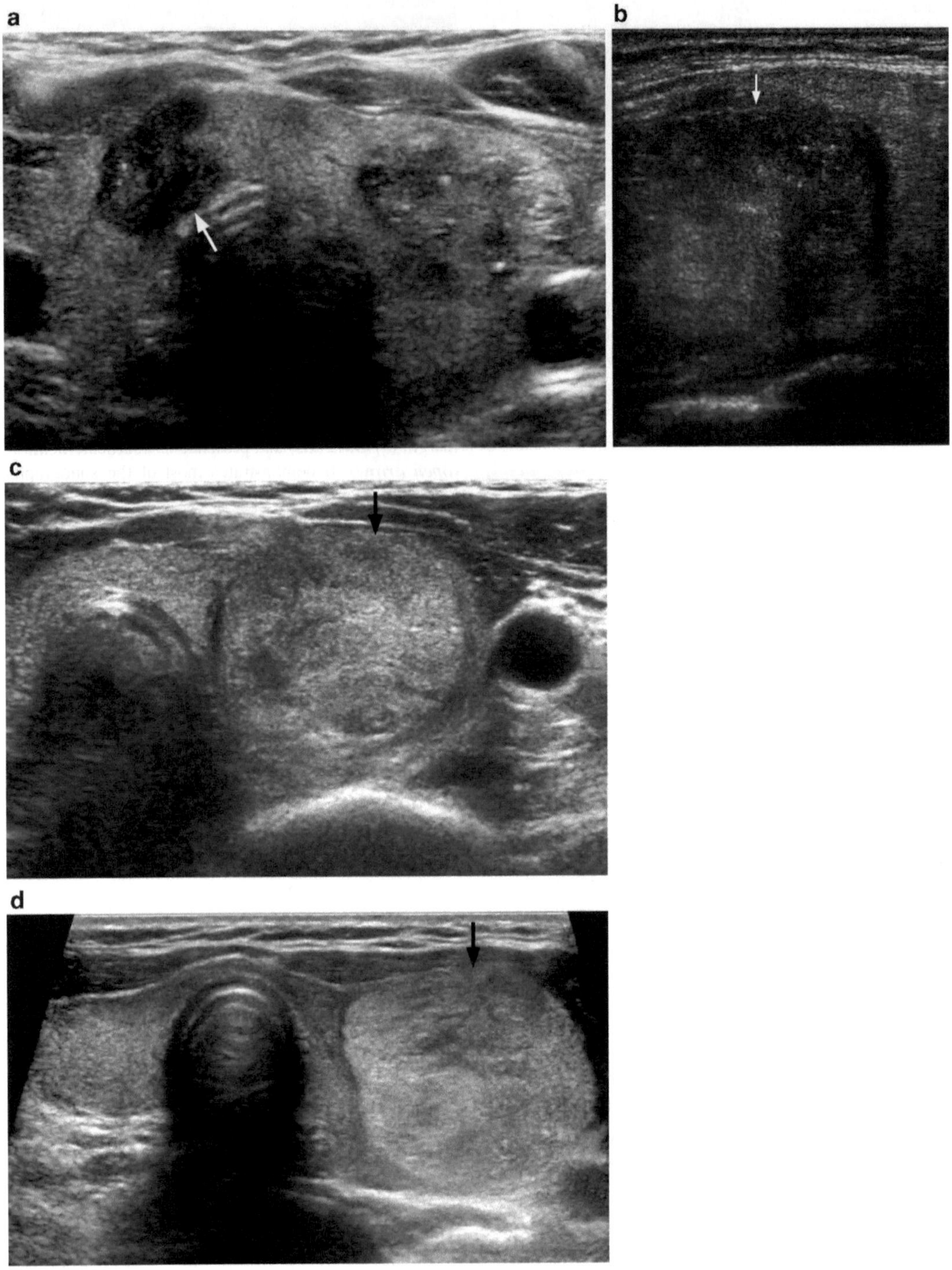

Fig. 6.17 Gray-scale ultrasound showing the spectrum of echogenicity of a thyroid nodule (*arrows*) (**a**) markedly hypoechoic, (**b**) hypoechoic, (**c**) isoechoic, and (**d**) hyperechoic. The risk of malignancy decreases as the echogenicity increases

and the majority of small benign nodules may be hypoechoic as well [32, 39, 43]. As benign nodules are much more commonly seen in routine practice, a large proportion of hypoechoic nodules will turn out to be benign rather than malignant.

- Marked hypoechogenicity is highly specific for a malignant nodule [39, 43] and is a more specific and reliable criterion for malignancy.

Vascularity

- Doppler ultrasound assesses the vascularity of a thyroid nodule to help determine the likelihood of a thyroid nodule being malignant.
- Color-flow Doppler provides information regarding both direction and velocity, whereas power Doppler does not provide any information regarding velocity or flow direction. However, it is more sensitive in the detection of flow, has less noise interference, and is less dependent on the angle of incidence between the ultrasound waves and the moving objects. Therefore, power Doppler is generally the preferred imaging technique for assessing vascularity of thyroid tissue [46].
- To adequately perform Doppler sonography of thyroid nodules, it is essential to calibrate the equipment for highest sensitivity in the detection of vascularity. The parameters for this include:
  - Pulse Repetition Frequency (PRF): 350–500–700 Hz
  - Persistence: medium
  - Wall filter: low
  - Color gain: Increase the color gain till color noise appears. Then gradually reduce it to a level to eliminate the color noise. This would be the correct level for color gain
  - Transducer pressure: light
- There are a variety of vascular patterns described; however, when the parameters are optimally set, three major patterns of vascularity are common in literature: Type I: complete absence of flow signal within the nodule, Type II: perinodular flow signal, and Type III: marked intranodular flow signal (Fig. 6.18) [106]. In routine clinical practice, the distribution of vessels related to a thyroid nodule is classified as central or peripheral. Most benign nodules have either absent vascularity (Type I) or its perinodular vascularity is greater than intranodular vascularity (Type II>Type III). In malignant nodules, the intranodular vascularity is greater than peripheral vascularity (Type III>Type II [32, 107]). In our experience, Type I vascularity is not often seen as most modern equipment (with their high Doppler sensitivity) are able to demonstrate small intranodular or perinodular vessels routinely. Therefore, the absence of vascularity in a thyroid nodule may be explained by equipment or technique used [108].
- Though solid hypervascular thyroid nodules have a high likelihood of malignancy (as high as 42% [37]), the Doppler characteristics of a thyroid nodule cannot be used to exclude malignancy because 14% of solid nonhypervascular nodules may be malignant [37].
- Type III vascularity is a significant criterion to suggest malignant disease; intranodular blood flow is observed in 91.7% of malignancy and in 65.3% of benign nodule ($p<0.005$) [41]. The combination of an absence of halo sign on gray-scale US and a Type III vascularity pattern has a higher sensitivity (83.3%) for malignancy with a specificity of 43.7% [41]. The combination of absent halo plus microcalcifications and a Type III vascularity pattern has sensitivity of 72.2% and specificity of 77.2% [41]. The combination of microcalcification and Type III vascularity has a sensitivity of 80.6% and specificity of 75.4% in identifying malignancy [41].
- Resistive index (RI) obtained from spectral Doppler analysis has been used to differentiate malignant and benign thyroid nodules [109, 110]. Malignant nodules have a mean RI of 0.72 ± 0.13 which is significantly higher than those associated with benign nodules (0.6 ± 0.08) [109]. The RI cutoff of 0.75 has a good accuracy (91%), specificity (97%), and negative predictive value (92%) in predicting malignancy, with relatively low sensitivity (40%) and positive predictive value (67%) [110].

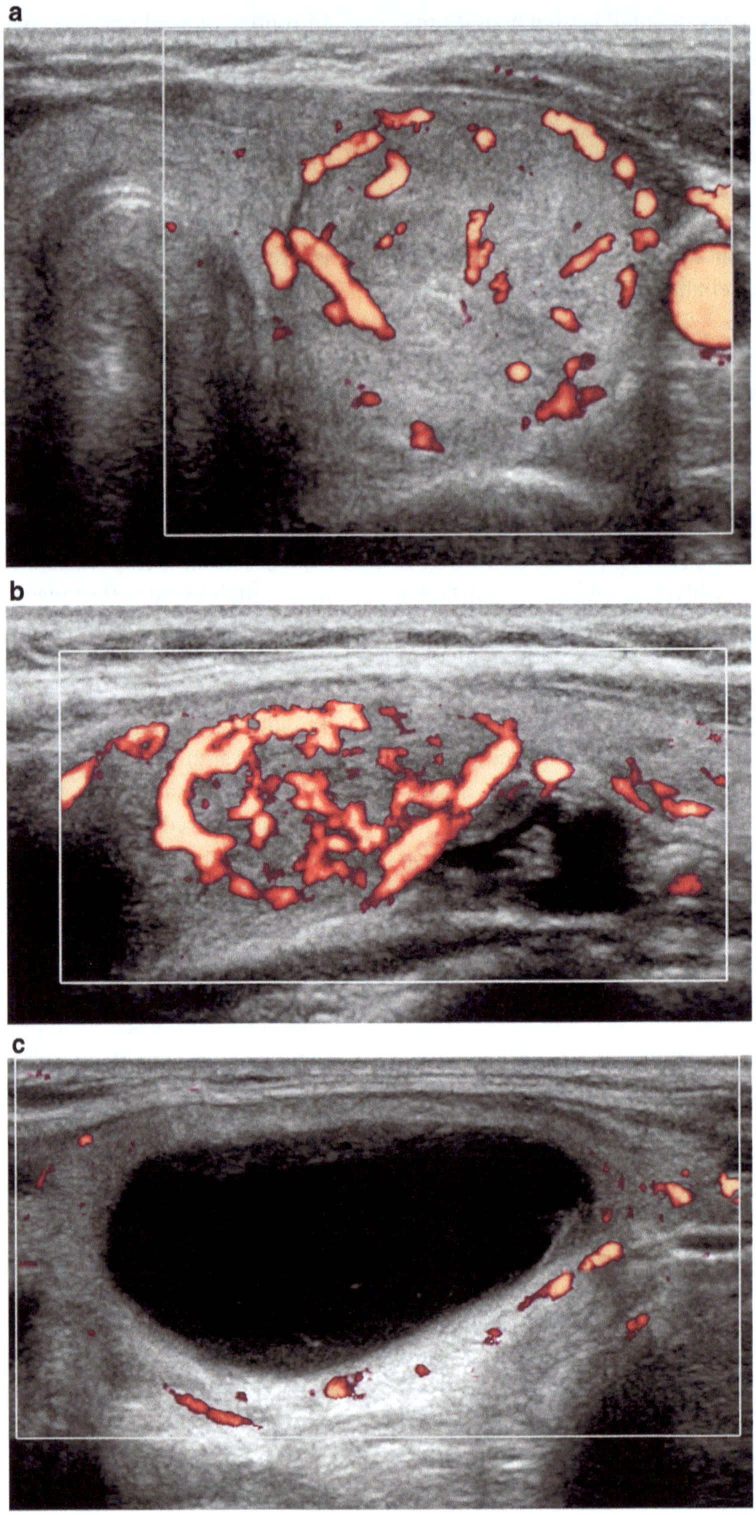

Fig. 6.18 Power Doppler ultrasound assessment of thyroid nodules with (**a**) Type II vascularity (perinodular vascularity > intranodular vascularity) and (**b**) Type III vascularity (marked intranodular chaotic vascularity). With modern equipment, Type I vascularity (avascular) is rarely seen in solid thyroid nodules. However, predominantly cystic nodule may show no obvious vascularity (**c**)

- Malignant nodules also have a higher pulsatility index (PI) (1.15 ± 0.33) than benign nodules (0.91 ± 0.19) [109].
- The use of maximal systolic velocity (MSV) in limited studies produced inconsistent results. Cerbone et al. reported cutoff value of 50 cm/s for predicting malignancy in thyroid nodules [46], while Tamsel et al. showed Doppler US characteristics are not useful parameters for distinguishing malignant from benign thyroid nodule [108].
- In our institution, we do not measure RI, PI, and MSV of intranodular vessels. The technique is time consuming, fraught with difficulty, does not obviate the need for FNA, and its accuracy has yet to be convincingly established
- The predictive value of Doppler may be stronger for nodules with previous follicular biopsy than for all unselected nodules as benign hyperplastic nodules (by the far the commonest nodules seen on US) often show increased intranodular vascularity. Absence of vascularity in a nodule with follicular biopsy makes malignancy less likely [111]. Follicular nodules with no intranodular flow have a 3% probability of malignancy rather than the 15–20% likelihood in unselected follicular nodules. Vascular follicular nodules have a 50% probability of malignancy [112].

Local Invasion and Lymph Node Metastases

- The presence of direct tumor invasion of adjacent soft tissue and metastases to regional lymph nodes are highly specific of thyroid malignancy [86].
- On ultrasound, direct tumor invasion of adjacent soft tissues may appear as a subtle extension of the tumor beyond the contours of the thyroid gland, or as frank invasion of adjacent structures (Fig. 6.19) [101].
- Although ultrasound is able to detect the presence of extracapsular spread, it may not be able to delineate its entire extent (particularly for large thyroid masses). Invasion of prevertebral muscle, esophagus and trachea are better demonstrated on cross-sectional imaging such as CT and MRI. Shadowing from the thyroid cartilage, trachea renders these areas sonographically invisible.

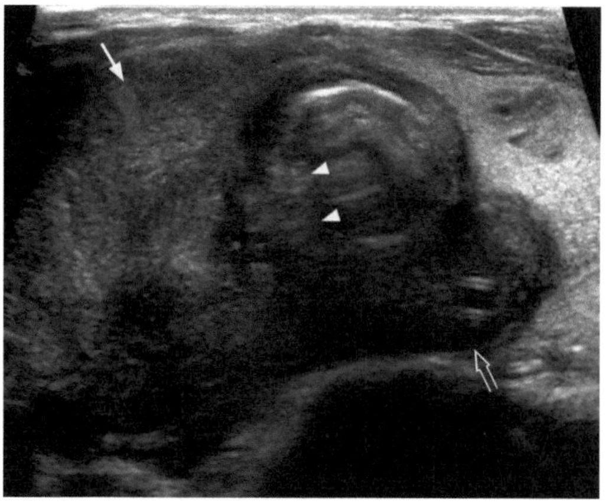

Fig. 6.19 Transverse gray-scale ultrasound of the right neck shows a large ill-defined, solid, hypoechoic mass (*arrow*) involving the entire right lobe of thyroid gland. Note the tumor infiltration to trachea (*arrowheads*) and cervical esophagus (*open arrow*). Often CT and MR better define the entire extent of a large thyroid tumor

- Regional nodal metastases have been reported to occur in 19.4% of all thyroid malignancies [32], most commonly seen in papillary carcinoma and medullary carcinoma. US features raising the suspicion of metastatic nodes include round shape, loss of echogenic hilum, heterogeneous internal architecture, presence of microcalcification, cystic necrosis, and abnormal peripheral vascularity on power Doppler [27, 113–116]. The sonographic features of abnormal nodes are discussed in a separate chapter in this book.
- Any sonographic examination of the thyroid must include a detailed examination of the neck for nodal disease. Metastatic nodes are frequently seen in thyroid cancers (especially papillary carcinoma and medullary carcinoma) and may affect overall prognosis and alter the surgical management of patients. If an elective neck dissection is performed for palpable lymph nodes, up to 90% of patients with papillary carcinoma will have regional nodal metastases. If no neck dissection is performed

when no nodes are palpable, metastatic nodes develop in 7–15% of patients, with a mean delay of 4.5 years [117].

Indication for FNAC of Thyroid Nodule

- The use of FNAC increases the rate of detection of thyroid cancer and reduces the number of unnecessary surgical procedures and overall cost of medical care [1, 118, 119].
- Performing FNAC on every thyroid nodule detected on USG is not cost-effective because of its high prevalence.
- No single ultrasound feature has a high positive predictive value for cancer detection that can be used to identify nodules that should be subjected to FNAC.
- Guidelines established to help select nodules for FNAC include:
  (a) Guideline from the Society of Radiologists in Ultrasound [27] – The criteria are based on size and ultrasound characteristics:
    - Nodule ≥1 cm in diameter if microcalcifications are present.
    - Nodule ≥1.5 cm in diameter if completely or almost entirely solid or if coarse calcifications are present.
    - Nodule ≥2 cm in diameter if mixed solid and cystic components are present or nodule is almost entirely cystic with a solid mural component.
    - Nodule has grown substantially since previous ultrasound examination.
    - Presence of abnormal lymph nodes regardless of the ultrasound features of the thyroid nodule.

  (b) Guideline by Kim et al. [39] – FNAC of thyroid nodule with any single suspicious ultrasound feature, regardless of nodule size, is recommended. Suspicious ultrasound features include:
    - Marked hypoechogenicity.
    - Irregular or microlobulated margins.
    - Microcalcifications.
    - Anteroposterior to transverse diameter ratio of 1 or greater (i.e., taller than wide).

  (c) Guideline from the American Association of Clinical Endocrinologists [70] – FNAC should be performed on all hypoechoic nodules with at least one of the following additional ultrasound features: irregular margins, intranodular vascular spots, taller-than-wide shape, or microcalcifications.
- A recent study compared the three sets of guidelines for FNAC of thyroid nodule [69] and concluded that Kim et al. (area under ROC curve = 0.868) and American Association of Clinical Endocrinologists (area under ROC curve = 0.850) criteria were more accurate than the Society of Radiologists in Ultrasound (area under ROC curve = 0.551) criteria.

Thyroid Malignancy

Imaging Features of Common Thyroid Cancer

Differentiated thyroid cancer, which includes papillary and follicular carcinoma, comprises the vast majority (90%) of thyroid cancers [120]. Other less common thyroid malignancies include Hurthle cell carcinoma, anaplastic carcinoma and medullary carcinoma. Metastases and lymphoma of the thyroid gland are also occasionally encountered.

Ultrasound provides the best morphological assessment of the primary tumor; metastatic cervical lymphadenopathy and some primary thyroid malignancies have specific ultrasound features which allow accurate preoperative diagnosis. Cross-sectional imaging, including CT, MRI and FDG-PET, is mainly used for detection of tumor extent, invasion of adjacent structures (e.g., trachea, esophagus, prevertebral muscle and recurrent laryngeal nerve) and presence of distant metastases.

From the morass of information available in literature, we have tried to consolidate the sonographic features of common thyroid cancers. These are discussed in the subsequent paragraphs.

Papillary Carcinoma

Papillary carcinoma accounts for 60–70% of all thyroid malignancies [121], with a peak incidence in the third and fourth decades. The majority of patients are female. It has an excellent prognosis with the 30-year survival rate as high as 95% [29]. Poor prognostic factors include male sex, increased age (> 45 years), large tumor size (>3 cm), presence of vascular invasion, presence of extraglandular extension and poor differentiation on histopathology. There is a well-known relationship between exposure to low-dose radiation and papillary thyroid cancer. The risk of papillary cancer also appears to be increased in familial adenomatous polyposis syndrome, including Gardner's and Cowden's syndrome [122].

The tumor commonly spreads along the rich lymphatics in and around the thyroid gland, accounting for the multifocal nature of the tumor within the thyroid gland and its propensity to metastasize to regional lymph nodes. Venous invasion occurs in 7% of papillary carcinomas, and distant metastases to bone and lung are seen in 5–7% [123].

Variants of papillary carcinoma:

- Diffuse sclerosing variant of papillary carcinoma accounts for 0.74–5.3% of all papillary carcinomas [124]. As compared with the usual type of papillary carcinoma, it affects younger patients and has a higher incidence of cervical lymph node involvement and lung metastases at presentation [124–127]. The overall survival is similar to the classic type but with higher risk of recurrence after surgical treatment. Histologically, the variant is characterized by diffuse involvement of one or both lobes, dense sclerosis, numerous psammoma bodies, typical papillary carcinoma elements, extensive squamous metaplasia and dense lymphocytic infiltration [128, 129].
- Follicular variant has a histologic pattern where neoplastic follicles constitute most of the cellular material. Its behavior and prognosis is similar to the classic variety.
- Tall cell variant represents <5% of all papillary carcinomas with frequent metastases, recurrence and poor prognosis [130–132]. The columnar cell variant is extremely rare and is similar to the tall cell variant except that the height of the cell is three times the width. It is an aggressive tumor with a poor prognosis [133–135].

Ultrasound features of papillary carcinoma [36, 136]:

Primary Tumor (Fig. 6.20):

- Predominantly hypoechoic (77–90%) [25, 137] due to the closely packed cell content and sparse colloid within the tumor.
- Mostly solid (70%). 13–26% have a cystic component, but a predominantly cystic appearance is uncommon [47, 93]. In cystic papillary tumors with septa or solid components, vascularity and punctate calcifications may be seen in the solid component/septa, contrary to the findings in benign cystic nodules where the solid portion/septa are usually avascular.
- Margin of nodule is ill-defined and irregular, indicating its infiltrative nature. 15–30% appears well-defined and haloed [98, 138–140]. Some of the tumors may be completely encapsulated (encapsulated variant) with small areas of capsular invasion.
- Presence of punctate microcalcifications is seen in 25–90% [25, 137] and corresponds to calcified psammoma bodies on histology. These punctate microcalcifications may not exhibit posterior acoustic shadowing, and increasing transducer frequency/scanning in fundamental mode may help to detect fine shadowing.
- 10–20% is multifocal on ultrasound [141].
- In diffuse sclerosing variant, apart from the primary papillary tumor, there are diffuse, scattered microcalcifications in both lobes with a "snowstorm" appearance (Fig. 6.21) [47, 129, 142].
- 90% shows chaotic intranodular vascularity within the tumor on power Doppler examination [137].

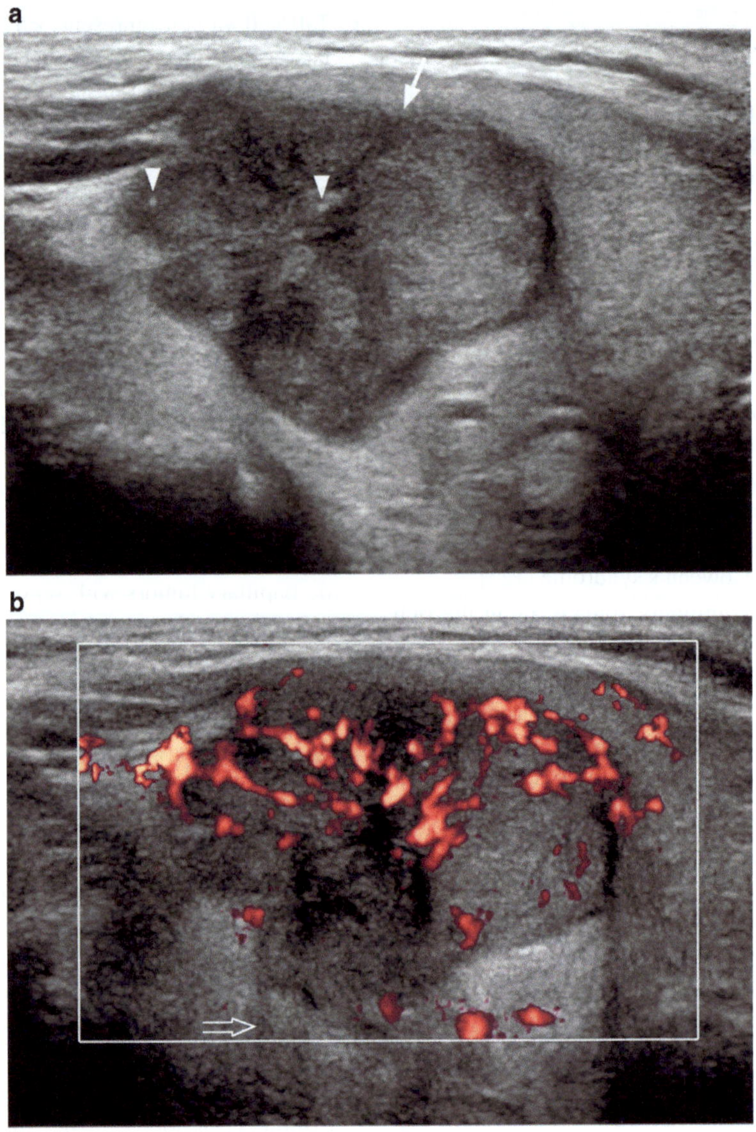

Fig. 6.20 (**a**) Longitudinal gray-scale ultrasound of the thyroid gland shows a solid, hypoechoic nodule (*arrow*) with ill-defined and lobulated margins with foci of microcalcifications (*arrowheads*). Note the absence of any shadowing from the microcalcifications. (**b**) Corresponding power Doppler ultrasound reveals marked chaotic intranodular vascularity. Note the true shadowing from microcalcification (*open arrow*) is clearly seen on this "fundamental" scan mode

- Absence of a well-defined margin with adjacent structures such as strap muscles, trachea, and esophagus are suspicious of early tumor infiltration. Frank tumor invasion ± vascular involvement is occasionally seen on ultrasound in locally advanced disease.

Metastatic regional lymphadenopathy (Fig. 6.22) [143]:

- Distribution in the pre/paratracheal regions and along the cervical chain.
- Lymph nodes are hyperechoic relative to muscle in 80%.
- Presence of punctate microcalcifications in 50%.
- Cystic necrosis in 25%. In some cases, the presence of a thick-walled cystic node or a

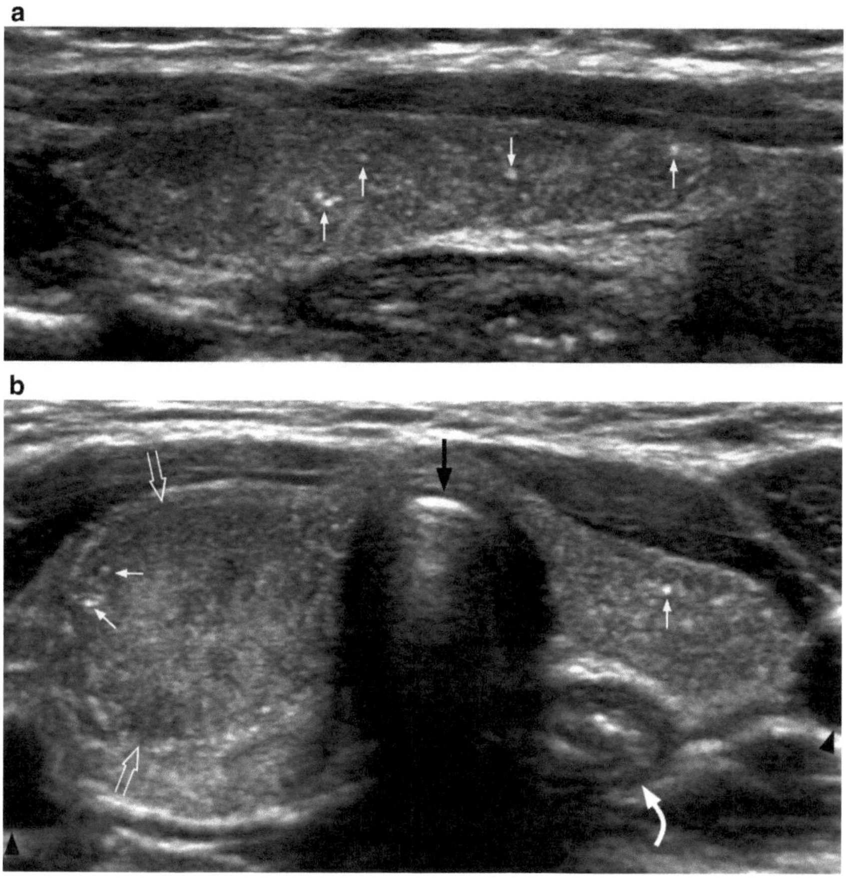

Fig. 6.21 (**a**) Longitudinal and (**b**) transverse gray-scale ultrasound of the thyroid showing scattered small echogenic foci (*arrows*) within the left thyroid parenchyma. These were associated with large ipsilateral metastatic paratracheal and pretracheal lymph nodes. Note a focal right papillary carcinoma with echogenic foci (*open arrows*). Metastatic nodes were also seen on the right. *Bold arrow*=Trachea, *arrowheads*=CCA and *curved arrow*=esophagus

cystic node with a solid component which demonstrates punctate calcifications and internal vascularity on power Doppler imaging (Fig. 6.23) may be the only clue to the presence of occult carcinoma in the thyroid gland.

Follicular Lesion

Follicular lesions of the thyroid comprise follicular carcinomas, follicular adenomas, hyperplastic/adenomatoid nodules, and follicular variant of papillary carcinoma (unencapsulated with psammoma bodies and characteristic nuclei) [144, 145].

It is not possible to distinguish a benign from a malignant follicular lesion with FNAC, core biopsy and frozen sections, as vascular and capsular invasion (which form the basis for the diagnosis of malignancy in these lesions) can only be evaluated on histological specimen. However, some suggest the accuracy in distinguishing them on FNAC can be improved by careful attention to cytologic features, skillful application of FNA techniques and using special staining by a panel of immunohistochemical markers (e.g., HBME-1, galectin-3, cytokeratin-19) [146, 147]. Therefore, the preferred collective term is "follicular lesion" for both a benign follicular adenoma and a malignant follicular carcinoma. Some believe

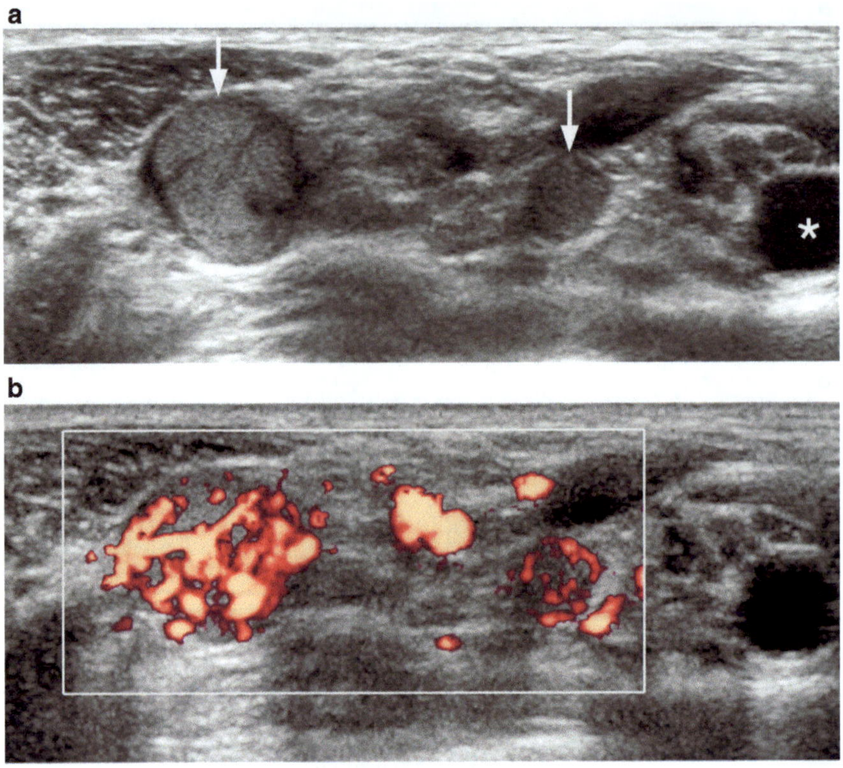

Fig. 6.22 (**a**) Transverse gray-scale ultrasound of the right neck shows two enlarged, round lymph nodes (*arrows*) with loss of normal echogenic hilum. Note the hyperechoic nature of the larger node (compared to adjacent muscle) which is commonly seen in a metastatic node from papillary thyroid carcinoma. *Asterisk* – right common carotid artery. (**b**) Corresponding power Doppler ultrasound reveals marked intranodular vascularity within the metastatic nodes

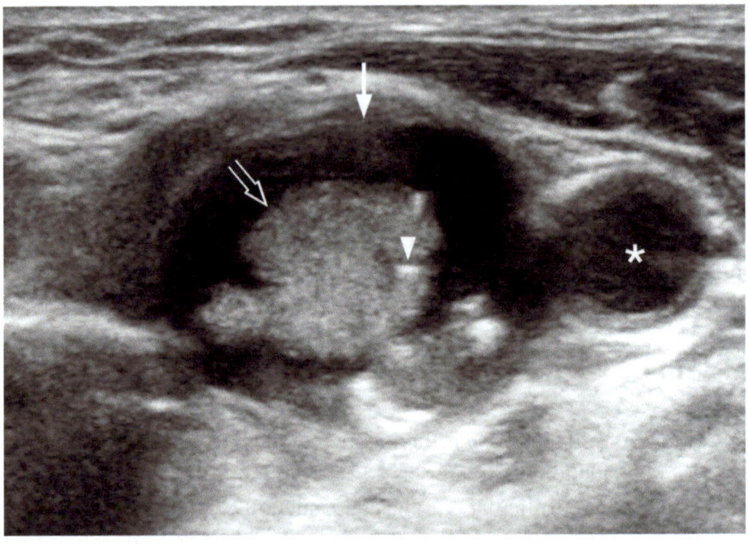

Fig. 6.23 Transverse gray-scale ultrasound of the left neck shows a cystic metastatic lymph node (*arrow*) from papillary carcinoma. Note the presence of microcalcifications (*arrowhead*) within the eccentric solid component (*open arrow*) of the metastatic node. The solid component is markedly vascular on power Doppler examination (not shown). *Asterisk* – left common carotid artery

in most cases follicular carcinoma develops from a preexisting adenoma [137]. 60–70% of follicular carcinomas are associated with adenomatous/hyperplastic nodules [137]. Identifying such carcinomas against a background of multinodularity is difficult on any imaging modality, unless frank signs of malignancy are present.

While the cytological differentiation between follicular adenoma and follicular carcinoma is contentious, some cytologists classify follicular lesions as either microfollicular or macrofollicular. A macrofollicular lesion has a low risk for malignancy, whereas a microfollicular lesion may carry a 20–25% risk of being a follicular carcinoma [148].

Follicular carcinoma accounts for 2–5% of all thyroid cancers [137] and is more prevalent (25–30%) in iodine-deficient areas [149]. Similar to papillary carcinoma, follicular carcinomas are commoner in females than males [150]. It has a propensity for hematogenous spread to the lungs, liver, bone, and brain. Although patients often present with distant metastases, nodal neck metastases at presentation are rare. Nodal spread: papillary (50%) >> follicular (10%), whereas for distant spread: follicular (20%) >papillary (5–10%).

There are two common histologic subtypes:

- Minimally invasive: encapsulated, invasion, or capsular penetration but no vascular involvement [123]. These tumors have a 3% fatality rate and rarely metastasize (8–10%) [137].
- Frankly invasive: obvious vascular and thyroid invasion [123]. They have a high fatality rate (50%) and 50–80% metastasize [137].

Ultrasound features of follicular neoplasm (Fig. 6.24) [36, 136]:

- Predominantly solid and homogeneous in 70%.
- Well-defined, haloed in 80%.
- Commonly isoechoic/hyperechoic to the adjacent thyroid parenchyma. Hypoechoic lesions are rare and have a higher risk of being malignant [151].
- Calcification is rare.
- Benign lesions have a Type II vascularity (perinodular > intranodular), whereas malignant lesions have a Type III vascularity (intranodular > perinodular) [110, 137] or only intranodular flow [152]. A follicular neoplasm without predominant intranodular flow has a low probability of being malignant [152].

In general, ultrasound cannot accurately distinguish a benign from malignant follicular lesion. The suspicion of malignancy is raised if the nodule is ill-defined, has a hypoechoic component in an otherwise iso/hyperechoic nodule and has a thick irregular capsule and chaotic intranodular vascularity. The certain signs of malignancy are frank vascular invasion (e.g. to adjacent internal jugular vein, common carotid artery), tumor spread beyond the thyroid capsule and distant metastases.

Hurthle Cell Lesions

Cells with abundant granular cytoplasm have been called oxyphils, Hurthle cells or Askanazy cells. They can be seen in multinodular goiter, Hashimoto's thyroiditis, follicular neoplasm, papillary carcinomas and in long-standing hyperthyroidism. Hurthle cell neoplasms are sometimes considered to be variants of follicular adenomas and carcinomas [153–159]. The criteria for distinguishing benign from malignant Hurthle cell neoplasms are similar to follicular neoplasms and also rely on capsular infiltration and angioinvasion [160]. As with follicular neoplasms, on FNAC, Hurthle cell lesions are designated Hurthle cell neoplasms with a potential for malignancy [161, 162]. However, patients with Hurthle cell carcinoma often have an aggressive tumor and generally a worse prognosis than those with papillary or follicular thyroid carcinomas [163].

It is an uncommon lesion and accounts for 2–3% of all thyroid malignancies. It is more common in females, with a female/male ratio of 2:1. These carcinomas are more likely to invade adjacent soft tissues of the neck compared to follicular carcinomas. The most common sites of metastases are lung and bone [164]. Nodal metastasis is commoner than follicular carcinomas but less than papillary carcinomas.

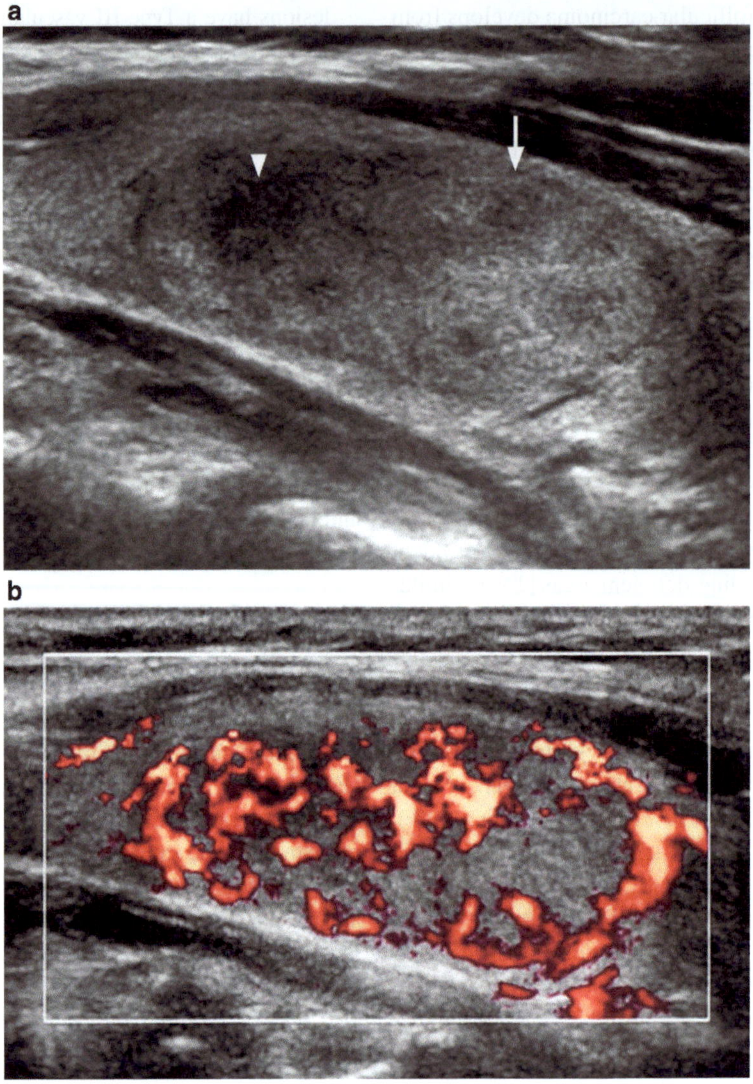

Fig. 6.24 (**a**) Longitudinal gray-scale ultrasound of the thyroid gland shows an ill-defined, solid, predominantly isoechoic nodule (*arrow*). Note the presence of hypoechoic areas (*arrowhead*) within the nodule with marked intranodular vascular flow on corresponding power Doppler examination (**b**). Hypoechoic, vascular areas in an otherwise isoechoic nodule should raise the suspicion of malignancy

Ultrasound features of Hurthle cell neoplasm (Fig. 6.25) [36, 136]:

- Predominantly solid.
- Mixed internal echogenicity with both hyperechoic and hypoechoic components.
- Ill-defined, partially haloed.
- Noncalcified.
- May show Type III chaotic intranodular vascularity on power Doppler USG. The overall Doppler characteristics are similar to follicular neoplasm.

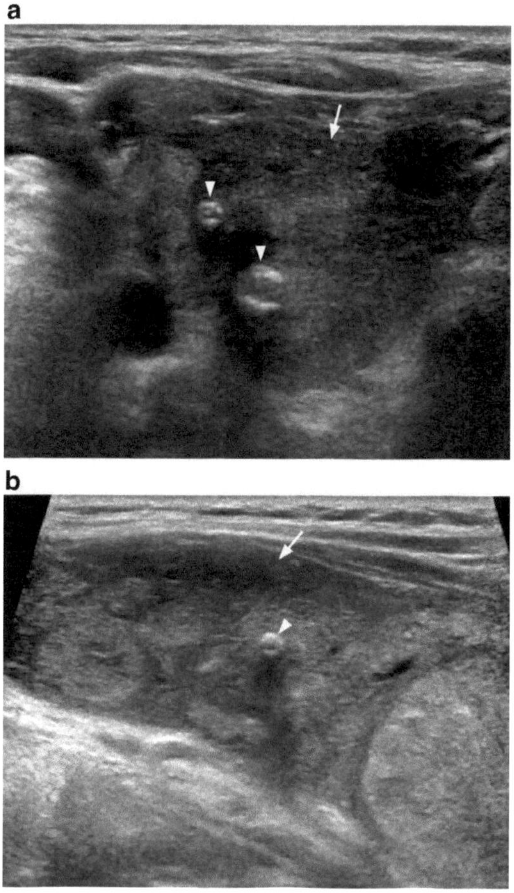

Fig. 6.25 (**a**) Transverse and (**b**) longitudinal gray-scale ultrasound of the thyroid gland shows a solid, hypoechoic nodule (*arrow*) with ill-defined margins and coarse interrupted curvilinear calcifications (*arrowheads*). Pathology – Hurthle cell carcinoma. Note that it demonstrates obvious sonographic features of malignancy

- Adjacent malignant nodes may be the only clue to the malignant nature of the thyroid nodule.

Anaplastic Carcinoma

It is one of the most aggressive head and neck cancers, has a poor prognosis (median survival of 6 months despite a variety of treatment modalities) and accounts for 2–5% of all thyroid cancers [165, 166]. These tumors commonly occur in older patients in the seventh decade of life, have a female predominance, and are usually large at presentation (>5 cm). It seems to occur more frequently in regions of endemic goiter, arise in long-standing goiter, and in some cases, residual papillary or follicular carcinomas can be identified.

They commonly present as a rapidly enlarging mass with compressive symptoms such as dyspnea, dysphagia and hoarseness of voice. Some patients may present with distant metastases at initial presentation (metastases are seen in lungs, bone, liver and brain). Most patients are euthyroid, but some may occasionally be hypothyroid or hyperthyroid. The hyperthyroidism is related to release of thyroid hormones into circulation due to the extensive parenchymal destruction. Most patients die due to extensive local tumor growth or complication of lung metastases.

Ultrasound features of anaplastic carcinoma (Fig. 6.26) [36, 136]:

- Hypoechoic tumor diffusely involving the entire lobe or gland.
- Presence of areas of necrosis in 78% and dense amorphous calcification in 58% [167]. The dense calcification is a reflection of long-standing MNG.
- Often seen against a background of nodular goiter (47%).
- Extracapsular spread (trachea, larynx, esophagus and recurrent laryngeal nerve) and vascular invasion (common carotid artery, IJV) in a third of patients [168].
- Multiple chaotic small vessels on color flow, however, necrotic tumors may be hypovascular (due to vascular infiltration and occlusion by tumor).
- Nodal or distant metastases in 80% of patients [168]. Metastatic hypoechoic lymph nodes with cystic necrosis are present in 50% [25] and may show abnormal vascularity.

The differential diagnosis includes malignant lymphoma, medullary carcinoma and thyroid metastases.

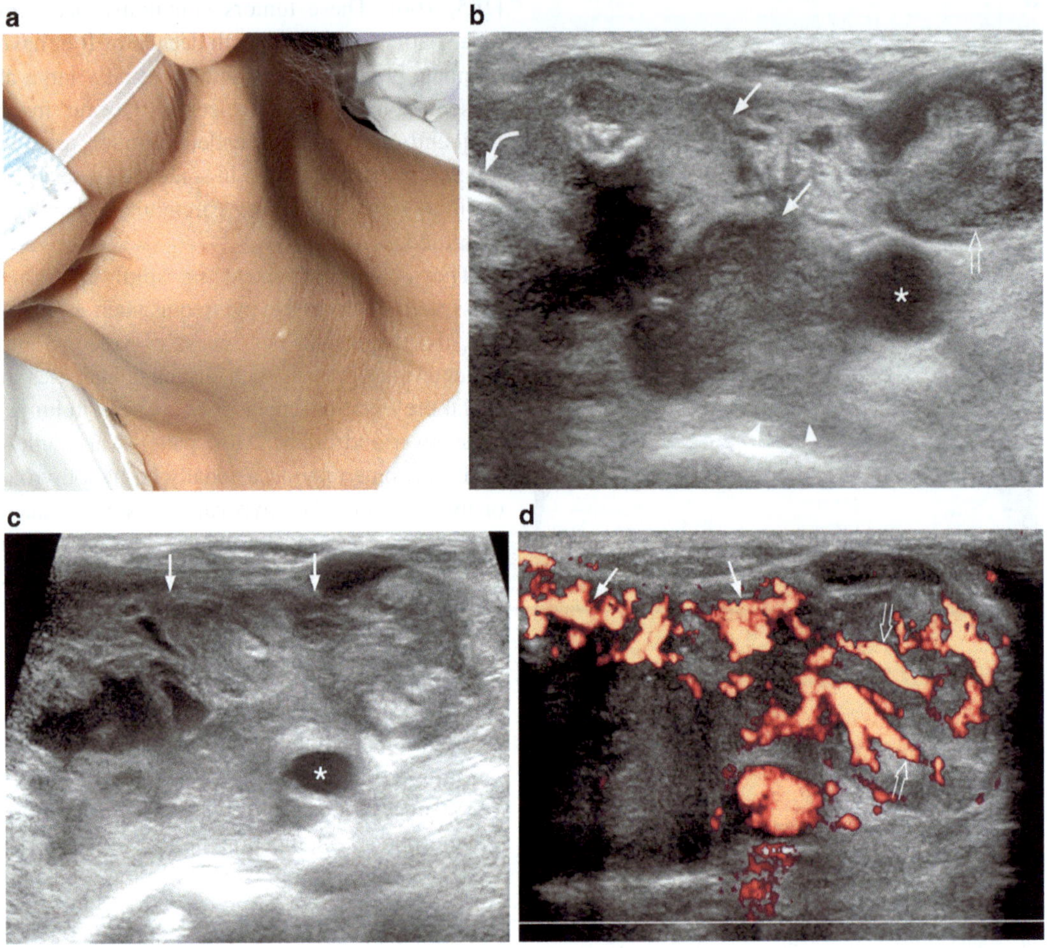

Fig. 6.26 (**a**) Clinical photograph of an elderly patient presenting with a rapidly enlarging left anterior neck mass. (**b**) Transverse and (**c**) oblique gray-scale ultrasound of the thyroid gland show a large, solid, heterogeneous, hypoechoic mass with calcification involving the entire left lobe of thyroid gland (*arrows*). Note the presence of extracapsular tumor spread beyond the posterior capsule of the left lobe (*arrowheads*) and metastatic lymphadenopathy (*open arrow*). *Asterisk* – left common carotid artery, *curved arrow* – trachea. (**d**) Corresponding power Doppler examination in oblique plane reveals chaotic intranodular vascularity within part of the thyroid tumor (*arrows*) and metastatic node (*open arrows*). Note part of the thyroid mass is avascular which may be due to occlusion of vessels by the malignancy

Medullary Carcinoma

Medullary carcinoma accounts for 3–5% of all thyroid cancer. It has a familial form which accounts for 10–20% of all cases and usually affects several family members. It is inherited as an autosomal dominant trait and associated with other endocrine neoplasm [169, 170]. Multiple endocrine neoplasms (MEN 2a and MEN 2b) may contain medullary carcinoma as one of their components [171]. MEN 1 and Wermer's syndrome are not associated with medullary carcinoma [171].

Medullary carcinoma is believed to be derived from C-cells and is thus associated with development of calcitonin [172–177]. The tumor contains stromal amyloid and arises in the lateral upper 2/3 of the thyroid gland. Elevated plasma calcitonin levels form the basis of diagnosis and follow-up of recurrent disease.

Sporadic medullary carcinomas are tumors of the middle age (~50 years) with a female predominance [178]. Patients with familial medullary carcinoma have a mean age of 50 years. Patients with MEN 2a-associated medullary carcinoma have a mean age of 20 years, and those with MEN 2b may develop tumor in childhood. The survival of patients with medullary carcinoma strongly correlates with stage at diagnosis: the 10-year overall survival rate for stage I and II is 90–100%, while it is 20–55% for stage IV patients [179–181].

Ultrasound features of medullary carcinoma (Figs. 6.27 and 6.28) [36, 136]:

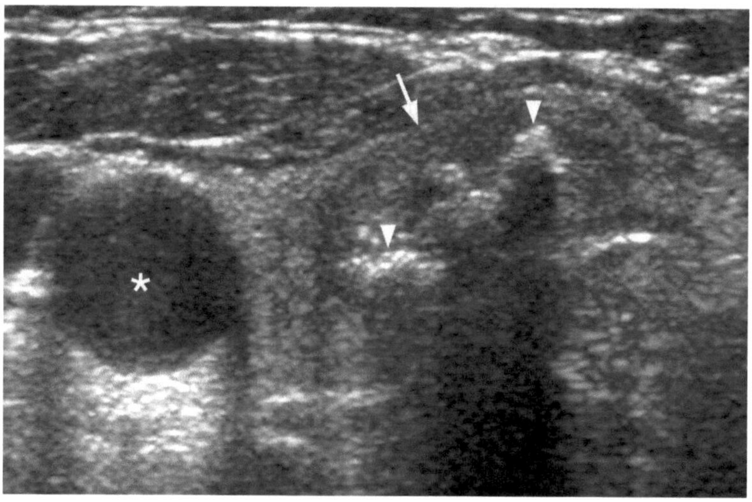

Fig. 6.27 Transverse gray-scale ultrasound of the thyroid gland shows an ill-defined, solid, hypoechoic nodule (*arrow*) with foci of coarse calcifications (*arrowheads*). The calcific foci represent a combination of amyloid and calcium deposition. Medullary carcinoma is often mistaken for papillary carcinoma, and the diagnosis is usually made on biopsy. *Asterisk* – right common carotid artery. Pathology – medullary carcinoma

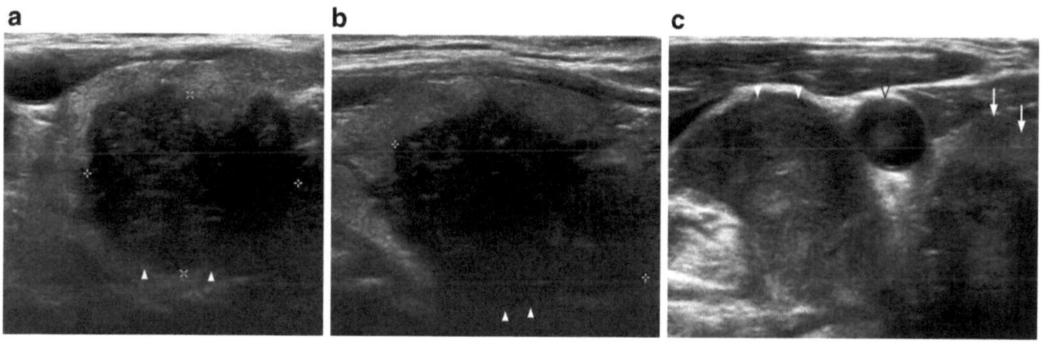

Fig. 6.28 Transverse (**a**) and longitudinal (**b**) gray-scale images of a medullary thyroid carcinoma. Note the ill-defined, hypoechoic, predominantly solid, tumor (calipers) within the thyroid. Posteriorly and inferiorly it appears to have an extrathyroid extension (*arrowheads*). In patients without a familial history, MTC is often mistaken for a papillary carcinoma as their ultrasound features are similar. The diagnosis is often made following FNAC/biopsy/surgery. (**c**) Along with the thyroid primary (*arrows*), there is an associated large, solid, hypoechoic metastatic node (*arrowheads*) lateral to the CCA (*open arrow*), low in the neck. Metastatic nodes in MTC tend to be hypoechoic compared to the hyperechoic nodes in papillary thyroid carcinoma

- Location: focal hypoechoic mass in lateral upper 2/3 of the gland (where C-cells are supposedly concentrated) in the sporadic form and diffuse involvement of both lobes in the familial form [121].
- Solid hypoechoic nodule.
- Frequently well-defined, may have ill-defined border.
- Presence of echogenic foci in 80–90% of tumors which represent deposits of amyloid and associated calcification [25, 121]. The calcifications are denser than in papillary carcinoma and many show frank posterior acoustic shadowing. Similar calcific deposits are also seen in 50–60% of associated nodal metastases.
- Chaotic vessels Type III vascularity within the tumor.

Metastatic regional lymphadenopathy (patients often have lymphadenopathy at presentation) (Fig. 6.28):

- Nodes along mid and low internal jugular chain and mediastinum.
- Predominantly hypoechoic (unlike papillary thyroid metastatic nodes) ± coarse shadowing calcification.

On initial ultrasound, a medullary carcinoma is invariably mistaken for a papillary carcinoma as their sonographic appearances are similar and papillary carcinoma is much more common. The diagnosis is often established on biopsy and based on clinical presentation (familial form and association with other endocrine neoplasia).

The distinguishing features of medullary carcinoma (from papillary carcinoma) include:

- Dense shadowing calcification in primary tumor and lymph nodes (rather than fine punctate calcification).
- Hypoechoic nodes (rather than hyperechoic nodes).
- More often larger than a papillary carcinoma, more cystic in nature, and the solid portion is commonly homogeneous in echotexture [182].

Thyroid Metastases

Metastases to the thyroid gland are uncommon, usually occurring late in the course of the disease and as part of disseminated metastases. The incidence in patients with a known primary is 2–17% [123]. Metastases to the thyroid are due to hematogenous spread commonly from the following primary sites: melanoma, breast, kidney, lungs and colon.

Metastatic involvement of the thyroid gland is often well circumscribed and nodular in appearance, though diffuse involvement is also a recognized pattern.

Secondary involvement of the thyroid may also occur due to direct extension of cancer from contiguous structures.

Ultrasound features of thyroid metastases (Figs. 6.29 and 6.30) [36, 136]:

- Solitary: homogeneous, hypoechoic, noncalcified, well-circumscribed mass predominantly in the lower pole.

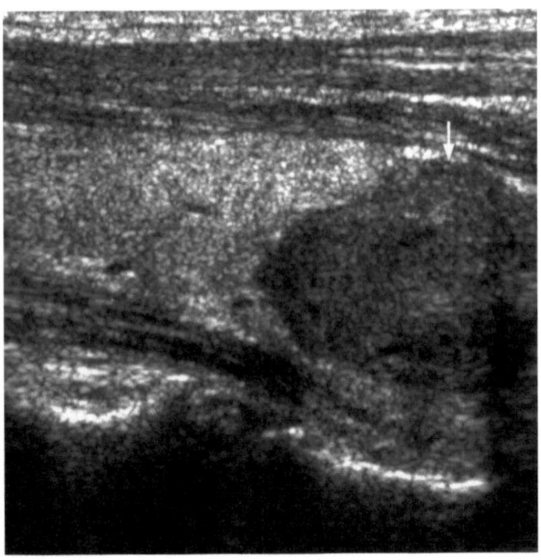

Fig. 6.29 Longitudinal gray-scale ultrasound in a patient with a known lung cancer showing a solid, hypoechoic, well-defined, noncalcified nodule (*arrow*) in the lower pole of the thyroid. The lower pole is a common location for large thyroid metastases, and the presence of such a nodule in a patient with known cancer suggests thyroid metastases unless proven otherwise

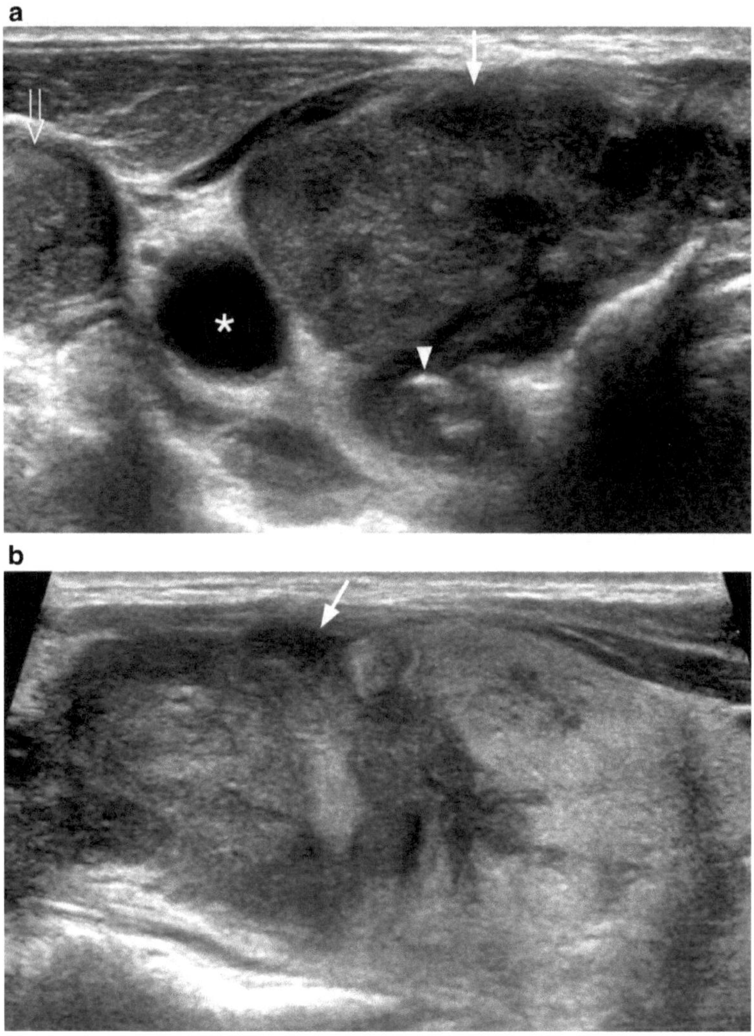

Fig. 6.30 (**a**) Transverse and (**b**) longitudinal gray-scale ultrasound in a patient with history of lung carcinoma. There is a large, solid, hypoechoic mass (*arrow*) in the right lobe of thyroid gland with tumor extension to the cervical esophagus (*arrowhead*). Note the presence of metastatic lymph node (*open arrow*) in adjacent right jugular chain. *Asterisk* – right common carotid artery. Metastases to the thyroid are invariably associated with other evidence of disseminated disease

- Multiple: hypoechoic, well-defined, solid, thyroid nodules.
- Metastatic nodules may show diffuse, disorganized vascularity.
- Diffuse: heterogeneous parenchymal echo pattern, ± thyroid enlargement.
- Invariably associated with disseminated metastatic disease (metastatic cervical lymphadenopathy, lung, liver, bone metastases).

Although a solitary metastasis may simulate a primary thyroid mass and diffuse involvement resembles thyroiditis or lymphoma, the clues to thyroid metastases include:

- Patient has a known history of a primary carcinoma.
- Thyroid involvement occurs as a part of disseminated disease and is often associated with abnormal lymphadenopathy and lung, bone, brain, liver metastases.

Thyroid Lymphoma

Lymphoma may arise primarily from the thyroid gland or involve the thyroid gland secondarily as part of a systemic lymphoma. Primary thyroid lymphoma is a rare tumor and accounts for 1–5% of thyroid malignancies and less than 2% of extranodal lymphomas.

A common presentation is of an elderly (sixth decade) female with a rapidly enlarging thyroid mass (unilateral or bilateral) with or without enlarged lymph nodes. The patient may have compressive symptoms such as dyspnea, dysphagia and hoarseness of voice. An antecedent history of Hashimoto's thyroiditis is commonly present [25, 121]. Although the majority of patients are euthyroid, some may be hypothyroid due to the associated Hashimoto's thyroiditis.

The clinical presentation of thyroid lymphoma as a rapidly enlarging mass is very similar to a patient with anaplastic carcinoma. Thyroid involvement may be focal or diffuse, and extrathyroid spread and vascular invasion are seen in 50–60% and 25% respectively [183, 184].

Ultrasound appearance of thyroid lymphoma [36, 136]:

Thyroid mass:

- Background evidence of Hashimoto's thyroiditis with bright fibrotic streaks in a lobulated hypoechoic gland.
- Focal nodule is usually hypoechoic, heterogeneous, noncalcified and solid.
- Nodule may be ill-defined or well-defined, solitary/multiple, unilateral/ bilateral.
- Nonspecific vascularity, ± prominent intranodular vessels.

Diffuse thyroid involvement (Fig. 6.31):

- Diffuse, thyroid enlargement, hypoechoic gland with lobulated contours.
- ± Prominent vascularity.
- Simple nonspecific glandular enlargement.

Lymphadenopathy:

- Unilateral/bilateral, enlarged, solid noncalcified nodes.
- Hypoechoic, reticulated echo pattern.
- Prominent central and peripheral vascularity.
- They displace vessels and soft tissues without infiltrating them.

The clinical presentation and sonographic appearance of thyroid lymphoma and anaplastic carcinoma (and to some degree diffuse thyroid metastases) are quite similar. The distinguishing features include:

- Anaplastic carcinoma is more infiltrative, whereas lymphoma is more compressive.
- Background evidence of MNG (+ calcification) is seen in anaplastic carcinoma, whereas in lymphoma of thyroid, one often has background evidence of Hashimoto's thyroiditis.
- Necrosis of tumor and heterogeneous architecture are seen in anaplastic carcinoma.
- Lymphomatous nodes are solid/reticulated, whereas anaplastic nodes may show evidence of necrosis.

Poorly Differentiated Carcinoma (Fig. 6.32)

This group of thyroid carcinomas includes tumors with a histologic pattern between differentiated and undifferentiated thyroid cancers [185–187]. Insular carcinoma is the best described tumor in this group and has a female predominance with a median age of 55 years. Patients commonly have distant (36%) and regional metastases (26%) at presentation [188].

On ultrasound, their appearances are similar to other thyroid cancers (i.e., solid, hypoechoic, ill defined with a heterogeneous echo pattern) (Figs. 6.32a, b). They may be associated with internal jugular vein thrombosis (Fig. 6.32c), malignant neck nodes (Fig. 6.32d), and chest (Fig. 6.32e), liver and bone metastases. The prognosis of insular carcinoma is poor [188], and the treatment of a pure insular carcinoma is similar to undifferentiated carcinomas.

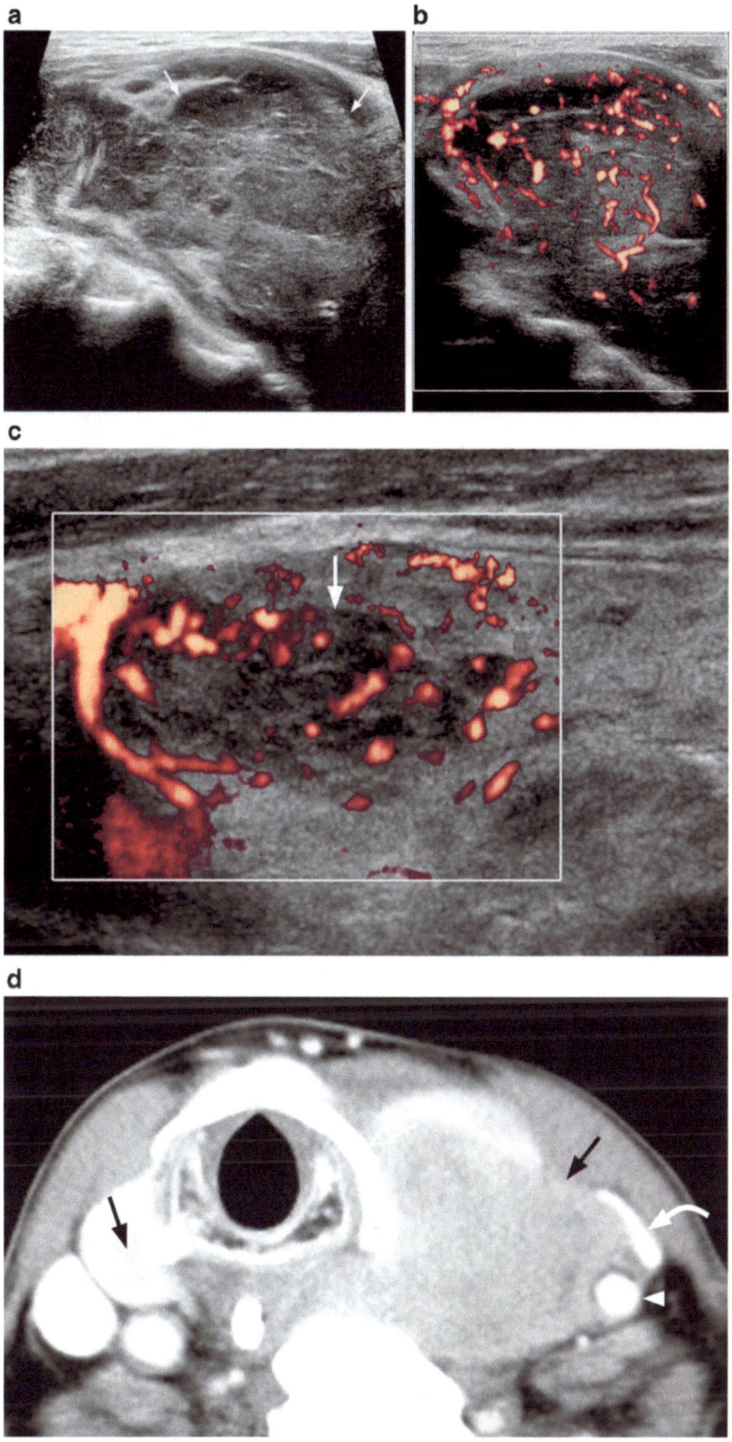

Fig. 6.31 (**a**) Transverse gray-scale ultrasound shows diffuse lymphomatous involvement of the left lobe of thyroid gland, which is replaced by a large solid, hypoechoic mass (*arrows*). (**b**) The mass is hypervascular on corresponding power Doppler examination. The differential diagnoses include anaplastic carcinoma. The presence of lymphomatous nodes and background of Hashimoto's thyroiditis are clues to diagnosis of lymphoma. (**c**) Longitudinal power Doppler ultrasound of the right lobe reveals another area of lymphomatous involvement (*arrow*) in the upper pole. Note the abnormal vascularity within the lesion. (**d**) Axial contrast-enhanced CT in the same patient better defines the extent of lymphomatous involvement in both lobes of thyroid gland (*arrows*) and its relationship to adjacent structures such as left common carotid artery (*arrowhead*), compressed left internal jugular vein (*curved arrow*), and thyroid cartilage (*open arrow*)

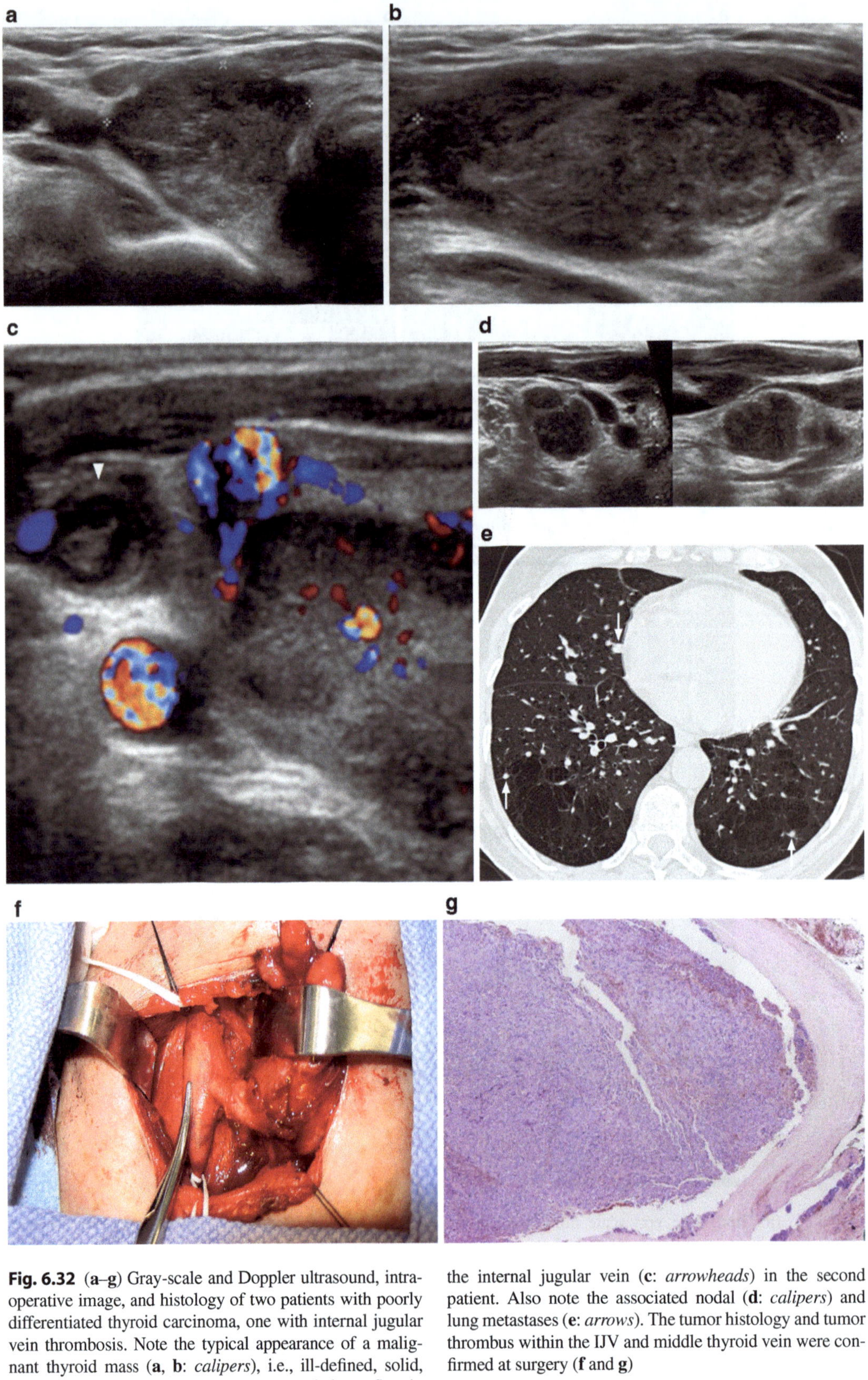

Fig. 6.32 (**a**–**g**) Gray-scale and Doppler ultrasound, intraoperative image, and histology of two patients with poorly differentiated thyroid carcinoma, one with internal jugular vein thrombosis. Note the typical appearance of a malignant thyroid mass (**a**, **b**: *calipers*), i.e., ill-defined, solid, markedly hypoechoic in the first patient and absent flow in the internal jugular vein (**c**: *arrowheads*) in the second patient. Also note the associated nodal (**d**: *calipers*) and lung metastases (**e**: *arrows*). The tumor histology and tumor thrombus within the IJV and middle thyroid vein were confirmed at surgery (**f** and **g**)

Postoperative Disease Surveillance

Accurate surveillance for possible tumor recurrence in patients treated with total thyroidectomy with/without lymph node dissection is the major goal of long-term follow-up in patients with thyroid cancer. Although differentiated thyroid cancer is typically an indolent disease with a high rate of cure, recurrence is common (15–30%), even in early-stage disease [189]. Patients with higher risk of recurrence are monitored more aggressively as early detection of recurrent disease is essential for effective treatment.

The risk of recurrence is stratified into (5):

Low-risk patients [190–192]:

- No local or distant metastases.
- All macroscopic tumor has been resected.
- No local / regional or vascular tumor infiltration.
- Tumor does not have an aggressive histology (such as tall cell, insular, columnar carcinoma).
- No ^{131}I uptake outside thyroid bed on first post–treatment whole body RAI scan.

Intermediate-risk patients [131, 193, 194]:

- Aggressive tumor histology or vascular invasion
- Microscopic perithyroidal tumor invasion
- Neck node metastases or ^{131}I uptake outside thyroid bed after thyroid remnant ablation

High-risk patients:

- Incomplete tumor excision.
- Macroscopic tumor invasion.
- Distant metastases.
- Thyroglobulinemia disproportionate to post-treatment scan [195].

Clinical examination is essential to detect any obvious tumor recurrence or raise the suspicion of probable recurrent tumor. This necessitates further investigations including biochemical markers (serum thyroglobulin for well-differentiated thyroid cancer, serum calcitonin for medullary thyroid carcinoma). Imaging plays an integral role in assessment of early recurrent tumor (local, regional nodal and metastatic disease) with ultrasound, radionuclide imaging including ^{18}FDG-PET among the most useful imaging tools for disease surveillance [189, 196, 197].

Ultrasound is a commonly utilized imaging modality (nonionizing, relatively inexpensive, readily combined with FNA, and easily done as an office-based examination) for disease surveillance for patients with thyroid cancer treated with thyroidectomy [189, 198]. Although in the postoperative state ultrasound may be difficult to perform (due to distorted anatomy and surface scar tissue); in experienced hands, it clearly evaluates the postoperative thyroid bed and the neck for presence or absence of any disease (Fig. 6.33). It also acts as a guidance system for directed fine needle aspiration of suspicious lesions. Remnant thyroid tissue, postoperative fibrosis, suture granuloma, strap muscle with a nodular contour, reactive lymph nodes, cysts, and fat necrosis [199] may mimic locally recurrent tumor with overlapping and nonspecific sonographic appearance. FNA under ultrasound guidance is often required to identify recurrent disease. A suture granuloma in the thyroid bed closely simulates recurrent disease, particularly papillary carcinoma. The echogenic focus seen in a suture granuloma is larger and denser and casts a posterior acoustic shadow.

In patients with well-differentiated cancers, serum thyroglobulin is a sensitive parameter to detect disease recurrence.

Radioiodine whole-body scan (WBS) is recommended for high-risk patients or those with elevated TSH-stimulated thyroglobulin level [16–18].

^{18}FDG-PET is indicated for detection and localization of recurrent tumor in thyroglobulin-positive, radioactive iodine (RAI) scan-negative patients [200].

Conclusion

The main aim in the management of a thyroid nodule is to identify the small group of patients in whom the nodule is malignant and warrants a timely definitive treatment (while avoiding unnecessary investigations and treatment in the majority of patients with benign nodules).

Ultrasound (combined with FNA) is a useful and widely available tool for the initial assessment of a thyroid nodule and cervical lymph nodes.

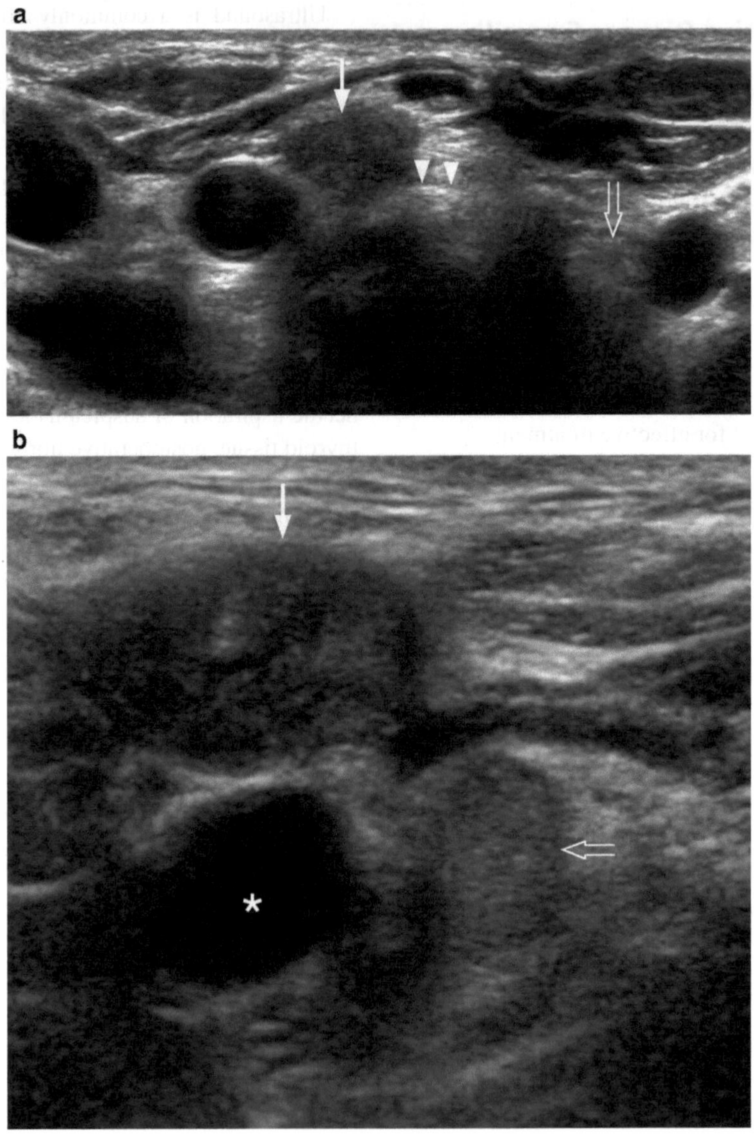

Fig. 6.33 (**a**) Transverse gray-scale ultrasound in a patient with history of total thyroidectomy for papillary carcinoma. Note the solid, ill-defined, hypoechoic nodule in the postoperative bed on the right (*arrow*). This is proven to be a nodal recurrence. Note its relationship to the trachea (*arrowheads*) and the empty left thyroid bed (*open arrow*). (**b**) Transverse gray-scale ultrasound in another patient with history of total thyroidectomy for papillary carcinoma. Note the solid, ill-defined, hypoechoic nodal recurrence (*arrow*) anterior to the right common carotid artery (*asterisk*). Also note the recurrence in the postoperative right thyroid bed (*open arrow*)

Apart from preoperative diagnosis, ultrasound also plays a pivotal role in post–treatment follow-up surveillance of thyroid cancer for early detection of recurrent tumor.

References

1. Hegedüs L. Clinical practice. The thyroid nodule. N Engl J Med. 2004;351:1764–71.
2. Mandel SJ. A 64-year-old woman with a thyroid nodule. JAMA. 2004;292:2632–42.
3. Curtis RE, Rowlings PA, Deeg HJ, et al. Solid cancers after bone marrow transplantation. N Engl J Med. 1997;336:897–904.
4. Pacini F, Vorontsova T, Demidchik E, et al. Post-Chernobyl thyroid carcinoma in Belarus children and adolescents: comparison with naturally occurring thyroid carcinoma in Italy and France. J Clin Endocrinol Metab. 1997;81:3563–9.
5. American Thyroid Association (ATA) Guidelines Taskforce on Thyroid Nodules and Differentiated Thyroid Cancer, Cooper DS, Doherty GM, Haugen BR, et al. Revised American Thyroid Association management guidelines for patients with thyroid nodules and differentiated thyroid cancer. Thyroid 2009;19:1167–1214.
6. Boelaert K, Horacek J, Holder RL, Watkinson JC, Sheppard MC, Franklyn JA. Serum thyrotropin concentration as a novel predictor of malignancy in thyroid nodules investigated by fine-needle aspiration. J Clin Endocrinol Metab. 2006;91:4295–301.
7. Walsh RM, Watkinson JC, Franklyn J. The management of the solitary thyroid nodule: a review. Clin Otolaryngol. 1999;24:388–97.
8. Campbell JP, Pillsbury HC. Management of the thyroid nodule. Head Neck. 1989;11:414–25.
9. Ashcroft MW, Van Herle AJ. Management of thyroid nodules. II Scanning techniques, thyroid suppressive therapy, and fine needle aspiration. Head Neck Surg. 1981;3:297–322.
10. The Papanicolaou Society of Cytopathology Task Force on Standards of Practice. Guidelines of the Papanicolaou Society of Cytopathology for examination of fine-needle aspiration specimens from thyroid nodules. Diagn Cytopathol. 1996;15:84–9.
11. Sabel MS, Haque D, Velasco JM, Staren ED. Use of ultrasound-guided fine needle aspiration biopsy in the management of thyroid disease. Am Surg. 1998;64:738–42.
12. Hatada T, Okada K, Ishii H, Ichii S, Utsunomiya J. Evaluation of ultrasound-guided fine-needle aspiration Biopsy for thyroid nodules. Am J Surg. 1998;175:133–6.
13. Newkirk KA, Ruigel MD, Jelinek J, et al. Ultrasound-guided fine needle aspiration and thyroid disease. Ootolaryngol Head Neck. 2000;123:700–5.
14. Alexander EK, Heering JP, Benson CB, et al. Assessment of nondiagnostic ultrasound-guided fine needle aspiration of thyroid nodules. J Clin Endocrinol Metab. 2002;87:4924–7.
15. Kwak JY, Koo H, Youk JH, et al. Value of US correlation of a thyroid nodule with initially benign cytologic results. Radiology. 2010;254:292–300.
16. Fatourechi V, Hay ID, Mullan BP, et al. Are post-therapy radioiodine scans informative and do they influence subsequent therapy of patients with differentiated thyroid cancer? Thyroid. 2000;10:573–7.
17. Sherman SI, Tielens ET, Sostre S, Wharam Jr MD, Ladenson PW. Clinical utility of posttreatment radioiodine scans in the management of patients with thyroid carcinoma. J Clin Endocrinol Metab. 1994;78:629–34.
18. Reynolds JC. Percent ^{131}I uptake and post-therapy ^{131}I scans: their role in the management of thyroid cancer. Thyroid. 1997;7:281–4.
19. Mitchell JC, Grant F, Evenson AR, Parker JA, Hasselgren PO, Parangi S. Preoperative evaluation of thyroid nodules with 18FDG-PET/CT. Surgery. 2005;138:1166–74. discussion 1174–5.
20. de Geus-Oei LF, Pieters GF, Bonenkamp JJ, et al. 18F-FDG PET reduces unnecessary hemithyroidectomies for thyroid nodules with inconclusive cytologic results. J Nucl Med. 2006;47:770–5.
21. Kim JM, Ryu JS, Kim TY, et al. 18F-fluorodeoxyglucose positron emission tomography does not predict malignancy in thyroid nodules cytologically diagnosed as follicular neoplasm. J Clin Endocrinol Metab. 2007;92:1630–4.
22. Sebastianes FM, Cerci JJ, Zanoni PH, et al. Role of 18F-fluorodeoxyglucose positron emission tomography in preoperative assessment of cytologically indeterminate thyroid nodules. J Clin Endocrinol Metab. 2007;92:4485–8.
23. Hales NW, Krempl GA, Medina JE. Is there a role for fluorodeoxyglucose positron emission tomography/computed tomography in cytologically indeterminate thyroid nodules? Am J Otolaryngol. 2008; 29:113–8.
24. King AD, Ahuja AT, To EWH, Tse GMK, Metreweli C. Staging of papillary carcinoma of the thyroid: magnetic resonance imaging vs ultrasound of the neck. Clin Radiol. 2000;55:222–6.
25. Yousem DM, Scheff AM. Thyroid and parathyroid. In: Som PM, Curtin HD, editors. Head and neck imaging. 3rd ed. St Louis: Mosby; 1996. p. 954–8.
26. Mazzaferri EL. Managing small thyroid cancers. JAMA. 2006;295:2179–82.
27. Frates MC, Benson CB, Charboneau JW, et al. Society of Radiologists in Ultrasound. Management of thyroid nodules detected at US: Society of Radiologists in Ultrasound consensus conference statement. Radiology. 2005;237:794–800.
28. Ross DS. Editorial: predicting thyroid malignancy. J Clin Endocrinol Metab. 2006;91:4253–5.

29. Jemal A, Murray T, Ward E, et al. Cancer statistics, 2005. CA Cancer J Clin. 2005;55:10–30. Erratum in: CA Cancer J Clin 2005;55:259.
30. Harach HR, Franssila KO, Wasenius VM. Occult papillary carcinoma of the thyroid. A "normal" finding in Finland. A systematic autopsy study. Cancer. 1985;56:531–8.
31. Are C, Hsu JF, Ghossein RA, Schoder H, Shah JP, Shaha AR. Histological aggressiveness of fluorodeoxyglucose positron-emission tomogram (FDG-PET)-detected incidental thyroid carcinomas. Ann Surg Oncol. 2007;14:3210–5.
32. Papini E, Guglielmi R, Bianchini A, et al. Risk of malignancy in nonpalpable thyroid nodules: predictive value of ultrasound and color-Doppler features. J Clin Endocrinol Metab. 2002;87:1941–6.
33. Hagag P, Strauss S, Weiss M. Role of ultrasound-guided fine-needle aspiration biopsy in evaluation of nonpalpable thyroid nodules. Thyroid. 1998;8: 989–95.
34. Nam-Goong IS, Kim HY, Gong G, et al. Ultrasonography-guided fine-needle aspiration of thyroid incidentaloma: correlation with pathological findings. Clin Endocrinol (Oxf). 2004;60:21–8.
35. Cronan JJ. Thyroid nodules: is it time to turn off the US machines? Radiology. 2008;247:602–4.
36. Wong KT, Ahuja AT. Ultrasound of thyroid cancer. Cancer Imaging. 2005;5:157–66.
37. Frates MC, Benson CB, Doubilet PM, Cibas ES, Marqusee E. Can color Doppler sonography aid in the prediction of malignancy of thyroid nodules? J Ultrasound Med. 2003;22:127–31.
38. Khoo ML, Asa SL, Witterick IJ, Freeman JL. Thyroid calcification and its association with thyroid carcinoma. Head Neck. 2002;24:651–5.
39. Kim EK, Park CS, Chung WY, Oh KK, Kim DI, Lee JT, et al. New sonographic criteria for recommending fine-needle aspiration biopsy of nonpalpable solid nodules of the thyroid. AJR Am J Roentgenol. 2002;178:687–91.
40. Peccin S, de Castsro JA, Furlanetto TW, Furtado AP, Brasil BA, Czepielewski MA. Ultrasonography: is it useful in the diagnosis of cancer in thyroid nodules? J Endocrinol Invest. 2002;25:39–43.
41. Appetecchia M, Solivetti FM. The association of colour flow Doppler sonography and conventional ultrasonography improves the diagnosis of thyroid carcinoma. Horm Res. 2006;66:249–56.
42. Cappelli C, Castellano M, Pirola I, et al. The predictive value of ultrasound findings in the management of thyroid nodules. QJM. 2007;100:29–35.
43. Moon WJ, Jung SL, Lee JH, et al. Thyroid Study Group, Korean Society of Neuro- and Head and Neck Radiology. Benign and malignant thyroid nodules: US differentiation – multicenter retrospective study. Radiology. 2008;247:762–70.
44. Rago T, Vitti P, Chiovato L, et al. Role of conventional ultrasonography and color flow-doppler sonography in predicting malignancy in 'cold' thyroid nodules. Eur J Endocrinol. 1998;138:41–6.
45. Brunese L, Romeo A, Iorio S, et al. A new marker for diagnosis of thyroid papillary cancer: B-flow twinkling sign. J Ultrasound Med. 2008;27: 1187–94.
46. Cerbone G, Spiezia S, Colao A, et al. Power Doppler improves the diagnostic accuracy of color Doppler ultrasonography in cold thyroid nodules: follow-up results. Horm Res. 1999;52:19–24.
47. Chan BK, Desser TS, McDougall IR, Weigel RJ, Jeffrey Jr RB. Common and uncommon sonographic features of papillary thyroid carcinoma. J Ultrasound Med. 2003;22:1083–90.
48. Solbiati L, Cioffi V, Ballarati E. Ultrasonography of the neck. Radiol Clin North Am. 1992;30:941–54.
49. Varverakis E, Neonakis E, Tzardi M, Chrysos E. Role of color Doppler ultrasonography in the preoperative management of cold thyroid nodules. Hormones (Athens). 2007;6:44–51.
50. Yuan WH, Chiou HJ, Chou YH, et al. Gray-scale and color Doppler ultrasonographic manifestations of papillary thyroid carcinoma: analysis of 51 cases. Clin Imaging. 2006;30:394–401.
51. Iannuccilli JD, Cronan JJ, Monchik JM. Risk for malignancy of thyroid nodules as assessed by sonographic criteria: the need for biopsy. J Ultrasound Med. 2004;23:1455–64.
52. Fobbe F, Finke R, Reichenstein E, Schleusener H, Wolf KJ. Appearance of thyroid diseases using colour-coded duplex sonography. Eur J Radiol. 1989;9:29–31.
53. Shimamoto K, Endo T, Ishigaki T, Sakuma S, Makino N. Thyroid nodules: evaluation with color Doppler ultrasonography. J Ultrasound Med. 1993; 12:673–8.
54. Spiezia S, Colao A, Assanti AP, et al. Usefulness of color echo Doppler with power Doppler in the diagnosis of hypoechoic thyroid nodules: work in progress. Radiol Med. 1996;91:616–21.
55. Stacul F, Bertolotto M, De Gobbis F, et al. US, colour-Doppler US and fine-needle aspiration biopsy in the diagnosis of thyroid nodules. Radiol Med. 2007;112:751–62.
56. Moon HJ, Kwak JY, Kim MJ, Son EJ, Kim EK. Can vascularity at power Doppler US help predict thyroid malignancy? Radiology. 2010;255:260–9.
57. Takashima S, Fukuda H, Nomura N, et al. Thyroid nodules: re-evaluation with ultrasound. J Clin Ultrasound. 1995;23:179–84.
58. Cappelli C, Castellano M, Pirola I, et al. Thyroid nodule shape suggests malignancy. Eur J Endocrinol. 2006;155:27–31.
59. Reading CC, Charboneau JW, Hay ID, Sebo TJ. Sonography of thyroid nodules: a "classic pattern" diagnostic approach. Ultrasound Q. 2005;21:157–65.
60. Bonavita JA, Mayo J, Babb J, et al. Pattern recognition of benign nodules at ultrasound of the thyroid: which nodules can be left alone? AJR Am J Roentgenol. 2009;193:207–13.
61. Frates MC, Benson CB, Doubilet PM, et al. Prevalence and distribution of carcinoma in patients

with solitary and multiple thyroid nodules on sonography. J Clin Endocrinol Metab. 2006;91:3411–7.
62. Moon WJ, Kwag HJ, Na DG. Are there any specific ultrasound findings of nodular hyperplasia ("leave me alone" lesion) to differentiate it from follicular adenoma? Acta Radiol. 2009;50:383–8.
63. Ahuja A, Chick W, King W, Metreweli C. Clinical significance of the comet tail artifact in thyroid ultrasound. J Clin Ultrasound. 1996;24:129–33.
64. Horvath E, Majlis S, Rossi R, et al. An ultrasonogram reporting system for thyroid nodules stratifying cancer risk for clinical management. J Clin Endocrinol Metab. 2009;94:1748–51.
65. Mihailescu DV, Schneider AB. Size, number, and distribution of thyroid nodules and the risk of malignancy in radiation-exposed patients who underwent surgery. J Clin Endocrinol Metab. 2008;93:2188–93.
66. Alexander EK, Hurwitz S, Heering JP, et al. Natural history of benign solid and cystic thyroid nodules. Ann Intern Med. 2003;138:315–8.
67. Asanuma K, Kobayashi S, Shingu K, et al. The rate of tumour growth does not distinguish between malignant and benign thyroid nodules. Eur J Surg. 2001;167:102–5.
68. Papini E, Petrucci L, Guglielmi R, et al. Long-term changes in nodular goiter: a 5-year prospective randomized trial of levothyroxine suppressive therapy for benign cold thyroid nodules. J Clin Endocrinol Metab. 1998;83:780–3.
69. Ahn SS, Kim EK, Kang DR, Lim SK, Kwak JY, Kim MJ. Biopsy of thyroid nodules: comparison of three sets of guidelines. AJR Am J Roentgenol. 2010;194:31–7.
70. Gharib H, Papini E, Valcavi R, et al. AACE/AME Task Force on Thyroid Nodules. American Association of Clinical Endocrinologists and Associazione Medici Endocrinologi medical guidelines for clinical practice for the diagnosis and management of thyroid nodules. Endocr Pract. 2006;12:63–102.
71. Filetti S, Durante C, Torlontano M. Nonsurgical approaches to the management of thyroid nodules. Nat Clin Pract Endocrinol Metab. 2006;2:384–94.
72. Quadbeck B, Pruellage J, Roggenbuck U, Hirche H, Janssen OE, Mann K, et al. Long-term follow-up of thyroid nodule growth. Exp Clin Endocrinol Diabetes. 2002;110:348–54.
73. Alexander EK, Marqusee E, Orcutt J, et al. Thyroid nodule shape and prediction of malignancy. Thyroid. 2004;14:953–8.
74. Roti E, degli Uberti EC, Bondanelli M, Braverman LE. Thyroid papillary microcarcinoma: a descriptive and meta-analysis study. Eur J Endocrinol. 2008; 159: 659–73.
75. Sugino K, Ito Jr K, Ozaki O, Mimura T, Iwasaki H, Ito K. Papillary microcarcinoma of the thyroid. J Endocrinol Invest. 1998;21:445–8.
76. Mazzaferri EL, de los Santos ET, Rofagha-Keyhani S. Solitary thyroid nodule: diagnosis and management. Med Clin North Am. 1988;72:1177–211.
77. Noguchi S, Yamashita H, Murakami N, Nakayama I, Toda M, Kawamoto H. Small carcinomas of the thyroid. A long-term follow-up of 867 patients. Arch Surg. 1996;131:187–91.
78. Berker D, Aydin Y, Ustun I, et al. The value of fine-needle aspiration biopsy in subcentimeter thyroid nodules. Thyroid. 2008;18:603–8.
79. Wada N, Duh QY, Sugino K, et al. Lymph node metastasis from 259 papillary thyroid microcarcinomas: frequency, pattern of occurrence and recurrence, and optimal strategy for neck dissection. Ann Surg. 2003;237:399–407.
80. Cappelli C, Castellano M, Braga M, et al. Aggressiveness and outcome of papillary thyroid carcinoma (PTC) versus microcarcinoma (PMC): a mono-institutional experience. J Surg Oncol. 2007; 95:555–60.
81. Popowicz B, Klencki M, Lewiński A, Słowińska-Klencka D. The usefulness of sonographic features in selection of thyroid nodules for biopsy in relation to the nodule's size. Eur J Endocrinol. 2009;161:103–11.
82. Lyshchik A, Drozd V, Demidchik Y, Reiners C. Diagnosis of thyroid cancer in children: value of gray-scale and power doppler US. Radiology. 2005;235:604–13.
83. Mazzaferri EL, Sipos J. Should all patients with subcentimeter thyroid nodules undergo fine-needle aspiration biopsy and preoperative neck ultrasonography to define the extent of tumor invasion? Thyroid. 2008;18:597–602.
84. Ito Y, Uruno T, Nakano K, et al. An observation trial without surgical treatment in patients with papillary microcarcinoma of the thyroid. Thyroid. 2003; 13:381–7.
85. Kwak JY, Kim EK, Youk JH, et al. Extrathyroid extension of well-differentiated papillary thyroid microcarcinoma on US. Thyroid. 2008;18:609–14.
86. Koike E, Noguchi S, Yamashita H, et al. Ultrasonographic characteristics of thyroid nodules: prediction of malignancy. Arch Surg. 2001;136:334–7.
87. Solbiati L, Osti V, Cova L, Tonolini M. Ultrasound of thyroid, parathyroid glands and neck lymph nodes. Eur Radiol. 2001;11:2411–24.
88. Kuma K, Matsuzuka F, Kobayashi A, et al. Outcome of long standing solitary thyroid nodules. World J Surg. 1992;16:583–7.
89. Komolafe F. Radiological patterns and significance of thyroid calcification. Clin Radiol. 1981;32: 571–5.
90. Taki S, Terahata S, Yamashita R, et al. Thyroid calcifications: sonographic patterns and incidence of cancer. Clin Imaging. 2004;28:368–71.
91. Yoon DY, Lee JW, Chang SK, et al. Peripheral calcification in thyroid nodules. J Ultrasound Med. 2007;26:1349–55.
92. Kim BM, Kim MJ, Kim EK, et al. Sonographic differentiation of thyroid nodules with eggshell calcifications. J Ultrasound Med. 2008;27:1425–30.

93. Watters DA, Ahuja AT, Evans RM, et al. Role of ultrasound in the management of thyroid nodules. Am J Surg. 1992;164:654–7.
94. Wienke JR, Chong WK, Fielding JR, Zou KH, Mittelstaedt CA. Sonographic features of benign thyroid nodules: interobserver reliability and overlap with malignancy. J Ultrasound Med. 2003;22: 1027–31.
95. Marqusee E, Benson CB, Frates MC, et al. Usefulness of ultrasonography in the management of nodular thyroid disease. Ann Intern Med. 2000;133:696–700.
96. Hegedüs L, Bonnema SJ, Bennedbaek FN. Management of simple nodular goiter: current status and future perspectives. Endocr Rev. 2003;24: |102–32.
97. Kunreuther E, Orcutt J, Benson CB, et al. *Prevalence and distribution of carcinoma in the uninodular and multinodular goiter*. Presented at the 76th Annual Meeting of the American Thyroid Association, Vancouver, British Columbia, Canada, September 29 – October 3, 2004.
98. Propper RA, Skolnick ML, Weinstein BJ, Dekker A. The nonspecificity of the thyroid halo sign. J Clin Ultrasound. 1980;8:129–32.
99. Lu C, Chang TC, Hsiao YL, Kuo MS. Ultrasonographic findings of papillary thyroid carcinoma and their relation to pathologic changes. J Formos Med Assoc. 1994;93:933–8.
100. Hayashi N, Tamaki N, Yamamoto K, et al. Real-time ultrasonography of thyroid nodules. Acta Radiol Diagn (Stockh). 1986;27:403–8.
101. Hoang JK, Lee WK, Lee M, Johnson D, Farrell S. US Features of thyroid malignancy: pearls and pitfalls. Radiographics. 2007;27:847–60.
102. Cappelli C, Pirola I, Cumetti D, et al. Is the anteroposterior and transverse diameter ratio of nonpalpable thyroid nodules a sonographic criteria for recommending fine-needle aspiration cytology? Clin Endocrinol (Oxf). 2005;63:689–93.
103. Stavros AT, Thickman D, Rapp CL, Dennis MA, Parker SH, Sisney GA. Solid breast nodules: use of sonography to distinguish between benign and malignant lesions. Radiology. 1995;196:123–34.
104. Yoon SJ, Yoon DY, Chang SK, et al. "Taller-than-wide sign" of thyroid malignancy: comparison between ultrasound and CT. AJR Am J Roentgenol. 2010;194:W420–4.
105. Brkljačić B, Cuk V, Tomić-Brzac H, Bence-Zigman Z, Delić-Brkljačić D, Drinković I. Ultrasonic evaluation of benign and malignant nodules in echographically multinodular thyroids. J Clin Ultrasound. 1994;22: 71–6.
106. Lagalla R, Cariso G, Midiri M, Cardinale AE. Echo-Doppler couleru et pathologie thyroidienne. J Echograph Med Ultrasons. 1992;13:44–7.
107. Berni A, Tromba L, Falvo L, Marchesi M, Grilli P, Peparini N. Malignant thyroid nodules: comparison between color Doppler diagnosis and histological examination of surgical samples. Chir Ital. 2002;54: 643–7.
108. Tamsel S, Demirpolat G, Erdogan M, et al. Power Doppler US patterns of vascularity and spectral Doppler US parameters in predicting malignancy in thyroid nodules. Clin Radiol. 2007;62:245–51.
109. Bakhshaee M, Davoudi Y, Mehrabi M, et al. Vascular pattern and spectral parameters of power Doppler ultrasound as predictors of malignancy risk in thyroid nodules. Laryngoscope. 2008;118: 2182–6.
110. De Nicola H, Szejnfeld J, Logullo AF, Wolosker AM, Souza LR, Chiferi Jr V. Flow pattern and vascular resistive index as predictors of malignancy risk in thyroid follicular neoplasms. J Ultrasound Med. 2005;24:897–904.
111. Levine RA. Doppler ultrasound. In: Baskin HJ, Duick DS, Levine RA, editors. Thyroid ultrasound and ultrasound-guided FNA. 2nd ed. New York: Springer Science; 2008. p. 30–5.
112. Levine RA. Value of Doppler ultrasonography in management of patients with follicular thyroid biopsy specimens. Endocr Pract. 2006;12:270–4.
113. Ahuja AT, Ying M, Ho SY, Antonio G, Lee YP, King AD, et al. Ultrasound of malignant cervical lymph nodes. Cancer Imaging. 2008;8:48–56.
114. Leboulleux S, Girard E, Rose M, et al. Ultrasound criteria of malignancy for cervical lymph nodes in patients followed up for differentiated thyroid cancer. J Clin Endocrinol Metab. 2007;92:3590–4.
115. Kuna SK, Bracic I, Tesic V, et al. Ultrasonographic differentiation of benign from malignant neck lymphadenopathy in thyroid cancer. J Ultrasound Med. 2006;25:1531–7.
116. Kessler A, Rappaport Y, Blank A, Marmor S, Weiss J, Graif M. Cystic appearance of cervical lymph nodes is characteristic of metastatic papillary thyroid carcinoma. J Clin Ultrasound. 2003;31:21–5.
117. McGregor GI, Luomo A, Jackson SM. Lymph node metastases from well-differentiated thyroid cancer: a clinical review. Am J Surg. 1985;149:610.
118. Hamberger B, Gharib H, Melton 3rd LJ, Goellner JR, Zinsmeister AR. Fine-needle aspiration biopsy of thyroid nodules. Impact on thyroid practice and cost of care. Am J Med. 1982;73:381–4.
119. Mittendorf EA, Tamarkin SW, McHenry CR. The results of ultrasound-guided fine-needle aspiration biopsy for evaluation of nodular thyroid disease. Surgery. 2002;132:648–53.
120. Jemal A, Murray T, Ward E, et al. Cancer statistics, 2008. CA Cancer J Clin. 2008;58:71–96.
121. Bruneton JN, Normand F. Thyroid gland. In: Bruneton JN, editor. Ultrasonography of the neck. Berlin: Springer; 1987. p. 22–50.
122. Rustgi AK. Hereditary gastrointestinal polyposis and nonpolyposis syndromes. N Engl J Med. 1994;331:1694–702.
123. LiVolsi VA. Pathology of thyroid disease. In: Flak SA, editor. Thyroid disease: endocrinology, surgery, nuclear medicine and radiotherapy. Philadelphia: Lippincott-Raven; 1997. p. 70–5.
124. Chow SM, Chan JK, Law SC, et al. Diffuse sclerosing variant of papillary thyroid carcinoma – clinical

features and outcome. Eur J Surg Oncol. 2003;29: 446–9.

125. Carcangiu ML, Bianchi S. Diffuse sclerosing variant of papillary thyroid carcinoma. Clinicopathologic study of 15 cases. Am J Surg Pathol. 1989;13:1041–9.
126. Fujimoto Y, Obara T, Ito Y, Kodama T, Aiba M, Yamaguchi K. Diffuse sclerosing variant of papillary carcinoma of the thyroid. Clinical importance, surgical treatment, and follow-up study. Cancer. 1990;66:2306–12.
127. Lam AK, Lo CY. Diffuse sclerosing variant of papillary carcinoma of the thyroid: a 35-year comparative study at a single institution. Ann Surg Oncol. 2006;13:176–81.
128. Vickery Jr AL, Carcangiu ML, Johannessen JV, Sobrinho-Simoes M. Papillary carcinoma. Semin Diagn Pathol. 1985;2:90–100.
129. Lee JY, Shin JH, Han BK, et al. Diffuse sclerosing variant of papillary carcinoma of the thyroid: imaging and cytologic findings. Thyroid. 2007;17:567–73.
130. Filie AC, Chiesa A, Bryant BR, Merino MJ, Sobel ME, Abati A. The Tall cell variant of papillary carcinoma of the thyroid: cytologic features and loss of heterozygosity of metastatic and/or recurrent neoplasms and primary neoplasms. Cancer. 1999;87:238–42.
131. Prendiville S, Burman KD, Ringel MD, et al. Tall cell variant: an aggressive form of papillary thyroid carcinoma. Otolaryngol Head Neck Surg. 2000; 122:352–7.
132. Ostrowski ML, Merino MJ. Tall cell variant of papillary thyroid carcinoma: a reassessment and immunohistochemical study with comparison to the usual type of papillary carcinoma of the thyroid. Am J Surg Pathol. 1996;20:964–74.
133. Putti TC, Bhuiya TA. Mixed columnar cell and tall cell variant of papillary carcinoma of thyroid: a case report and review of the literature. Pathology. 2000;32:286–9.
134. Jayaram G. Cytology of columnar-cell variant of papillary thyroid carcinoma. Diagn Cytopathol. 2000;22:227–9.
135. Sobrinho-Simões M, Nesland JM, Johannessen JV. Columnar-cell carcinoma. Another variant of poorly differentiated carcinoma of the thyroid. Am J Clin Pathol. 1988;89:264–7.
136. Ahuja AT. The thyroid and parathyroids. In: Ahuja AT, Evans RM, editors. Practical head and neck ultrasound. London: Greenwich Medical Media Limited; 2000. p. 35–64.
137. Solbiati L, Livraghi T, Ballarati E, Ierace T, Crespi L. Thyroid gland. In: Solbiati L, Rizzatto G, editors. Ultrasound of superficial structures. London: Churchill Livingstone; 1995. p. 49–85.
138. Simeone JF, Daniels GH, Mueller PR, et al. High resolution real time sonography of the thyroid. Radiology. 1982;145:431–5.
139. Solbiati L, Volterrani L, Rizzatto G, et al. The thyroid gland with low uptake lesions: evaluation with ultrasound. Radiology. 1985;155:187–91.
140. Noyek AM, Finkelstein DM, Witterick IJ, Kirsch JC. Diagnostic imaging of the thyroid gland. In: Falk SA, editor. Thyroid disease: endocrinology, surgery, nuclear medicine, and radiotherapy. New York: Raven Press; 1997. p. 137–9.
141. McIvor NP, Freeman JL, Salem S. Ultrasonography of the thyroid and parathyroid glands. ORL J Otorhinolaryngol Relat Spec. 1993;55:303–8.
142. Kim HS, Han BK, Shin JH, et al. Papillary thyroid carcinoma of a diffuse sclerosing variant: ultrasonographic monitoring from a normal thyroid gland to mass formation. Korean J Radiol. 2010;11:579–82.
143. Ahuja AT, Chow L, Chick W, et al. Metastatic cervical nodes in papillary carcinoma of the thyroid: ultrasound and histological correlation. Clin Radiol. 1995;50:229–31.
144. DeMay RM. Follicular lesions of the thyroid. W(h)ither follicular carcinoma? Am J Clin Pathol. 2000;114:681–3.
145. Baloch ZW, LiVolsi VA. Our approach to follicular-patterned lesions of the thyroid. J Clin Pathol. 2007;60:244–50.
146. Greaves TS, Olvera M, Florentine BD, et al. Follicular lesions of thyroid: a 5-year fine-needle aspiration experience. Cancer. 2000;90:335–41.
147. Saggiorato E, De Pompa R, Volante M, et al. Characterization of thyroid 'follicular neoplasms' in fine-needle aspiration cytological specimens using a panel of immunohistochemical markers: a proposal for clinical application. Endocr Relat Cancer. 2005;12:305–17.
148. Tombouret R, Szefelbein WM, Pitman MB. Ultrasound-guided fine-needle aspiration biopsy of the thyroid. Cancer. 1999;87:299–305.
149. Williams ED, Doinach I, Bjanarson O, Michie W. Thyroid cancer in an iodide rich area. Cancer. 1977;39:215–22.
150. Lang W, Choritz H, Hundeshagen H. Risk factors in follicular thyroid carcinomas. A retrospective follow-up study covering a 14-year period with emphasis on morphological findings. Am J Surg Pathol. 1986;10:246–55.
151. Lin JD, Hsueh C, Chao TC, Weng JF, Huang BY. Thyroid follicular neoplasms diagnosed by high-resolution ultrasonography with fine needle aspiration cytology. Acta Cytol. 1997;41:687–91.
152. Iared W, Shigueoka DC, Cristófoli JC, et al. Use of color Doppler ultrasonography for the prediction of malignancy in follicular thyroid neoplasms: systematic review and meta-analysis. J Ultrasound Med. 2010;29:419–25.
153. Bondeson L, Bondeson AG, Ljungberg O, Tibblin S. Oxyphil tumors of the thyroid: follow-up of 42 surgical cases. Ann Surg. 1981;194:677–80.
154. Caplan RH, Abellera RM, Kisken WA. Hürthle cell tumors of the thyroid gland. A clinicopathologic review and long-term follow-up. JAMA. 1984;251:3114–7.
155. Chesky VE, Dreese WC, Hellwig CA. Hürthle cell tumors of the thyroid gland: a report on 25 cases. J Clin Endocrinol Metab. 1951;11:1535–48.

156. Frazell EL, Duffy Jr BJ. Hürthle-cell cancer of the thyroid; a review of forty cases. Cancer. 1951;4:952–6.
157. Gosain AK, Clark OH. Hürthle cell neoplasms. Malignant potential. Arch Surg. 1984;119:515–9.
158. Horn Jr RC. Hürthle-cell tumors of the thyroid. Cancer. 1954;7:234–44.
159. Saull SC, Kimmelman CP. Hürthle cell tumors of the thyroid gland. Otolaryngol Head Neck Surg. 1985;93:58–62.
160. Phitayakorn R, McHenry CR. Follicular and Hürthle cell carcinoma of the thyroid gland. Surg Oncol Clin N Am. 2006;15:603–23.
161. Thompson NW, Dunn EL, Batsakis JG, Nishiyama RH. Hürthle cell lesions of the thyroid gland. Surg Gynecol Obstet. 1974;139:555–60.
162. Gundry SR, Burney RE, Thompson NW, Lloyd R. Total thyroidectomy for Hürthle cell neoplasm of the thyroid. Arch Surg. 1983;118:529–32.
163. Yutan E, Clark OH. Hürthle cell carcinoma. Curr Treat Options Oncol. 2001;2:331–5.
164. Tollefsen HR, Shah JP, Huvos AG. Hürthle cell carcinoma of the thyroid. Am J Surg. 1975;130:390–4.
165. Chiacchio S, Lorenzoni A, Boni G, Rubello D, Elisei R, Mariani G. Anaplastic thyroid cancer: prevalence, diagnosis and treatment. Minerva Endocrinol. 2008;33:341–57.
166. Are C, Shaha AR. Anaplastic thyroid carcinoma: biology, pathogenesis, prognostic factors, and treatment approaches. Ann Surg Oncol. 2006;13:453–64.
167. Takashima S, Morimoto S, Ikezoe J, et al. CT evaluation of anaplastic thyroid carcinoma. Am J Roentgenol. 1990;154:61–3.
168. Compagno J. Diseases of the thyroid. In: Barnes L, editor. Surgical pathology of the head and neck. New York: Marcel Dekker; 1985. p. 1435–86.
169. LiVolsi VA. Calcitonin: the hormone and its significance. Prog Surg Pathol. 1980;1:71–103.
170. Steiner AL, Goodman AD, Powers SR. Study of a kindred with pheochromocytoma, medullary thyroid carcinoma, hyperparathyroidism and Cushing's disease: multiple endocrine neoplasia, type 2. Medicine (Baltimore). 1968;47:371–409.
171. LiVolsi VA. Medullary carcinoma. In: LiVolsi VA, editor. Surgical pathology of the thyroid. Philadelphia: WB Saunders Co.; 1990. p. 217–20.
172. Hazard JB, The C. Cells (parafollicular cells) of the thyroid gland and medullary thyroid carcinoma. A review. Am J Pathol. 1977;88:213–50.
173. Mendelsohn G, Eggleston JC, Weisburger WR, Gann DS, Baylin SB. Calcitonin and histaminase in C-cell hyperplasia and medullary thyroid carcinoma. A light microscopic and immunohistochemical study. Am J Pathol. 1978;92:35–52.
174. Wolfe HJ, Melvin KE, Cervi-Skinner SJ, et al. C-cell hyperplasia preceding medullary thyroid carcinoma. N Engl J Med. 1973;289:437–41.
175. Aliapoulios MA, Kacoyanis GP. Primary and metastatic medullary thyroid carcinoma. Determination of thyrocalcitonin content by bioassay. Arch Surg. 1973;106:105–8.
176. Deftos LJ. Radioimmunoassay for calcitonin in medullary thyroid carcinoma. JAMA. 1974;227:403–6.
177. Dubé WJ, Bell GO, Aliapoulios MA. Thyrocalcitonin activity in metastatic medullary thyroid carcinoma. Further evidence for its parafollicular cell origin. Arch Intern Med. 1969;123:423–7.
178. Rosai J, Carcangiu ML, DeLellis RA. Tumors of the thyroid gland. Atlas of tumor pathology. Washington, DC: Armed Forces Institute of Pathology; 1992. p. 207–9.
179. Kebebew E, Ituarte PH, Siperstein AE, Duh QY, Clark OH. Medullary thyroid carcinoma: clinical characteristics, treatment, prognostic factors, and a comparison of staging systems. Cancer. 2000;88:1139–48.
180. Pelizzo MR, Boschin IM, Bernante P, et al. Natural history, diagnosis, treatment and outcome of medullary thyroid cancer: 37 years experience on 157 patients. Eur J Surg Oncol. 2007;33:493–7.
181. Roman S, Lin R, Sosa JA. Prognosis of medullary thyroid carcinoma: demographic, clinical, and pathologic predictors of survival in 1252 cases. Cancer. 2006;107:2134–42.
182. Lee S, Shin JH, Han BK, Ko EY. Medullary thyroid carcinoma: comparison with papillary thyroid carcinoma and application of current sonographic criteria. AJR Am J Roentgenol. 2010;194:1090–4.
183. Anscombe AM, Wright DH. Primary malignant lymphoma of the thyroid – a tumour of mucosa associated lymphoid tissue: review of seventy-six cases. Histopathology. 1985;9:81–7.
184. Burke JS, Butler JJ, Fuller LM. Malignant lymphomas of the thyroid. Cancer. 1977;39:1587–602.
185. Sakamoto A, Kasai N, Sugano H. Poorly differentiated carcinoma of the thyroid. A clinicopathologic entity for a high-risk group of papillary and follicular carcinomas. Cancer. 1983;52:1849–55.
186. Carcangiu ML, Zampi G, Rosai J. Poorly differentiated ("insular") thyroid carcinoma. A reinterpretation of Langhans' "wuchernde Struma". Am J Surg Pathol. 1984;8:655–68.
187. Papotti M, Botto Micca F, Favero A, Palestini N, Bussolati G. Poorly differentiated thyroid carcinomas with primordial cell component. A group of aggressive lesions sharing insular, trabecular, and solid patterns. Am J Surg Pathol. 1993;17:291–301.
188. Burman KD, Ringel MD, Wartofsky L. Unusual types of thyroid neoplasms. Endocrinol Metab Clin North Am. 1996;25:49–68.
189. Johnson NA, Tublin ME. Postoperative surveillance of differentiated thyroid carcinoma: rationale, techniques, and controversies. Radiology. 2008;249:429–44.
190. Schlumberger M, Berg G, Cohen O, et al. Follow-up of low-risk patients with differentiated thyroid carcinoma: a European perspective. Eur J Endocrinol. 2004;150:105–12.
191. Toubeau M, Touzery C, Arveux P, et al. Predictive value for disease progression of serum thyroglobulin levels measured in the postoperative period and after

(131)I ablation therapy in patients with differentiated thyroid cancer. J Nucl Med. 2004;45:988–94.
192. Rouxel A, Hejblum G, Bernier MO, et al. Prognostic factors associated with the survival of patients developing loco-regional recurrences of differentiated thyroid carcinomas. J Clin Endocrinol Metab. 2004;89:5362–8.
193. Wenig BM, Thompson LD, Adair CF, Shmookler B, Heffess CS. Thyroid papillary carcinoma of columnar cell type: a clinicopathologic study of 16 cases. Cancer. 1998;82:740–53.
194. Akslen LA, LiVolsi VA. Prognostic significance of histologic grading compared with subclassification of papillary thyroid carcinoma. Cancer. 2000;88:1902–8.
195. Kim TY, Kim WB, Kim ES, et al. Serum thyroglobulin levels at the time of 131I remnant ablation just after thyroidectomy are useful for early prediction of clinical recurrence in low-risk patients with differentiated thyroid carcinoma. J Clin Endocrinol Metab. 2005;90:1440–5.
196. Aygun N. Imaging of recurrent thyroid cancer. Otolaryngol Clin North Am. 2008;41:1095–106.
197. Lind P, Kohlfürst S. Respective roles of thyroglobulin, radioiodine imaging, and positron emission tomography in the assessment of thyroid cancer. Semin Nucl Med. 2006;36:194–205.
198. Sheth S, Hamper UM. Role of sonography after total thyroidectomy for thyroid cancer. Ultrasound Q. 2008;24:147–54.
199. Shin JH, Han BK, Ko EY, Kang SS. Sonographic findings in the surgical bed after thyroidectomy: comparison of recurrent tumors and nonrecurrent lesions. J Ultrasound Med. 2007;26:1359–66.
200. Wong KT, Choi FP, Lee YY, Ahuja AT. Current role of radionuclide imaging in differentiated thyroid cancer. Cancer Imaging. 2008;8:159–62.

Ultrasound Surveillance

7

Robert A. Sofferman

Single Nodules

Determining the size and character of a single nodule within the thyroid gland is dependent on both ultrasound and fine needle aspiration cytology. Although ultrasound can provide a strong index of suspicion of benignity or malignancy, the actual examination of adequate groups of cells under the eyes and expertise of an experienced cytopathologist is more definitive. As previously mentioned, there are specific targets which the clinician should consider to obtain the most representative sample. In spite of adherence to these principles, a false negative rate of nearly 5% can occur [1, 2].

In addition, in large nodules greater than 4 cm with proven benign cytology, a false negative rate even greater than 5% has been reported [3]. Thus, single nodules should be followed over time with sequential ultrasound examination. Even this process is not foolproof. One report of small nodules followed for 38 months with ultrasound and measurement of nodule growth indicated that errors are still unavoidable [4]. Regardless, any nodule which demonstrates significant increase in size should be suspect and considered for re-biopsy. What constitutes a "significant increase" worthy of resampling? Does change in volume of a nodule represent the most accurate measurement to be followed, or are there other simpler parameters? Measurement of the mean nodule diameter has been recommended as a considered dimension for following a nodule. A 20% increase in diameter of the nodule with at least 2-mm increase in two or more dimensions has been suggested by some authors [5, 6]. These values were considered prior to application of FNA cytology when TSH suppression was a clinical means of determining which nodules might be observed and others submitted to surgical intervention.

Just for historical interest, TSH suppression may still be considered in nodules in areas of the world where iodine intake is insufficient with the expectation that existing nodules may shrink and new nodules may not develop. However, in patients with normal dietary intake of iodine, only 17–25% of thyroid nodules shrink more than 50% in volume on suppressive dosages of levothyroxine [7–9]. This is no longer a recommended practice and has been replaced by ultrasound-guided FNA.

Brauer et al. and others [10–12] have strongly urged volume changes to be the most important measurements to be applied to long-term follow-up. They suggest that volume changes of 50% or greater are worthy of statistical significance in either growth or shrinkage.

The revised ATA guidelines [13] for following benign thyroid nodules suggest repeat ultrasound

R.A. Sofferman (✉)
Division of Otolaryngology-Head and Neck Surgery, University of Vermont School of Medicine, Fletcher Allen Health Care, 111 Colchester Ave., Burlington, VT 05401, USA
e-mail: robert.sofferman@vtmednet.org

R.A. Sofferman and A.T. Ahuja (eds.), *Ultrasound of the Thyroid and Parathyroid Glands*,
DOI 10.1007/978-1-4614-0974-8_7,

examinations at 6–18 months after the initial fine needle aspiration. If the nodule size is relatively unchanged over this time frame according to the just described parameters, the interval to the next examination can be extended to 3–5 years. If a lesion has mixed solid and cystic areas, the solid component is the volume/dimension to be measured.

Of course, if there are other clinical symptoms such as local pain or hoarseness and vocal cord dysfunction, the nodule should be sampled or removed regardless of the stability of the nodule dimensions. On the other hand, if the nodule has enlarged by palpation and preferably measured with ultrasound (more than a 50% change in volume or a 20% increase in at least 2 nodule dimensions with at least 2-mm increase in the solid component), repeat FNA should be performed [13].

ATA guidelines Recommendation B: "The recommendation is based on fair evidence that the service or intervention can improve health outcomes. However, the strength of the evidence is limited by the number, quality, of consistency of individual studies."

Benign cystic nodules frequently demonstrate recurrence after initial significant aspiration and reduction in size. In selected cases, either surgical removal via hemithyroidectomy or percutaneous alcohol injection may be considered. Whereas re-aspiration has a low rate of long-term control (7–38%), alcohol injection is considerably more successful (75–80%) [14, 15].

Thyroid Nodules in Children

Thyroid nodules are less common in children and have always been considered more at risk of malignancy. This concept may no longer be axiomatic. A malignancy rate for a single nodule in children below 18 years has been identified at 15–20% in some series [16–18].

Other studies have indicated that the frequency of thyroid cancer in nodules identified in children is the same as that of adults [17–19]. In fact, these statistics are irrelevant to the concepts of initial management and follow-up with ultrasound examination and guided FNA. Significant nodules must be sampled in the same way adults have been managed. There may be little evidence that all childhood solid thyroid nodules require surgical intervention, although a lifetime ahead of follow-up and potential resampling may suggest that thyroid lobectomy is the most practical approach.

Thyroid Nodules Detected During Pregnancy

Thyroid nodules during pregnancy can similarly be managed with guided FNA. Papillary carcinoma behaves in a similar manner to age-matched women with the disease who are not pregnant [20, 21]. If a nodule is identified early in pregnancy and is proven to be malignant, it should be followed with ultrasound monthly until the 24th week of gestation. If there has been significant enlargement of the nodule with ultrasound surveillance or new lymphadenopathy develops, a thyroidectomy and appropriate neck surgery would be a serious consideration during this second trimester. If the disease is stable on sequential ultrasound, surgery can be delayed until after delivery.

Ultrasonography in Surveillance After Surgical Management of Well-Differentiated Thyroid Carcinoma

There are certain circumstances where a total thyroidectomy may not have been performed as part of the initial management. A small papillary carcinoma less than 1 cm may have had a planned thyroid lobectomy alone. A follicular lesion which has been managed with a thyroid lobectomy may demonstrate capsular invasion on formal histopathology. This lesion would be technically classified as a follicular carcinoma but may not require a completion total thyroidectomy. The usual postoperative process of follow-up of

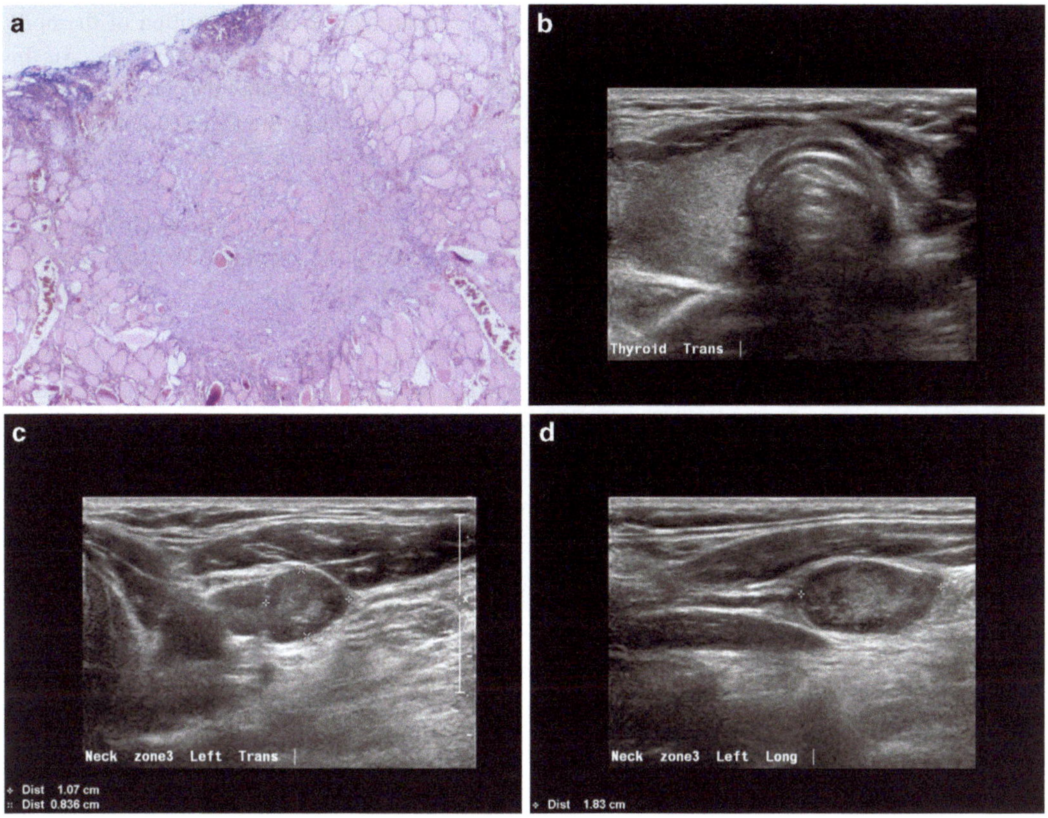

Fig. 7.1 The importance of lymph node surveillance is illustrated by this case of a patient with a mass in one lobe of the thyroid. The mass proved to be benign, and an incidental 3-mm micropapillary carcinoma was found (**a**). Five years later, the patient presented for a survey ultrasound. Although the remaining thyroid lobe was unremarkable (**b**), a complete lymph node survey demonstrated a malignant metastatic lymph node in zone III ipsilateral to the original microcarcinoma as demonstrated in these transverse (**c**) and sagittal images (**d**)

thyroid cancer with or without radioactive iodine ablation of remnant or microscopic disease involves assessment of serum thyroglobulin. The use of thyroglobulin for identification of recurrence or persistent disease requires that all thyroid tissue has been removed. In circumstances of lesser malignancy where a total thyroidectomy has not been performed, serum thyroglobulin cannot be used for surveillance. When there is potential for the development of cancer in the opposite lobe either as a second focus or lymphatic spread from the original tumor, the remaining lobe would be examined indefinitely with ultrasound on an annual basis. Any suspicious change is usually amenable to aspiration cytology.

The use of whole body RAI scans versus stimulated thyroglobulin assessment is the current important method of surveillance. The debate concerning which of these methods is preferred is beyond the purpose of this discussion, but there is a place for either concurrent or additional use of screening ultrasound of the thyroid and cervical node basins. High-resolution ultrasound is an effective means of systematically examining cervical lymph nodes. In addition, the sonographic identification of nodal metastasis in differentiated thyroid cancer has been recognized as a simple and advantageous means of follow-up [22–24]. An interesting representative case of a microcarcinoma with delayed cervical node metastasis illustrates many of these discussed elements of surveillance (Fig. 7.1).

The elements which indicate suspicion for malignancy in cervical nodes have already been characterized in this text. Interpreting the cytologic details which determine malignant cells is the responsibility of the cytopathologist, but there is still a false negative rate which can occur. The presence of thyroglobulin in cervical lymph nodes in the setting of a known prior differentiated thyroid cancer is diagnostic of metastasis. A relatively new and excellent advance in this field has amplified the ability to identify metastatic differentiated thyroid cancer [25, 26]. When a lymph node is sampled with ultrasound-guided FNA with cytology, a simple washout of the needle with 0.5 cc of saline should be performed and submitted for thyroglobulin assessment. Any thyroglobulin regardless of its concentration is abnormal and confirmatory, and this should be recognized as complimentary to the cytologic investigation.

In fact, even in circumstances where stimulated serum thyroglobulin is undetectable, cervical ultrasound can detect metastatic cervical lymphadenopathy [27].

One real and appropriate quandary is to determine the significance of microscopic metastasis to one or more lymph nodes. As this is still a question in the process of evolution, the most appropriate position is to review the current revised ATA guidelines for the use of ultrasound in search of lymph node metastasis [13]:

(a) Both the central and lateral cervical node regions should be examined with ultrasound at 6–12 months after surgery and then periodically. If a positive aspirate would alter management, suspicious nodes greater than 5–8 mm should be sampled with both cytology and Tg washout assessment.
(b) Suspicious lymph nodes less than 5–8 mm in greatest dimension may not require biopsy but should be followed with subsequent ultrasound. If there is growth or vital structures are threatened, aspiration biopsy should be performed.
(c) Lastly, the decision of just how to manage identification of one or more metastatic lymph nodes usually falls within the purview of a surgical process. This depends on many factors such as tumor stage, original surgical management of the lateral neck and central compartment, size and position of the node, and many other important issues. At this point, surgery remains the most appropriate option for addressing metastatic nodes as the efficacy of radioactive iodine has not been proven [28].

Other creative techniques which depend on prior ultrasound localization are radiofrequency and ethanol ablation [29, 30]. The challenges will be to determine when they will replace simple surgical excision or regional node dissection and how to guarantee safety for surrounding structures.

References

1. Carmeci C, Jeffrey RB, McDoughall IR, Nowels KW, Weigel RJ. Thyroid. 1998;8:283–9.
2. Ylagan LR, Farkas T, Dehner LP. Fine needle aspiration of the thyroid: a cytohistologic correlation and study of discrepant cases. Thyroid. 2004;14:35–41.
3. McCoy KL, Jabbour N, Ogilvie JB, Ohori NP, Carty SE, Yim JH. The incidence of cancer and rate of false-negative cytology in thyroid nodules greater than or equal to 4 cm in size. Surgery. 2007;142:837–44.
4. Asanuma K, Kobayashi S, Shingu K, Hama Y, Yokoyama S, Fujimori M, et al. The rate of tumour growth does not distinguish between malignant and benign thyroid nodules. Eur J Surg. 2001;167:102–5.
5. Alexander EK, Hurwitz S, Heering JP, Benson CB, Frates MC, Doubilet PM, et al. Natural history of benign solid and cystic thyroid nodules. Ann Int Med. 2003;138:315–8.
6. Papini E, Petrucci L, Guglielmi R, Panunzi C, Rinaldi R, Bacci V, et al. Long-term changes in nodular goiter: a 5-year prospective randomized trial of levothyroxine suppressive therapy for benign cold thyroid nodules. J Clin Endocrinol Meat. 1998;83:780–3.
7. Zelmanovitz F, Genro S, Gross JL. Suppressive therapy with levothyroxine for solitary thyroid nodules: a double-blind controlled clinical study and cumulative meta-analyses. J Clin Endocrinol Metab. 1998; 83:3881 5.
8. Wemeau JL, Caron P, Schvartz C, Schlienger JL, Orgiazzi J, Cousty C, et al. Effects of thyroid-stimulating hormone suppression with levothyroxine in reducing the volume of solitary thyroid nodules and improving extranodular nonpalpable changes: a randomized, double-blind, placebo-controlled trial by the French Thyroid Research Group. J Clin Endocrinol Metab. 2002;87:4928–34.
9. Castro MR, Caraballo PJ, Morris JC. Effectiveness of thyroid hormone suppressive therapy in benign solitary thyroid nodules: a meta-analysis. J Clin Endocrinol Metab. 2002;87:4154–9.

10. Brauer VF, Eder P, Miehle K, Wiesner TD, Hasenclever H, Pashke R. Interobserver variation for ultrasound determination of thyroid nodule volumes. Thyroid. 2005;15:1169–75.
11. Brander AE, Viikinkoski VP, Nickels JI, Kivisaari LM. Importance of thyroid abnormalities detected at US screening: a 5-year follow-up. Radiology. 2000;215:801–6.
12. Oertel YC, Miyahara-Filipe L, Mendoza MG, Yu K. Value of repeated fine needle aspirations of the thyroid: an analysis of over ten thousand FNAs. Thyroid. 2007;17:1061–6.
13. Cooper D et al. Revised American Thyroid Association Management Guidelines for patients with thyroid nodules and differentiated thyroid cancer. Thyroid. 2009;19(11):1–48.
14. Bennedbaek FN, Hegedus L. Treatment of recurrent thyroid cysts with ethanol: a randomized double-blind controlled trial. J Clin Endocrinol Metab. 2003;88: 5773–7.
15. Valcavi R, Frasoldati A. Ultrasound-guided percutaneous ethanol injection therapy in thyroid cystic nodules. Endocr Pract. 2004;10:269–75.
16. Raab SS, Silverman JF, Elsheikh TM, Thomas PA, Wakely PE. Pediatric thyroid nodules: disease demographics and clinical management as determined by fine needle aspiration biopsy. Pediatrics. 1995;95: 46–9.
17. Corrias A, Einaudi S, Chiorboli E, Weber G, Crino A, Andrea M, et al. Accuracy of fine needle aspiration biopsy of thyroid nodules in detecting malignancy in childhood: comparison with conventional clinical, laboratory, and imaging approaches. J Clin Endocrinol Metab. 2001;86:4644–8.
18. Hung W. Solitary thyroid nodules in 93 children and adolescents, a 35-years experience. Horm Res. 1999; 52:15–8.
19. Gharib H, Zimmerman D, Goellner JR, Bridley SM, LeBlanc SM. Fine-needle aspiration biopsy: use in diagnosis and management of pediatric thyroid diseases. Endo Pract. 1995;1:9–13.
20. Moosa M, Mazzaferri EL. Outcome of differentiated thyroid cancer diagnosed in pregnant women. J Clin Endocdrinol Metab. 1997;82:2862–6.
21. Herzon FS, Morris DM, Segal MN, Rauch G, Parnell T. Coexistent thyroid cancer and pregnancy. Arch Otolaryngol Head Neck Surg. 1994;120:1191–3.
22. Kouvaraki MA, Shapiro SE, Fornage BD, Edeiken-Monro BS, Sherman SI, Vassilopoulou-Sellin R, et al. Role of preoperative ultrasonography in the surgical management of patients with thyroid cancer. Surgery. 2003;134:946–54.
23. Torlontano M, Crocetti U, Augello G, D'Aloiso L, Bonfitto N, Varraso A, et al. Comparative evaluation of recombinant human thyrotropin-stimulated thyroglobulin levels, I 131 whole-body scintigraphy, and neck ultrasonography in the follow-up of patients with papillary thyroid microcarcinoma who have not undergone radioiodine therapy. J Clin Endocrinol Metab. 2006;91:60–3.
24. Pacini F, Molinaro E, Castagna MG, Agate L, Elisei R, Ceccarelli C, et al. Recombinant human thyrotropin-stimulated serum thyroglobulin combined with neck ultrasonography has the highest sensitivity in monitoring differentiated thyroid carcinoma. J Clin Endocrio Metab. 2003;88:3668–73.
25. Snozek CL, Chambers EP, Reading CC, Sebo TJ, Sistrunk JW, Singh RJ, et al. Serum thyroglobulin, high resolution ultrasound, and lymph node thyroglobulin in diagnosis of differentiated thyroid carcinoma nodal metastases. J Clin Endocrinol Metab. 2007;92:4278–81.
26. Cunha N, Rodrigues F, Curado F, Ilheu O, Cruz C, Naidenov P, et al. Thyroglobulin detection in fine-needle aspirates of cervical lymph nodes: a technique for the diagnosis of metastatic differentiated thyroid cancer. Eur J Endocrinol. 2007;157:101–7.
27. Bachelot A, Cailleux AF, Klain M, Baudin E, Ricard M, Bellon N, et al. Relationship between tumor burden and serum thyroglobulin level in patients with papillary and follicular thyroid carcinoma. Thyroid. 2002;12:707–11.
28. Van Nostrand D, Atkins F, Yeganeh F, Acio E, Bursaw R, Wartofsky L. Dosimetrically determined doses of radioiodine for the treatment of metastatic thyroid carcinoma. Thyroid. 2002;12:121–34.
29. Dupuy DE, Monchik JM, Decrea C, Pisharodi L. Radiofrequency ablation of regional recurrence from well-differentiated thyroid malignancy. Surgery. 2001;130:971–7.
30. Lewis BD, Hay ID, Charboneau JW, McIver B, Reading CC, Goellner JR. Percutaneous ethanol injection for treatment of cervical lymph node metastases in patients with papillary thyroid carcinoma. Am J Roentgenol. 2002;178:699–704.

Parathyroid Ultrasound

8

Robert A. Sofferman

Before delving into a comprehensive discussion of parathyroid ultrasound, the embryology, anatomy, and particularly vascular supply of the parathyroid glands are relevant and important to review. This information will permit the sonographer/clinician to differentiate lymphadenopathy and thyroid pathology from true parathyroid lesions. As with any imaging study, the history and laboratory data will influence the expectations of the pathobiology and often whether one or more glands are enlarged. As an example, patients with renal failure or those with MEN syndromes are likely to demonstrate multiple-gland enlargement. The patient with extreme elevation in calcium and parathyroid hormone levels may be suspect for parathyroid carcinoma. The importance of linking clinical information to the concepts of parathyroid ultrasound cannot be overemphasized.

Embryology

The parathyroid glands arise from the dorsal aspect of branchial pouches 3 and 4. In a seeming paradox, the inferior parathyroid glands arise from the more rostral third branchial apparatus, and the superior glands, from the more distal fourth branchial system (Figs. 8.1 and 8.2). In the formation of the thyroid gland where there is fusion of the medial and lateral anlage, occasionally, the parathyroid tissue can be trapped within the mature thyroid gland. Exactly how this occurs and which glands are most likely to be involved are unclear, but it is a real entity and must be considered in the search for the elusive parathyroid at certain surgical interventions. A recent study of 178 surgically confirmed patients with primary hyperparathyroidism indicates a 3.4% rate of this condition [1].

In this series, two entrapped glands were of superior origin, and four involved the inferior gland. When the gland is intrathyroidal, the parathyroid retains its vascular pattern. In contrast, the thyroid adenoma does not demonstrate the same single vascular pattern as its vascularity is more diffuse from the surrounding thyroid tissues and too small for Doppler identification.

Normal Anatomy

Gilmour studied the parathyroid glands in a study of 428 cadavers. In 87% of individuals, four parathyroid glands were identified. In 6.3%, only three parathyroid glands were found, and in 5.8% of cadavers, five parathyroids were proven. However, there may be even larger numbers of parathyroid glands than one usually considers. In that study, 0.5% of cadavers revealed six parathyroid glands, and there were 8 and 12

R.A. Sofferman (✉)
Division of Otolaryngology-Head and Neck Surgery, University of Vermont School of Medicine, Fletcher Allen Health Care, 111 Colchester Ave., Burlington, VT 05401, USA
e-mail: robert.sofferman@vtmednet.org

R.A. Sofferman and A.T. Ahuja (eds.), *Ultrasound of the Thyroid and Parathyroid Glands*,
DOI 10.1007/978-1-4614-0974-8_8, © Springer Science+Business Media, LLC 2012

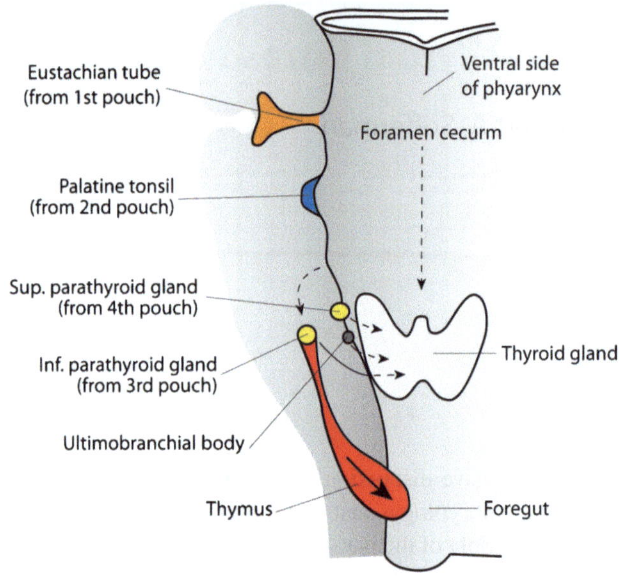

Fig. 8.1 Embryology of the parathyroid glands demonstrates the third and fourth branchial pouch relationships

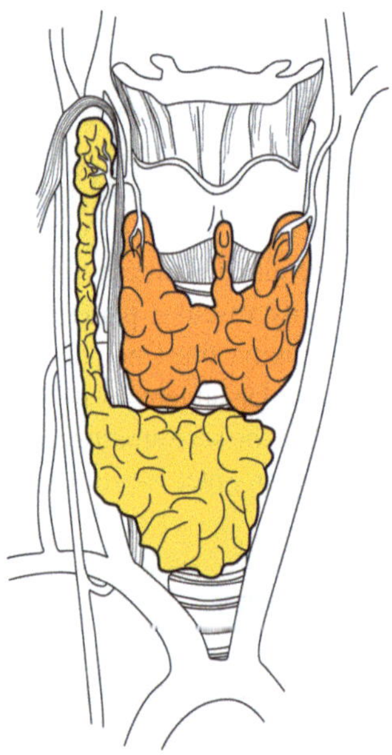

Fig. 8.2 The inferior parathyroid gland may not descend and remain in the upper cervical region along with the "parathymus"

parathyroid glands, respectively, in two studied individuals [2].

The cardinal parathyroid position is peri- or subcapsular, and the normal glands are the size of a flattened pea. The normal gland weighs approximately 40–60 mg and has ovoid dimensions of $4 \times 2 \times 6$ mm. When enlarged, they vary considerably in size and color. Most commonly, a single adenoma is ovoid in shape and nearly anechoic in appearance (Fig. 8.3a, b). Occasionally, the large adenoma is a mixture of solid and cystic elements which can alter this echogenic pattern (Fig. 8.3c). Whether normal or enlarged, the inferior parathyroid gland is usually found at or near the posterior aspect of the inferior thyroid pole. The superior glands are generally found adjacent to the posterosuperior aspect of the thyroid gland and generally located within 2 cm of the junctional crossing of the inferior thyroid artery and recurrent laryngeal nerve (Fig. 8.4).

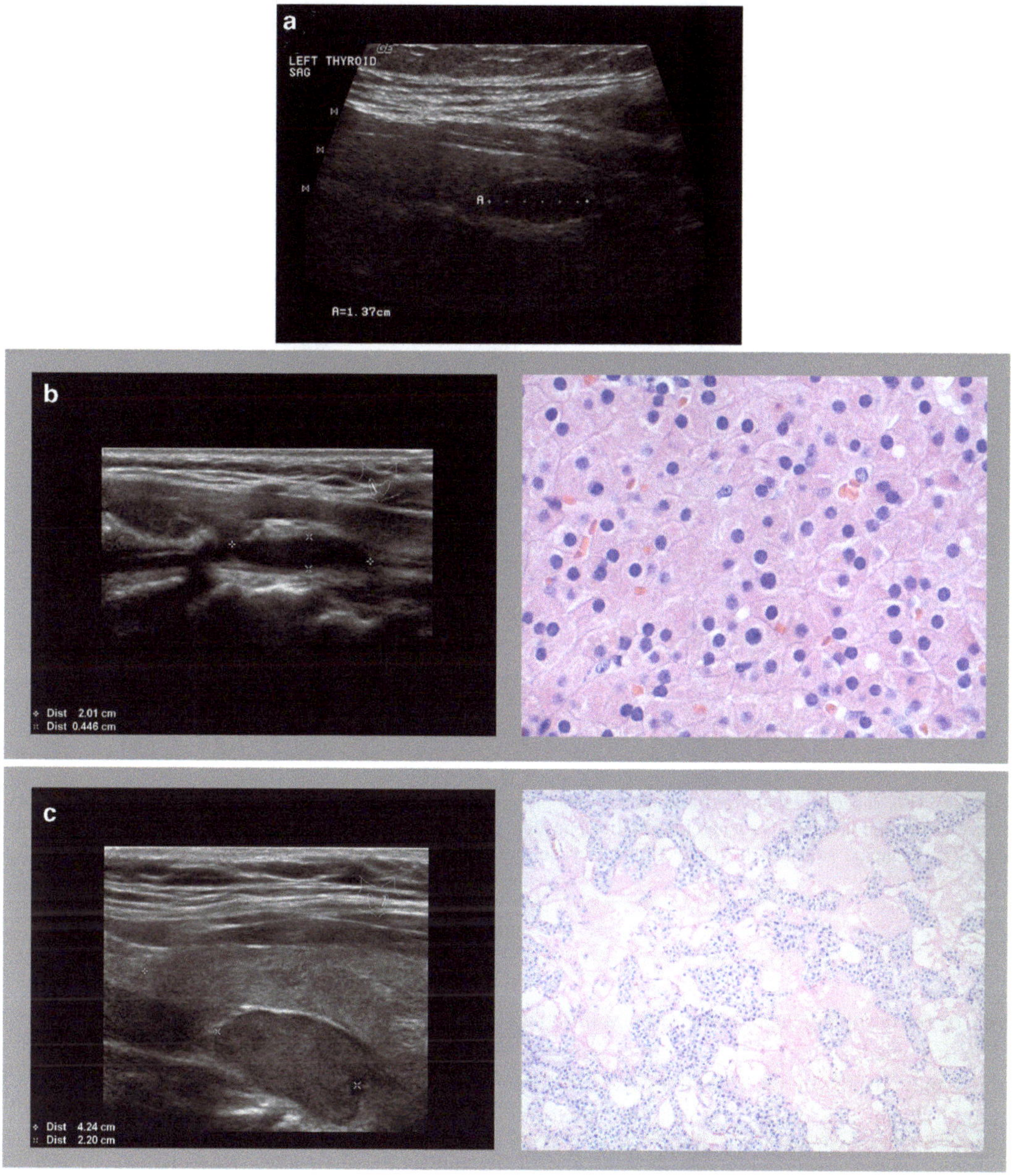

Fig. 8.3 A typical inferior parathyroid adenoma is demonstrated in the sagittal plane (**a**).The dense, uniform cellular structure may reflect the nearly anechoic appearance of the ultrasound image (**b**). This parathyroid adenoma demonstrates a heterogeneous cellular and fluid-like composition, likely the basis of its less echogenic appearance (**c**)

Ectopic Position

Ectopy of parathyroid location is linked to variations in embryologic development. For example, the thymus, as well as the inferior parathyroid glands, derives from the third branchial pouch. Thus the ectopic inferior parathyroid is often found in the thyrothymic ligament or further down in the anterior mediastinum, imbedded within the thymus (Figs. 8.2, 8.5–8.6). Ectopic superior parathyroid glands are dorsal to the recurrent nerve and other fourth arch structures.

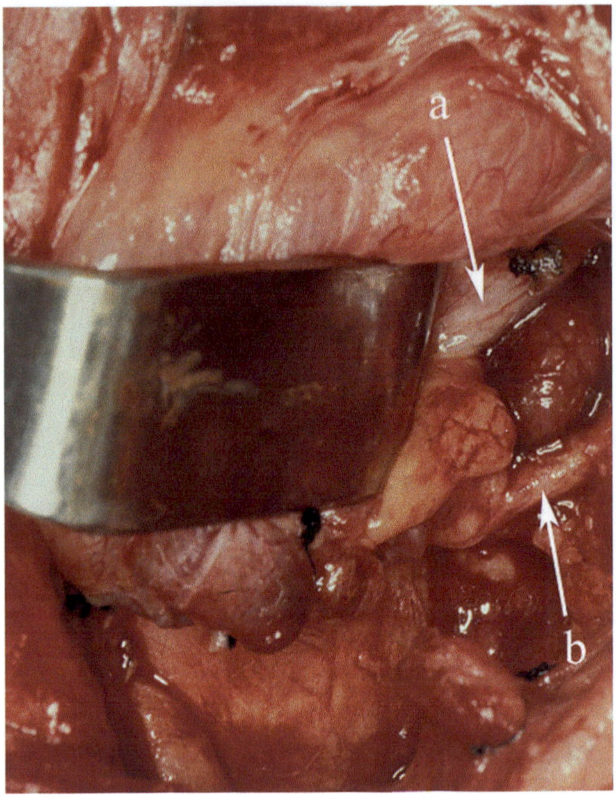

Fig. 8.4 This superior parathyroid adenoma is demonstrated as the thyroid gland is rotated toward the opposite side. The adenoma is dorsal to the recurrent laryngeal nerve (**a**) which thus determines that it is of superior origin. The relationship to the inferior thyroid artery is demonstrated (**b**)

Thus, these parathyroids' out-of-normal position may be retroesophageal and can descend into the posterior mediastinum. The ectopic superior gland may reside in the lateral neck, and the carotid sheath may harbor the ectopic superior gland. The parathyroid adenoma may reside entirely within the thyroid gland in 2–5% of cases [3, 4]. Lastly, the inferior parathyroid glands may never descend properly and remain in zone I of the neck along with the parathymus (Figs. 8.2, 8.7–8.9). On occasion, normal parathyroid tissue may be identified adherent to the apex of a Zenker's diverticulum or pyriform sinus (Fig. 8.10a, b). This may be one position of an undescended superior parathyroid gland.

Vascular Pattern

The parathyroid glands have a distinct and often dual blood supply. A study of 357 parathyroid vascular pedicles by Flament et al. demonstrates a single artery in 80%, two distinct arteries in 15%, and three distinct vessels in 4% of studied parathyroid glands [5]. The inferior thyroid artery is the principal supplier to both the superior and inferior parathyroid glands. However, the superior parathyroid may have its sole vascular supply from the superior thyroid artery. The superior parathyroid gland receives its dominant blood supply from the inferior thyroid artery in 80% of

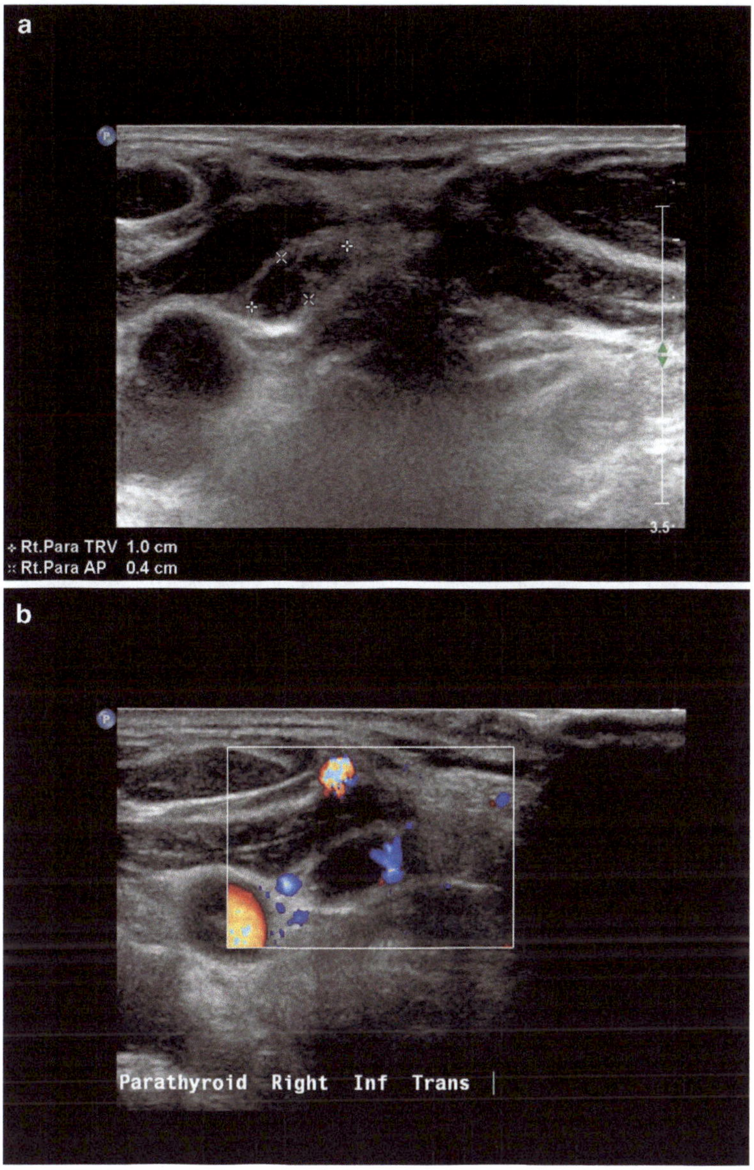

Fig. 8.5 A thymic parathyroid adenoma is demonstrated in transverse plane (**a**), often the only view possible due to the medial clavicular heads and sternal manubrium. Note that no thyroid gland is seen in this low transverse scan. Doppler shows the characteristic vascularity of an adenoma (**b**). This is helpful in differentiating a lymph node from an enlarged ectopic parathyroid gland

analyzed glands, from the superior thyroid artery in 15%, and an anastomosis of both vessels in only 5%. The inferior parathyroid gland receives its primary vascular supply solely from the inferior thyroid artery in 90% of analyzed glands, and only 10% of inferior parathyroids receive the dominant vessel from the superior parathyroid artery.

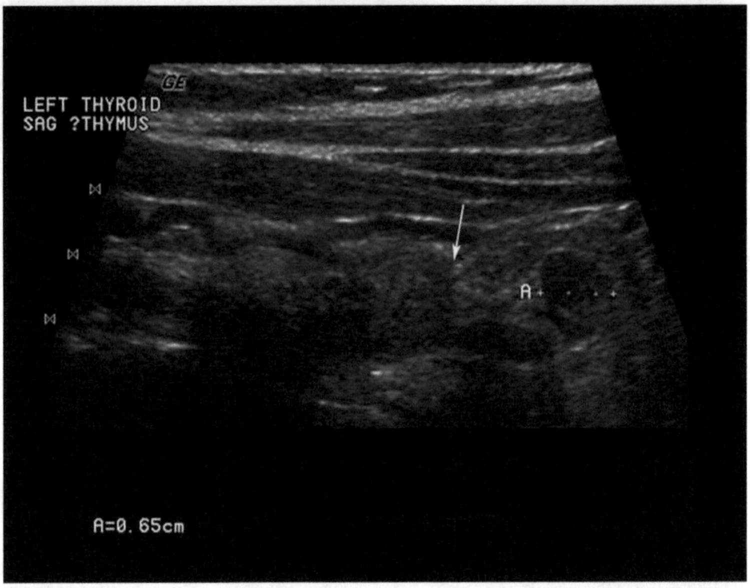

Fig. 8.6 In this sagittal view of a thymic parathyroid adenoma, the *arrow* demonstrates the lower border of the thyroid gland which is well separated from the adenoma

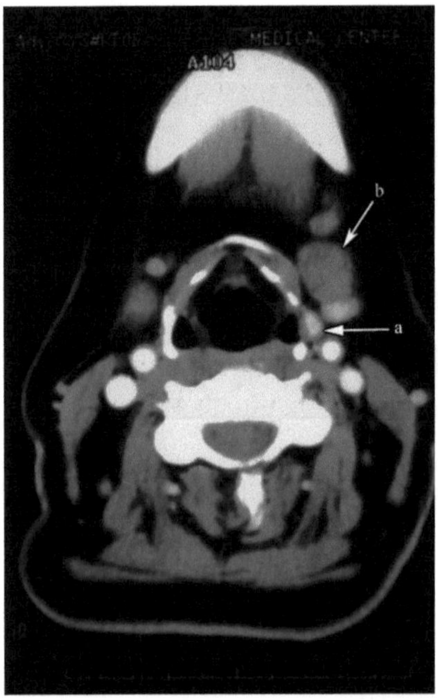

Fig. 8.7 This patient was evaluated after a failed parathyroid exploration. Sestamibi scan was interpreted as negative, and no preoperative ultrasound was performed in this early case. CT scan demonstrates a small mass adjacent to the left pyriform sinus (**a**). The submandibular gland is defined (**b**)

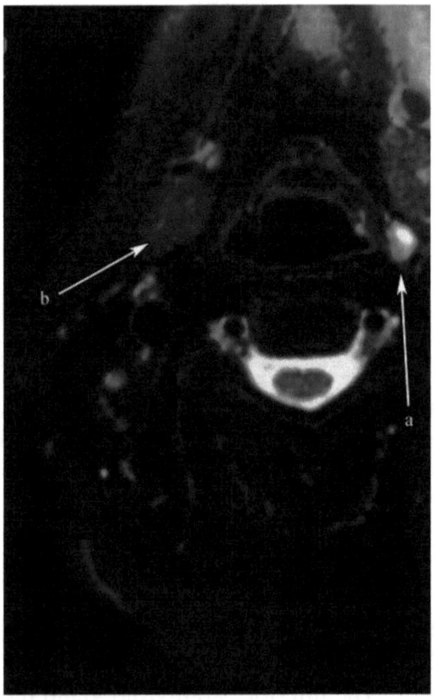

Fig. 8.8 MRI scan confirms the findings on previous CT scan. The undescended parathyroid gland/adenoma is demonstrated (**a**), as is the opposite submandibular gland (**b**)

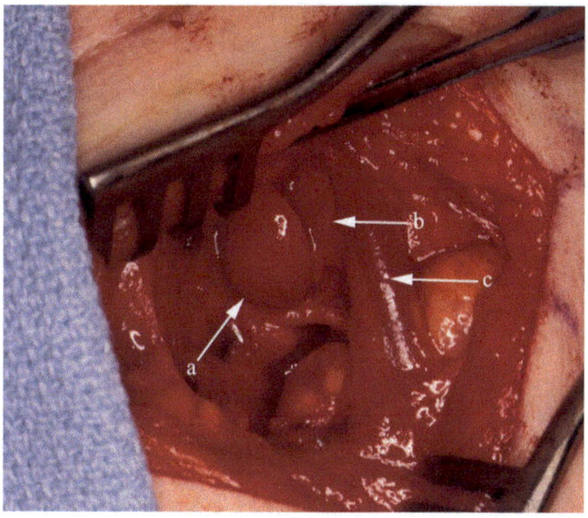

Fig. 8.9 Operative view demonstrates the adenoma (**a**) within zone I adjacent to the submandibular gland (**b**) and common facial vein (**c**). These operative photographs are from the patient demonstrated in Figs. 8.7 and 8.8

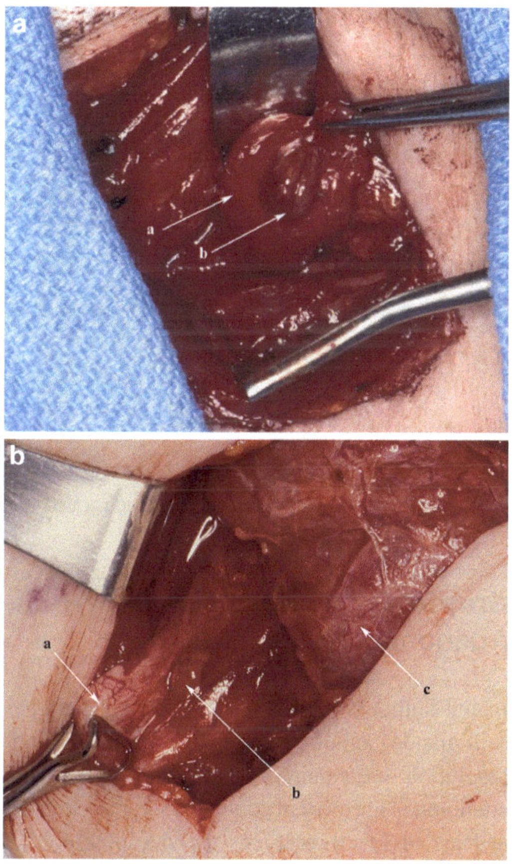

Fig. 8.10 Parathyroid glands can be ectopic in unusual locations. These two separate intraoperative cases demonstrate normal parathyroid glands (**b**) on the surface of the Zenker's diverticulum (**a**). The thyroid gland (**c**) is demonstrated for reference

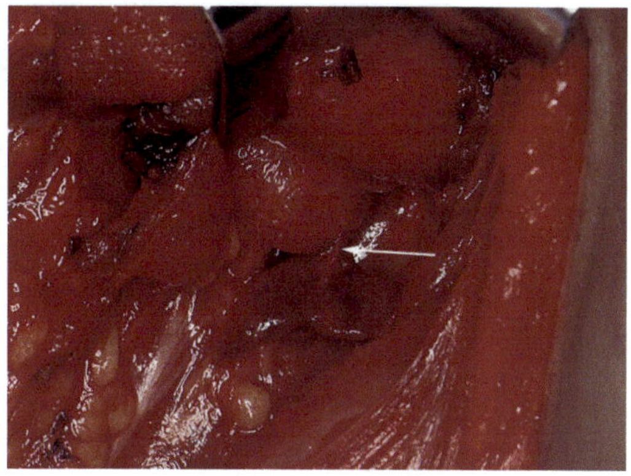

Fig. 8.11 A single vessel to a parathyroid adenoma is demonstrated in an operative image

Regardless, each parathyroid gland has a dominant single vessel as a generous branch from its larger-named parent artery, and this can be readily appreciated with Doppler when a gland is enlarged as an adenoma (Figs. 8.11–8.12). It is important to emphasize that there is a limited contribution to the parathyroid gland from the adjacent thyroid capsule or parenchyma. Of course, the venous outflow and lymphatic supply accompany the parathyroid tributaries and main artery.

Technical Considerations

One principal consideration in ultrasound imaging of enlarged parathyroid glands is body habitus and thyroid position. A patient with excessive neck adiposity or dense dermis may have impairment of ideal penetration and reflection of sound waves with resultant reduction in image resolution. The low thyroid may preclude adequate sagittal imaging due to mechanical interference from the clavicular heads. An elderly patient or individual with kyphosis or other anatomical abnormality may not allow adequate neck extension, thus limiting investigation of the parathyroid regions of interest. The shape of the transducer may determine the ease or difficulty of ultrasound recognition of an enlarged parathyroid gland. High-frequency transducers of 10–12 MHz allow

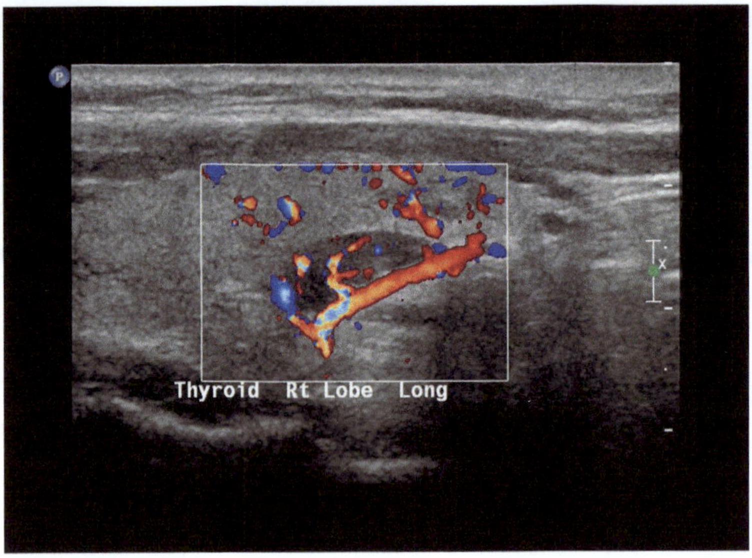

Fig. 8.12 Doppler demonstrates the characteristic dominant parathyroid artery conforming to the surface of the parathyroid adenoma

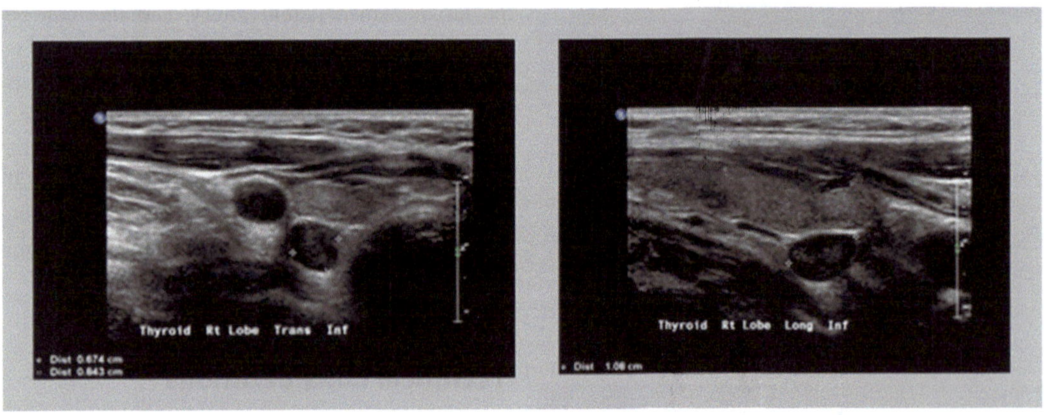

Fig. 8.13 Typical transverse and sagittal ultrasound images of an inferior parathyroid adenoma are demonstrated

best axial resolution. Power Doppler examines low-flow vascularity of small vessels, a process which is very helpful in distinguishing parathyroid from lymph node. In contrast, color Doppler may readily determine flow volumes and directionality in large vessels, but this process is irrelevant to virtually every aspect of parathyroid anatomy and pathophysiology. Some color Doppler machines image in broadband, which produce excellent image quality of even the smallest vessels of interest and serve as an adequate alternative to power Doppler.

Gray Scale Imaging of a Parathyroid Adenoma

In the author's experience, the normal parathyroid glands cannot be visualized with even high-resolution ultrasound. The typical parathyroid adenoma is uniform in echogenicity, hypoechoic, at least two to three times the size of a normal gland, and teardrop in shape [6]. The inferior adenoma is usually immediately adjacent to the posterolateral thyroid capsule (Fig. 8.13). The

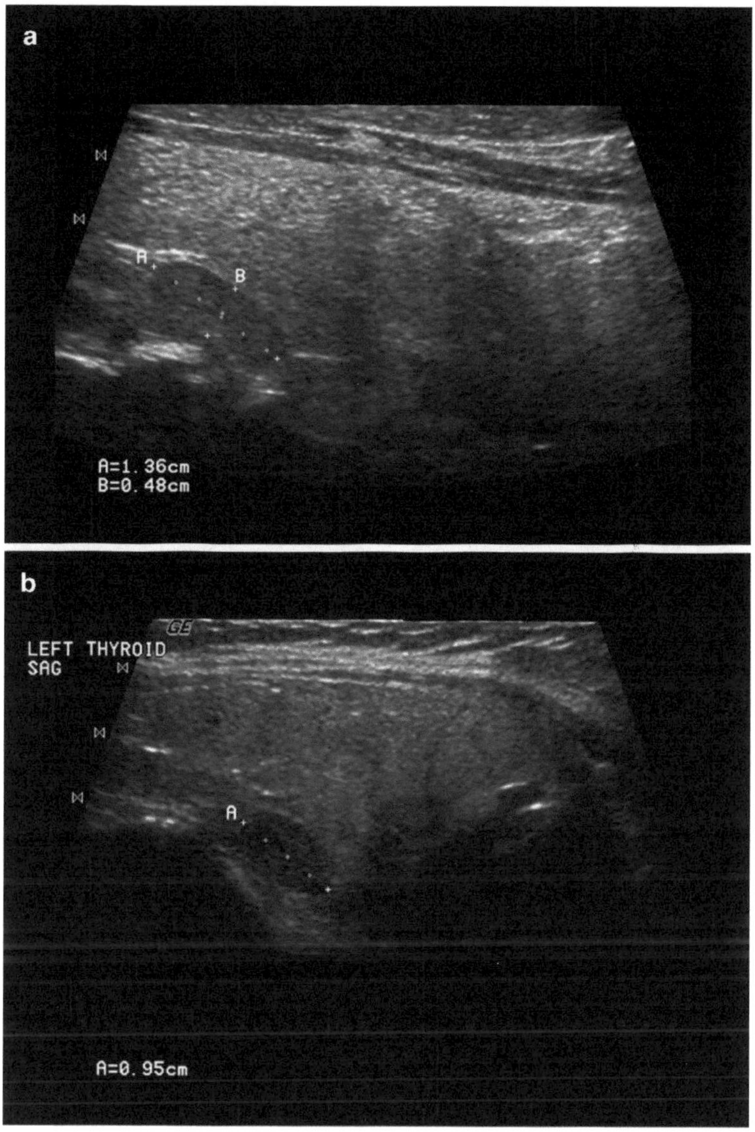

Fig. 8.14 A superior parathyroid adenoma is illustrated in two separate patients illustrated with sagittal thyroid ultrasound

superior adenoma in the cardinal position is ovoid in shape and similarly enlarged and resides posterior to the superior thyroid capsule (Fig. 8.14). In each of these circumstances, the adenoma capsule is distinct and hyperechoic relative to its parenchyma [7]. Larger adenomas may be cystic, lobulated, contain calcification, or demonstrate increased echogenicity [8] (Fig. 8.15a, b). In some circumstances, the superior parathyroid may actually be below the level of the enlarged inferior parathyroid gland (Fig. 8.16a). This would be an ectopic superior gland and is one of the many variations identified with parathyroid hyperplasia or MEN I (Fig. 8.16b).

Ectopic superior parathyroids are otherwise difficult to visualize posterior to the esophagus (Fig. 8.17a, b) and, of course, when in the chest, may not be identified by ultrasound. Ultrasound may identify more than the usual four glands in hyperplasia when Tc-99 m sestamibi cannot be

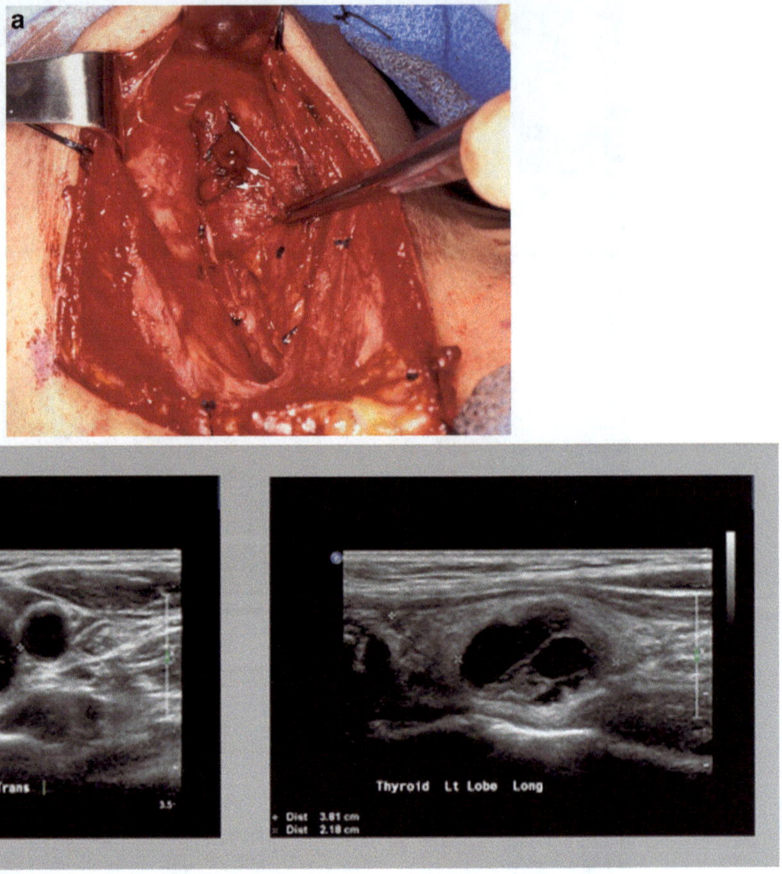

Fig. 8.15 An enlarged, lobulated parathyroid gland (denoted by *arrows*) is demonstrated intraoperatively and suggests diffuse hyperplasia (**a**). This is an important finding at surgery and may be identifiable at preoperative ultrasound. A cystic intrathyroidal adenoma is demonstrated in both transverse and sagittal images (**b**)

relied upon to provide preoperative imaging information. When an inferior parathyroid adenoma is ectopic in the upper anterior mediastinum, it may be properly imaged with the transducer in the transverse orientation and angled downward. With the option of changing ultrasound frequency, occasionally a lower-frequency setting can allow deeper penetration and idealized imaging. A subcapsular adenoma is not truly intrathyroidal. Although rare, a true intrathyroidal parathyroid adenoma should be suspected and usually formally identified with preoperative ultrasound (Fig. 8.18a, b). The intrathyroidal adenoma so imaged may be impossible to differentiate from a thyroid adenoma in gray scale alone (Fig. 8.19). In order to qualify as a true intrathyroidal adenoma, it must be completely surrounded by thyroid tissue (Fig. 8.20). When a parathyroid adenoma cannot be imaged in the usual locations, a complete ultrasound survey must then ensue. The entire neck must be examined systematically with specific inspection of the full carotid sheath (Figs. 8.21–8.23), upper neck and paraesophagus, and as much of the mediastinum as the anatomy will allow.

Power Doppler

Ultrasonographic display of the vascular supply of a parathyroid adenoma is a little recognized advantage [9]. There is always a large vessel in

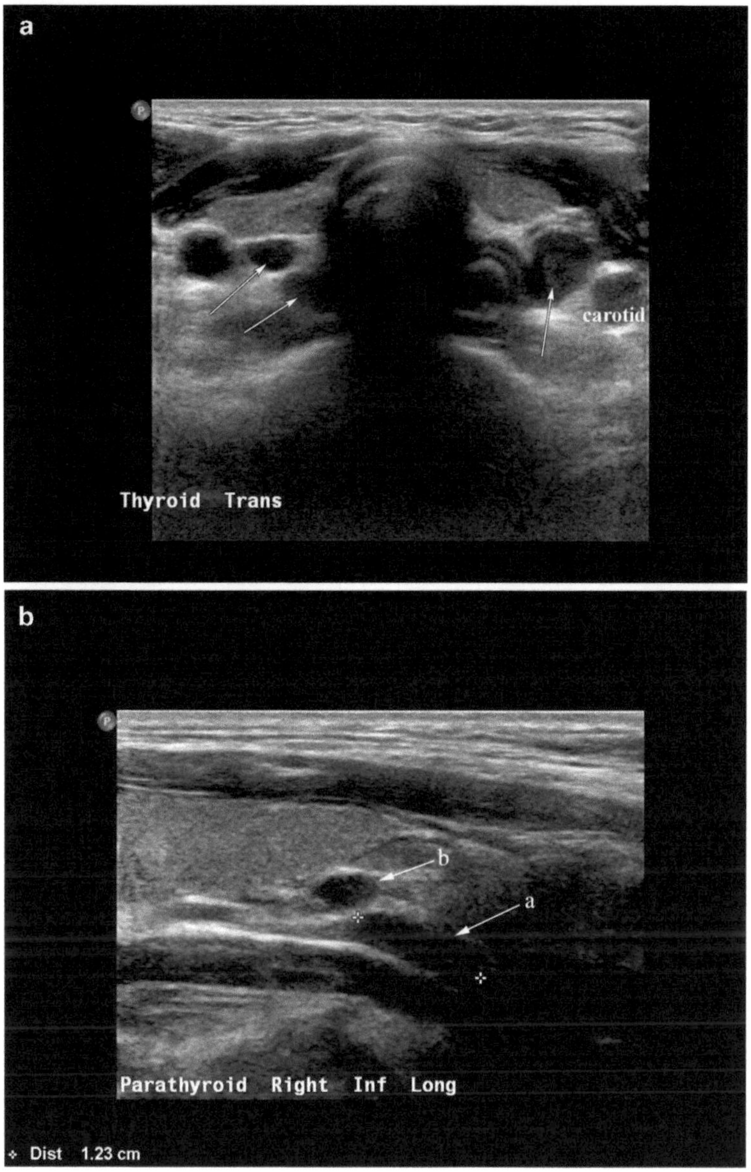

Fig. 8.16 (**a**) This transverse thyroid view of a patient with MEN I demonstrates three enlarged parathyroid glands, as designated by the *arrows* (**b**) Sagittal view of the same patient with MEN I. Both superior and inferior parathyroid glands can be below the midsagittal point of the thyroid gland. The superior parathyroid gland (*a*) is more inferior in position than the adjacent inferior hyperplastic parathyroid (*b*) in this particular patient

close proximity to the lesion [10], usually contributing to the end artery which enters the adenoma from an anterior and superior position (Fig. 8.24). The most important characteristic on power Doppler is a reproducible blunt termination of the vessel a few millimeters after it enters the parenchyma of the adenoma (Fig. 8.25). In contrast, the vascular supply of a lymph node within its parenchyma is quite different in distribution. The primary vessel arborizes into smaller arteries which may be properly demonstrated with appropriate manipulation of the Doppler

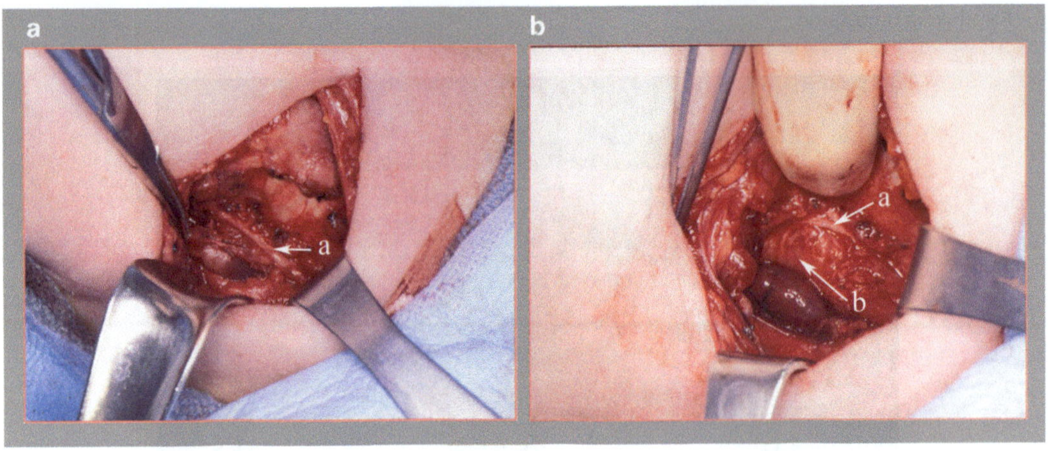

Fig. 8.17 A retroesophageal parathyroid adenoma is demonstrated as it has been retrieved after identification with digital palpation. This patient has had a thyroid lobectomy at the same procedure demonstrating the recurrent laryngeal nerve (**a**) and esophagus (**b**). This adenoma was not able to be identified with ultrasound

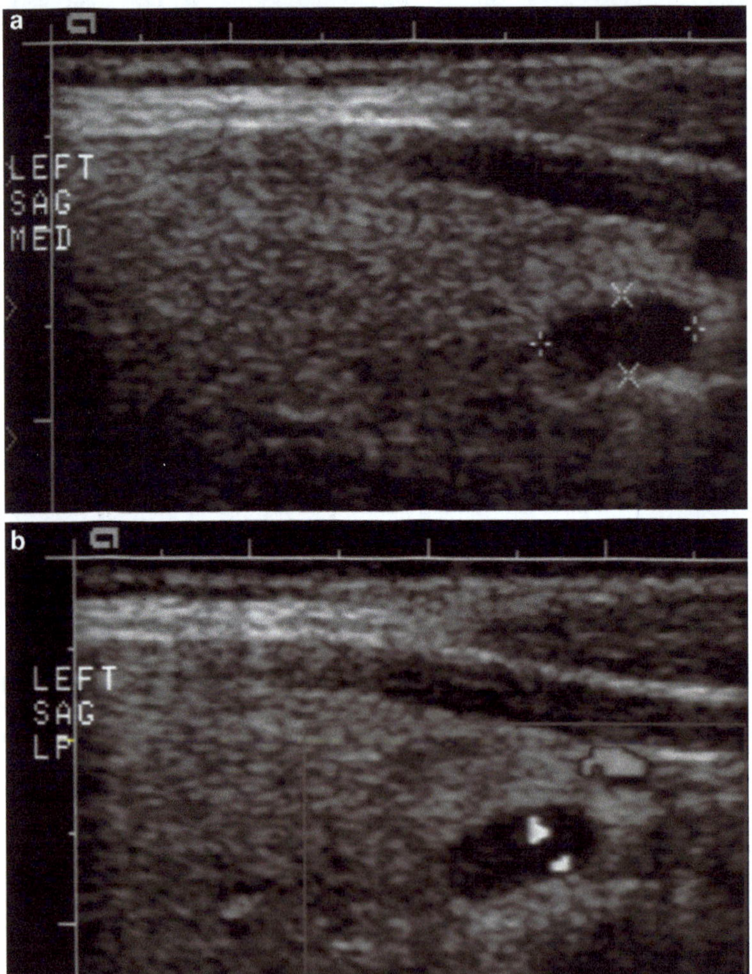

Fig. 8.18 This proven intrathyroidal parathyroid adenoma is completely surrounded by thyroid tissue (**a**). Doppler in gray scale demonstrates its unique singular blood supply (**b**)

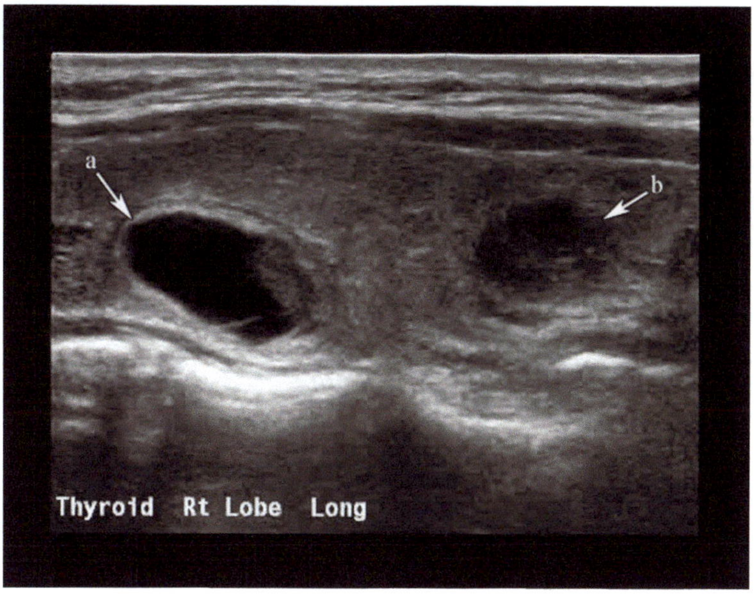

Fig. 8.19 This sagittal ultrasound demonstrates two potential intrathyroidal parathyroid adenomas. The superior lesion proved to be a colloid cyst (**a**), and the inferior less distinct mass, the actual parathyroid adenoma (**b**) proven on FNA for PTH

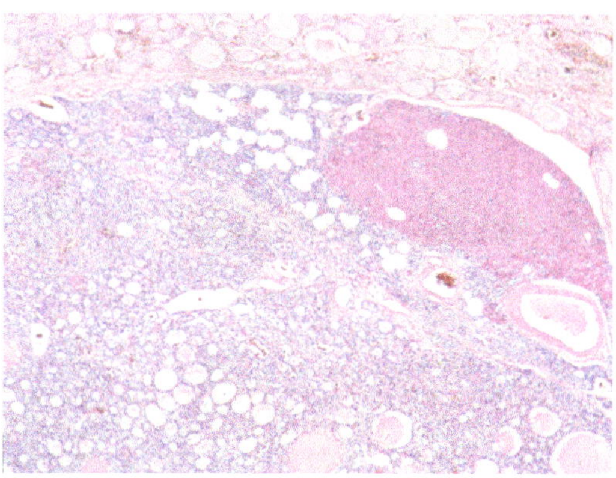

Fig. 8.20 A partial view of the histology of an intrathyroidal parathyroid adenoma demonstrates the full perimeter of enveloping thyroid tissue

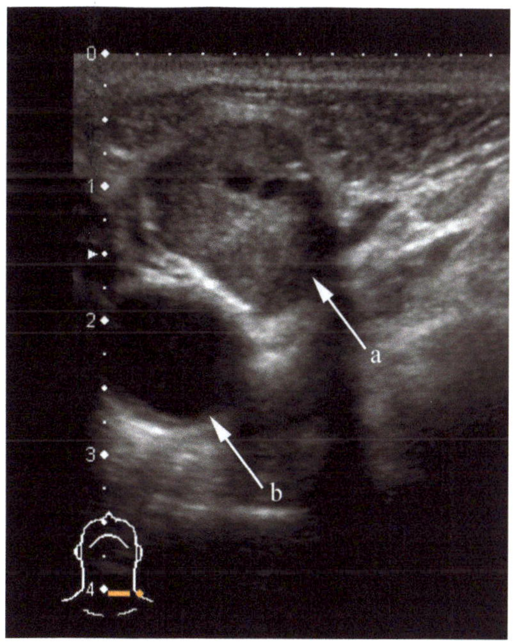

Fig. 8.21 A parathyroid adenoma (**a**) ectopic to the carotid sheath (**b**) is demonstrated with ultrasound (Courtesy: Dr. Asif Momin, Mumbai, India)

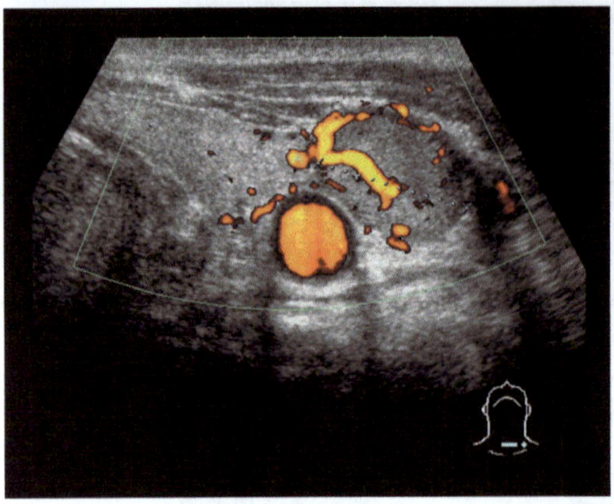

Fig. 8.22 Power Doppler of carotid sheath parathyroid adenoma. Note the typical blunt termination of the single vessel into the parenchyma (Courtesy: Dr. Asif Momin, Mumbai, India)

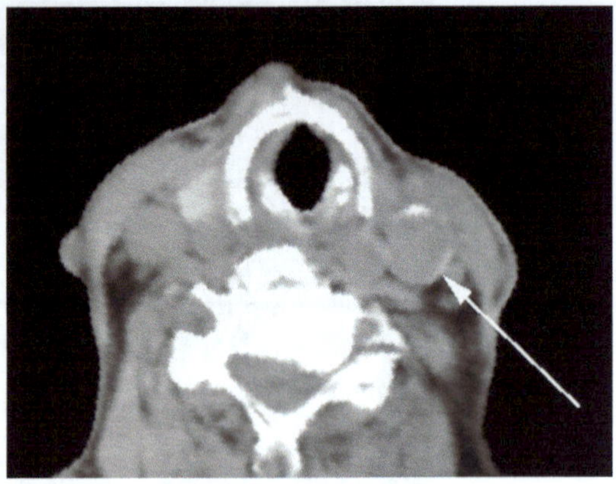

Fig. 8.23 *Arrow* demonstrates the carotid sheath parathyroid adenoma, as noted on CT scan (Courtesy: Dr. Asif Momin, Mumbai, India)

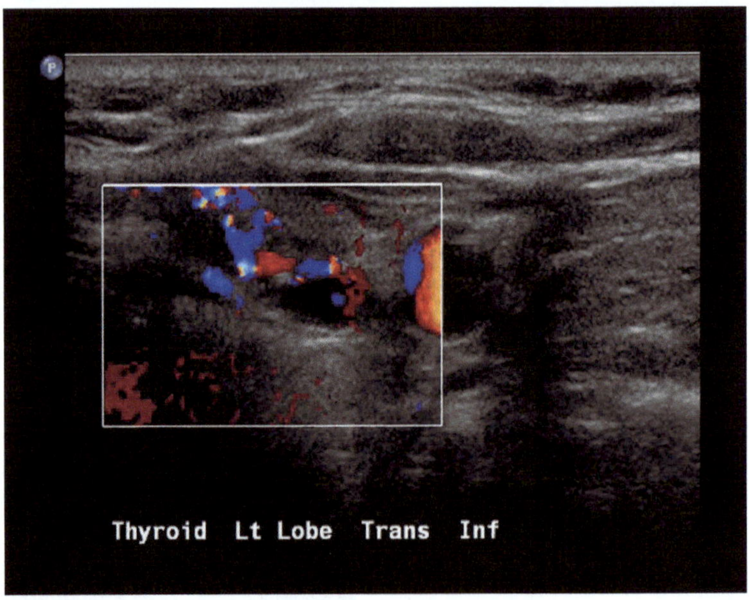

Fig. 8.24 Doppler demonstrates the parathyroid artery entering an inferior parathyroid adenoma from an anterosuperior direction

gain and changes in transducer orientation (Fig. 8.26). This issue is particularly important when an adenoma is ectopic to the thymus and anterior mediastinum, and the clinician must differentiate adenoma from lymph node, especially when the Tc sestamibi scan is negative. For this reason, Doppler resolution should be an important consideration when determining purchase of an ultrasound machine. Smaller adenomas may not demonstrate sestamibi uptake while ultrasound is often the only imaging study which defines the proper preoperative location of the offending gland (Fig. 8.27a, b, c). In a study of 28 parathyroid adenomas, 100% of gray

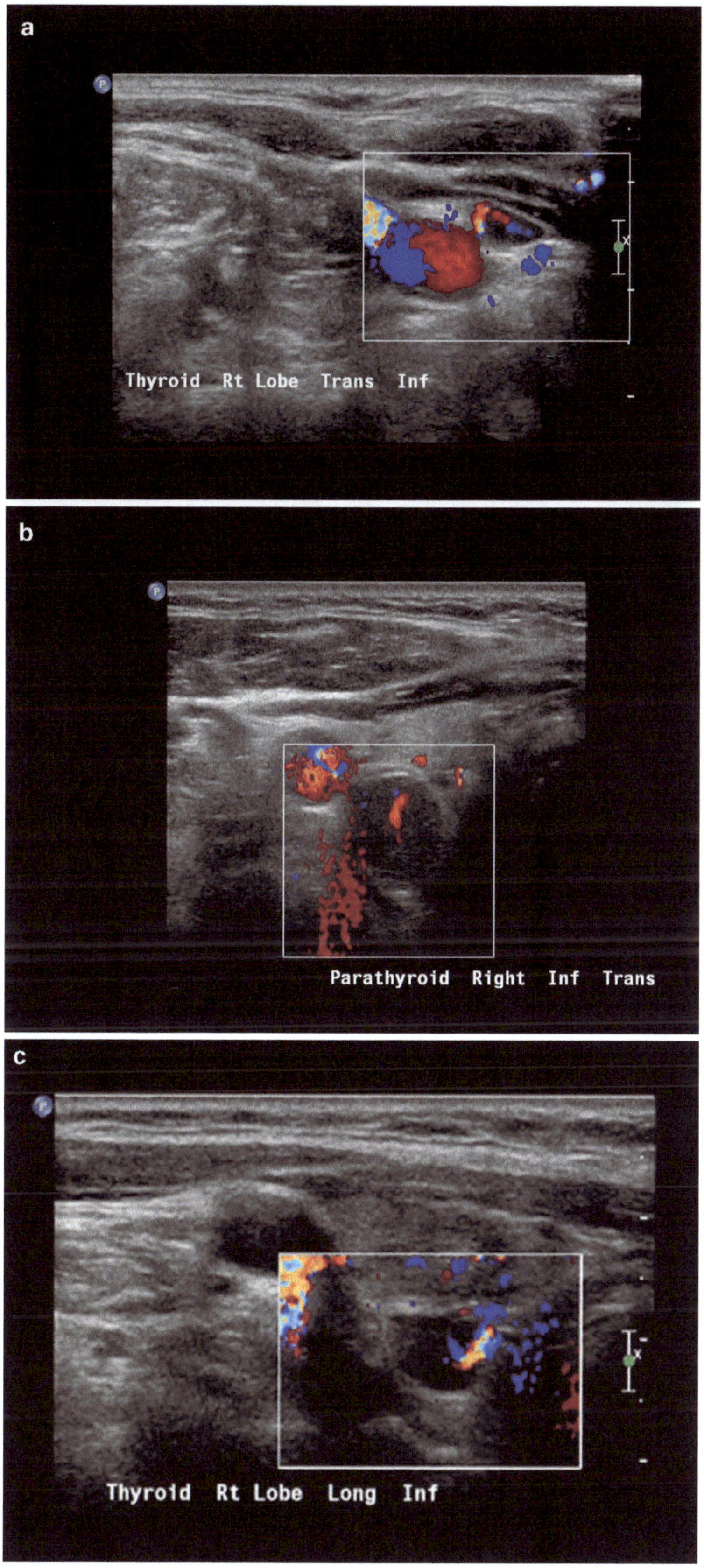

Fig. 8.25 The primary artery to the adenoma ends bluntly in its parenchyma (**a**, **b**, **c**)

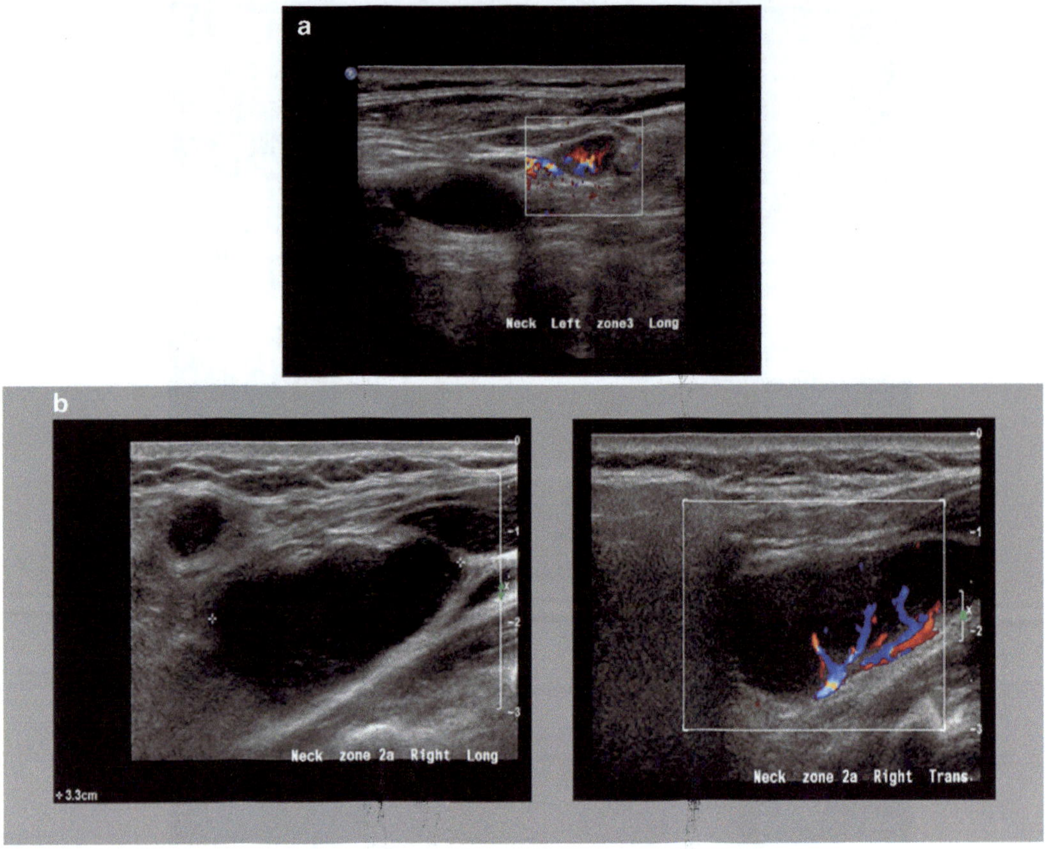

Fig. 8.26 Doppler imaging of a hyperplastic lymph node demonstrates a pattern of internal arborization within the lymph node (**a**, **b**).This pattern is different from that of a parathyroid adenoma which generally shows a blunt end to the larger defined internal vessel

scale images defined the specific enlarged gland when it was greater than 1 cm in longest dimension. However, only 11% of adenomas were appropriately identified with gray scale ultrasound when the gland was less than 1 cm in size. Additionally, sestamibi uptake may not occur in certain defined histology such as lesions which have a predominance of water-clear cells rather than mitochondria-rich oxyphil cells. In 25 of 28 adenomas, the addition of Doppler aided in proper demonstration of the enlarged gland [11]. Another study of 42 parathyroid adenomas identified a specific extrathyroidal artery in 35 masses, and in five cases, the Doppler study was the only process which allowed proper identification of the actual adenoma [12]. Thus, Doppler imaging is extremely important to preoperative localization.

Aspiration PTH

Ultrasound-guided FNA is a fundamental element of assessment of thyroid nodules. In circumstances where a patient with primary hyperparathyroidism has an undetected adenoma in the usual expected position and an ipsilateral thyroid nodule demonstrated, an intrathyroidal parathyroid adenoma is to be considered [13]. This is the perfect scenario for ultrasound-guided aspiration for PTH and needle rinse with 0.5 cc of saline. Even moderate elevation of PTH

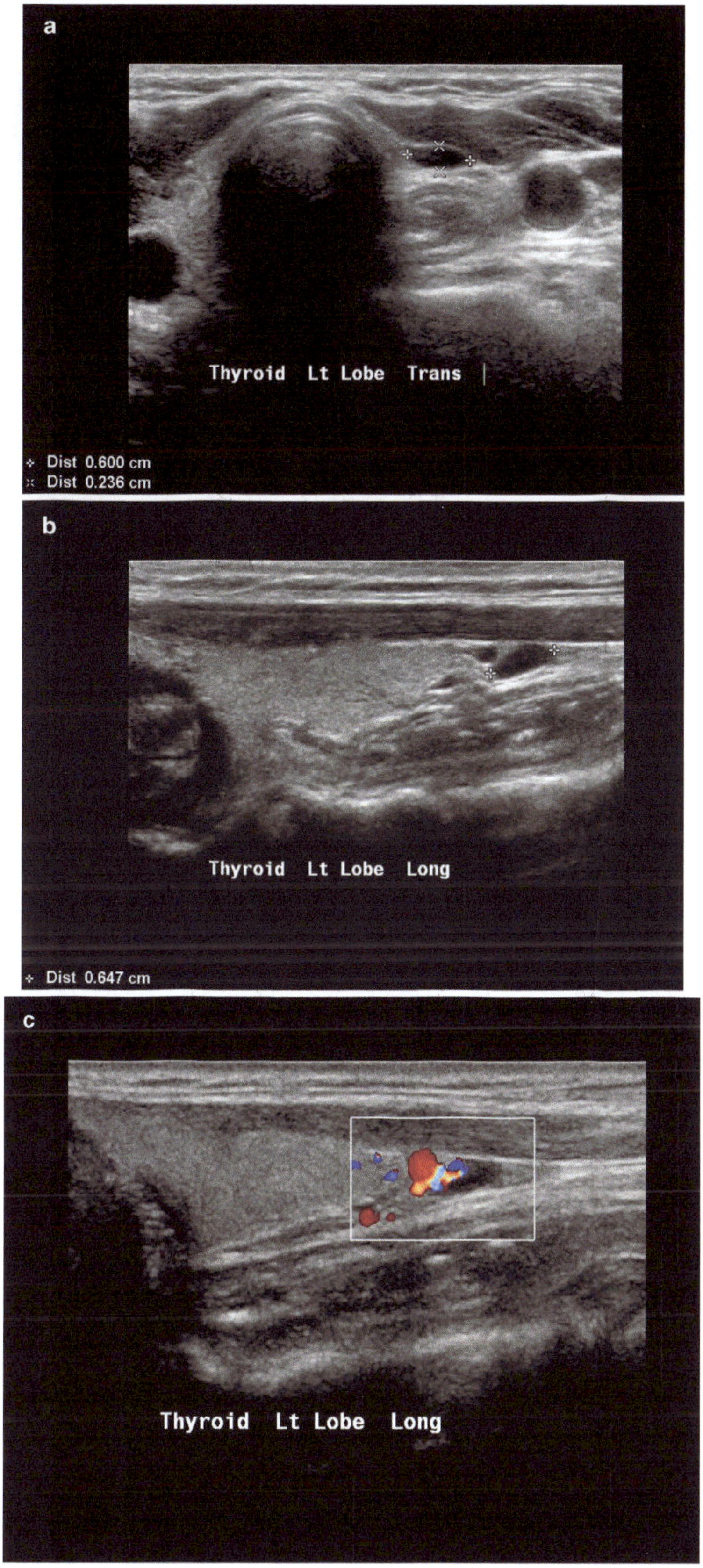

Fig. 8.27 Three views (**a**, **b**, **c**) including Doppler denote a small parathyroid adenoma

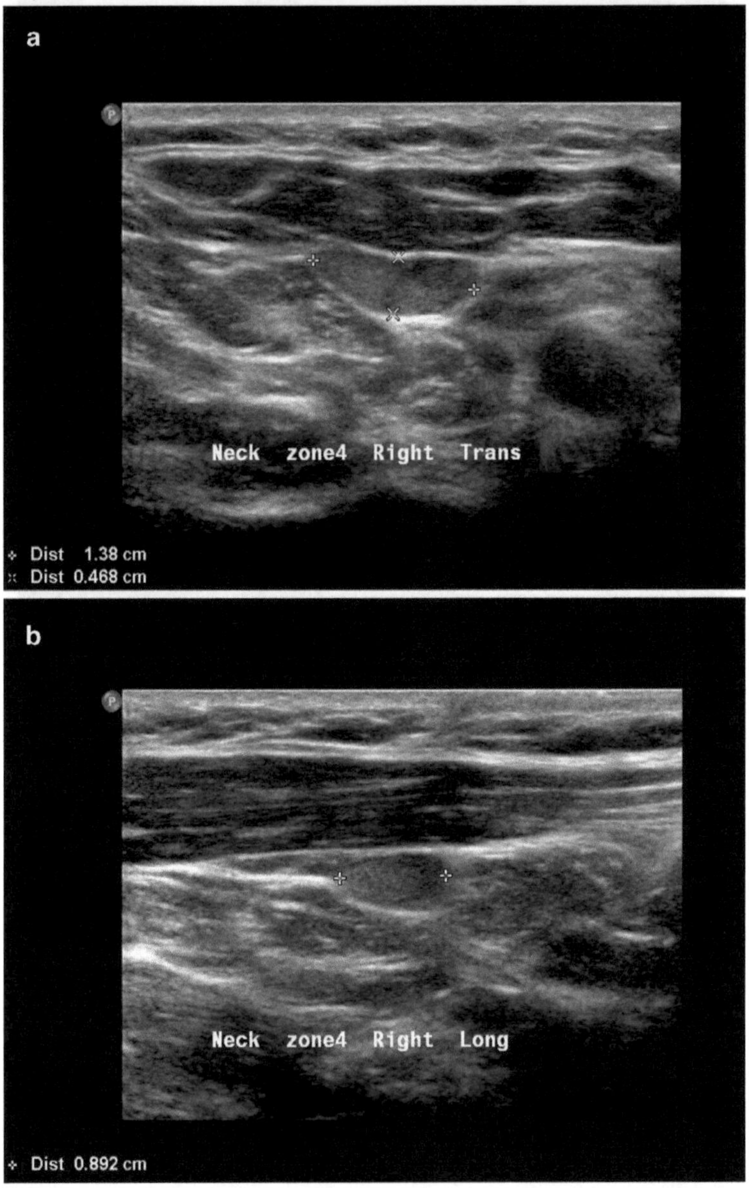

Fig. 8.28 An ectopic parathyroid adenoma in zone III in the midlateral neck is proven as such with FNA for parathyroid hormone (**a**, **b**)

from the aspirate is supportive of an intrathyroidal parathyroid adenoma, and often the values are excessive measured in the thousands. Similarly a hypoechoic nodule in the lateral neck can be aspirated for PTH (Fig. 8.28a, b). The cytology is less likely to be definitive, and in this circumstance, the chemical value is all important. This concept adds significantly to the evolving opportunities to image hyperplastic parathyroid glands. To illustrate this point, 17 patients with discordant scintigraphy and ultrasound were studied [14]. In 11 patients, the scintigraphy was negative. Of the 17 patients, 13 demonstrated a positive value for adenoma on aspiration of PTH, and two of these 13 lesions were intrathyroidal.

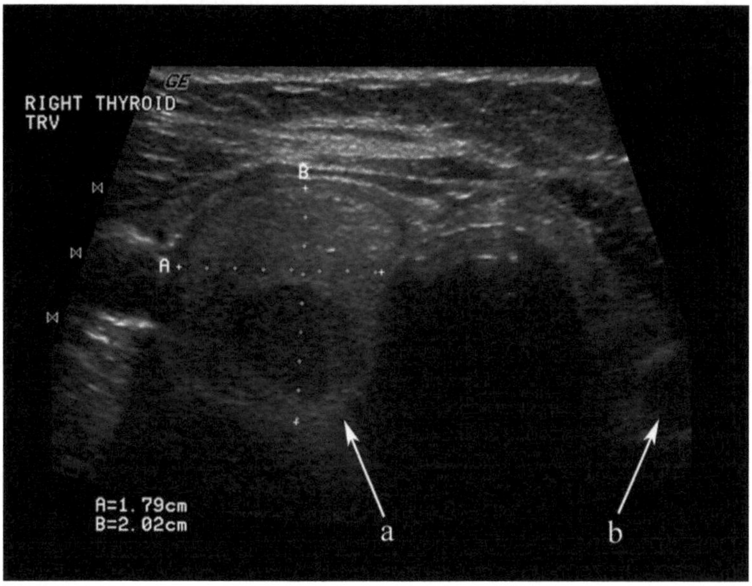

Fig. 8.29 This ultrasound demonstrates a concurrent papillary carcinoma of the thyroid gland (**a**) and a contralateral parathyroid adenoma (**b**)

Other Issues

The gold standard of parathyroid localization has been technetium sestamibi, and now with the addition of SPECT scan, the identification rate is amplified even further. The use of intraoperative PTH has allowed surgeons to terminate surgery after focused exploration with confidence that single-gland excision will be effective in eliminating the hyperparathyroid state. Gwande and colleagues [15] have examined the issue of concordance of high-resolution ultrasound and preoperative Tc sestamibi scanning. When in agreement as to precise location, the two studies predict a 99% cure rate with focused single-gland excision. In fact, these authors argue that intraoperative PTH becomes superfluous and elect to omit this process from their surgical framework. The two primary reasons for performing parathyroid ultrasound are to identify the possibility of both an intrathyroidal adenoma and unexpected concurrent thyroid pathology. Adler et al. [16]. have described their experience in 312 patients with hyperparathyroidism. Of those, 29% had identified concurrent thyroid pathology, and 2%, thyroid malignancy. We have identified several circumstances when occult papillary thyroid carcinomas are identified during ultrasonographic evaluation of the neck in patients with hyperparathyroidism (Figs. 8.29–8.30). This is not only an important step for the patient at the primary setting since both the thyroid and parathyroid problems can be addressed at the same surgical procedure, but it also eliminates a failure to identify a malignancy when it may be earlier in evolution. This spares the patient a second procedure into the same operative site with potential risks to the recurrent laryngeal nerve and remaining ipsilateral parathyroid gland. Up to this point, primary hyperparathyroidism has been the main element of discussion, whether it be diffuse hyperplasia, single or double adenoma, or asymmetrical hyperplasia in MEN. Secondary hyperparathyroidism also produces enlargement of all parathyroid tissue, and Tc sestamibi is rarely utilized. Ultrasound is simple, noninvasive, and does not suffer from inadequate sestamibi uptake. All enlarged glands are usually demonstrated with transverse and sagittal ultrasound

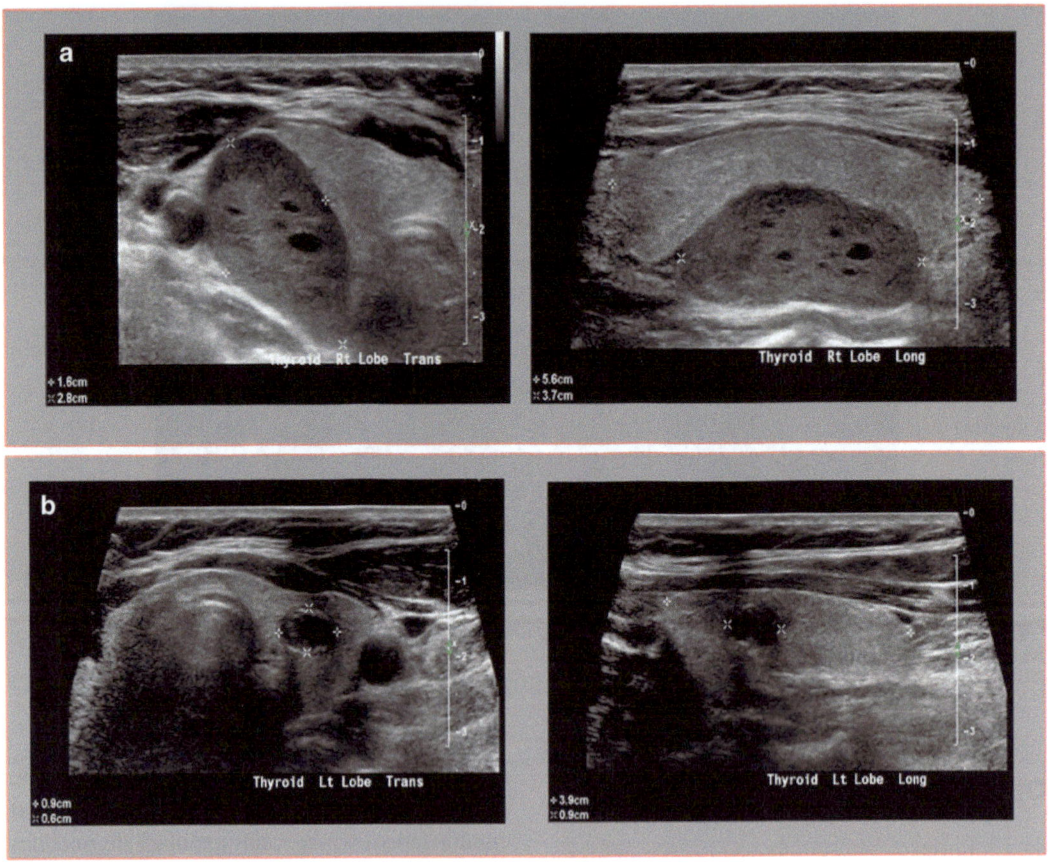

Fig. 8.30 This patient with primary hyperparathyroidism demonstrates a very large parathyroid adenoma (**a**) which draws the sonographer's eye. A second nodule in the opposite thyroid lobe is identified and although small has interrupted rim calcification (**b**). Subsequent FNA demonstrates papillary carcinoma, all of which underscores the importance of performing ultrasound in every case of hyperparathyroidism

(Figs. 8.31–8.32). Enlarged supernumerary parathyroid tissue within the upper mediastinum may occasionally be demonstrated. Limited access parathyroidectomy, whether done with an endoscope, a gamma probe, or a smaller incision focused over the presumed site of the enlarged single gland, requires a more precise understanding of its vertical and lateral position in the neck. Preoperative ultrasound is the perfect venue to identify the offending gland, and the skin can be marked just prior to surgery to relay this information (Fig. 8.33). Lastly, intraoperative ultrasound may have a role in the setting of the "failure to locate" gland or in reoperative parathyroidectomy [17]. The low transverse incision limits direct surgical access and palpation of the upper neck. Careful, orderly intraoperative ultrasound of the upper neck and carotid sheath is one additional option, especially if a preoperative study has not been performed.

Special Cases

Lingual Thyroid

Ultrasound offers the opportunity for the clinician to be creative in considering unconventional applications in the office setting. While there are other imaging tools which can allow one to arrive at a proper diagnosis, the initial study is often a simple gray scale ultrasound. For example, a patient

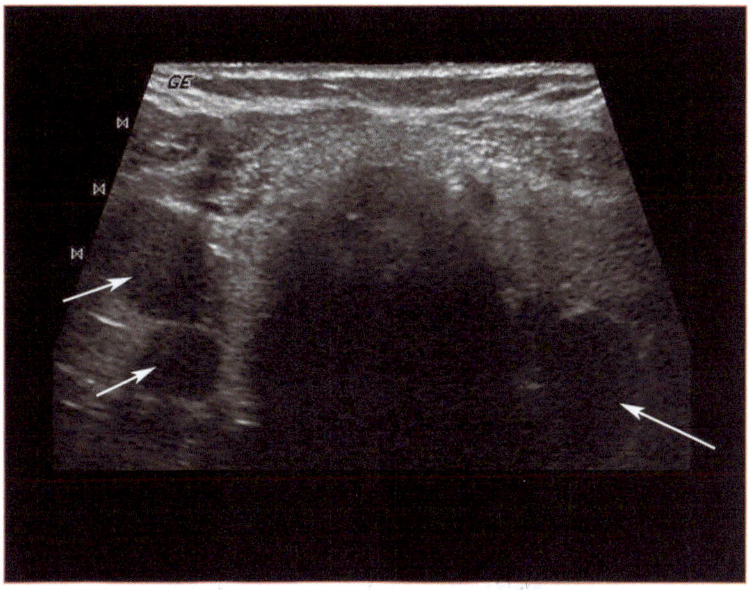

Fig. 8.31 Secondary hyperparathyroidism is associated with large parathyroid glands which may vary in size. This transverse view demonstrates three enlarged glands in the same plane

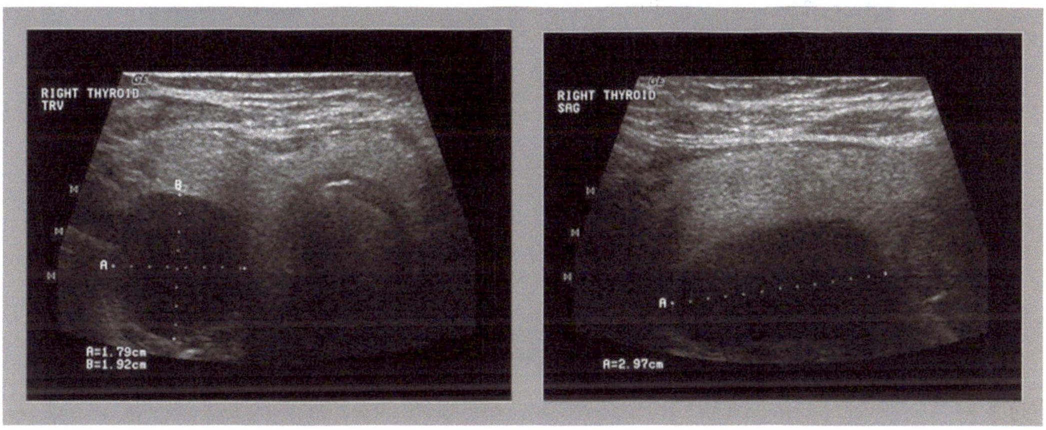

Fig. 8.32 The parathyroid glands in secondary hyperparathyroidism can be quite large and rounded

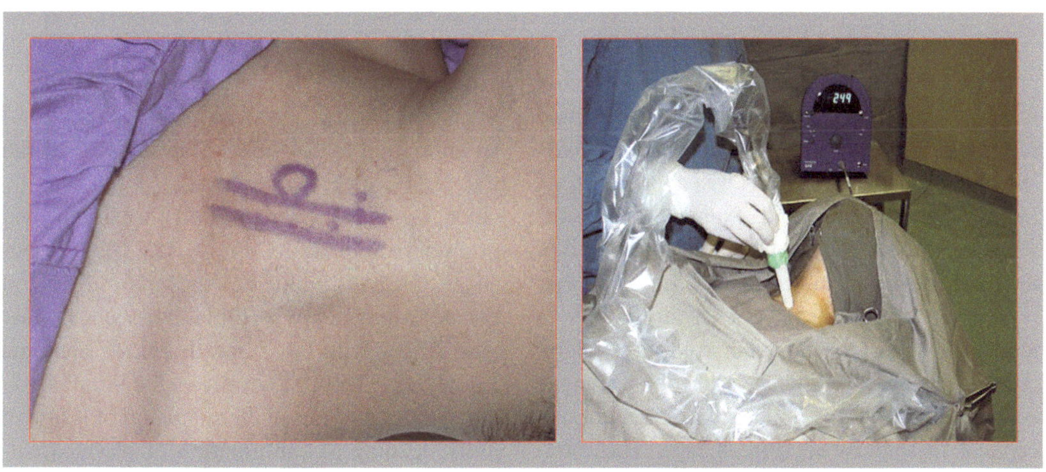

Fig. 8.33 The location of a parathyroid adenoma prior to surgery, as seen on ultrasound, can be marked for limited access surgery

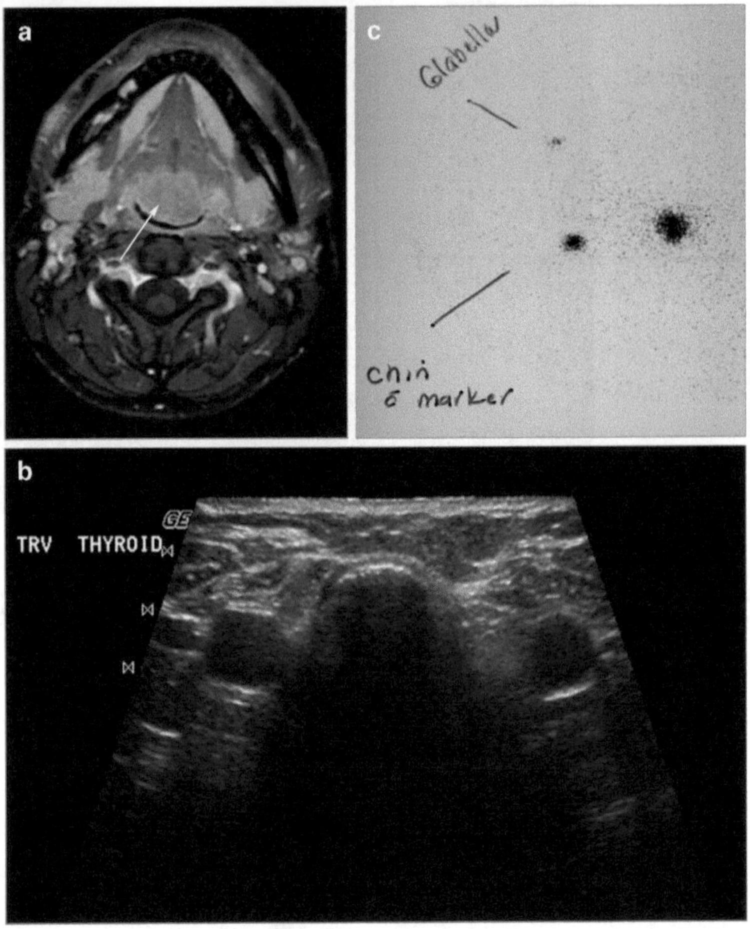

Fig. 8.34 This patient presented with a reddish submucosal tongue base mass on physical examination, and MRI demonstrates this finding, as denoted by the *arrow* (**a**). A cervical ultrasound performed on the initial consultation visit demonstrated absent thyroid tissue in the neck (**b**). Thus, a lingual thyroid was suspected and later confirmed with a nuclear scan (**c**)

presented on self-referral for a second opinion regarding a planned general anesthesia and base of tongue biopsy of a submucosal reddish mass (Fig. 8.34a). Indeed the mass was appreciated on indirect laryngoscopy and examination of the tongue and hypopharynx. However, ultrasound of the full neck demonstrated that there was no thyroid tissue overlying the trachea, leading to a tentative diagnosis of lingual thyroid (Fig. 8.34b). A subsequent I 123 nuclear scan of the tongue base demonstrated the lingual thyroid and absent cervical thyroid tissue (Fig. 8.34c). The ultrasound averted a general anesthetic and the morbidity of a wedge biopsy of the tongue base.

Brown Tumor

An immigrant to the United States from Somalia presented with a painful mass in the maxilla which was demonstrated both on external and intraoral examinations (Fig. 8.35a, b). A cervical ultrasound including the thyroid region revealed a large extrathyroidal hypoechoic mass consistent with a parathyroid adenoma (Fig. 8.36). The ultrasound was the initial study which indirectly raised the suspicion of a Brown tumor, leading to confirmation of elevated calcium and intact parathyroid hormone levels. A subsequent CT scan of the maxilla (Fig. 8.37)

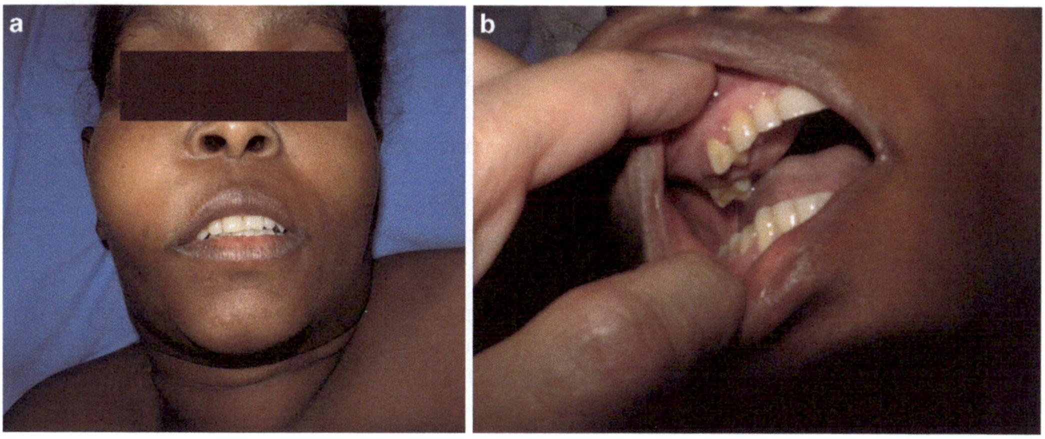

Fig. 8.35 This Somalian woman presented with a painful right maxillary swelling. This was noted both on external (**a**) and intraoral (**b**) examination

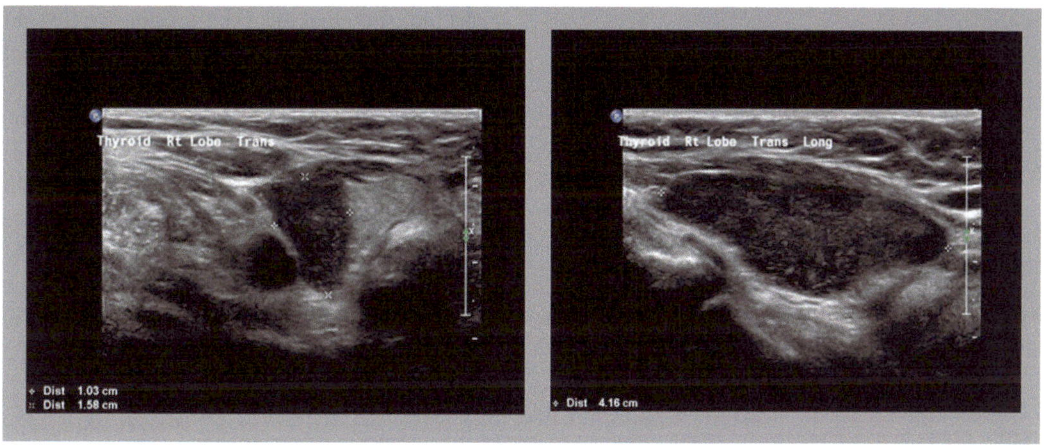

Fig. 8.36 A cervical ultrasound on initial consultation demonstrated a large parathyroid adenoma which directed attention toward the diagnosis of Brown tumor rather than an ominous malignancy

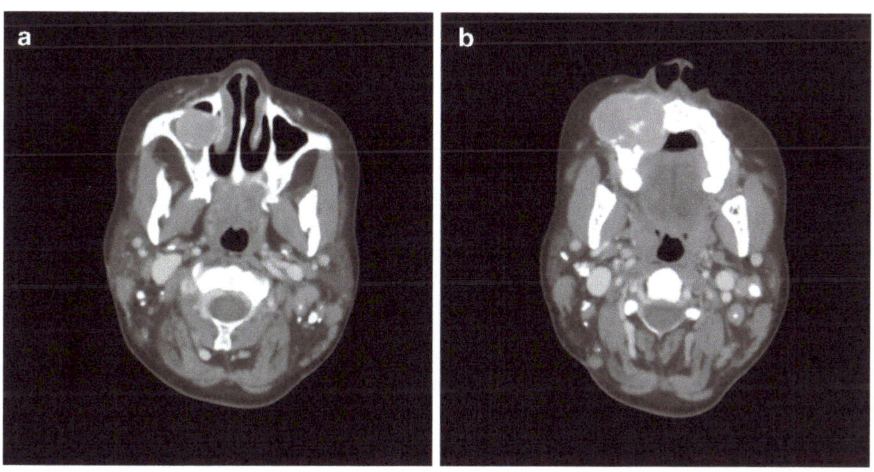

Fig. 8.37 Subsequent CT scans (**a**, **b**) were consistent with Brown tumor. Subsequently, a large 4.65-g, 3.5 × 1.5 × 1.5-cm adenoma was removed

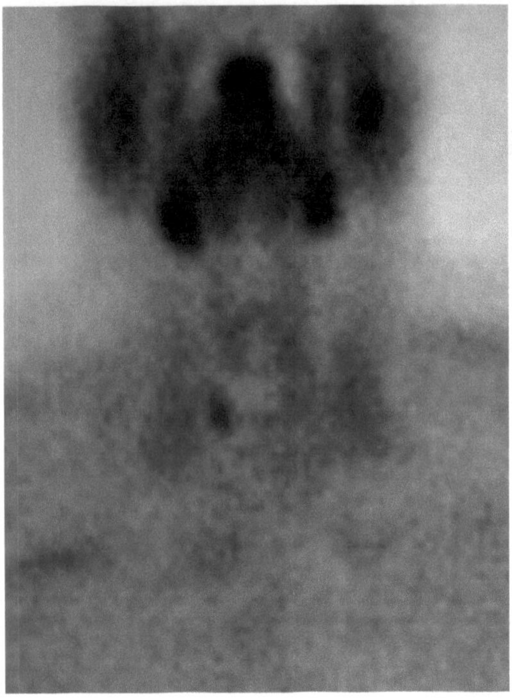

Fig. 8.38 This patient with previous thyroid lobectomy for a benign nodule underwent implantation of a devascularized parathyroid into the ipsilateral SCM muscle. She developed hyperparathyroidism, and the biplanar sestamibi demonstrates uptake slightly lateral to the usual parathyroid position

demonstrates the destructive expansile process which partially resolved one year after parathyroidectomy.

Parathyroid Reimplantation

A patient with primary hyperparathyroidism demonstrates persistent uptake in the right lower neck on this earlier biplanar T-99 m sestamibi scan (Fig. 8.38). The lesion appears slightly lateral to the normal parathyroid position. Several years earlier, the patient had undergone right thyroid lobectomy for a mass which proved to be a benign thyroid adenoma. Review of the operative report indicated that the right inferior parathyroid gland had become devascularized. It was diced and reimplanted into the lower ipsilateral sternocleidomastoid muscle (SCM). Returning to the current problem at hand and planned parathyroidectomy, an ultrasound was performed with specific interest in the SCM. A discrete hypoechoic mass was identified (Fig. 8.39). At surgery, after baseline PTH was obtained, the nodule within the muscle was removed, and the values then dropped by 70% and normalized. The

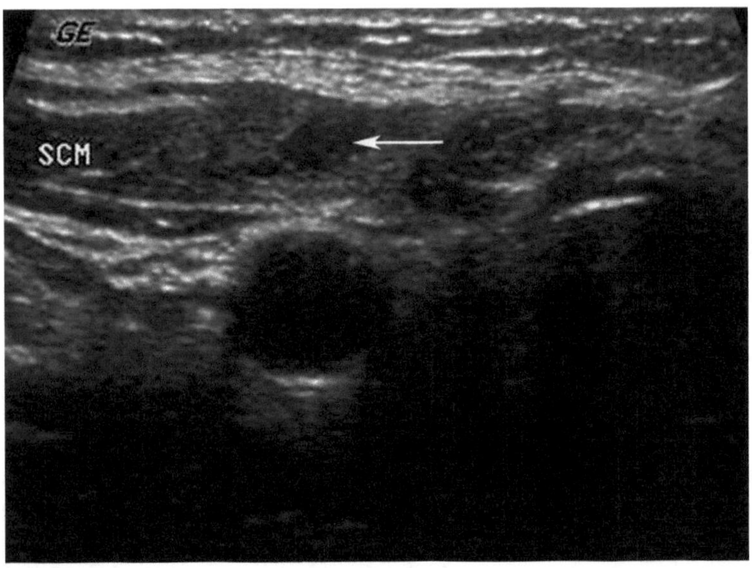

Fig. 8.39 Ultrasound of the SCM demonstrates a discrete hypoechoic mass. This was removed after baseline PTH levels were obtained with appropriate resolution of the hyperparathyroid state

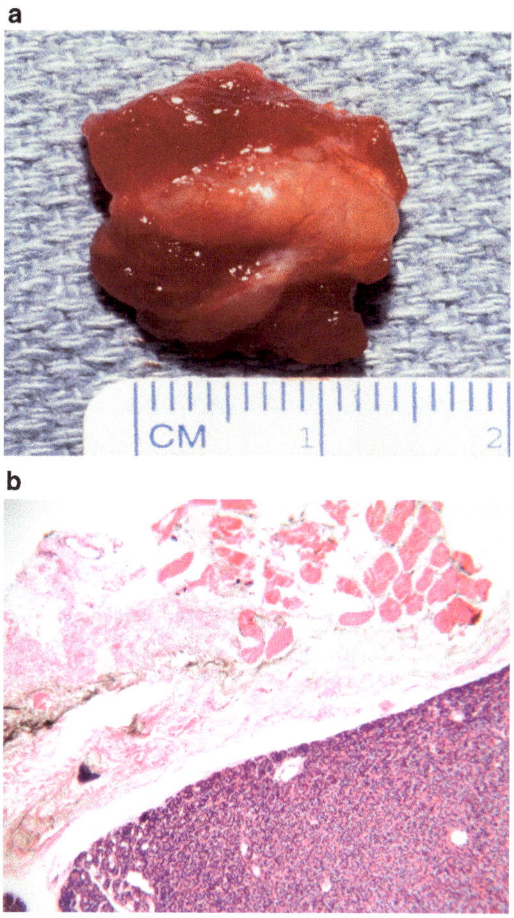

Fig. 8.40 The gross (a) and histologic images (b) are demonstrated. Compact hyperplasia of the parathyroid tissue is demonstrated

procedure was terminated without the need to reexplore the prior scarred operative site and risks to the recurrent laryngeal nerve. Formal histology demonstrates that this implanted parathyroid tissue had become hyperplastic within the muscle (Fig. 8.40).

A second patient with reimplantation issues deserves discussion. This patient has had several prior procedures for parathyroid hyperplasia and recurrent hypercalcemia even after well-documented four-gland excision. During the last procedure as the presumed final gland was excised, a portion of the parathyroid tissue was reimplanted into the brachioradialis muscle of the forearm. Fusion sestamibi, SPECT scans, and MRI failed to demonstrate any parathyroid enlargement in the neck, and cervical ultrasound was negative. With isolation of the forearm in question from the peripheral blood with application of a 5-min venous tourniquet, the systemic PTH value dropped appropriately, suggesting that the implanted parathyroid was the incriminating problem. An ultrasound of the brachioradialis muscle of the forearm confirmed a defined area at the reimplantation site which was iso- to hyperechoic (Fig. 8.41). In comparison, the previously discussed case of parathyroid tissue which was reimplanted into the sternocleidomastoid muscle demonstrates a nodule of decidedly lower echogenicity. Perhaps the compact,

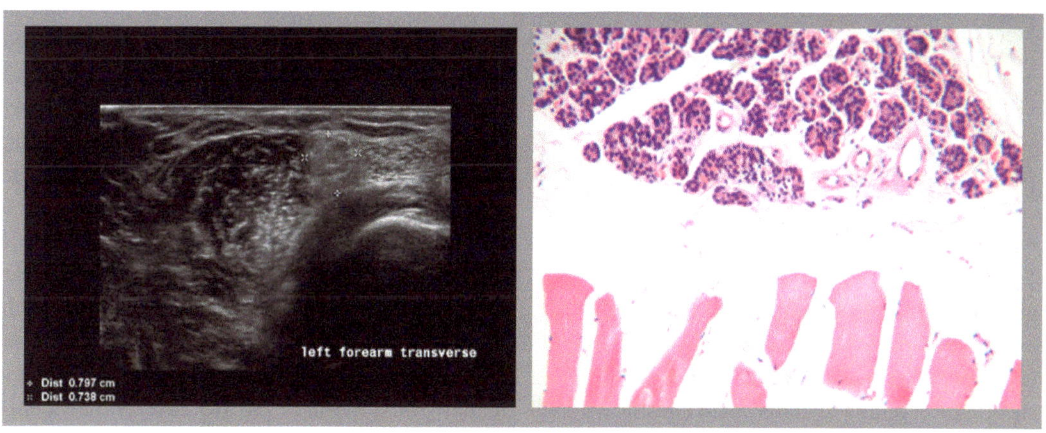

Fig. 8.41 A hypoechoic area in the left brachioradialis muscle of the forearm is the site of prior reimplantation of segments of hyperplastic parathyroid gland. The corresponding normal parathyroid histology is relatively less compact than the usual parathyroid adenoma. This may explain its relatively isoechoic appearance on ultrasound in comparison with the nearly anechoic parathyroid nodule demonstrated in Figure 8.42 appearance on ultrasound

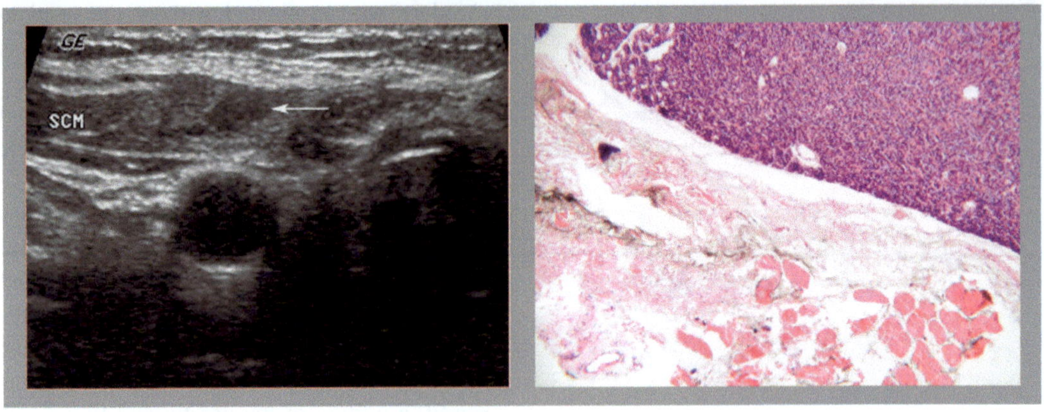

Fig. 8.42 The previously discussed reimplanted tissue into the sternocleidomastoid muscle demonstrates a hypoechoic area similar to a parathyroid adenoma. The corresponding histology shows a compact uniform complex of cells. This histology may be reflected in the reduced echogenicity of the lesion

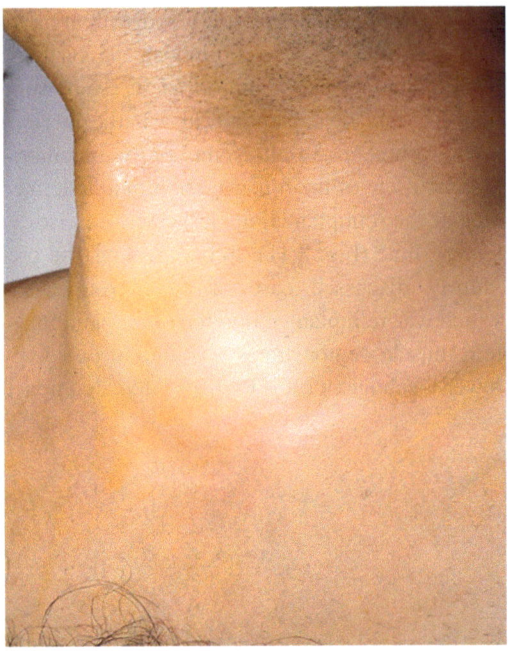

Fig. 8.43 A mass is demonstrated in the left lower neck

uniform, hyperplastic implanted tissue produces ultrasound images that are more similar to the usual parathyroid adenoma (Fig. 8.42). It was successfully removed under local anesthesia, and histopathology demonstrated the parathyroid hyperplasia. The serum calcium and parathyroid hormone levels have remained normal for the past year, suggesting that there is still active, functional parathyroid tissue somewhere in the neck or mediastinum.

Parathyroid Cysts

Parathyroid cysts [18] are curious masses in the lower neck in the paramedian position (Fig. 8.43). They do not produce hyperparathyroidism, nor are they particularly symptomatic. Ultrasound displays a thin-walled cyst below but immediately adjacent to the thyroid gland. The cysts demonstrate typical posterior enhancement (Fig. 8.44). On sagittal view (Fig. 8.45) and at surgery (Fig. 8.46), the parathyroid cyst is noted to be separate from the thyroid gland. In contradistinction, a large parathyroid adenoma may undergo complete or partial cystic degeneration, but there is usually a solid component, and the patient has typical laboratory confirmation of the hyperparathyroid state. The clue to the proper diagnosis of parathyroid cyst is retrieval of clear fluid on aspiration and identification of a high intact PTH value. In fact, a lower neck cyst extending into the anterior mediastinum may actually be a thymic cyst. Because of their common embryological origins, thymic and parathyroid cysts may have similar histologic patterns with Hassel's corpuscles and parathyroid tissue. The only differentiating point is the elevated PTH

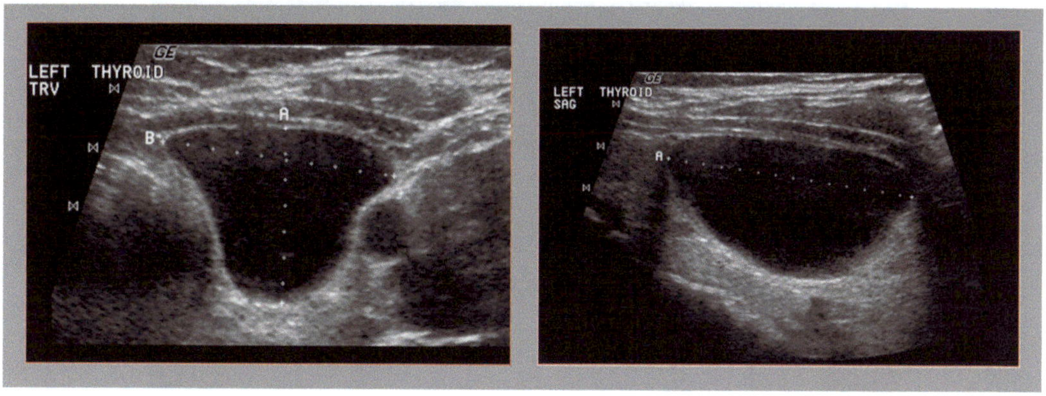

Fig. 8.44 Transverse and sagittal ultrasonographic images demonstrate the cystic nature of the mass with posterior enhancement

Fig. 8.45 A different sagittal view demonstrates the relationship of the cyst (**b**) to the thyroid gland (**a**) extending into the upper anterior mediastinum

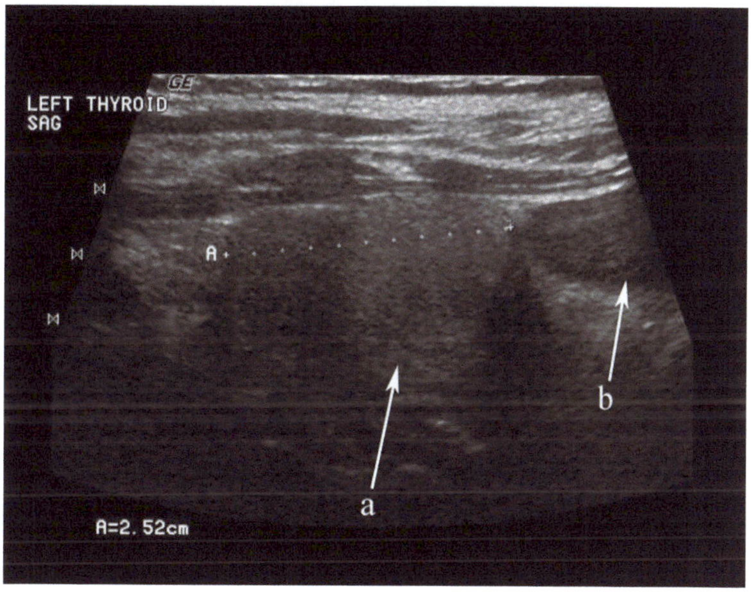

Fig. 8.46 An operative image indicates that these cysts are usually associated with the inferior aspect of the thyroid gland; the cyst has been drained, and only its envelope remains before it is excised

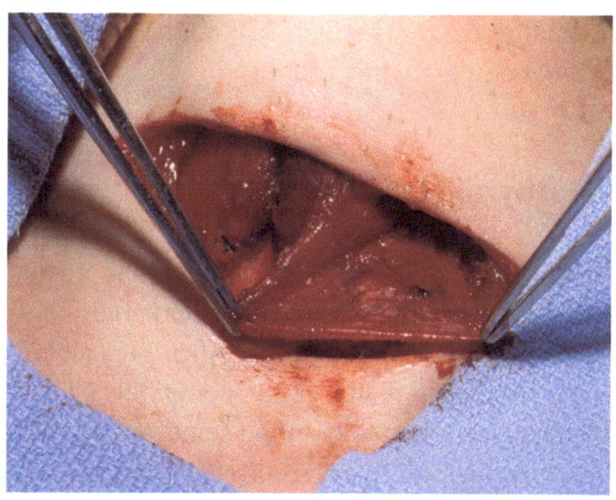

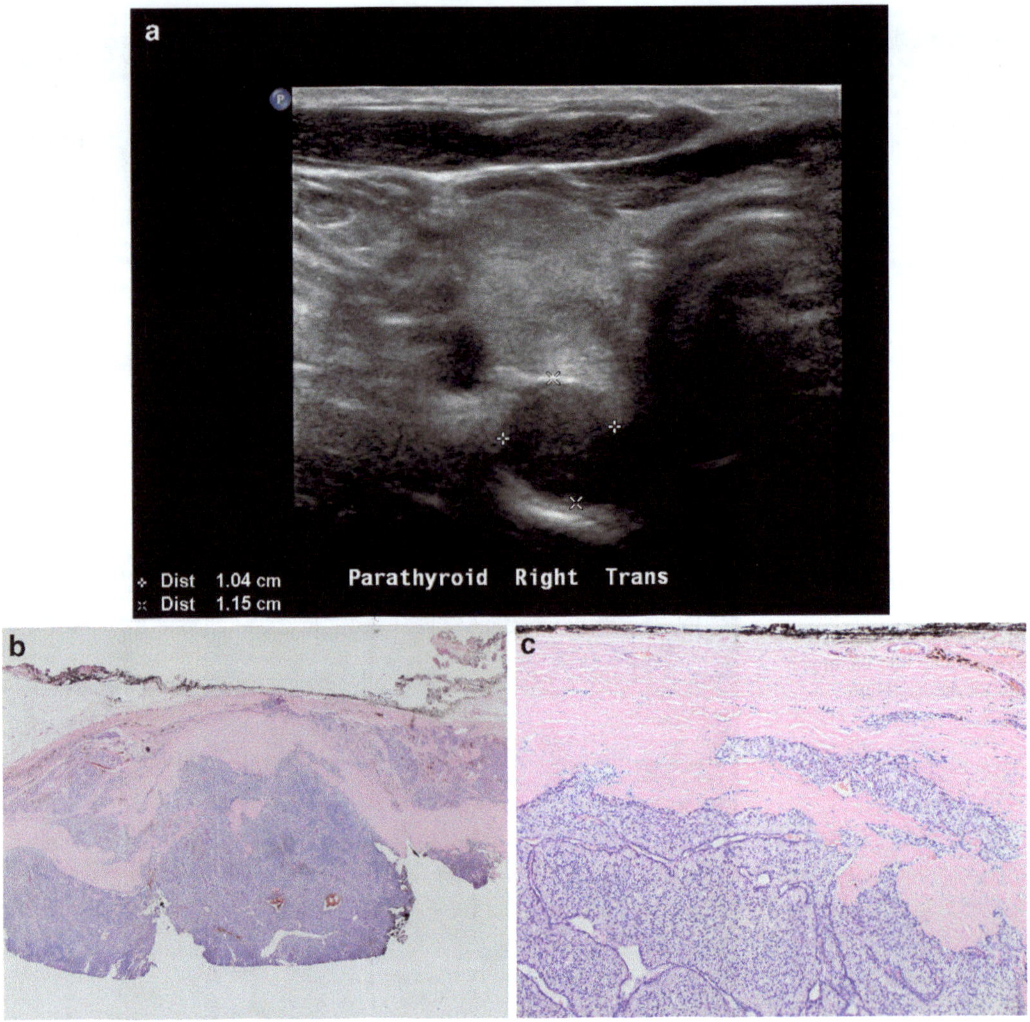

Fig. 8.47 Parathyroid carcinoma does not usually demonstrate specific features on ultrasound. This transverse image (**a**) is rather nonspecific. Representative histology is presented from this same patient's mass (**b, c**), and the confirmed diagnosis is that of a parathyroid carcinoma. Often, this may be suspected based on extremely high calcium levels or surgical findings of adherence and invasion rather than any imaging parameter

in parathyroid cysts which will not be present in cysts of purely thymic origin.

Parathyroid Carcinoma

Parathyroid carcinoma is uncommon and occurs in less than 1% of patients with hyperparathyroidism. It is most often suspected when the calcium levels are abnormally high, commonly above 14–15 pg/mL. Certainly in the setting of primary hyperparathyroidism and recurrent laryngeal nerve paralysis, parathyroid carcinoma must be suspected. In addition, cervical node metastasis is not nearly as often noted as in patients with papillary or medullary carcinoma. Even cytology or open biopsy is not particularly helpful. The disease is usually diagnosed clinically at the time of open surgery as the tumor is locally infiltrative and the parathyroid mass is adherent to surrounding structures. Preoperative ultrasound is not particularly helpful except in the rare circumstance when a metastatic lymph node is sampled, revealing parathyroid tissue or positive PTH values (Fig. 8.47).

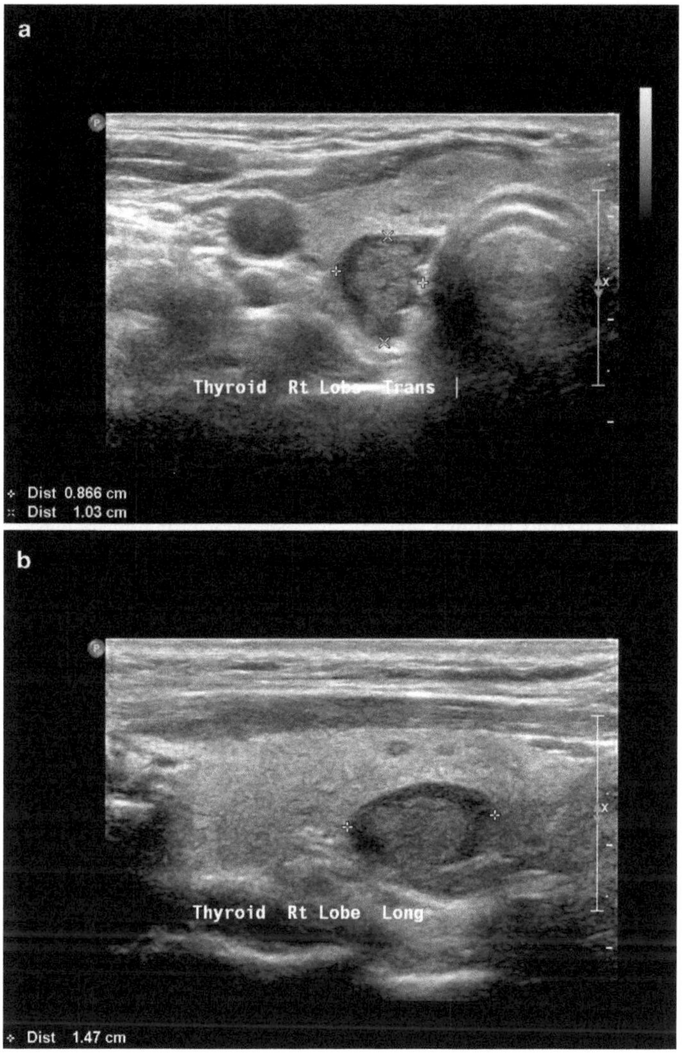

Fig. 8.48 The patient with normocalcemic hyperparathyroidism has a negative sestamibi scan. The transverse (**a**) and sagittal (**b**) images are typical of a parathyroid adenoma although it does extend significantly into the thyroid parenchyma as noted in this sagittal view

Normocalcemic Hyperparathyroidism

There are many circumstances in which the calcium may be normal but the parathyroid hormone level is elevated. Hypovitaminosis D is probably the most common explanation, especially in areas where people live indoors throughout the winter months and do not have sun exposure for months at a time. Benign familial hypocalciuric hypercalcemia is another condition in which the calcium level may not be strongly elevated in spite of increasing PTH. In these circumstances, neither ultrasound nor sestamibi scan will demonstrate evidence of an enlarged parathyroid gland. Occasionally patients will present with symptoms of hyperparathyroidism but no calcium elevation. Parathyroid hormone may be slightly elevated in early or mild cases. This entity is designated normocalcemic hyperparathyroidism. A representative ultrasound demonstrates significant enlargement of an inferior parathyroid gland in spite of a negative sestamibi scan. This problem is relatively rare, and the imaging profile is not as yet well defined (Fig. 8.48).

In summary, high-resolution ultrasound is an indispensible tool in the ideal management of surgical hyperparathyroidism. With many of the adjunctive concepts outlined above, the clinician/surgeon will have several unique opportunities to more accurately locate aberrant enlarged parathyroid glands either prior to or during the surgical exercise. Most importantly, the operating surgeon has a vested interest in the accuracy of localization and will be more motivated than anyone to find the offending pathology before entering the operating room. Lastly, there are false-positive lesions which can be misinterpreted by the uninitiated starting out with ultrasound or with instruments of either low resolution or without Doppler capability. Thyroid nodules, accessory thyroid tissue, lymph nodes, the esophagus, longus colli muscle, and perithyroidal vessels may be inappropriately identified as adenomas. In order for this technology to be worthwhile, it is critical for the clinician embarking on the use of this technology to continue to study image recognition and to have a skilled mentor to work with until appropriate ultrasound experience has evolved.

References

1. Abboud B et al. Intrathyroid parathyroid adenoma in primary hyperparathyroidism: can it be predicted preoperatively? World J Surg. 2007;31:817–23.
2. Gilmour JR. The gross anatomy of the parathyroid glands. J Pathol. 1938;46:133.
3. Andre V, Andre M, LeDreff P, Granier H, Forlodou P, Garcia JF. Intrathyroidal parathyroid adenoma. J Radiol. 1999;80:591–2.
4. McIntyre Jr R, Eisenach J, Pearlman N, Ridgeway C, Liechty RD. Intrathyroidal parathyroid glands can be a cause of failed cervical exploration for hyperparathyroidism. Am J Surg. 1997;174:750–4.
5. Flament JB, Delattre JF, Pluot M. Arterial supply to the parathyroid glands: implications for thyroid surgery. Anat Clin. 1982;3:279.
6. Abboud B et al. Ultrasonography: highly accuracy technique for preoperative localization of parathyroid adenoma. Laryngoscope. 2008;118:1574–8.
7. Baskin J, Duick D, Levine R. Thyroid ultrasound and ultrasound guided FNA. 2nd ed. New York: Springer; 2008. p. 139.
8. Randel SB, Gooding GA, Clark OH, et al. Parathyroid variants: US evaluation. Radiology. 1987;165:191–4.
9. Mazzeo S et al. Usefulness of echo color Doppler in differentiating parathyroid lesions from other cervical masses. Eur Radiol. 1997;7:90–5.
10. Lane MJ, Desser TS, Weigel RJ, Jeffrey Jr RB. Use of color and power Doppler sonography to identify feeding arteries associated with parathyroid adenomas. Am J Roentgenol. 1998;171:818–23.
11. Reeder SB, Desser TS, Weigel RJ, Jeffrey RB. Sonography in primary hyperparathyroidism: review with emphasis on scanning technique. J Ultrasound Med. 2002;21:539–52.
12. Lane MJ et al. Use of color and power Doppler sonography to identify feeding arteries associated with parathyroid adenomas. Am J Roentgenol. 1998;171:819–23.
13. Marcocci C et al. Preoperative localization of suspicious adenomas by assay of parathyroid hormone in needle aspirates. Eur J Endocrinol. 1998;139:72–7.
14. Marcocci C et al. Preoperative localization of suspicious parathyroid adenoma by assay of parathyroid hormone in needle aspirates. Eur J Endocrinol. 1999;139:72–7.
15. Gwande A et al. Reassessment of parathyroid hormone monitoring during parathyroidectomy for primary hyperparathyroidism after two preoperative localization studies. Arch Surg. 2006;141:381–4.
16. Adler JT, Chen H, Schaefer S, Sippel RS. Does routine use of ultrasound result in additional thyroid procedures in patients with primary hyperparathyroidism? J Am Coll Surg. 2010;221:536–9.
17. Ghaheri BA, Koslin DB, Wood AH, Cohen JI. Preoperative ultrasound is worthwhile for reoperative parathyroid surgery. Laryngoscope. 2004;114:2168–71.
18. Ihm P, Dray T, Sofferman R, Nathan M, Hardin N. Parathyroid cyst: diagnosis and management. Laryngocope. 2006;111:1406–9.

Fine Needle Aspiration Cytology

9

Robert A. Sofferman

The application of fine needle aspiration cytology to the management of thyroid disorders has an interesting practical history. The first clinical uses of aspiration cytology evolved from Scandinavia in the 1950s [1]. Martin and Ellis utilized this technique in 1930 to diagnose a variety of masses at Memorial Hospital in New York [2]. Stewart then reported 2,500 tumors in 1933 [3]. Subsequently, other European publications began to emphasize the utility of this method to more accurately characterize thyroid nodules [4–7]. How did the interest in cytology polarize to Scandinavia in those early years? At that time, pathologists in the United States were reluctant to accept this technique due to various reasons. They were interested in tissue diagnosis and used hematoxylin and eosin (Papanicolaou) stains to advantage in frozen section assessment. The Scandinavian pathologists did not perform frozen sections at that time and sought other methods of assessment. Their hematology colleagues were used to looking at preparations with Giemsa stains and were recruited into the adaptation of their skills to examination of aspirated materials before surgery (Gladwyn Leiman, personal communication).

R.A. Sofferman (✉)
Division of Otolaryngology-Head and Neck Surgery, University of Vermont School of Medicine, Fletcher Allen Health Care, 111 Colchester Ave., Burlington, VT 05401, USA
e-mail: robert.sofferman@vtmednet.org

In the 1970s interest in FNA cytology was published in the Canadian literature, and there was some early interest in large needle biopsy methods in Cleveland and Boston [8–10]. The first American study was published in 1979, emphasizing a combination of small and large needle samples [11]. Within short order, aspiration cytology became universal in its application, although the experience in Scandinavia over so many years before afforded their cytopathologists with a substantial experiential advantage [12].

Sudha Kini at Henry Ford Hospital in Detroit, Michigan, has published a text devoted to thyroid cytopathology, currently in its 3rd edition, and has recently described her experience with 4,500 satisfactory aspirates (1975–1985) along with 1,100 correlations with surgical specimens [13]. Besides the efficiency and simplicity of the procedure, they have cited the economic advantages of this method which has halved the number of open surgical procedures and doubled the number of cancers identified at formal pathologic examination [14].

Thyroid nodules are common. Ultrasound identifies nodules in 50% of individuals beyond the fifth decade. Five to six percent of single nodules are malignant, and this incidence increases to 12% if there is a preexisting exposure to ionizing radiation [15]. The goal of aspiration cytology is to select out of this pool the lesions which are benign and can be observed and those which are either suspicious or diagnostic of malignancy. Although thyroid cancer is

R.A. Sofferman and A.T. Ahuja (eds.), *Ultrasound of the Thyroid and Parathyroid Glands*,
DOI 10.1007/978-1-4614-0974-8_9, © Springer Science+Business Media, LLC 2012

less common than other malignancies and often cited as a more "favorable" type, it is still a question which can be readily answered in most clinical circumstances. There are about 20,000 new thyroid cancers and 1,300 cancer-related deaths in the United States annually. This accounts for only 1.5% of new cancer cases and 0.4% of cancer deaths. The most common form, papillary carcinoma, is often readily diagnosed on aspiration cytology, and it often appears in young individuals. The clinically suspicious nodule and one which should be considered for cytologic sampling is as follows [15, 16]:

1. Male gender
2. <20 and >70 years of age
3. Prior exposure to ionizing radiation during childhood or adolescence
4. Family history of thyroid disease, especially papillary thyroid cancer and medullary cancer
5. Family or personal history of multiple endocrine neoplasia (MEN)
6. Prior hemithyroidectomy with finding of micro- or macropapillary carcinoma in the specimen
7. FDG-PET-positive thyroid nodule, usually identified incidental to investigation of other lesions outside of the thyroid
8. Defined hoarseness, local pain, dysphagia
9. Certain physical characteristics, i.e., firm and/or fixed thyroid mass, nodule greater than 4 cm, suspicious metastatic cervical lymphadenopathy

Many would argue that aspiration by palpation is adequate for sampling thyroid nodules, and indeed the large, obvious mass can be addressed in this manner. However, the use of ultrasound guidance allows more specific sampling within a nodule or determining which of several nodules should be submitted to this analysis. Thus, both nondiagnostic and false-negative results can be better avoided, and this has been documented in retrospective studies [17, 18].

There are sonographic changes in addition to the pure cyst which are likely to be predictive of a benign process. The spongiform nodule in which more than 50% of its volume is microcystic in appearance is nearly always benign with a reported negative predictive value of 98.5% [19, 20].

Technical Issues Pertaining to the Aspirate

Prior to consideration for aspiration cytology, the single nodule must indeed be a candidate for sampling. From a diagnostic standpoint, there is little reason to do this procedure on a small anechoic nodule with a discrete envelope, absolutely no solid component, and the sonographic characteristics of a cyst. Patients may be anxious about a larger, palpable cyst and the psychological advantage of eliminating it with aspiration may be important, but these often recur and cytology will usually be inadequate. If the goals of aspiration and reaspiration are understood, this may be a warranted procedure. A TSH should be obtained in advance of FNA. If the patient has a suppressed TSH in the face of a single thyroid nodule, it is likely to be a hyperfunctioning nodule and not malignant. In this circumstance, FNA with cytology will not be necessary. A radionuclear scan may more definitively answer this question to the point where the patient may undergo a therapeutic lobectomy [21, 22].

Fine needle aspiration cytology may be a misnomer. The first formal recommendation for use of a capillary technique was published in 1988, and others have embraced the idea. A lot of attention has been directed at methods which produce less bleeding, and those who perform needle aspiration on a routine basis are mystified by the strong feelings and bias which surround this issue. It is clear that cells will readily ascend into a 25- or 27-gauge needle without the need for suction, as more often than not the needle hub will fill with blood and aspiration material. Whether applied suction or a larger-gauge needle will by physical effects produce more bleeding is really conjectural. However, the reduction in bleeding within the aspirate is an important issue. The 95% alcohol which is used in the Papanicolaou technique lyses red cells, and this hemolysis interferes with stain resolution [23]. At the present time there are no defined proven methods which reduce bleeding into the aspirate. Most of the time a capillary method will allow sufficient material to be sampled and satisfy cytopathologic criteria. On occasion, a more fibrotic nodule or one with more cohesive characteristics will not produce a good capillary aspirate, requiring either suction or a larger-bore needle. Lastly there are circumstances where a very inferior or deep nodule is identified or the neck/thyroid tissues are so large that sampling with the usual 1.5-in.-long needle will be problematic. In fact, many times the most superficial aspect of a target nodule is more than 2 cm from the surface, suggesting that conventional aspiration techniques will not be possible. The skin and subcutaneous tissues can often be compressed to allow deeper penetration of the 1.5-in. needle for adequate nodule entry. There are some circumstances where a 4–6-cm or even longer distance must be traversed to target a lesion. A 22-gauge spinal needle may then be utilized to accomplish this goal. The larger-bore needle is required as the thinner long needles are too flexible and are more difficult to accurately direct. The stylet is retained until the nodule is entered, and aspiration may be applied to the hub after the stylet is removed.

The use of lidocaine into the skin, subcutaneous tissues, and occasionally strap or sternocleidomastoid muscles is a helpful adjunct to aspiration cytology as several needle entries are usually required. If the local anesthetic avoids the thyroid gland or nodule, no distortion of the nodule or interference with the aspirated cells will occur. The application of local anesthesia provides comfort and allows all efforts at the task at hand rather than dealing with the discomforts and anxieties of the patient. Alternative agents such as Carbocaine or Benadryl can be used for patients with alleged lidocaine allergy. Inherent in the capillary technique is a subtle but practical procedural advantage. The individual performing the aspirate grasps the needle at its hub which allows the hand to be stabilized on the patient's skin and body. This shorter "instrument" is much easier to direct than when a syringe is attached and the hand more distant from the needle tip. In addition, the authors prefer to use an aspiration method which simulates the advantages of the capillary method. A short length of sterile tubing can be inserted between the needle and syringe, and an assistant on request at the proper time can provide suction while the operator continues to grasp the needle hub region. It must be emphasized that when the capillary method is used, no syringe is attached to the needle. Otherwise the capillary flow into the needle may not occur.

Cytology

It is instructive to review some basics of cytologic preparation [13].

In the procurement of cytologic material, it is critical to make certain that the patient's name and identifying information are placed on each slide. Of course, prior to beginning the procedure, the patient must be queried about his/her name, date of birth, and site to be sampled. Whether the transferred information about the clinical condition is done by paper or electronic means, the patient name, medical record number, lab accession number, precise site, and size and character of the lesion are important details for the cytopathologist.

Smear methods in which the cells are spread over the receptor slide by the leading edge of another glass slide or a "pull apart" method where the material is sandwiched between two slides and then they are separated are common methods of initial preparation. The material should be fixed immediately, either by insertion into 95% ethyl alcohol or application of a spray fixative. Some technicians use 80% isopropyl alcohol. Even a slight delay can produce air-drying artifact. A separate planned air-dried specimen is often obtained as it readily demonstrates colloid and other advantages which supplement the wet specimen. There are some disadvantages to the use of ethyl alcohol. Red cells are lysed and the cytoplasm of epithelial cells may be destroyed. As indicated earlier, the precipitate after red cell hemolysis may produce a background eosinophilia which interferes with staining resolution. Occasionally thyroid aspirates "fall" off the glass slide. Precoating the slide with albumin can prevent this, but this material imparts an eosinophilia to the cells.

There are several basic cytologic preparation techniques which are used by cytopathologists in assessment of thyroid aspirates:

1. Papanicolaou stained smears. This is the most popular method. This is a polychrome stain for differentiating components of the cell. The hematoxylin stains the nucleus, and the 3-acid dyes (eosin, light green, orange G) stain the cytoplasm. The nucleus stains dark blue; the nucleolus red; and the cytoplasm eosinophilic, cyanophilic, or orange.
2. Cell block. This is a sediment obtained from the preservative solution where needles are rinsed. It contains cells, blood clots, and visible tissue flecks that are processed by paraffin embedding and staining by hematoxylin and eosin.
3. Cytospin. This is a centrifugation method for amplifying poorly cellular samples. The collected cells are retrieved from a filter placed over a "well" etched on a special glass slide made for this procedure. A monolayer is produced for subsequent staining.

There are some adjunctive techniques which are used depending on lab preference. Saponin is an enzyme which lyses red cells, but the excess may destroy the cellular component if it is not applied in the proper concentration. The Saccomanno fixative (2% Carbowax or polyethylene glycol in 50% ethylene ethyl alcohol) may be used for aspirates which are performed in some centers away from the primary laboratory. Advantages are limited fear of cell deterioration or air-drying and no need for production of a thin prep. Its disadvantages are significantly longer time for cytopreparation, lysis of red cells with background precipitation, and nuclear shrinkage.

Another popular method is the use of the Romanowsky-type stain. This is useful for determining the adequacy of a sample for follicular cell groups. It is a combination of an acid and basic dye in the same solution. When applied, it produces a "neutral salt" which reacts with cellular components. The included methylene blue (basic dye) and eosin (acidic dye) stain the nucleus purple and nucleolus and cytoplasm blue. This is useful for evaluating background substances which show up as a magenta pink (mucin, colloid, chondroid tissue, basement membrane tissue).

Adequacy of Sample

This is a crucial part of fine needle aspiration cytology. It is a multifaceted process and depends on factors such as quality of the specimen (fixation and preparation), quantity and quality of diagnostic cells, interpreter skill and experience, and comfort level of the cytopathologist in rendering a definitive opinion. The cytopathologist is motivated to give the clinician as much accurate information as possible so that a proper surgical or observational decision can be presented. If the cytopathologist cannot arrive at a cytologic decision with confidence over time, patients are submitted to an unreasonable number of reaspirations with its costs and discomforts. On the other hand, if the pathologist is too aggressive in making decisions based on inadequate sampling, inappropriate surgery may result. So an important dialog and trust must evolve between the clinician and cytopathologist. In the clinical setting where a large volume of patients with thyroid disorders present, an efficiency of providing ultrasound availability and corresponding FNA sampling must be developed. If there is knowledge up front that several patients will require FNA, a proper timing schedule can be developed. In the experience of the authors, simple procurement of appropriately defined FNA samples under ultrasound guidance can be obtained within 10 min. On the other hand, samples procured with the cytopathologist on site, who must examine the specimens for adequacy at the same time, add significant time to the process. In review of sampling diagnostic rate in the setting with sampling alone, an approximate 20% nondiagnostic rate occurs. One could argue that this "failure" rate could be reduced to a negligible value if each case were examined concurrently with the cytopathology review. It is simply a matter of preference for the clinician and availability of the cytopathologist or technician who may be the emissary reviewing the sample for adequacy. One alternative is to accrue "nondiagnostic" aspirate patients into one expanded clinic time-slot with the pathologist in attendance to examine each specimen for adequacy.

Several criteria for "adequacy" have evolved. Although there are variations in what cytopathologists recognize when they examine a specimen through the microscope, an attempt to standardize this process has been developed at a national and even international level. At Henry Ford Hospital, the same criteria remain today as those published in 1985, and this is based on a single institutional experience with over 3,000 specimens. They require identification of 8–10 fragments of follicular cells on each of at least two smears [24]. These criteria are rather rigid, and thus a high unsatisfactory rate of 20% is inherent in their results. They argue that this requirement reduces their false-negative rate. There are several exceptions to the numeric requirement of benign follicular cells. Any specimen that contains abundant colloid is considered adequate (and benign), even if six groups of follicular cells are not identified. A sparsely cellular specimen with abundant colloid is by implication a predominantly macrofollicular nodule and thus almost certainly benign. When a specific diagnosis (i.e., lymphocytic thyroiditis) can be rendered and whenever there is atypia, the specimen is considered adequate for evaluation. Other experts at the Mayo Clinic and Ohio State have published their requirements which appear more liberal. These authors require 5–6 groups of well-preserved follicular cells, each group requiring 10–15 cells [25, 26]. In fact, the recently published guidelines from the ATA suggest that sample adequacy of six follicular groups of 10–15 cells from at least two aspirates of a nodule are sufficient for specimen adequacy [16].

When samples are nondiagnostic or inadequate, the clinician must not assume that the lesion is benign. There are certain circumstances in which the patient can be observed with delayed repeat ultrasound rather than submitted to repeat biopsy, but this concept thus assumes that no biopsy has ever been taken. The reasons for this approach may be secondary to patient preference and low index of suspicion of malignancy on ultrasound. Most of the time a repeat FNA cytology is required. In this circumstance it is preferable to make provisions for the cytopathologist to be in attendance to review the specimen for adequacy. Seventy-five percent of these nodules will then be converted into a diagnostic category [27].

With lesions of mixed solid and cystic composition, the sample target should always be the more solid areas under ultrasound direction. In spite of these efforts, nondiagnostic results may be reported. In this circumstance, the sonographic characteristics may determine whether this patient should have a repeat sample, undergo surgical excision, or prefer to be followed with ultrasound surveillance. With certain single nodules identified on ultrasound, cytologic findings may not be definitive in spite of adequacy of sampling. Two common aspirates in this category are "follicular neoplasm" or "Hurthle cell lesion" and are reported in 15–30% of specimens along with a 20–30% risk of malignancy [28, 29]. Occasionally, an aspirate has so many cells with nuclear grooves and cytoplasmic inclusions that a diagnosis of papillary carcinoma is definitive and certain. The alert cytopathologist must consider the possibility that this lesion may be a hyalinizing trabecular tumor. An immunohistochemical stain with MIB-1 should be requested in this circumstance. An article from the Mayo Clinic by Carney et al. from 2008 describes their experience with 119 cases of this tumor [30]. Nineteen of 24 specimens which they reviewed from outside consultation were submitted to them with a tentative diagnosis of highly suspicious or overt papillary carcinoma which in retrospect was incorrect. In their entire series with this tumor, MIB-1 was positive in 71% and another 13% were equivocal whereas papillary carcinoma does not demonstrate uptake of this stain. This is an important process to identify before surgery as this tumor is actually benign, noninvasive, nonrecurring, and does not metastasize. Of these 119 cases, 118 have remained benign with the aforementioned characteristics. The surgical implications are important as the only procedure required would be a thyroid lobectomy. A representative

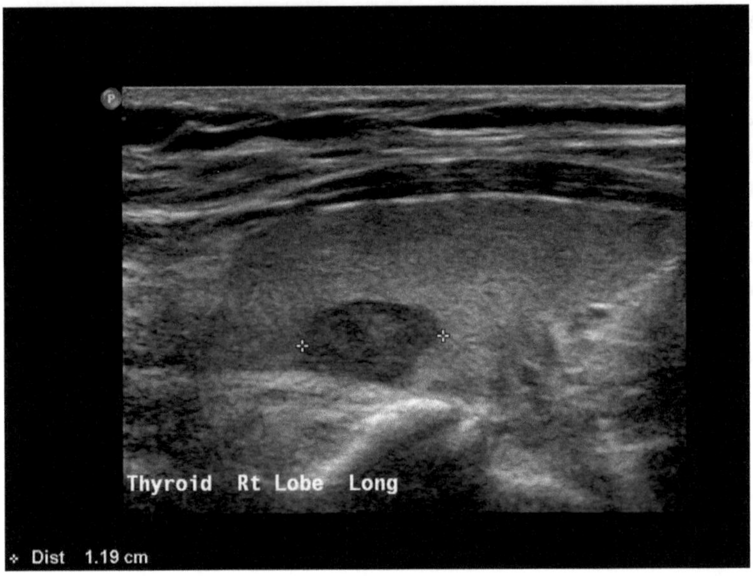

Fig. 9.1 A hypoechoic nodule is noted on sagittal gray scale ultrasound. It has no specific characteristics suggesting malignancy but subsequent FNA demonstrates abundant nuclear inclusions and grooves suggestive of papillary carcinoma. Immunohistochemical stain with MIB-1 of the fine needle aspirate suggests a diagnosis of hyalinizing trabecular tumor, a generally benign lesion. This was confirmed at definitive histology demonstrated in Fig. 9.2d, e

ultrasound and other cytologic/histologic details are illustrated (Figs. 9.1 and 9.2).

The issues of which lesions have a higher malignant potential and which can be observed are as yet indeterminate, and patients with these cytologic diagnoses are recommended for surgical intervention and assessment for both capsular and vascular invasion. There is some promise in molecular markers to improve the diagnostic accuracy of the cytologic specimens and assist in making these decisions. Prospective studies evaluating genetic markers such as BRAF, RAS, and RET/PTC and protein markers such as galactin-3 have been completed, but their clinical applications are as yet in the early development phase [31–33].

Another ultrasound sampling issue surrounds the problem of multinodular goiter and which nodules to submit to biopsy. A multinodular thyroid has the same risk of malignancy as a gland containing a single solitary nodule [34, 35]. However, one study with large sample size determined that a solitary nodule does indeed carry a statistically greater likelihood of malignancy than multiple nodules [36]. These authors recommend diagnostic ultrasound with delineation of the size and characteristics of each nodule, but caution that if only the dominant nodule is sampled, thyroid cancer may be overlooked.

Recommendation 12 from the revised ATA guidelines 2009 addresses this issue in the following ways [16]:

(a) In the presence of two or more thyroid nodules >1 cm, those with a suspicious sonographic appearance should be aspirated preferentially. Recommendation rating: B. ("The recommendation is based on fair evidence that a service or intervention can improve important health outcomes, but the strength of the evidence is limited by the number, quality or consistency of the individual studies; generalizability to routine practice; or indirect nature of the evidence on health outcomes.")

(b) If none of the nodules has a suspicious sonographic appearance and multiple sonographically similar coalescent nodules with no intervening normal parenchyma are present, the likelihood of malignancy is low and it is reasonable to aspirate the largest nodules only and observe the others with serial US examinations. Recommendation rating: C. ("The recommendation is based on expert opinion.")

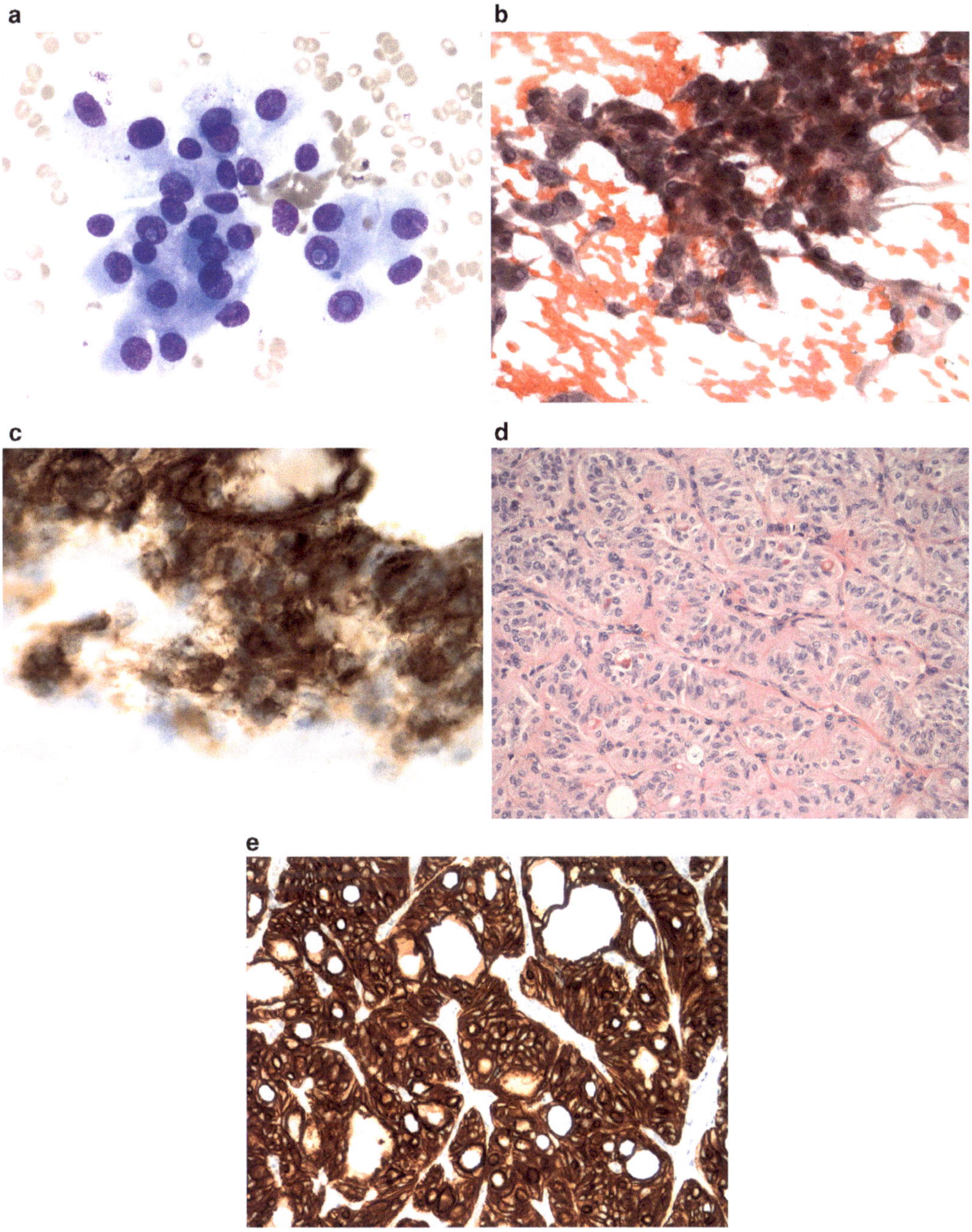

Fig. 9.2 After FNA of the nodule, routine cytology demonstrates abundant intranuclear inclusions and nuclear grooves (**a**, **b**). Immunohistochemical stain reveals positive cytoplasmic concentration of MIB-1 (**c**). H and E histology demonstrates the typical compact trabecular pattern, hyaline matrix, and nests of benign cells (**d**). MIB-1 stain of the tissue sample designates intense uniform cytoplasmic stain throughout the specimen (**e**)

Cytologic Criteria

Now that the process of procurement of samples and adequacy of cellular material has been covered, the specific elements that the cytopathologist employs to render a diagnosis should be described. There are some variations on this schema, but most employ something relatively similar to the six categories outlined below. This will allow the reader to understand just what the cytopathologist means when reporting one of these six broad diagnoses [13]:

1. Unsatisfactory – No follicular cells are identified.
2. Inadequate – Follicular cells are present, but there are insufficient numbers below the criteria established for adequacy. There may be abundant colloid with no follicular cells but some histiocytes. Some of the follicular cells may be atypical but still inadequate to advance to a higher diagnostic level. Cysts are commonly placed in this category.

   Both 1 and 2 would be determined to represent "nondiagnostic" aspirates. Ten to twenty percent of samples fall into the nondiagnostic category depending on which of the aforementioned criteria for adequacy is adhered to [13, 37, 38].
3. Negative – Cellular detail consistent with benign, nonneoplastic disorder. The processes which routinely fall into this category are benign adenomatous nodule, goiter, and thyroiditis. There may be isolated groups of mildly atypical follicular cells in a background of multinodular goiter or Hashimoto thyroiditis where cellular atypia is common. Sixty to seventy percent of diagnoses fall into this category.
4. Abnormal – Benign neoplasms such as follicular adenoma or Hurthle cell neoplasm fall into this category.
5. Suspicious – There are three subsets which are as follows (a) adequate cellularity with cytology suggestive but not diagnostic of malignancy, (b) adequate cellularity with most but not all features of malignancy, and (c) inadequate cellularity but nuclear details strongly favor malignancy. Eleven to twenty-one percent of cases fall into the "suspicious" category [26, 37, 39, 40].
6. Positive – The cytologic details are confirmatory of malignancy with adequacy of sample. Four percent of specimens fall into this category. The false-positive rate varies between 0 and 7.7%, and papillary carcinoma is the most common presumed diagnosis [26]. The sensitivity of malignancy ranges from 65% to 98% with an average of 83%. The specificity is higher with a range of 72–100% and average 92% [37].

Techniques of Ultrasound-Guided FNA

The specific methodology of fine needle aspiration has been left for the end of the chapter to better emphasize the information gleaned from the technique and the goals which the clinician must have in mind prior to sampling. There are many ways to arrive at the same place, and the details of the aspiration techniques are simply the way both authors perform the procedure. Some of the elements of FNA have been discussed in other portions of the chapter for reasons of association, but it will be helpful to describe the technique in an orderly manner as if the sample is being obtained as we proceed through the dialog.

Decision to proceed or defer the procedure – To begin, the clinician must decide whether circumstances are reasonable to proceed at the initial visit or invite the patient to return for the procedure at a future date. These decisions will depend on whether or not the physician is on time with his/her clinic schedule and perhaps more importantly how much the patient will be inconvenienced by a return for the procedure. Patients who have traveled several hours for the visit including ultrasound really appreciate the efforts to accomplish everything at the same time. Some patients have comorbidities which include anticoagulation with Coumadin. In this situation, it may be preferable to perform the procedure with the cytopathologist in attendance to minimize extra aspiration passes. It is rarely necessary to ask the patient to discontinue Coumadin for fine needle aspiration.

Preliminaries – Regardless of the method, the patient must understand the goals of the procedure, and this should be rediscussed if this has been done at a previous visit. The patient should sign an operative consent and understand the risks to include bleeding, hematoma, and inadequate sample requiring repeat FNA at some future date. Every patient is apprehensive about having needles penetrate into the neck, and it is helpful to emphasize that the procedure is painless after local anesthesia is initiated. In fact, local anesthesia is very helpful to allow the clinician to concentrate on the work ahead rather than have a squirming patient and the very real problem of vasovagal response.

Position – The patient should be placed into a recumbent position either with a static table or motorized chair which can be changed in its positioning. The patient should be at the waist level of the physician performing the procedure who himself is positioned at the patient's right side if the aspiration is performed by a right-handed individual. In most circumstances, the physician will use the left hand to manipulate the transducer and dominant right hand for the biopsy. Occasionally the hands are reversed especially if a long axis technique is performed with needle entry from the left of the transducer. The ultrasound console is above the patient's right shoulder and the nurse or assistant to the left of the patient.

Setup – This is perhaps one of the most important and underemphasized parts of the procedure. The solutions into which the slides will be placed should be organized before the procedure is initiated. It is helpful to use partitioned trays into which the receptor jars with slots for the slides are placed. The transducer with a layer of gel can be covered with saran wrap which does not interfere with the projected images at all (Fig. 9.3). This allows generous application of alcohol to both the covered transducer and the skin. Using this technique, the authors have never encountered a postprocedure infection. Alcohol is injurious to the components of the transducer, and the saran wrap cover both prevents alcohol contact and allows a sterile field for entry. The local anesthetic has been prepared, and a marking pen is easily accessed.

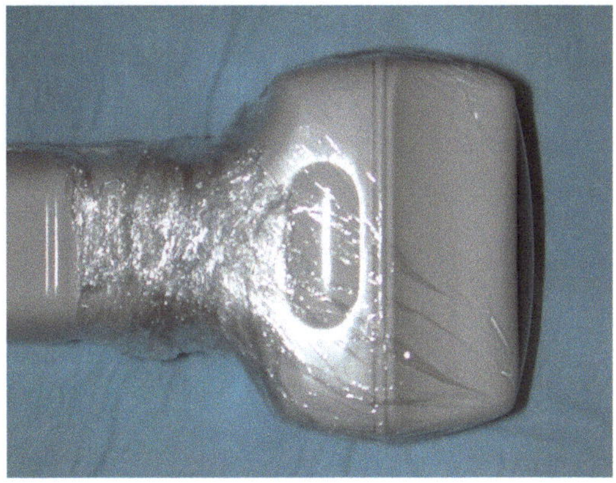

Fig. 9.3 Saran wrap is an excellent barrier to alcohol which can degrade materials covering the transducer. Gel must be placed on the transducer footprint before applying saran wrap which should as well cover the connecting cable

Local Anesthesia – Regardless of the problem at hand and previous ultrasounds, a formal basic ultrasound examination is repeated to obtain a fresh look at the lesion. If the short axis technique is employed, the target is positioned in the exact midportion of the display screen. A mark is placed 5 mm superior to the midpoint of the transducer which essentially bisects the thyroid lesion (Fig. 9.4). After the skin is marked, the transducer can be removed and the local anesthesia infiltrated. An area about the size of a quarter is infiltrated just at the level of dermis/subcutaneous tissues (Fig. 9.5). If the strap or SCM muscles are well developed, they can be infused secondarily under ultrasound guidance. If a long axis technique is employed, the entry site at the appropriate side of the transducer is anesthetized and then the tract to the lesion can be secondarily anesthetized under ultrasound guidance.

Needle Insertion – The short axis or vertical technique is generally preferred by the authors for most FNA samples. There are several reasons for this preference (1) the distance to be traversed is shorter, and (2) the needle tracks in a direction parallel to the trachea and great vessels,

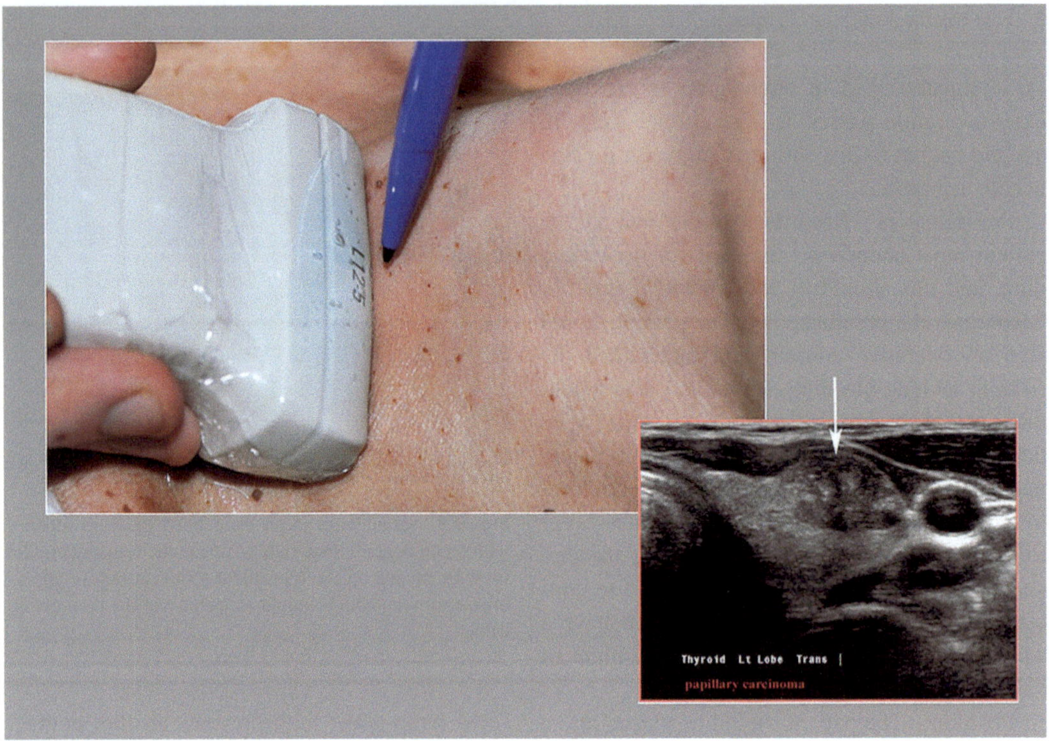

Fig. 9.4 With the short axis method of FNA, it is preferable to position the transducer in a transverse orientation. The transducer is moved to a position where the lesion is in the exact center of the field and a dot with marking pen placed approximately 5 mm craniad to the transducer at the midpoint

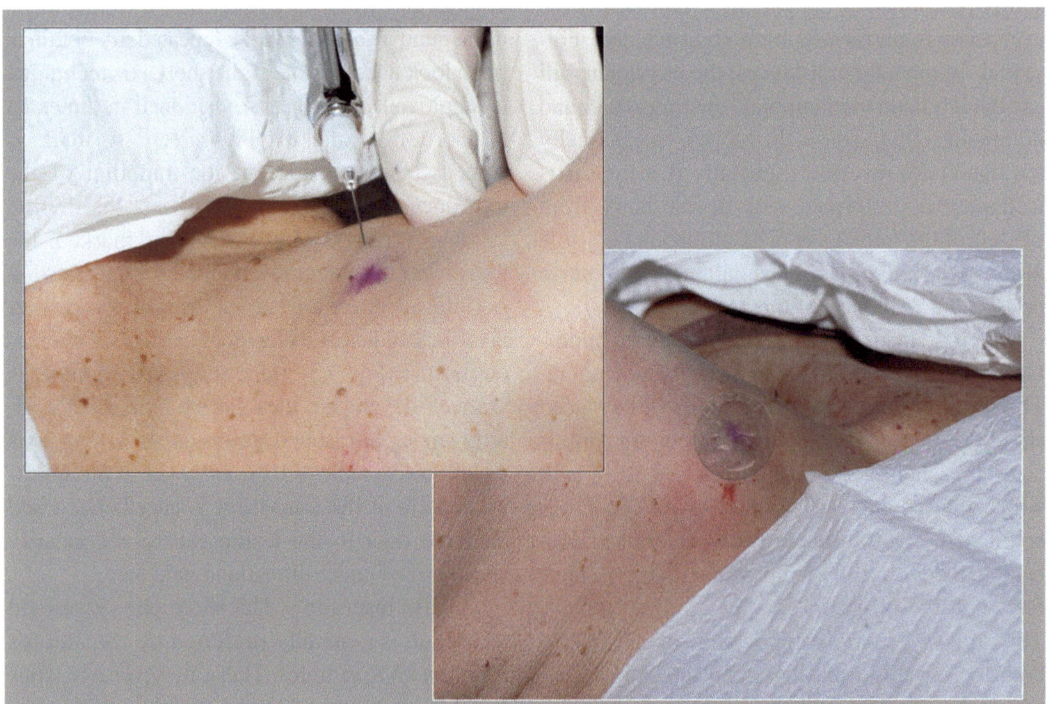

Fig. 9.5 The transducer is then removed and the skin cleansed with alcohol and infiltrated at the marked point and for a quarter-sized vicinity which includes the subcutaneous tissues and occasionally strap and SCM muscles. This provides a wide field for needle entry which always provides adequate analgesia for multiple insertions

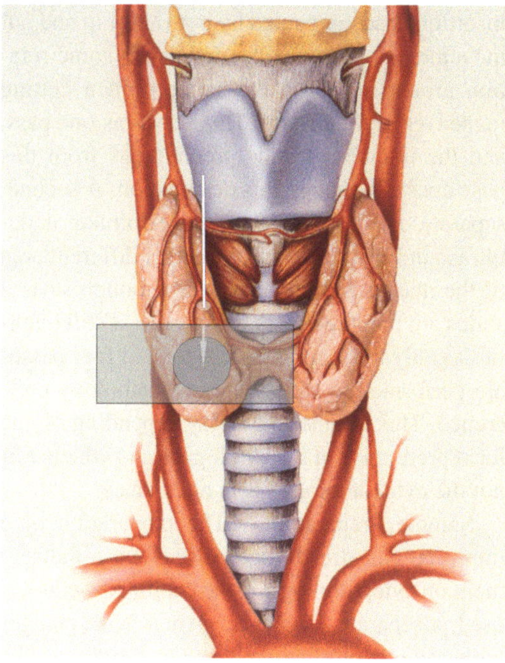

Fig. 9.6 The needle path in the short axis technique parallels both the trachea and vessels within the carotid sheath

minimizing potential penetration of those structures (Fig. 9.6). An example of this advantage is portrayed in a case of a narrow thyroid gland where the combination of a transverse transducer position along with a long axis technique becomes problematic (Fig. 9.7). In this circumstance the trachea or carotid artery cannot be avoided without using either the short axis method or turning the transducer to a sagittal orientation with long axis FNA.

With the short axis method, the path of the needle cannot be visualized. The tip of the needle is seen as a hyperechoic spot (Figs. 9.8 and 9.9). As with every method, the needle is oscillated so that it can be determined to be within, superficial, or deep to the lesion. With practice, the depth of the lesion can be matched with the proper angle of entry into the tissues, and usually the initial needle entry is into the mass proper (Fig. 9.10). Although this technique is more difficult to master initially as the entire needle cannot be seen, with commitment and practice it may become the

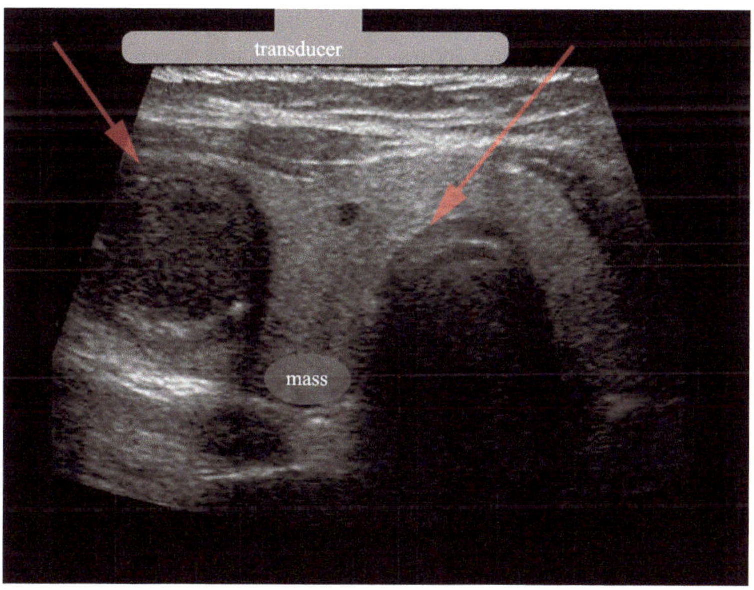

Fig. 9.7 In circumstances where the thyroid gland is narrow, it may not be possible to avoid the carotid artery or trachea without either a short axis method or rotation of the transducer to a sagittal orientation for long axis needle biopsy

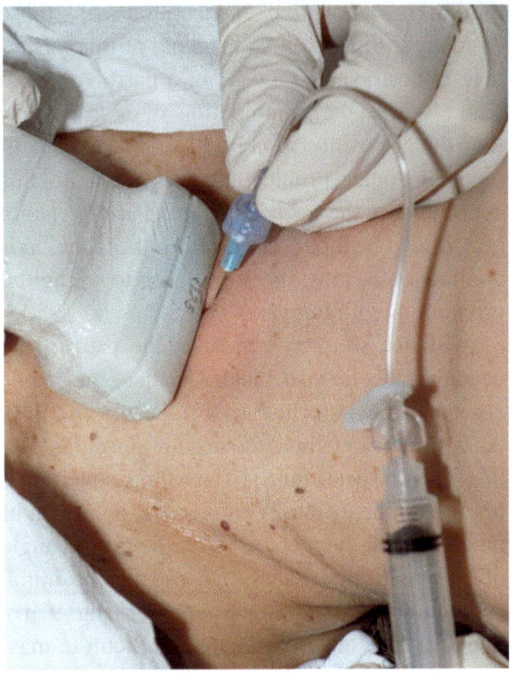

Fig. 9.8 A short length of tubing can be used between the aspirating syringe and the needle. This requires an assistant to perform aspiration on request

preferred technique. One technical tip concerning superficial lesions should be mentioned. In this circumstance, the needle entry should be further away from the transducer to allow a more appropriate superficial angle to the mass. If the long or longitudinal axis technique is employed, the needle must enter exactly at the midpoint of the side of the transducer and the penetration path must maintain an axis parallel to the long axis of the transducer (Fig. 9.11). From there, the only variation in needle position is to determine if the path is superficial or deep to the lesion. Corrective repositioning of the needle can then be performed. Occasionally the needle tip in the long axis method is beyond the lesion, and it is critical to make certain that the needle is withdrawn to a proper intralesional position before samples are taken. Again, the advantage of the long axis method is that the entire needle path can be visualized into the target (Fig. 9.12).

An important distinction must be examined regarding the number of samples. The initial needle insertion is accompanied by both short in and out movements of the needle along with some rotation around its long axis to perform a cutting maneuver of the tissues. This serves as one pass, and the number of slide preparations from this pass does not change this designation. A second, separate needle insertion is performed under ultrasound guidance, and usually a different area of the mass is sampled. Again, although several slides are prepared from this needle, it still qualifies as only the second pass. A total of four passes are performed to satisfy the cytopathology preference. This number may vary depending on the local preference of the cytologists and whether or not the cytopathologist is in attendance.

Sample Preparation – The preparation of a thin prep has already been discussed in the segment on cytopathology. If the capillary method is used, a separate 3- or 5-cc syringe with plunger withdrawn is used to expel the material onto the slide. If an aspiration method is employed and the syringe or tubing remains attached, some technicians recommend prewithdrawing the plunger halfway such that the material can automatically be expressed after the needle is removed from the tissue. The most important part of this process is to efficiently and immediately place the slide into the alcohol bay to avoid air-drying artifact. There is no need to worry or change strategies if the sample has an inordinate amount of blood. This simply cannot be avoided, and the only option is to sample a different area and hope that representative cells can be obtained. Air-dried samples are also important to obtain, as well as insertion of some samples into Cytolyte solution for preparation of a cell block if the cytopathologist chooses to add this to the methodology. Occasionally lymphoma is suspected on the basis of ultrasound and possibly adjacent lymphadenopathy. In this circumstance, specimens should also be placed in RPMI solution for subsequent flow cytometry. There are circumstances where thyroglobulin (Tg) identification is important, usually from lymph nodes in attempts to identify metastatic papillary carcinoma. This method of assessment is quite simple. After the material is expressed onto the slide, 0.5 cc of saline are flushed through the needle into

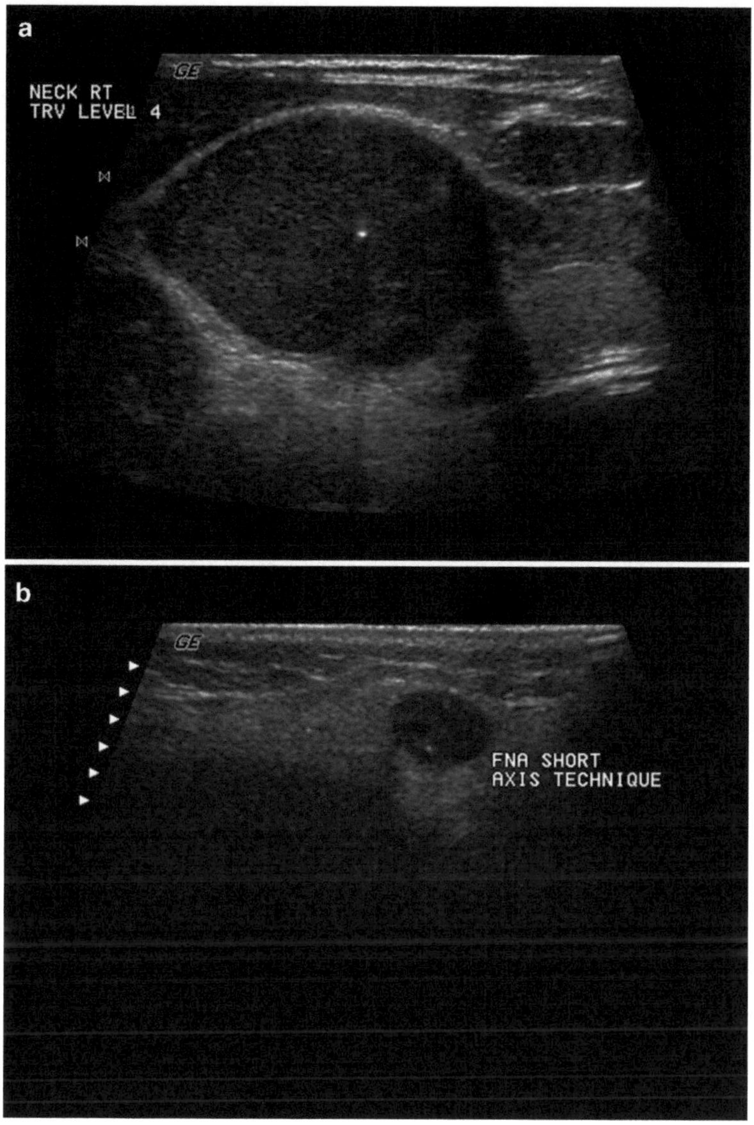

Fig. 9.9 With the short axis technique, the full length of the needle is not visible. These images demonstrate the appearance of the tip in static mode (**a**, **b**)

an appropriate vacuum tube for thyroglobulin determination. It is not important to have a precise quantitative assessment; the presence of thyroglobulin is enough to render the correct information. If preferred, an entire separate aspirate for thyroglobulin can be performed along with saline rinse. Similarly, there are circumstances when parathyroid hormone (PTH) is important to identify. Intrathyroidal lesions suspect for ectopic parathyroid adenoma or sonographically suspect masses in ectopic locations in the thymus, upper neck, carotid sheath, or lateral neck may be good candidates for PTH sampling. This material is handled in the same manner with saline rinse, and the specimen should be placed on ice. Usually if positive for an ectopic parathyroid

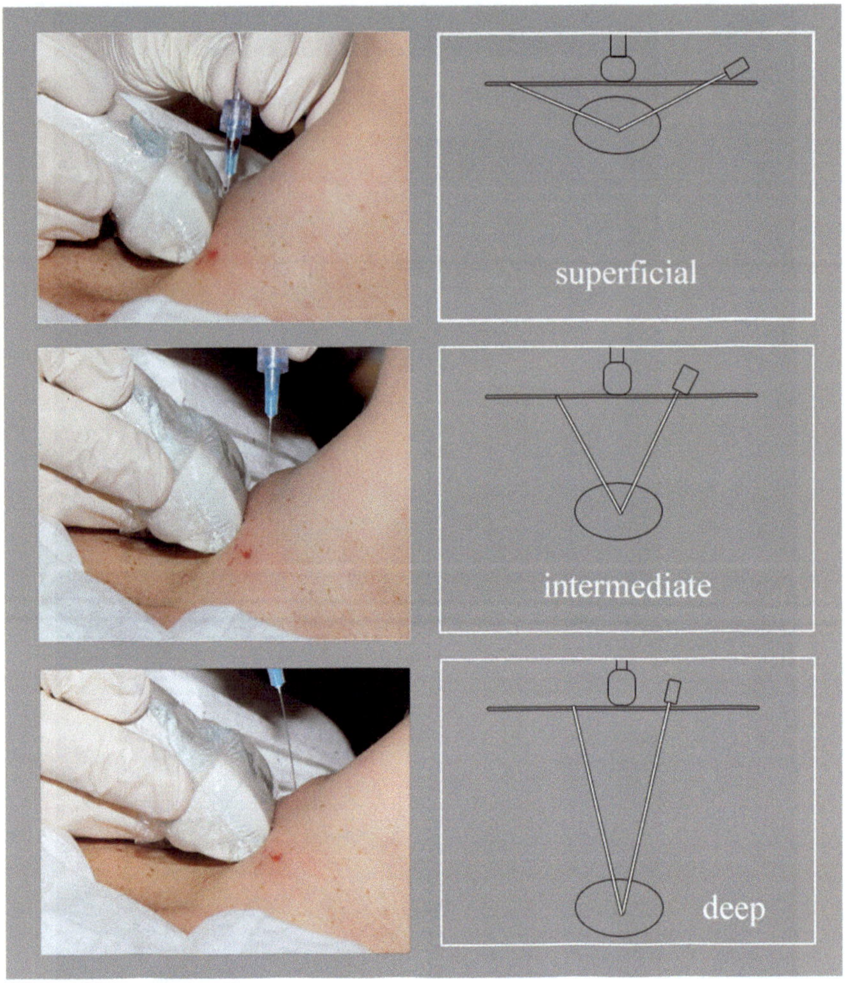

Fig. 9.10 The short axis technique of FNA is performed without a guide attached to the transducer. Appropriate angulation and insertion distance from the edge of the transducer is dependent on the depth of the lesion

lesion, the values will be quite abnormally elevated, in the thousands pg/ml. This is an extremely important concept since cytology may not be too helpful. Of course, immunohistochemistry can be applied to cytologic specimens for special circumstances.

Core Biopsy – Although this is not a commonly used method, in certain circumstances it is a pivotal technique. The Bard Magnum System is one of many tools to perform this sample (Figs. 9.13 and 9.14). Usually, it requires a larger than average mass and careful planning. The circumstances that are most often considered for core biopsy are lymphoma, large fixed neck masses, very fibrotic masses which do not yield cells for cytology such as Riedel thyroiditis, and occasionally poorly differentiated or anaplastic carcinoma (Fig. 9.15). There are a few steps which are somewhat different from FNA. The first requirement is to determine the depth of the mass from the surface and the depth of the lesion itself (Fig. 9.16). This is one circumstance where

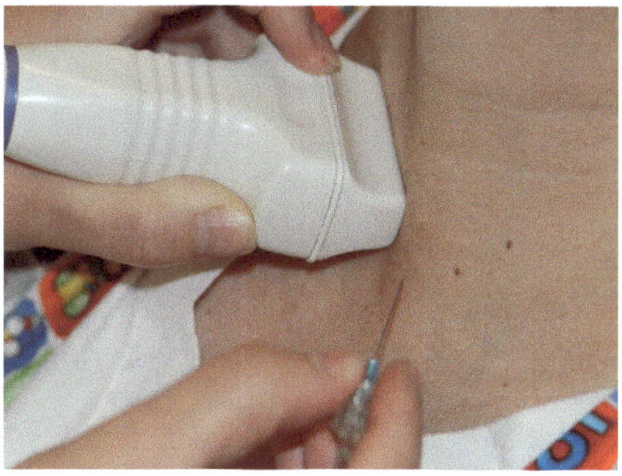

Fig. 9.11 In the long axis technique, the needle insertion is 1–2 cm lateral to the edge of the transducer for shallow lesions and closer for deep targets. The entire length of the needle beneath the transducer is identified. The needle must be exactly coaxial with the center of the long dimension of the transducer, and the angle of insertion depends on whether the needle will pass superficial, deep, or directly into the target

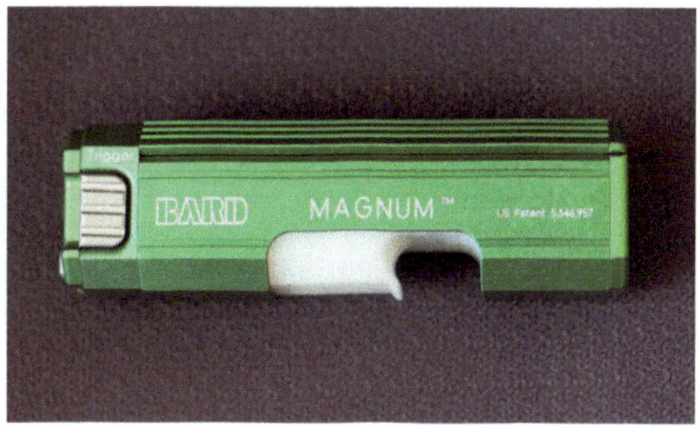

Fig. 9.13 Core biopsies may be obtained with a special triggering apparatus

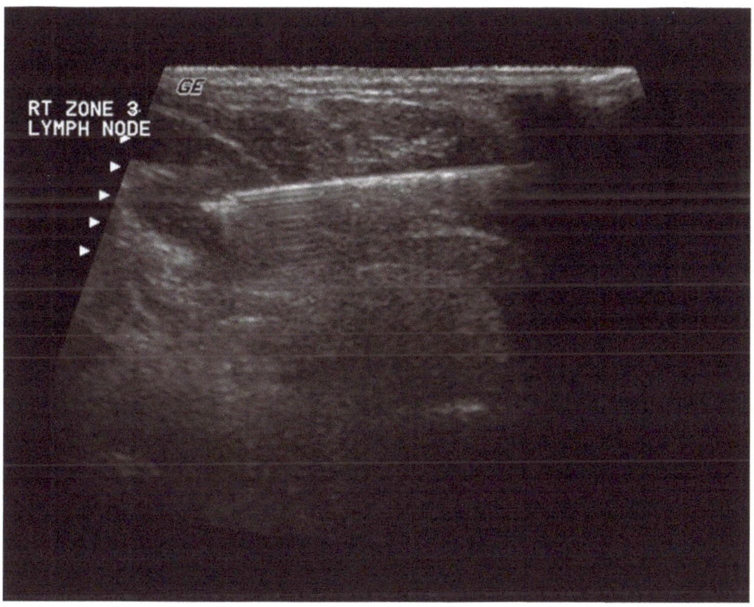

Fig. 9.12 The full length of the needle can be tracked with the long axis method. Reverberation artifact beneath the needle is commonly seen

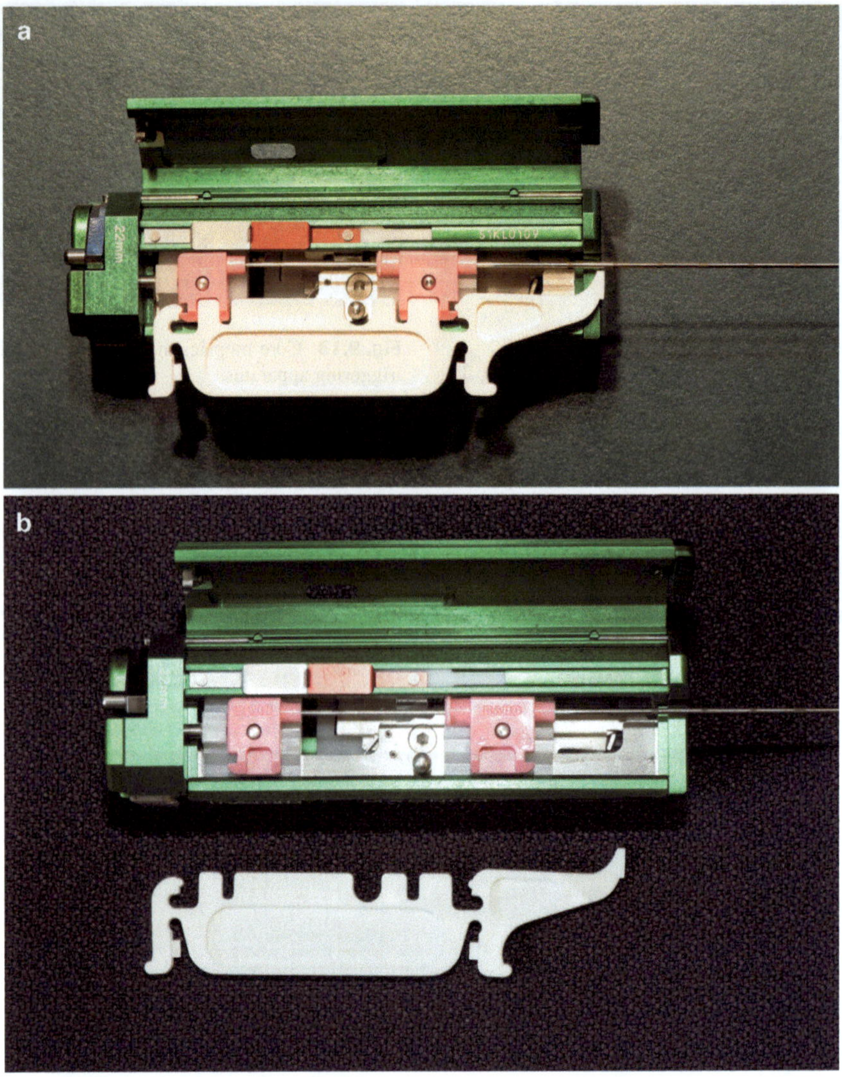

Fig. 9.14 The device holds sterile packaged core needles from 14 to 18 gauge. The core needle is placed in the device with a special element (**a**) which releases it (**b**) avoiding any contact with the shaft or needle tip

the short axis technique is preferable in order to maximize safety vis-a-vis the carotid artery and internal jugular vein. The sampling needle movements are parallel to the great vessels. The core needles have a measureable extension or "throw" from the tip. With the Bard Magnum Biopsy System, a setting on the body of the unit designates whether the needle extends either 15 or 22 mm beyond the resting tip (Fig. 9.17). When the trigger is depressed, a series of movements happen almost simultaneously. The stylet in the needle extends the specific additional distance from its resting length. In an instant later, the cutting sheath slides over the depression in the stylet, completing construction of the core (Fig. 9.18). If the lesion is substantially deeper in an AP or superior to inferior plane than this measured "throw," the technique has little risk. If the

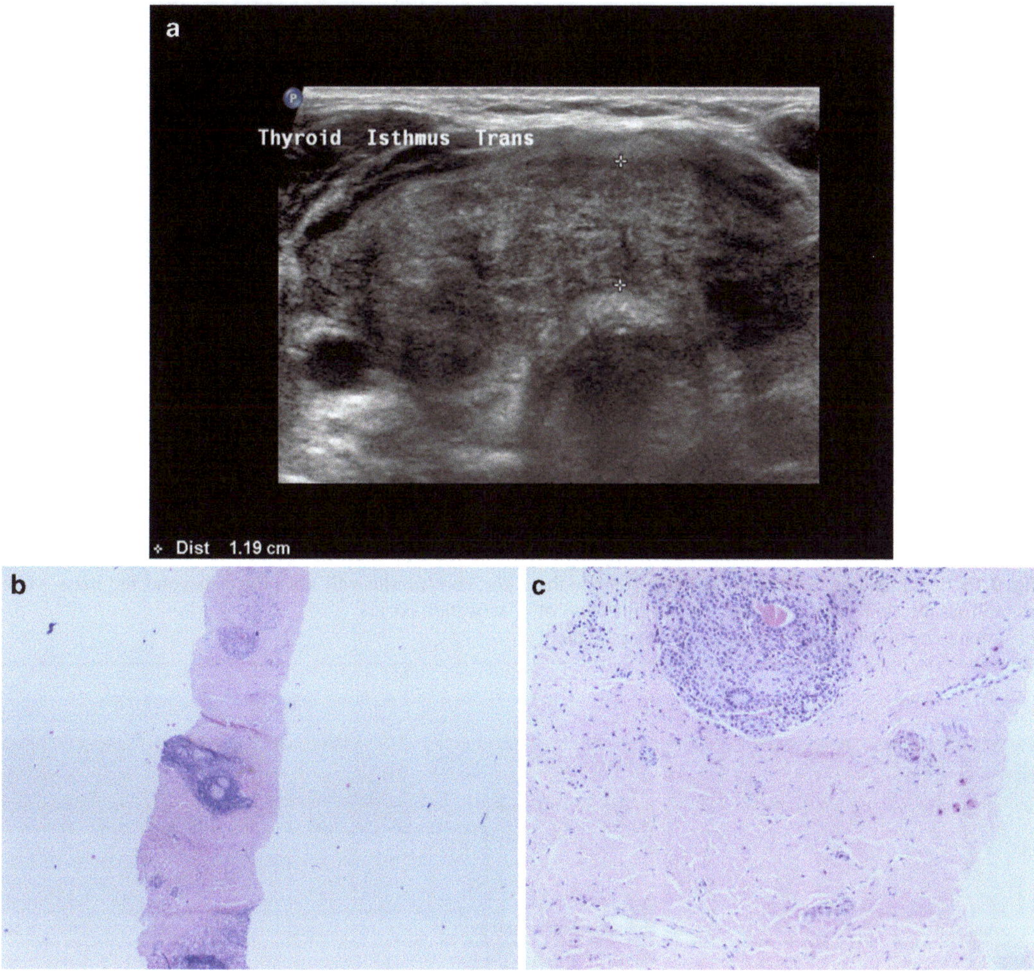

Fig. 9.15 A core biopsy was performed after two previous failed FNA attempts to retrieve any cells from this rock-hard thyroid gland and isthmus (**a**). The core sample demonstrates near-complete replacement of the gland with fibrosis and only occasional, scattered groups of follicular cells (**b**, **c**)

mass is smaller, then these measurements are more critical, and one needs to know just how far the needle can safely be inserted into the mass before extension beyond it can occur. Since a tissue core is obtained, vessels or nerves can be significantly injured if these details are not understood. These specimens are placed in formaldehyde or perhaps split to include solutions for flow cytometry if lymphoma is suspected. Finally, the patient is retained for at least 10–15 min after the sample and late ultrasound obtained to make certain that a hematoma is not developing, and a 10-min postcore biopsy ultrasound is an additional safety measure.

An alternative to large-bore core biopsy is the procurement of a microcore with the Franseen needle. In fact, there are significant arguments in favor of proceeding directly to this type of core in lieu of a side-cutting conventional core just described. The Franseen needle used for thyroid sampling is 9 cm in length and either sized 18 or 20 gauge. Local anesthesia is required and a small

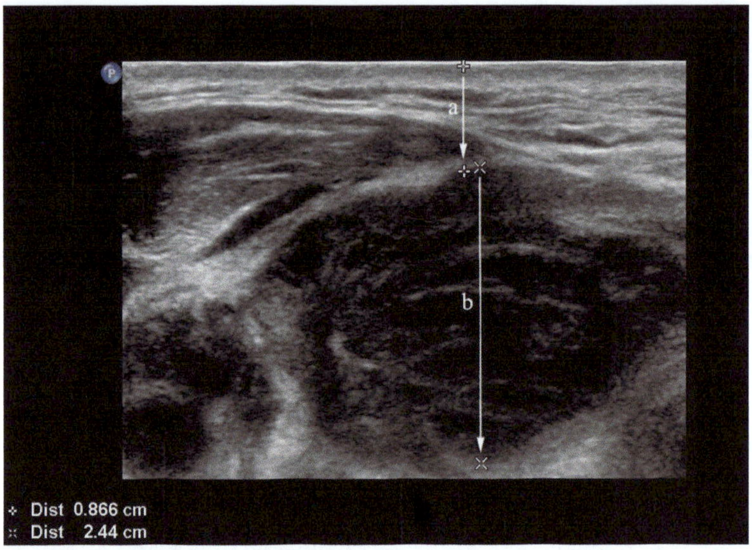

Fig. 9.16 It is important to measure both the depth to the lesion from the skin surface (**a**) and the full thickness of the lesion to be biopsied (**b**) to make certain that the tip of the core needle will not project beyond the mass when activation occurs

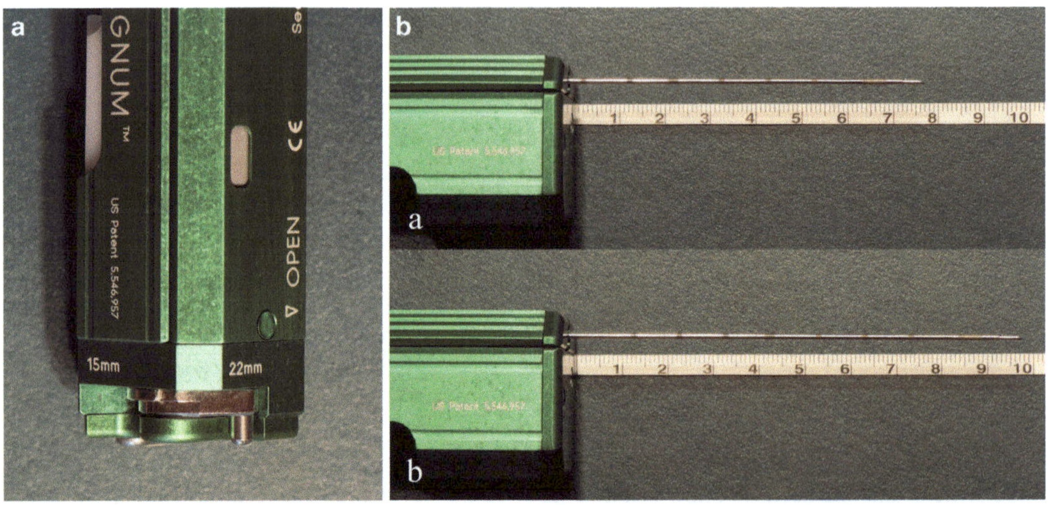

Fig. 9.17 The distance of needle penetration beyond the core resting length can be programmed for either 15 or 22 mm with this Bard device (**a**). This is illustrated with the needle in the handle device before and after the trigger is activated (**b**). Note the 22 mm extension of the needle beyond the ready length after the unit has been triggered

puncture of the skin allows proper entry of the outer trocar and its stylet into the deeper tissue planes (Fig. 9.19a). Once the needle/stylet combination is at the target under ultrasound guidance, the stylet is withdrawn and an extension of suction tubing with attached syringe is applied to the needle hub. The tip of the trocar is serrated (Fig. 9.19b), and when advanced with suction, it is rotated allowing a core to enter the needle. The needle is then withdrawn with continuous applied

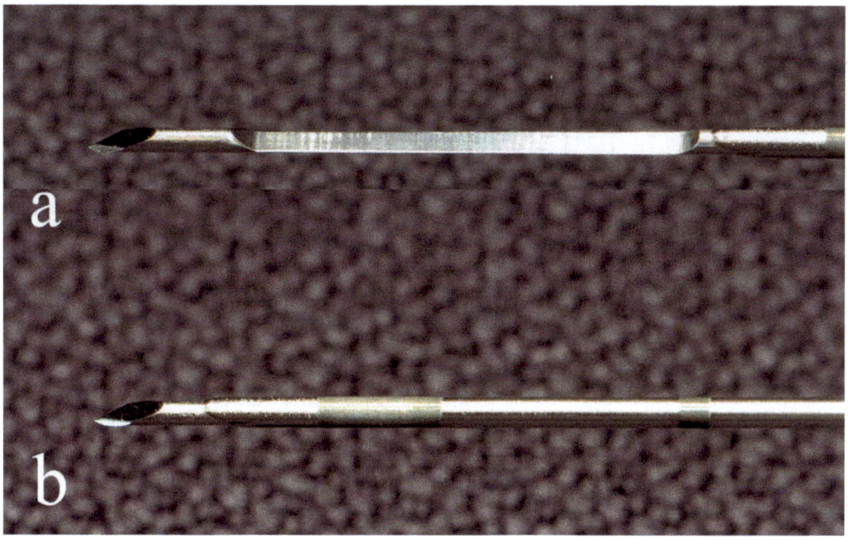

Fig. 9.18 In dynamic core mode, the internal stylet with depression extends into the tissues at the designated distance (**a**) and the cutting sheath shears the core (**b**) all in a fraction of a second when the device is triggered at the handle

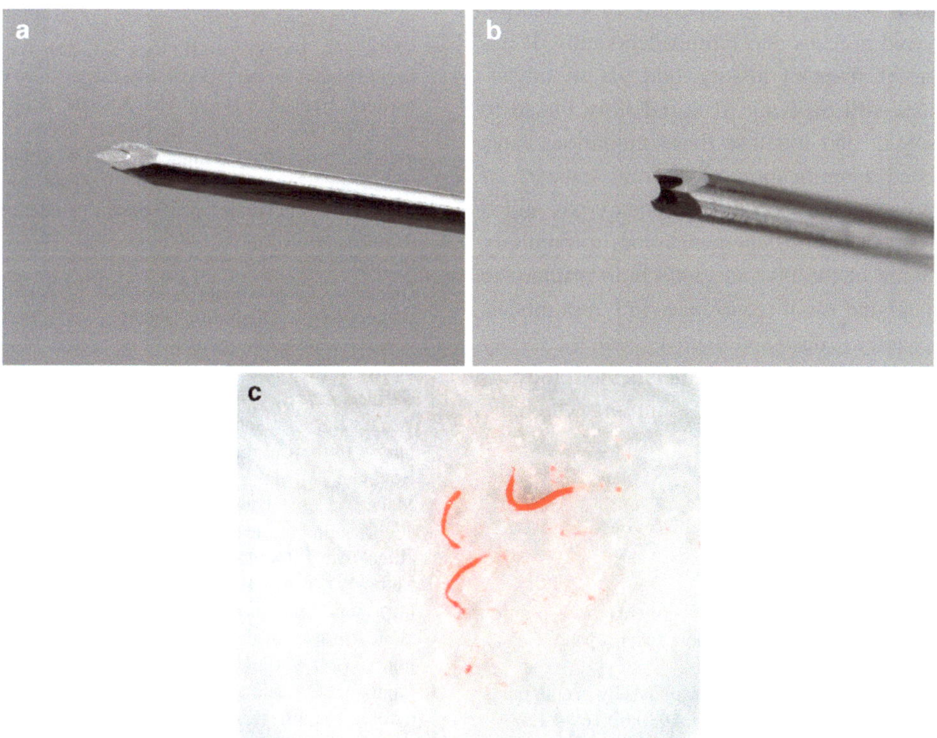

Fig. 9.19 (**a**) Franseen needle and stylet are illustrated. (**b**) The serrated end of the outer trocar is the cutting element. (**c**) The minicore samples are demonstrated

suction. The core sample can either be expressed by reinsertion of the stylet or saline rinse (Fig. 9.19c). These microcore specimens are handled in a similar way to large core samples. The principal advantages of this technique are safety of surrounding or adjacent structures since there is no "throw" or extension of the needle beyond that which is noted on the display, and there is less risk of bleeding. Whereas large core biopsies must be used for large lesions, this technique has the added advantage of its relative safety for smaller nodules and nodes. In fact, Yuen, Wong, and Ahuja have employed this technique as a conventional first option after one nondiagnostic sample in lieu of repeated FNA [41].

Summary

Fine needle aspiration cytology under ultrasound guidance is the current mainstay of evaluation of thyroid nodules and lymphadenopathy. It has a near 60 years of history, and yet its advantages are still evolving. It is indelibly linked to ultrasound, and together these modalities have permitted identification of thyroid cancers of 5 mm or less. In fact, this efficiency has added new ethical and management issues to papillary carcinoma of the thyroid gland both primary to the gland and small recurrences in lymph nodes. This chapter is designed to cover both the theory and literature surrounding the methodology as well as practical methods of sampling which are well defined and proven.

References

1. Soderstrom N. Puncture of goiters for aspiration biopsy. A preliminary report. Acta Med Scand. 1952;144:235–44.
2. Martin HE, Ellis B. Biopsy diagnosis by needle puncture and aspiration. Ann Surg. 1930;62:169–81.
3. Stewart FW. The diagnosis of tumors by aspiration. Am J Pathol. 1933;9:801–13.
4. Einhorn J, Franzen S. Thin needle biopsy in the diagnosis of thyroid diseases. Acta Radiol. 1962; 90:1619–25.
5. Lowhagen T, Zajicek J. In: Weid GL, editor. Thyroid in aspiration biopsy cytology. Part I. Cytology of supradiaphragmatic organs in monographs in clinical cytology, vol 4. Basel: S.Karger; 1974.
6. Lowhagen T, Granberg P, Lundell G, et al. Aspiration biopsy cytology (ABC) on nodules of the thyroid gland suspected to be malignant. Surg Clin North Am. 1979;59:3–18.
7. Akerman M, Tennvall J, Bjorklund J, et al. Sensitivity and specificity of fine needle aspiration cytology in the diagnosis of tumours of the thyroid gland. Acta Cytol. 1985;29:850–5.
8. Crockford PM, Bain GO. Fine needle aspiration biopsy of the thyroid. Can Med Assoc. 1974;110: 1029–32.
9. Crile Jr G, Hawk Jr WA. Aspiration biopsy of thyroid nodules. Surg Gyn Obst. 1973;136:241–5.
10. Wang CA, Vickery Jr AL, Maloof F. Needle biopsy of the thyroid. Surg Gyn Obst. 1976;143:365–8.
11. Miller JM, Hamburger JI, Kini SR. Diagnosis of thyroid nodules by fine needle aspiration and needle biopsy. JAMA. 1979;241:481–6.
12. Ashcraft MW, Van Herle AJ. Management of thyroid nodules II. Scanning techniques, thyroid suppression therapy, and fine needle aspiration. Head Neck Surg. 1981;3:297.
13. Sudha R, Kini SR. Thyroid cytopathology. Philadelphia: Lippincott Williams and Wilkins; 2008. pp. 1, 2, 21–26.
14. Miller JM, Hamburger JI, Kini SR. The impact of needle biopsy on the preoperative diagnosis of thyroid nodules. Henry Ford Hosp Med J. 1980;28:145.
15. Randolph GW. Surgery of the thyroid and parathyroid glands. Philadelphia: Saunders; 2003. p. 139–40.
16. American Thyroid Association. Revised American Thyroid Association management guidelines for patients with thyroid nodules and differentiated thyroid cancer. Thyroid. 2009;19(11):8–9.
17. Danese D, Sciacchitano S, Farsetti A, Andreoli M, Pontecorvi A. Diagnostic accuracy of conventional versus sonography-guided fine-needle aspiration biopsy of thyroid nodules. Thyroid. 1998;8:15–21.
18. Carmeci C, Jeffrey RB, McDougall IR, Nowels KW, Weigel RJ. Ultrasound-guided fine-needle aspiration biopsy of thyroid masses. Thyroid. 1998;8:283–9.
19. Bonavita JA, Mayo J, Babb J, Bennett G, Oweity T, Macari M, et al. Pattern recognition of benign nodules at ultrasound of the thyroid: which nodules can be left alone? Am J Roentgenol. 2009;193:207–13.
20. Moon WJ, Kwag HJ, Na DG. Are there any specific ultrasound findings of nodular hyperplasia ("leave me alone" lesion) to differentiate it from follicular adenoma? Acta Radiol. 2009;50:383–8.
21. Santos JEC, Leiman G. Nonaspiration fine needle cytology: application of a new technique to nodular thyroid disease. Acta Cytol. 1988;32:353–6.
22. Mair S, Dunbar F, Becker PJ, et al. Fine needle cytology: is aspiration suction necessary? A study of 100 masses in various sites. Acta Cytol. 1989;33:809–13.
23. Lowhagen T, Williams JS, Lundell G, et al. Aspiration biopsy cytology in diagnosis of cancer. World J Surg. 1981;5:61–73.

24. Kini SR, Miller JM, Hamburger JI, et al. Cytopathology of follicular lesions of the thyroid gland. Diagn Cytopathol. 1985;1:123–32.
25. Goellner JR, Gharib H, Grant CS, et al. Fine needle aspiration cytology of the thyroid 1980–86. Acta Cytol. 1987;31:587–90.
26. Caruso D, Mazzaferri EL. Fine needle aspiration biopsy in the management of thyroid nodules. Endocrinologist. 1991;1:194–202.
27. Alexander EK, Heering JP, Benson CB, Frates MC, Doubilet PM, Cibas ES, et al. Assessment of non-diagnostic ultrasound-guided fine needle aspiration of thyroid nodules. J Clin Endocrinol Metab. 2002; 87:4924–7.
28. Hegedus L. Clinical practice. The thyroid nodule. N Engl J Med. 2004;351:1674–771.
29. Baloch ZW, LiVolsi VA, Asa SL, Rosai J, Merino MJ, Randolph G, et al. Diagnostic terminology and morphologic criteria for cytologic diagnosis of thyroid lesions: a synopsis of the National Cancer Institute Thyroid Fine-Needle Aspiration State of the Science Conference. Diagn Cytopathol. 2008;36:425–37.
30. Carney JA et al. Hyalinizing trabecular tumors of the thyroid gland are almost all benign. Am J Surg Pathol. 2008;32:1877–89.
31. Bartolazzi A, Orlandi F, Saggiorato E, et al. Italian Cancer Study Group (ITCSG) Galectin-3 expression analysis in the surgical selection of follicular thyroid nodules with indeterminate fine-needle aspiration cytology: a prospective multicenter study. Lancet Oncol. 2008;9:543–9.
32. Nikiforov YE, Steward DL, Robinson-Smith TM, et al. Molecular testing for mutations in improving the fine-needle aspiration diagnosis of thyroid nodules. J Clin Endocrinol Metab. 2009;94:2092–8.
33. Franco C, Martinez V, Allamand JP, et al. Molecular markers in thyroid fine-needle aspiration biopsy: a prospective study. Appl Immunhistochem Mol Morphol. 2009;17:211–5.
34. Marqusee E, Benson CB, Frates MC, et al. Usefulness of ultrasonography in the management of nodular thyroid disease. Ann Intern Med. 2000;1339:696–700.
35. Papini E, Guglielme R, Bianchini A, et al. Risk of malignancy in nonpalpable thyroid nodules: predictive value of ultrasound and color-Doppler features. J Clin Endocrinol Metab. 2002;87:1941–6.
36. Frates MC, Benson CB, Doubilet PM, et al. Prevalence and distribution of carcinoma in patients with solitary and multiple thyroid nodules on sonography. J Clin Endocrinol Metab. 2006;91:3411–7.
37. Gharib H, Goellner JR. Fine needle aspiration biopsy of the thyroid: an appraisal. Ann Intern Med. 1993;118:282–9.
38. Hamburger JI. Extensive personal experience. Diagnosis of thyroid nodules by fine needle biopsy: use and abuse. J Clin Endocrinol Metab. 1994; 79:335–9.
39. Gharib H, Goellner JR, Johnson DA. Fine-needle aspiration cytology of the thyroid. A 12 year experience with 11,000 biopsies. Clin Lab Med. 1993;13:699–709.
40. Gharib H. Changing trends in thyroid practice: understanding nodular thyroid disease. Endocr Pract. 2004;10:31–9.
41. Yuen HY, Wong KT, Ahuja AT. Use of end-cutting needles in ultrasound-guided biopsy of neck lesions. In press.

Section III

Lymph Nodes and the Neck

Lymph Nodes

10

Michael T.C. Ying, Carmen C.M. Cho, and
Anil T. Ahuja

Introduction

Sonographic examination of neck nodes is an essential part of a routine complete ultrasound examination of head and neck lesions. It is therefore necessary for all sonologists to be familiar with the location and sonographic appearance of normal and abnormal lymph nodes.

Although there are more than 300 lymph nodes (ranging in size from 3 to 30 mm) in the head and neck, most are within 1–2 cm of the skin surface. This superficial location of neck nodes makes them readily accessible by ultrasound and amenable to a guided aspiration/biopsy.

The use of modern high-resolution transducers makes it possible for a detailed, high-quality sonographic examination to be carried out. Gray scale ultrasound evaluates nodal morphology, and Doppler ultrasound examines the intranodal vasculature. The sonologist must therefore be familiar with gray scale and Doppler features that help to distinguish a normal from an abnormal node.

M.T.C. Ying (✉)
Department of Health Technology and Informatics, The Hong Kong Polytechnic University, Hung Hom, Kowloon, Hong Kong, People's Republic of China
e-mail: htmying@polyu.edu.hk

C.C.M. Cho • A.T. Ahuja
Department of Imaging and Interventional Radiology, The Chinese University of Hong Kong, Prince of Wales Hospital, Shatin (NT), Hong Kong (SAR), China

Lymph Node Anatomy

Understanding the normal anatomy of a lymph node helps us to identify the changes in nodal morphology and vasculature during malignant transformation.

A cervical lymph node is divided into a cortex and medulla. The cortex is composed of densely packed lymphocytes, whereas the medulla consists of medullary trabeculae, medullary cords, and medullary sinuses. The afferent lymphatics enter the periphery of the lymph node and leave via the efferent lymphatic at the hilum. Cervical lymph nodes are also permeated by blood vessels. The main artery enters the lymph node at the hilum, where it branches into smaller arteries and arterioles towards the periphery of the node. Conversely, venules and small veins from the periphery converge to form the main vein, which leaves the lymph node at the hilum (Fig. 10.1) [1–3].

Classification of Lymph Nodes

Lymphatic groups in the neck form a continuous network through which lymph drains from the head and neck into the central thoracic ducts. The consistent location of lymph nodes in the head and neck helps the sonologist to systematically examine all areas in the neck. Although nodes in many areas may not be involved with thyroid and parathyroid lesions (e.g. facial, parotid, submandibular, submental), for the sake of completion, these are included in this chapter. Also, clinicians

R.A. Sofferman and A.T. Ahuja (eds.), *Ultrasound of the Thyroid and Parathyroid Glands*,
DOI 10.1007/978-1-4614-0974-8_10, © Springer Science+Business Media, LLC 2012

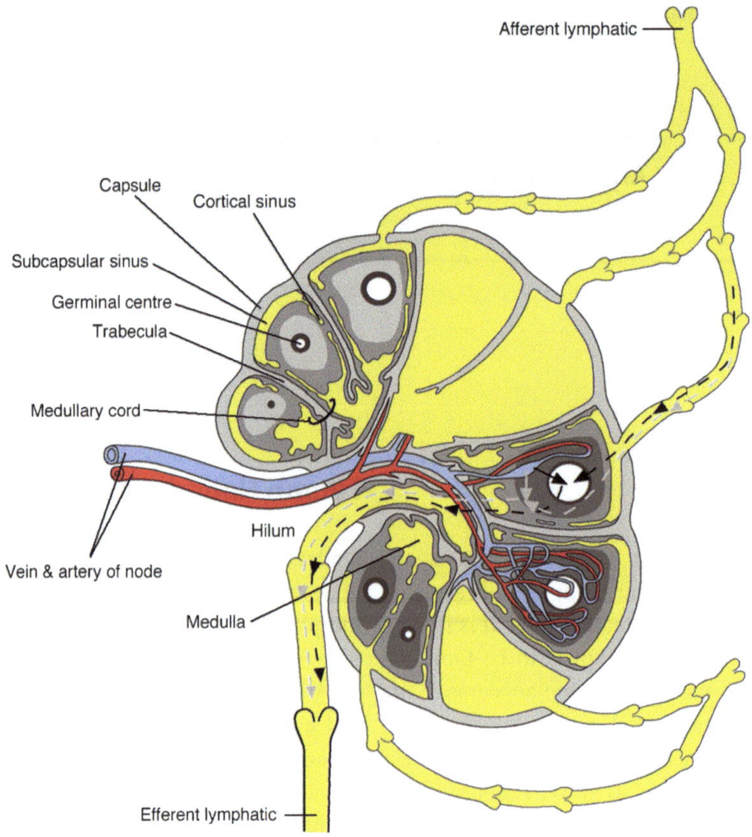

Fig. 10.1 Normal lymph node anatomy

involved with staging other head and neck cancers using ultrasound may find such information useful in their routine clinical practice.

Submental Group

Submental lymph nodes are situated behind the chin, between the anterior bellies of two digastric muscles, and superficial to the mylohyoid muscle. The number of nodes in the submental region varies from one to eight. These nodes may be distributed asymmetrically with a cluster of nodes found only on one side. Submental nodes receive lymph from the chin, lips, cheeks, floor of mouth and anterior tongue. Efferent lymph from submental nodes drains to the submandibular nodes and then into the deep cervical chain.

Submandibular Group

The submandibular gland is the key structure in identifying submandibular nodes. The submandibular gland undergoes early encapsulation during its embryonic development, and thus, most of the submandibular nodes are extraglandular. Occasionally, subcapsular nodes may be present but these are not true intraglandular nodes. Nodes are usually found at the superior and anterior aspects of the gland. Some of them are located in the submandibular niche, the space between the mylohyoid muscle and the medial surface of the mandible. There are about three to six nodes in this region. Submandibular nodes drain the anterior facial structures, floor of mouth and anterior oral cavity. Lymph from these nodes drains into the deep cervical chain.

Parotid Region

The parotid gland undergoes encapsulation late in its embryonic development. Nodes are therefore found both deep to the capsule (subcapsular) and within the parenchyma of the gland (predominantly in the superficial lobe). Thus, there are three groups of parotid nodes: nodes superficial to the parotid gland (extraparotid), subcapsular (extraglandular), and intraparenchymal (intraglandular). Extraparotid nodes (superficial parotid or preauricular nodes) are usually found in the region between the posterior parotid and the ear. There are usually three to four extraparotid nodes. Extraglandular nodes are often located at the preauricular region and the tail of the parotid gland. There are about one to two extraglandular preauricular nodes and up to three or four nodes in the tail of the parotid gland. Intraglandular nodes are usually within the superficial lobe of the parotid gland and within the fascia between the superficial and deep lobes. Normally, there are about three to four intraglandular nodes. The parotid nodes are particularly well seen in children. Their bilateral, symmetric nature and the presence of an echogenic hilus and hilar vascularity on Doppler help to distinguish them from intraparotid neoplasms. The parotid nodes drain the forehead, temporal region, external auditory canal and buccal region. These nodes in turn drain into the deep cervical chain.

Facial Region

Facial nodes are usually found anterior to the masseter muscle and superficial to the buccinator muscle in the buccal space. These nodes tend to be very small and are rarely seen on ultrasound. Lymph from the lips and maxillary region drains into the facial nodes, which then drains into the submandibular nodes.

Deep Cervical Chain

The deep cervical or internal jugular chain is the main lymphatic channel of the neck. Lymph nodes in the deep cervical chain are usually located adjacent to the internal jugular vein (IJV), predominantly at its anterolateral aspect. The deep cervical chain may be divided into upper, middle, and lower groups by the hyoid bone and cricoid cartilage (or cricothyroid membrane). There are 15–40 lymph nodes in the deep cervical chain. The jugulodigastric node (the largest node in the neck) is the most superior lymph node in the deep cervical chain, situated inferior to the posterior belly of the digastric muscle. The deep cervical nodes receive lymph from the parotid, retropharyngeal and submandibular nodes. They either empty into the IJV or subclavian vein or drain directly into the thoracic duct on the left or the right lymphatic duct on the right which then empties into the junction of the IJV and subclavian vein.

Spinal Accessory Chain

The spinal accessory chain forms a triangle with the deep cervical chain anteriorly and transverse cervical chain inferiorly. There are about 4–20 nodes in the spinal accessory chain. Lymph nodes in the spinal accessory chain run along a line drawn from the mastoid tip to the acromion and lie superficial to the scalene muscles. Looking for the fat plane between the sternomastoid muscle and the underlying scalene and levator scapulae muscles is the key to identifying these lymph nodes. At the apex of the triangle, where the sternomastoid muscle overlies the posterior belly of the digastric muscle, it is not possible to differentiate a node in the spinal accessory chain from a node in the deep cervical chain. The spinal accessory chain drains the mastoid and occipital nodes, parietal scalp, and lateral neck. It then drains into the deep cervical chain superiorly and the transverse cervical chain inferiorly.

Transverse Cervical Chain

The transverse cervical chain or supraclavicular nodes can be identified along the plane of the transverse cervical vessels. There are up to ten lymph nodes in this group. The transverse cervical chain receives lymph from the deep cervical chain medially and the spinal accessory chain laterally. It also drains the upper anterior chest wall and the anterolateral neck. The transverse cervical chain empties in a manner similar to the deep cervical chain, i.e. the left transverse cervical chain empties into the IJV or subclavian vein, or drains directly into the thoracic duct, whereas the right transverse cervical chain drains into the right lymphatic duct which then empties into the junction of the IJV and subclavian vein. Primary tumors from the chest and abdomen may metastasize to the transverse cervical chain.

Anterior Cervical Nodes

There are two main subgroups in the anterior cervical nodes that may be identified on ultrasound: the pretracheal nodes and the paratracheal nodes. The prelaryngeal (Delphian node) and prethyroid nodes are rarely seen on ultrasound. The pretracheal nodes are situated superficially and anterior to the trachea. They drain the thyroid gland and the muscles and skin of the anterior neck. They then drain into the thoracic duct on the left and into the lowest node of the deep cervical chain or upper thoracic node on the right. The paratracheal or recurrent laryngeal nodes are located lateral to the trachea in the tracheoesophageal groove and medial to the common carotid artery. These nodes may be situated behind the thyroid, between the thyroid and longus colli. On ultrasound, these nodes are often obscured by air in the trachea and esophagus and therefore cannot be adequately assessed, unless they are enlarged. The paratracheal nodes drain the larynx, piriform fossae, thyroid gland, esophagus, and trachea. They then drain into the thoracic duct on the left and the deep cervical chain on the right (Table 10.1).

Equipment and Settings

A 7.5-MHz linear transducer is the minimum requirement for ultrasound of neck lymph nodes. A higher-frequency transducer (>10 MHz) allows better resolution of the lymph node architecture. A 5-MHz convex transducer may be occasionally useful for the assessment of deeper lesions. The use of a standoff gel block may allow better visualization of large masses (using lower-frequency transducer) or very superficial mass (using a high-frequency transducer). Color and power Doppler are now routinely available on most ultrasound systems. Although power Doppler ultrasound does not provide information about

Table 10.1 Terminology of different groups of cervical lymph nodes

Common terms	Alternative terms/description
Jugulodigastric node	"Sentinel" (highest) node of internal jugular chain
Deep cervical chain	Internal jugular chain Lateral cervical chain
Omohyoid node	Deep cervical chain lymph node just superior to omohyoid (where it crosses jugular vein)
Virchow's node	"Signal" node Lowest node of deep cervical chain
Transverse cervical chain	Supraclavicular chain
Troisier's node	Most medial node of transverse cervical chain can be involved in carcinoma of the stomach
Spinal accessory chain	Posterior triangle chain Dorsal cervical chain Superficial cervical chain
Anterior cervical chain	Includes prelaryngeal, pretracheal, and paratracheal nodes
Prelaryngeal nodes	Delphian node – important in carcinoma of larynx
Paratracheal nodes	Recurrent laryngeal nodes
Retropharyngeal nodes	Lateral nodes are nodes of Rouviere

the flow direction, it is more desirable for the assessment of vasculature within lymph nodes because of its higher sensitivity in detecting small and low-flow blood vessels. When using power Doppler ultrasound, the Doppler settings should be optimized for detecting small vessels, i.e.:

- High sensitivity
- Low wall filter
- Pulse repetition frequency (PRF) 700 Hz
- Medium persistence
- The color gain is initially increased to a level which shows color noise and then gradually decreased to the level where the noise just disappears

If one would like to measure the resistance indices (resistive index, RI; pulsatility index, PI) of the intranodal vessels, the more prominent vessels should be selected. Measurements are obtained from the average of three consecutive Doppler spectral waveforms in order to get a more accurate value. The smallest sample volume should be chosen. If blood flow velocity (peak systolic velocity, PSV; and end-diastolic velocity, EDV) is measured, angle correction should be applied (angle of 60° or less).

An adjustable and mobile examination table is essential in ultrasound of neck lymph nodes, as it allows easy positioning such that the patient's neck is at the level of the ultrasound monitor and within the scanning range of the sinologist's arms.

Scanning Technique and Normal Sonographic Appearance

The patient should be positioned supine with the neck extended/hyperextended. (This may not always be possible in the old and infirm. In such cases, the neck is scanned with the patient supine and in the most comfortable position). A pillow or triangular soft pad is placed under the shoulders and lower neck for support. Each side of the neck is scanned with the chin turned toward the contralateral side. A standard examination consists of a series of scans starting in the submental region and working through the submandibular region, intraparotid area, along the cervical/deep cervical chain, followed by the transverse cervical chain/supraclavicular fossa, and culminating with examination of the accessory chain/posterior triangle. Using such a systematic scanning approach on both sides of the neck, the majority of neck lymph nodes are comprehensively evaluated.

Submental Region

The submental region is best examined with the transducer in a transverse plane. Identify the two heads of the anterior belly of the digastric muscles which come off the back of the mandibular symphysis menti. At the floor of the submental triangle is the mylohyoid muscle. Scanning downwards towards the hyoid bone, submental nodes are usually seen anterior to the mylohyoid, behind the mandible, and between the digastric muscles. Further inferiorly, nodes may be seen on, or just medial to, the digastric muscles. Submental nodes may be asymmetrically distributed with a cluster of nodes on one side only.

On high-resolution ultrasound, submental nodes are usually hypoechoic (94%), oval-shaped (short to long axis, $S/L<0.5$; 72%), with an echogenic hilus (80%) and have hilar vascularity (90%; the remaining appear apparently avascular) [4, 5].

Submandibular Region

The transducer is then swept laterally to one side of the neck with the patient's head turned towards the opposite side to allow free manipulation of the transducer. The submandibular region is examined with the transducer in a transverse plane along the inferior border of the mandibular body. The transducer should be angled cranially as some of the submandibular nodes are located in the submandibular niche behind the mandibular body. The mylohyoid and hyoglossus muscles form the floor of the submandibular region on which rests the submandibular gland (seen as a gland with fine, bright parenchymal echoes and linear echogenic lines representing intraglandular ducts). Using the submandibular gland as a reference point, submandibular nodes should be seen anterior, superior, or posterior to the gland.

Small nodes are commonly seen anterior to the submandibular gland between the mandible and the digastric muscle. Superiorly, nodes can also be found adjacent to the facial artery. Occasionally, nodes may be present posterior to the submandibular gland. Rarely, a node may lie deep to the posterior aspect of the gland.

Normal submandibular nodes tend to be hypoechoic (97%), round in shape (S/L >0.5; 95%), with an echogenic hilus (98%) and demonstrate hilar vascularity (93%; the remaining appear apparently avascular) [4, 5].

Parotid Region

The parotid region is assessed with the transducer in longitudinal and transverse planes along the ramus of the mandible. With the parotid gland as the reference point (the gland shows a fine, bright parenchymal echopattern with intraglandular linear echogenic lines representing intraglandular ducts), one must carefully examine the area between the posterior parotid and the ear, where the extraparotid nodes (superficial parotid or preauricular nodes) are found. Extraglandular nodes are usually found at the area anterior to the tragus (preauricular nodes) or posteriorly within the tail of the parotid (infraauricular nodes). Intraglandular nodes lie within the superficial lobe and in the fascia between superficial and deep lobes.

Parotid nodes are normally hypoechoic (91%), round in shape (59%), with echogenic hilus (86%) and either show hilar vascularity (48%) or appear apparently avascular (52%) [4, 5].

Facial Region

With the transducer moving anteriorly from the anterior aspect of the superficial lobe of the parotid, along a line drawn to the corner of the mouth, one visualizes the buccal region where the facial nodes should be found if they are present. Facial nodes are subcutaneous and usually lie along the plane of the facial artery and vein. There are two main groups of facial nodes: the inferior maxillary group and the buccinator or buccal group. The inferior maxillary nodes are usually found along the anterior border of the masseter muscle. The most inferior node of this group may lie on the inferior border of the mandible. The buccal nodes lie in the fat pad anterior to the masseter muscle and superficial to the buccinator muscle.

On high-resolution ultrasound, facial nodes are usually very small, hypoechoic with an echogenic hilus.

Deep Cervical Chain

The deep cervical chain is predominantly examined with the transducer in a transverse plane, scanning inferiorly along the IJV and common carotid artery (CCA), starting from the tail of parotid gland to the junction between IJV and the subclavian vein. Deep cervical nodes are readily identified adjacent to the IJV (predominantly at its anterolateral aspect). The jugulodigastric node (the largest node in the neck) is often oriented along the line of the posterior belly of digastric muscle. To differentiate the jugulodigastric node from the posterior belly of the digastric muscle, one can angle the transducer obliquely across the tail of the parotid and identify the posterior belly as it runs obliquely from deep to the sternomastoid down to the hyoid bone.

Rotate the transducer to a longitudinal plane and confirm the anatomy. Lymph node is seen as an oval or round structure, whereas muscle, IJV, and CCA are demonstrated as long, tubular structures.

On high-resolution ultrasound, normal deep cervical nodes are usually hypoechoic (94–100%), oval-shaped (S/L <0.5, 95–100%), with an echogenic hilus (79–100%) and show hilar vascularity (61–89%, with the remaining appearing apparently avascular) [4, 5].

Transverse Cervical Chain

After scanning the deep cervical chain, from the sternal end of the clavicle, the transducer (held in a transverse plane) is then swept laterally along the upper border of the clavicle towards the acromion to examine the transverse cervical chain. With the transducer angled caudally, the transverse cervical chain lymph nodes are usually located superior to the subclavian vessels. The most medial node of the transverse cervical chain is known as Troisier's node which may be involved in carcinoma of the stomach.

Normal transverse cervical chain nodes are rarely seen on ultrasound (<1%). However, if visualized, the lymph node is usually hypoechoic (100%), oval in shape (S/L <0.5, 75%), and with an echogenic hilus (75%) [4].

Spinal Accessory Chain

The spinal accessory chain is examined with the transducer in a transverse plane scanning along an imaginary line drawn from the mastoid tip to the acromion (the course and location of the spinal accessory nodes). Look for the plane between the sternomastoid and the underlying scalene and levator scapulae muscles because spinal accessory nodes are identified in this superficial plane.

Normal spinal accessory chain nodes are predominantly hypoechoic (99%), oval in shape (S/L <0.5, 98%), with an echogenic hilus (81%) and appear apparently avascular (60%, with the remaining showing hilar vascularity) [4, 5].

Anterior Cervical Nodes

After evaluating the spinal accessory chain, the transducer (in the transverse plane) is then placed back to the midline to look for the hyoid bone, and this is the starting point for examining the anterior cervical nodes. Scanning transversely from the hyoid, sweep inferiorly to identify the thyroid cartilage of the larynx, cricoids, trachea, thyroid isthmus, and then trachea again until it disappears into the mediastinum – the anterior cervical region should then be covered.

The anterior cervical nodes are often obscured by air in the trachea and esophagus and therefore cannot be adequately assessed, unless they are enlarged.

Sonographic Criteria of Malignancy

Distribution

Anyone performing ultrasound must be aware that on high-resolution ultrasound, normal cervical lymph nodes are invariably found in submandibular, parotid, upper cervical chain, and posterior triangles [6].

Metastatic cervical nodes from head and neck cancers are site specific, and this typical distribution helps with identifying neck node metastases and tumor staging [7–9]. In patients with no known primary tumor, the distribution of metastatic nodes may provide a clue to the site of the primary tumor. Table 10.2 summarizes the distribution of metastatic cervical lymph nodes from common head and neck primary tumors.

Size

In a patient with known head and neck primary, larger lymph nodes have a greater likelihood of malignancy. However, reactive nodes may be as large as malignant nodes. Minimal axial diameter is the most accurate dimension for predicting malignancy [10, 11]. Lymph nodes in the upper

Table 10.2 Common distribution of metastatic lymph nodes from head and neck primary tumors

Primary tumors	Nodal group(s) that commonly involved
Oropharynx, hypopharynx, larynx	Deep cervical chain Prelaryngeal/Delphian
Oral cavity	Submandibular Upper deep cervical chain
Nasopharyngeal carcinoma	Upper deep cervical chain Spinal accessory chain
Papillary carcinoma of the thyroid	Deep cervical chain Pretracheal Paratracheal
Non-head and neck (infraclavicular)	Transverse cervical chain Spinal accessory chain (low)

neck, including those in the submandibular and subdigastric region, tend to be larger than those in the lower neck [4, 12, 13]. van den Brekel et al. [14] suggested that a minimal axial diameter of 9 mm for subdigastric nodes and 8 mm for all other cervical nodes yielded a sensitivity, specificity and overall accuracy of 75%. If a lower cutoff is used, the sensitivity increases but the specificity diminishes. If a higher cutoff is used, the sensitivity is reduced but the specificity rises. However, one must note that the threshold for suspicion may be much lower (4 mm) in patients with known head and neck primary, with nodes in the appropriate drainage sites [15]. In our experience, size of lymph nodes alone cannot be used for identifying malignant nodes. However, in a patient with a known head and neck carcinoma, the serial change in nodal size is useful. Increasing size of lymph nodes on serial examinations is highly suspicious for metastases. Monitoring the progressive change of nodal size is also useful to assess treatment response [16, 17], particularly as many patients are now treated nonsurgically.

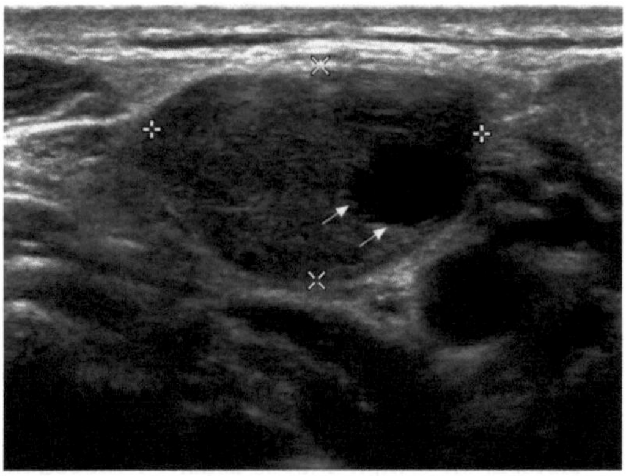

Fig. 10.2 Transverse gray scale ultrasound shows a round metastatic lymph node from a primary head and neck squamous cell carcinoma. Note the intranodal cystic necrosis which appears as an echolucent area within the lymph node (*arrows*)

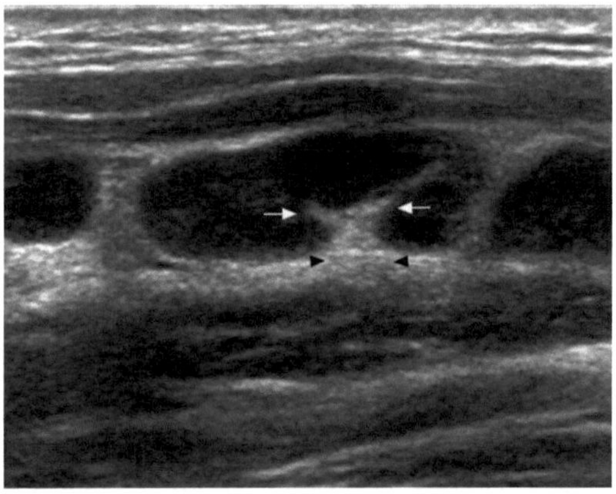

Fig. 10.3 Longitudinal gray scale ultrasound of an elliptical, hypoechoic reactive lymph node with an echogenic hilus (*arrows*). Note the continuity of the hilus with the adjacent fat (*arrowheads*)

Shape

Malignant nodes tend to be round in shape (Fig. 10.2), whereas normal or reactive nodes are usually oval or fusiform (Figs. 10.3 and 10.4) [9, 18–20]. A short to long axis (S/L) or long to short axis (L/S) ratio can be used to assess the nodal shape. An S/L ratio less than 0.5 (or L/S ratio greater than 2) indicates an oval- or fusiform-shaped node, while S/L ratio greater than 0.5 (or L/S ratio smaller than 2) indicates a round lymph node [21, 22]. Although round lymph nodes are more likely to be malignant, one must note that normal submandibular and parotid nodes are usually round. Therefore, one must be cautious in using nodal shape to distinguish malignant and reactive nodes in these regions. Another useful sign for identifying malignant nodes is the presence of eccentric cortical hypertrophy, which indicates focal cortical tumor infiltration within the lymph node (Fig. 10.5) [23]. For accurate diagnosis and nodal sampling, in nodes with focal/eccentric cortical hypertrophy, the needle (during FNAC or biopsy) must be guided into the site of hypertrophy.

Echogenic Hilus

The echogenic hilus is closely associated with the medullary sinuses in the lymph node. These act as multiple acoustic interfaces reflecting the ultrasound waves and producing an echogenic structure. Fatty deposition only makes the hilus more obvious on ultrasound [19, 24, 25].

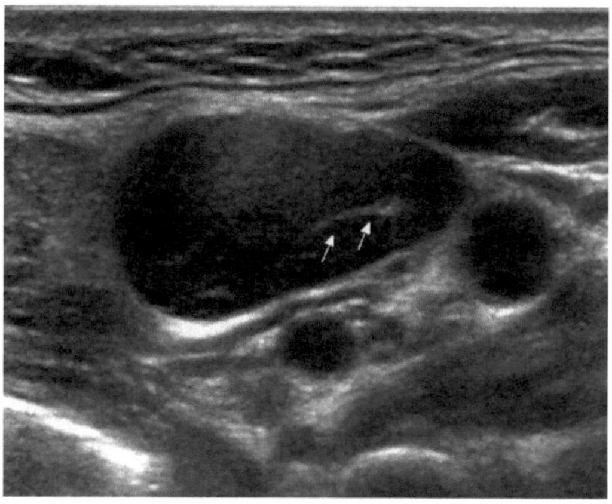

Fig. 10.4 Transverse gray scale ultrasound of an oval, hypoechoic reactive lymph node with an echogenic hilus (*arrows*). Note the concentric hypertrophy of the node

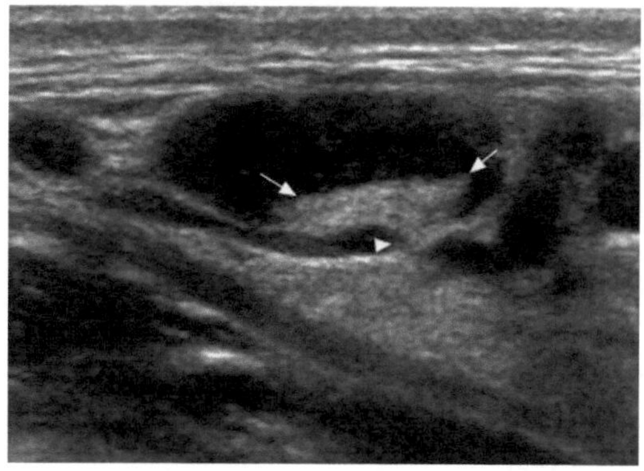

Fig. 10.6 Longitudinal gray scale ultrasound of an elliptical, hypoechoic reactive node with prominent echogenic hilus (*arrows*) continuous with the adjacent fat (*arrowheads*)

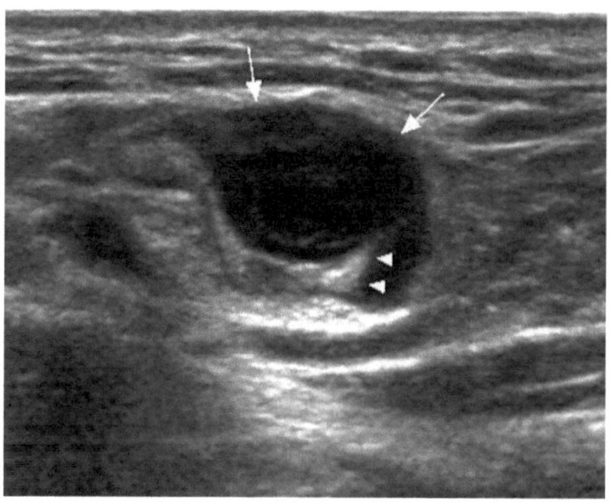

Fig. 10.5 Transverse gray scale ultrasound of a round, hypoechoic malignant node with eccentric cortical hypertrophy (*arrows*) due to focal tumor infiltration. Note the normal echogenic hilus (*arrowheads*) is displaced by the intranodal tumor mass. During FNAC of such a node, the needle tip should be directed towards the hypertrophied part of the node

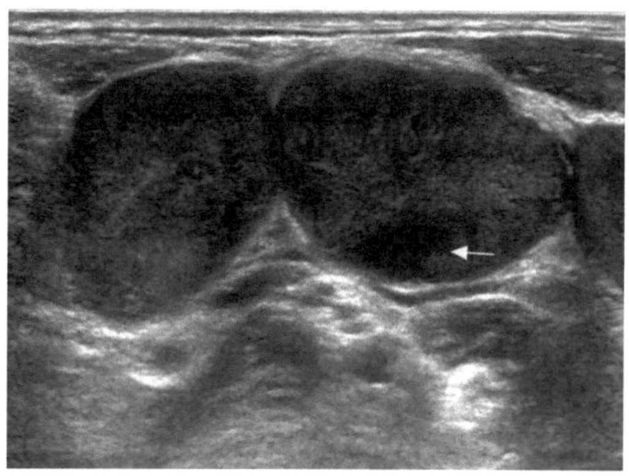

Fig. 10.7 Transverse gray scale ultrasound shows multiple round, hypoechoic malignant lymph nodes without the echogenic hilus. Note the intranodal cystic necrosis (*arrow*)

The echogenic hilus appears as a hyperechoic linear structure within the node and is continuous with the adjacent subcutaneous fat (Figs. 10.3 and 10.6) [24–26]. In the normal neck, 90% of nodes with a maximum transverse diameter greater than 5 mm show an echogenic hilus on high-resolution ultrasound [27]. Malignant nodes usually do not show an echogenic hilus (Figs. 10.7 and 10.8), and the presence of an echogenic hilus was once considered as a sign of benignity [19, 28]. However, lymph nodes with early metastatic infiltration may still demonstrate the echogenic hilus before the medullary sinuses are completely disrupted [25]. Therefore, the presence of an echogenic hilus should not be used as the sole criterion for benignity. Vassallo et al. [23] evaluated the width of the hilus and the cortex of lymph nodes and suggested that an absent hilus or a narrowed hilus with associated eccentric cortical hypertrophy is suspicious for malignancy.

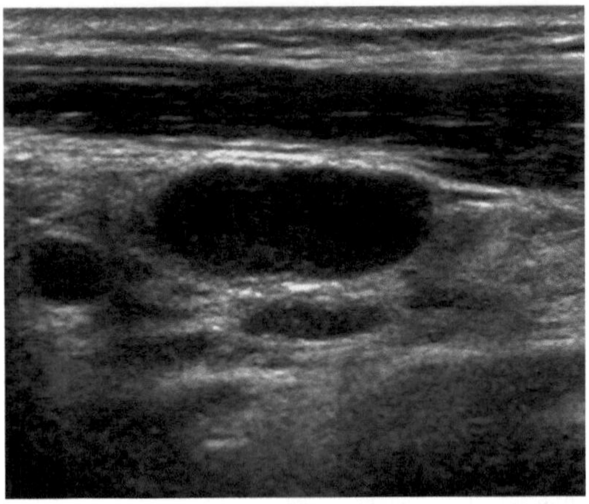

Fig. 10.8 Longitudinal gray scale ultrasound of an oval, hypoechoic malignant lymph node without an echogenic hilus. In this patient with a known head and neck carcinoma, despite its oval shape, the intranodal architecture points towards a malignant node

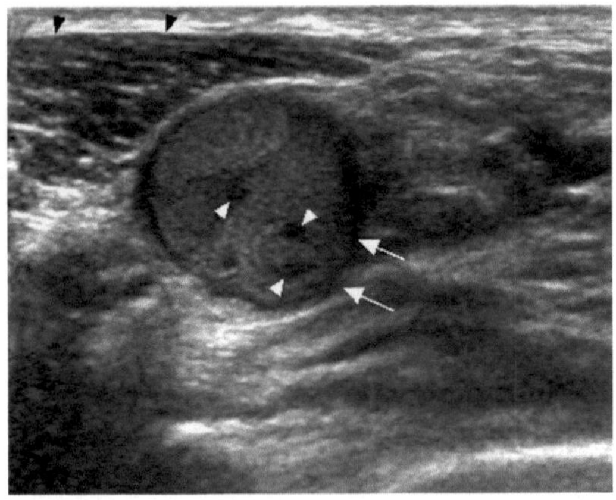

Fig. 10.9 Transverse gray scale ultrasound shows a round metastatic node (*arrows*) from papillary carcinoma of the thyroid. Note the lymph node is hyperechoic when compared to the adjacent muscle (*black arrowheads*). White arrowheads indicate intranodal cystic necrosis which is often seen in metastatic nodes from papillary carcinoma of the thyroid

Echogenicity

On high-resolution ultrasound, metastatic lymph nodes tend to be hypoechoic when compared to adjacent muscles [7, 10, 18, 20]. Exceptionally, metastatic nodes from papillary carcinoma of the thyroid are usually hyperechoic (87%) (Figs. 10.9 and 10.10) [29, 30]. As the presence of hyperechoic lymph nodes is strongly associated with papillary carcinoma of the thyroid, one should carefully examine the thyroid gland for any tumors when hyperechoic neck nodes are detected.

A "pseudocystic" appearance (solid, homogeneous, and hypoechoic node with posterior enhancement) of lymph nodes was previously suggested to be a specific feature for non-Hodgkin's lymphoma [31, 32]. However, with the use of newer transducers, this "pseudocystic" appearance is less commonly seen, and instead, lymphomatous nodes demonstrate a micronodular or reticulated pattern (Fig. 10.11) [33].

Necrosis

The presence of necrosis within lymph nodes is pathologic, regardless of the size of lymph nodes. In patients with a known primary tumor, intranodal necrosis is a very strong sign of malignancy.

Intranodal necrosis can be categorized into cystic and coagulation necrosis. Cystic necrosis is relatively more common than coagulation necrosis, and the two may be seen within the same node. On high-resolution ultrasound, cystic necrosis is seen as a truly cystic area (anechoic/hypoechoic area) within a lymph node (Figs. 10.2 and 10.7), whereas coagulation necrosis appears as a central, ill-defined, hyperechoic area (not as echogenic as the hilus) in the node (Fig. 10.12). Unlike the echogenic hilus, coagulation necrosis is not continuous with the adjacent fat, and the two are readily differentiated.

Intranodal necrosis is common in papillary carcinoma of the thyroid (Figs. 10.9, 10.13 and 10.14) and squamous cell carcinoma (SCC) (Fig. 10.2) [8, 29, 34–36]. Intranodal necrosis is also often seen in tuberculous nodes [20, 37]. Therefore, in the presence of intranodal cystic necrosis, wherever applicable, tuberculous lymphadenitis should always be considered in the differential diagnosis, and needle aspiration is needed for cytology and microbiology. Tuberculous nodes tend to be clumped together (matted) and associated with adjacent soft tissue edema. In our experience, they are predominantly found in supraclavicular and posterior triangle regions [20, 37].

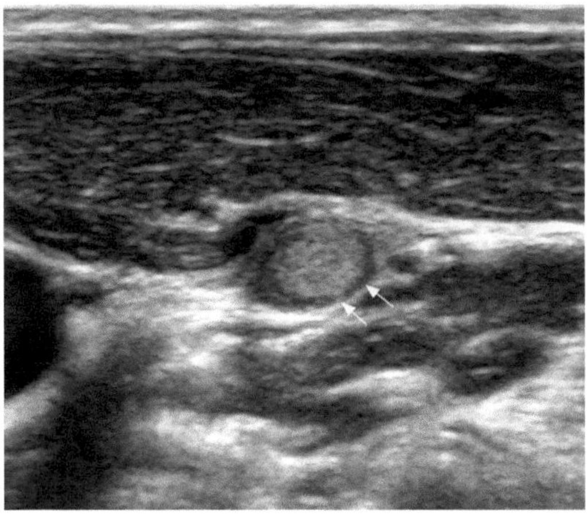

Fig. 10.10 Transverse gray scale ultrasound of a small, round, hyperechoic metastatic node (*arrows*) from papillary carcinoma of the thyroid. Despite its small size, its hyperechogenicity should suggest the location of the primary papillary tumor within the thyroid

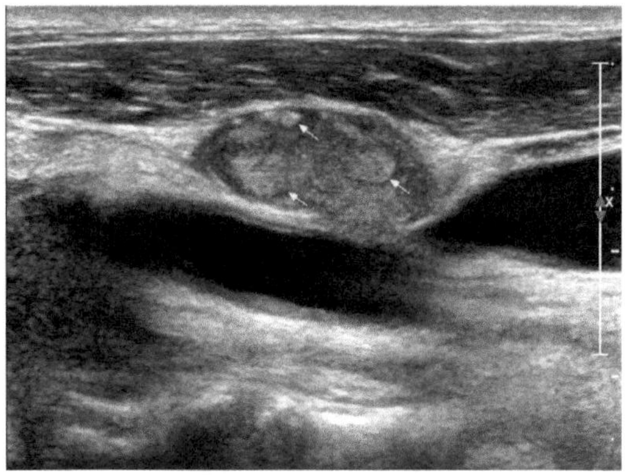

Fig. 10.12 Longitudinal gray scale ultrasound of an oval, hypoechoic malignant lymph node with intranodal coagulation necrosis (*arrows*). Note coagulation necrosis appears as intranodal hyperechogenic foci which are not continuous with the surrounding fat (distinguishing it from the echogenic hilum)

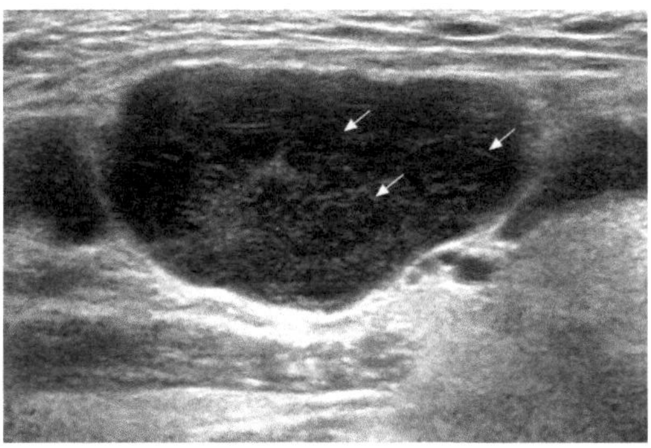

Fig. 10.11 Transverse gray scale ultrasound with high-resolution transducer showing a lymphomatous node with intranodal reticulation, i.e. micronodular pattern (*arrows*). In the past, such nodes frequently demonstrated a "pseudocystic" appearance

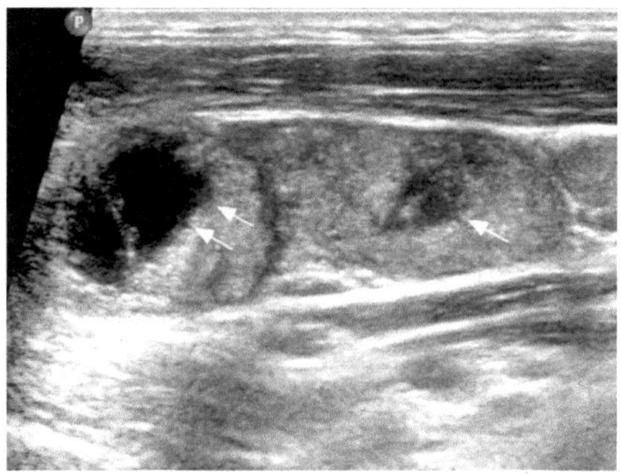

Fig. 10.13 Longitudinal gray scale ultrasound showing multiple round, hyperechoic metastatic nodes from papillary carcinoma of the thyroid with intranodal cystic necrosis (*arrows*). Note the combination of hyperechogenicity and cystic necrosis is strongly suggestive of a metastasis from papillary thyroid carcinoma

Calcification

Metastatic nodes from papillary (calcification represents calcified psammoma bodies) and medullary (represents amyloid + Ca^{++}) carcinoma of the thyroid tend to show calcification [8, 29, 30, 38, 39]. The calcification in metastatic nodes from papillary carcinoma is usually punctate and shows fine acoustic shadowing when a high-frequency transducer (>10 MHz) is used (Figs. 10.15–10.17). Although metastatic nodes from medullary carcinoma may also show fine punctate calcification, the calcification is usually coarse, dense, with strong acoustic shadowing. In addition, metastatic nodes from medullary carcinoma of the thyroid are hypoechoic, whereas those from papillary carcinoma of the thyroid are hyperechoic when compared to adjacent muscles. The relatively high incidence of fine/microcalcification in

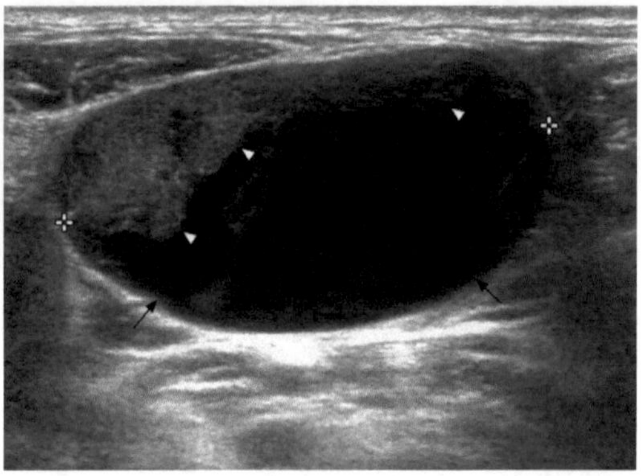

Fig. 10.14 Longitudinal gray scale ultrasound of a metastatic node from papillary carcinoma of the thyroid with both cystic (*arrows*) and solid (*arrowheads*) intranodal components. Figure 10.23 shows the vascularity within the solid component of the node

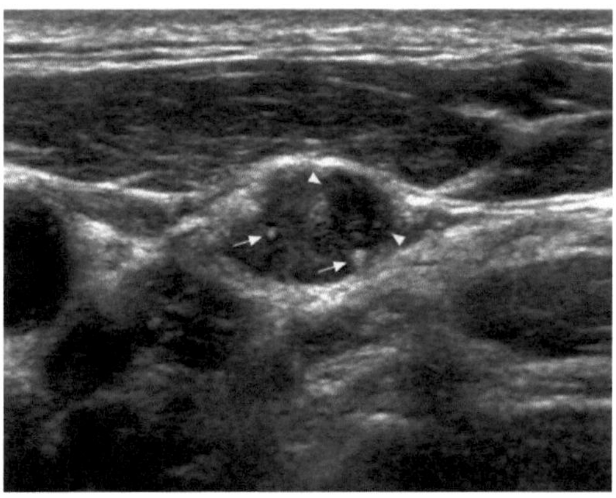

Fig. 10.15 Transverse gray scale ultrasound of a round metastatic node from papillary carcinoma of the thyroid with multiple punctate calcification (*arrows*). Note the intranodal cystic necrosis is also demonstrated (*arrowheads*)

metastatic nodes from papillary carcinoma of the thyroid makes it a useful diagnostic feature.

Calcification may also be seen in post-treatment lymphomatous and tuberculous nodes. However, the calcification in these nodes is usually dense and shows strong acoustic shadowing.

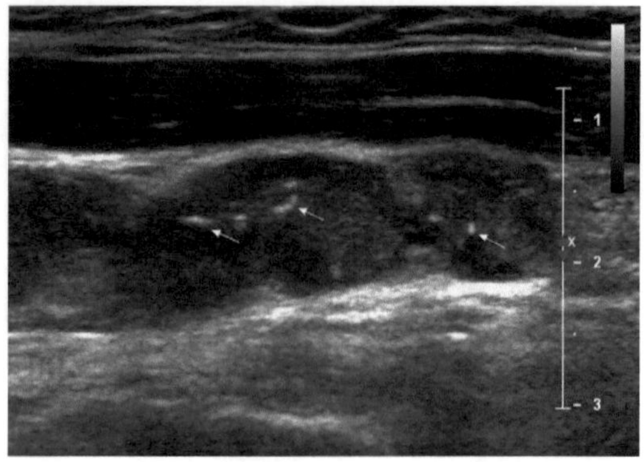

Fig. 10.16 Longitudinal gray scale ultrasound of multiple round, hyperechoic metastatic nodes from papillary carcinoma of the thyroid with multiple echogenic foci representing punctate calcifications (*arrows*). These microcalcifications represent psammoma bodies

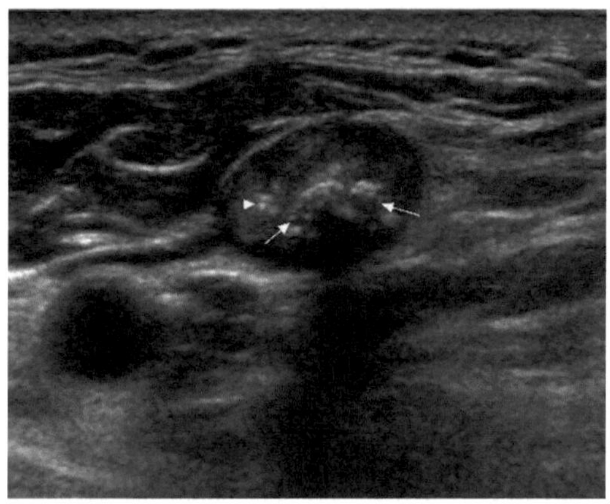

Fig. 10.17 Transverse gray scale ultrasound of a round, hyperechoic metastatic node from papillary carcinoma of the thyroid with both dense (*arrows*) and punctate (*arrowhead*) calcifications. Note the acoustic shadowing is better demonstrated posterior to the dense calcification. To demonstrate the fine shadowing from punctate calcification it may be necessary to use a higher-frequency transducer (as ↑ frequency leads to ↑ attenuation)

Nodal Border

Metastatic nodes usually have a sharp border due to a sharp attenuating interface between malignant tissue and surrounding soft tissues. Inflammatory nodes tend to have ill-defined

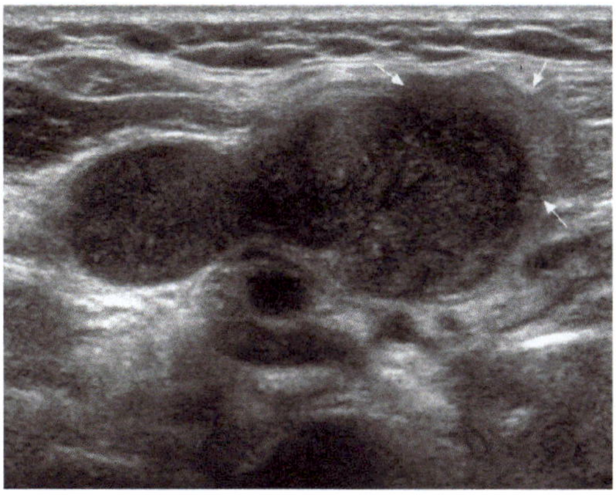

Fig. 10.18 Transverse gray scale ultrasound of a round, hypoechoic malignant node with ill-defined margins suggesting adjacent soft tissue involvement due to extracapsular spread (*arrows*). Any malignant-looking node with ill-defined margins should be viewed with a high degree of suspicion for extracapsular spread. Most malignant nodes have well-defined margins

borders due to the associated periadenitis. However, when a proven malignant node (or a node with other obvious malignant sonographic features) shows ill-defined borders, one must strongly suspect extracapsular spread (Fig. 10.18). This has a major significance as the 2-year survival rate drops by 50% [40]. Invasion of adjacent structures such as muscle, soft tissues is also an indicator of extracapsular spread. Presence of multiple nodes with extracapsular spread has a regional recurrence rate of 58% and distant metastases rate of 33%, with a median survival rate of less than 1 year [41]. The size of lymph node is related to the presence of extracapsular spread. Larger lymph nodes have a greater likelihood of extracapsular spread than smaller nodes [36].

Vascularity

Using high-resolution ultrasound, 90% of lymph nodes with a maximum transverse diameter >5 mm will demonstrate intranodal vascularity (hilar vascularity), and the remaining appear apparently avascular [27].

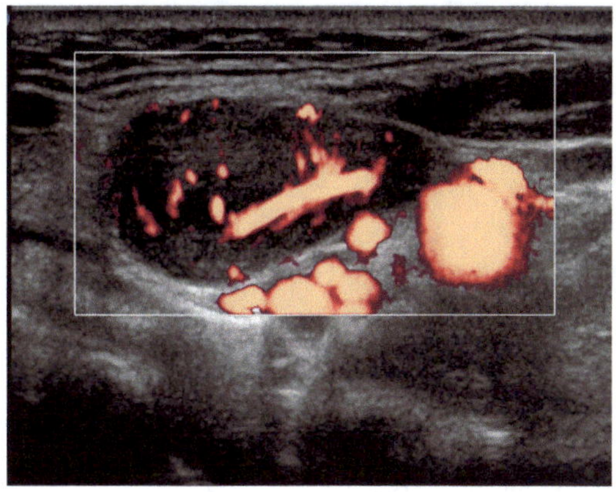

Fig. 10.19 Power Doppler ultrasound of a reactive lymph node showing hilar vascularity

Evaluation of intranodal vascularity involves:

- assessing the presence and distribution of intranodal vessels
- evaluating resistance indices within intranodal vessels

Evaluating resistance indices is time-consuming and fraught with difficulty as these vessels are very small and difficult to assess (particularly if the patient is uncooperative or the node is adjacent to the pulsatile carotid artery).

On the other hand, assessment of the vascular pattern of lymph nodes is more reliable, is less time-consuming, and provides adequate information for diagnosis and management. Thus, measurement of vascular resistance indices is usually not necessary in routine clinical practice [42, 43].

Benign lymph nodes tend to have a central hilar vascular pattern (Figs. 10.19–10.21) [5, 42, 44–46]. Peripheral vascularity is commonly found in metastatic nodes (Figs. 10.22–10.23) and is related to angiogenesis that induces recruitment of peripheral vessels into the lymph nodes [39, 42, 44–47]. Hilar vascularity may be present together with peripheral vascularity in metastatic nodes (mixed vascularity, Figs. 10.24 and 10.25). Such mixed vascularity is usually found in early metastases where the peripheral vessels are induced, but the normal hilar vessels are

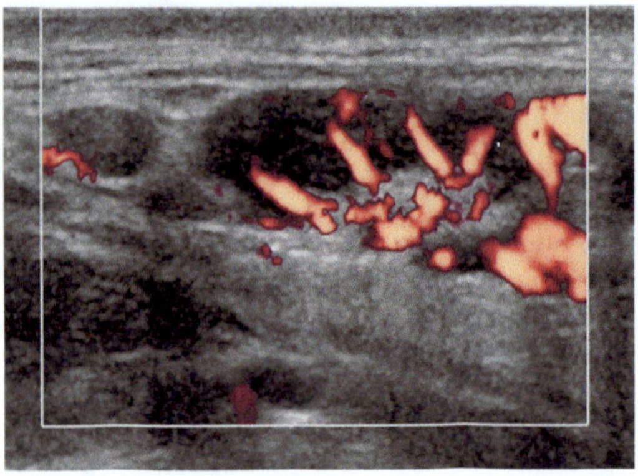

Fig. 10.20 Power Doppler ultrasound of a reactive node showing hilar vascularity branching out from the echogenic hilus

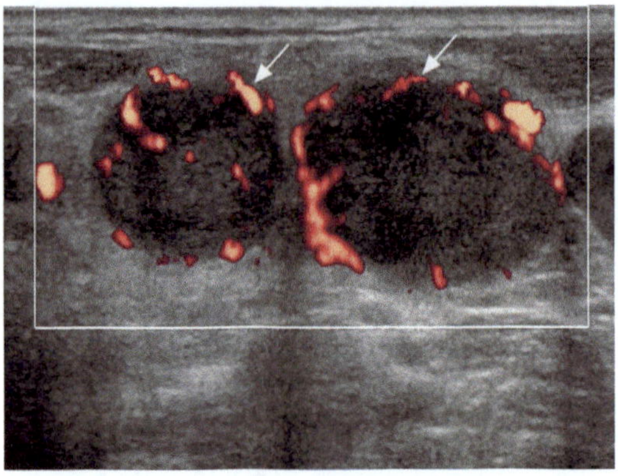

Fig. 10.22 Power Doppler ultrasound shows multiple round malignant lymph nodes with peripheral vascularity (*arrows*). Note the absence of an echogenic hilus and hilar vascularity

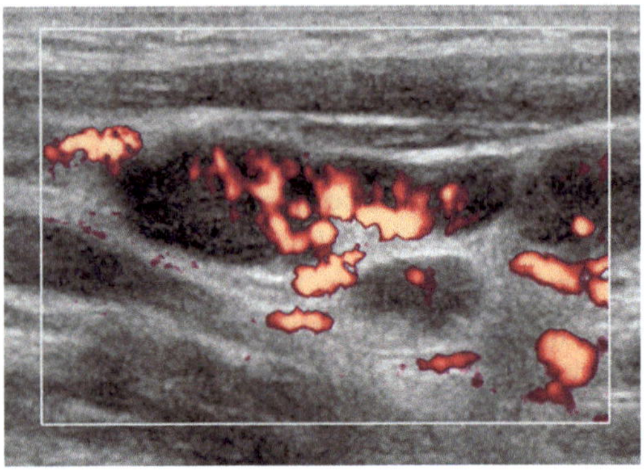

Fig. 10.21 Power Doppler ultrasound shows multiple reactive nodes. Note the hilar vascularity radiates outward from the echogenic hilus. Sometimes, such hilar radiating vessels may extend towards the periphery of the node and should not be confused with peripheral vascularity of malignant nodes

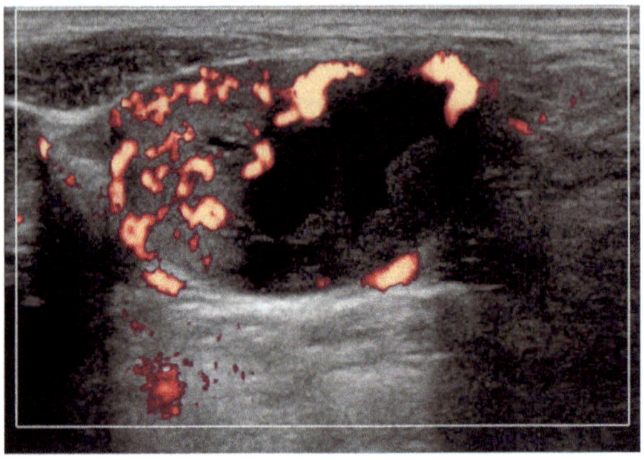

Fig. 10.23 Power Doppler ultrasound of a metastatic node from papillary carcinoma of the thyroid. Note the prominent vascularity in the solid component of the lymph node. Same case as Fig. 10.14

preserved, which may be destroyed by the tumor cells at a later stage [44].

A combination of gray scale sonographic features (round shape, presence of intranodal necrosis and absent hilus) and peripheral vascularity has a sensitivity and specificity of 100% in differentiating benign from malignant nodes [43]. These are quick, simple parameters to evaluate and provide a high degree of accuracy.

Besides pre-treatment assessment, evaluation of intranodal vascularity is also useful in monitoring treatment response of malignant lymph nodes. On color/power Doppler sonography, reduction of intranodal vascularity is a sensitive sign of positive treatment response and is useful in predicting patient prognosis [48, 49].

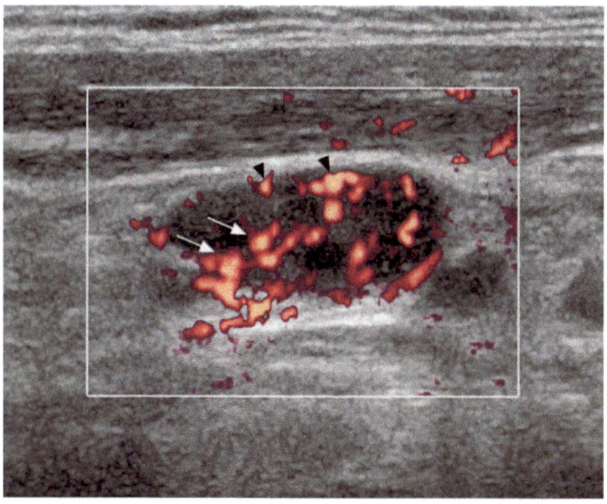

Fig. 10.24 Power Doppler ultrasound of a malignant lymph node with radiating hilar (*arrows*) and peripheral (*arrowheads*) vascularity

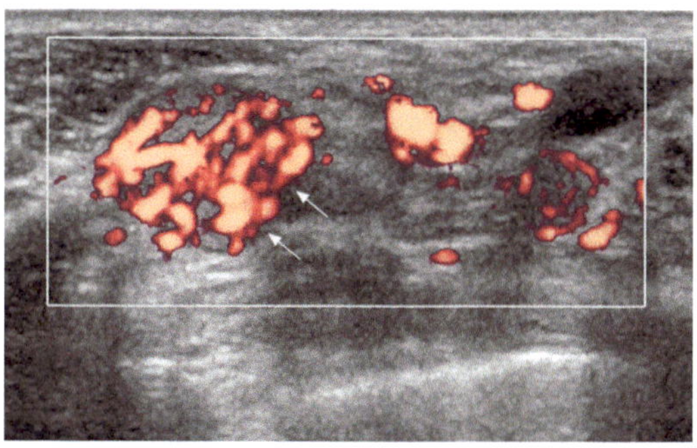

Fig. 10.25 Power Doppler ultrasound of a metastatic node from papillary carcinoma of the thyroid with exaggerated intranodal vascularity (*arrows*), both hilar and peripheral. Same case as Fig. 10.9

Contrast Enhancement

Contrast-enhanced ultrasound, using microbubble-based contrast agent, is increasingly used. However, the value of this technique in the assessment of cervical lymph nodes is controversial. It has been reported that contrast enhancement increases the sensitivity in detecting intranodal vessels, and thus improves the accuracy in distinguishing benign and malignant nodes [50–52]. However, Zenk et al. [53] compared the color Doppler ultrasound signals before and after contrast enhancement. They found that lymph nodes with low pre-contrast Doppler signals followed by a steep increase in post-contrast Doppler signals are more likely to be benign, whereas other contrast enhancement parameters are of limited value in differentiating benign and malignant nodes. Zenk et al. [54] also evaluated the value of contrast-enhanced ultrasound, in comparison with gray scale and Doppler ultrasound, in differentiating benign from malignant nodes, and found that contrast-enhanced ultrasound did not improve the accuracy of gray scale and Doppler ultrasound in predicting malignancy.

Although contrast-enhanced ultrasound may provide additional information in the assessment of lymph node, its value in routine clinical practice is limited (particularly as it is expensive, increases the examination time, and does not obviate the need for FNAC).

Application of Sonographic Criteria in Routine Clinical Practice

Once a sonographic examination of neck nodes is complete, it is time to evaluate the criteria and establish the diagnosis. How does one do that?

No single sonographic criteria will accurately distinguish a benign from malignant node. Sonologists often get stuck on the size of the node. In our experience, one should get beyond that and evaluate the other more relevant criteria such as increasing size on serial examinations, shape, cortical hypertrophy, intranodal necrosis, calcification, the presence of abnormal vascularity, and the node in the known drainage site of the primary tumor. These will be more useful in differentiating benign from malignant node. The probability of malignancy is higher if many of the above criteria are present in the same node [55].

Once ultrasound identifies a suspicious node, the next step invariably is a guided FNAC to confirm the nature. The superficial location of nodes and the superb visualization by high-resolution ultrasound make it readily amenable to a guided FNAC (irrespective of its size, and if it can be seen on ultrasound, it can invariably be FNAed). Ultrasound-guided FNAC is an accurate method of neck node evaluation with a sensitivity of 89–98%, specificity of 95–98%, and overall accuracy of 95–97% [56, 57]. Thyroglobulin measurement in the washout of fine-needle aspirates in cervical lymph nodes is another accurate technique for detecting nodal metastases from papillary carcinoma of the thyroid. Using a cutoff value of 10 ng/ml for thyroglobulin measurement, the sensitivity and specificity of the detection were 100% [58].

Not only does ultrasound-guided FNAC accurately stage the tumor and aid in treatment planning [57, 59–61], it is also a useful modality in post-operative neck node surveillance [62]. It is a safe and accurate procedure with a short learning curve and adds only a couple of minutes to a routine neck ultrasound: A complete sonographic examination of both sides of the neck (including a guided FNAC) should not take more than 15 min. It is ideally served as an office-based technique and provides the surgeon/physician with an accurate diagnosis and all the relevant information required for tumor staging, treatment planning and postoperative monitoring.

References

1. Castenholz A. Architecture of the lymph node with regard to its function. In: Grundmann E, Vollmer E, editors. Reaction patterns of the lymph node. Part 1. Cell types and functions. New York: Springer; 1990. p. 3–9.
2. Hall FG. The functional anatomy of lymph nodes. In: Stansfeld AG, d'Ardenne AJ, editors. Lymph node biopsy interpretation. 2nd ed. London: Churchill Livingstone; 1992. p. 10–3.
3. Papadimitriou CS, Kittas CN. Normal structure and function of lymph nodes. In: Pangalis GA, Polliack A, editors. Benign and malignant lymphadenopathies. Chur: Harwood Academic; 1993. p. 113–26.
4. Ying M, Ahuja A, Brook F, Brown B, Metreweli C. Sonographic appearance and distribution of normal cervical lymph nodes in a Chinese population. J Ultrasound Med. 1996;15:431–6.
5. Ying M, Ahuja A, Brook F, Metreweli C. Power Doppler sonography of normal cervical lymph nodes. J Ultrasound Med. 2000;19:511–7.
6. Ying M, Ahuja A, Brook F. Gray scale and power Doppler sonography of normal cervical lymph nodes: comparison between Chinese and white subjects. J Ultrasound Med. 2002;21:59–65.
7. Ahuja A, Ying M, King W, Metreweli C. A practical approach to ultrasound of cervical lymph nodes. J Laryngol Otol. 1997;111:245–56.
8. Som PM. Lymph nodes of the neck. Radiology. 1987;165:593–600.
9. Ahuja A, Ying M. Sonography of neck lymph nodes. Part II: abnormal lymph nodes. Clin Radiol. 2003;58:359–66.
10. van den Brekel MW, Stel HV, Castelijns JA, Nauta JJ, van der Waal I, Valk J, et al. Cervical lymph node metastasis: assessment of radiologic criteria. Radiology. 1990;177:379–84.
11. Som PM. Detection of metastasis in cervical lymph nodes: CT and MR criteria and differential diagnosis. Am J Roentgenol. 1992;158:961–9.
12. Bruneton JN, Balu-Maestro C, Marcy PY, Melia P, Mourou MY. Very high frequency (13 MHz) ultrasonographic examination of the normal neck: detection of normal lymph nodes and thyroid nodules. J Ultrasound Med. 1994;13:87–90.
13. Swartz JD, Yussen PS, Popky GL. Imaging of the neck: nodal disease. Crit Rev Diagn Imaging. 1991;31:413–69.
14. van den Brekel MW, Castelijns JA, Stel HV, Golding RP, Meyer CJ, Snow GB. Modern imaging techniques and ultrasound-guided aspiration cytology for the assessment of neck node metastases: a prospective comparative study. Eur Arch Otorhinolaryngol. 1993;250:11–7.
15. van den Brekel MW, Stel HV, Castelijns JA, Croll GJ, Snow GB. Lymph node staging in patients with clinically negative neck examinations by ultrasound and ultrasound-guided aspiration cytology. Am J Surg. 1991;162:362–6.
16. Ahuja A, Ying M, Leung SF, Metreweli C. The sonographic appearance and significance of cervical metastatic nodes following radiotherapy for nasopharyngeal carcinoma. Clin Radiol. 1996;51:698–701.
17. Ahuja A, Leung SF, Ying M, Metreweli C. Echography of metastatic nodes treated by radiotherapy. J Laryngol Otol. 1999;113:993–8.
18. Chan JM, Shin LK, Jeffrey RB. Ultrasonography of abnormal neck lymph nodes. Ultrasound Q. 2007;23:47–54.
19. Vassallo P, Edel G, Roos N, Naguib A, Peters PE. In-vitro high-resolution ultrasonography of benign and malignant lymph nodes. A sonographic-pathologic correlation. Invest Radiol. 1993;28:698–705.
20. Ying M, Ahuja AT, Evans R, King W, Metreweli C. Cervical lymphadenopathy: sonographic differentiation between tuberculous nodes and nodal metastases from non-head and neck carcinomas. J Clin Ultrasound. 1998;26:383–9.
21. Solbiati L, Rizzatto G, Bellotti E, Montali G, Cioffi V, Croce F. High-resolution sonography of cervical lymph nodes in head and neck cancer: criteria for differentiation of reactive versus malignant nodes. Radiology. 1988;169:113.
22. Tohnosu N, Onoda S, Isono K. Ultrasonographic evaluation of cervical lymph node metastases in esophageal cancer with special reference to the relationship between the short to long axis ratio (S/L) and the cancer content. J Clin Ultrasound. 1989;17:101–6.

23. Vassallo P, Wernecke K, Roos N, Peters PE. Differentiation of benign from malignant superficial lymphadenopathy: the role of high-resolution US. Radiology. 1992;183:215–20.
24. Rubaltelli L, Proto E, Salmaso R, Bortoletto P, Candiani F, Cagol P. Sonography of abnormal lymph nodes in vitro: correlation of sonographic and histologic findings. Am J Roentgenol. 1990;155:1241–4.
25. Evans RM, Ahuja A, Metreweli C. The linear echogenic hilus in cervical lymphadenopathy–a sign of benignity or malignancy? Clin Radiol. 1993;47: 262–4.
26. Sakai F, Kiyono K, Sone S, Kondo Y, Oguchi M, Watanabe T, et al. Ultrasonic evaluation of cervical metastatic lymphadenopathy. J Ultrasound Med. 1988;7:305–10.
27. Ying M, Ahuja A, Brook F, Metreweli C. Vascularity and grey-scale sonographic features of normal cervical lymph nodes: variations with nodal size. Clin Radiol. 2001;56:416–9.
28. Solbiati L, Cioffi V, Ballarati E. Ultrasonography of the neck. Radiol Clin North Am. 1992;30:941–54.
29. Ahuja AT, Chow L, Chick W, King W, Metreweli C. Metastatic cervical nodes in papillary carcinoma of the thyroid: ultrasound and histological correlation. Clin Radiol. 1995;50:229–31.
30. Rosario PW, de Faria S, Bicalho L, Alves MF, Borges MA, Purisch S, et al. Ultrasonographic differentiation between metastatic and benign lymph nodes in patients with papillary thyroid carcinoma. J Ultrasound Med. 2005;24:1385–9.
31. Ahuja A, Ying M, Yang WT, Evans R, King W, Metreweli C. The use of sonography in differentiating cervical lymphomatous lymph nodes from cervical metastatic lymph nodes. Clin Radiol. 1996;51: 186–90.
32. Ishii J, Fujii E, Suzuki H, Shinozuka K, Kawase N, Amagasa T. Ultrasonic diagnosis of oral and neck malignant lymphoma. Bull Tokyo Med Dent Univ. 1992;39:63–9.
33. Ahuja AT, Ying M, Yuen HY, Metreweli C. 'Pseudocystic' appearance of non-Hodgkin's lymphomatous nodes: an infrequent finding with high-resolution transducers. Clin Radiol. 2001;56:111–5.
34. Landry CS, Grubbs EG, Busaidy NL, Staerkel GA, Perrier ND, Edeiken-Monroe BS. Cystic lymph nodes in the lateral neck are an indicator of metastatic papillary thyroid cancer. Endocr Pract. 2010;16:1–16.
35. King AD, Tse GM, Ahuja AT, Yuen EH, Vlantis AC, To EW, et al. Necrosis in metastatic neck nodes: diagnostic accuracy of CT, MR imaging, and US. Radiology. 2004;230:720–6.
36. Gor DM, Langer JE, Loevner LA. Imaging of cervical lymph nodes in head and neck cancer: the basics. Radiol Clin North Am. 2006;44:101–10.
37. Ahuja A, Ying M, Evans R, King W, Metreweli C. The application of ultrasound criteria for malignancy in differentiating tuberculous cervical adenitis from metastatic nasopharyngeal carcinoma. Clin Radiol. 1995;50:391–5.
38. Som PM, Brandwein M, Lidov M, Lawson W, Biller HF. The varied presentations of papillary thyroid carcinoma cervical nodal disease: CT and MR findings. Am J Neuroradiol. 1994;15:1123–8.
39. Leboulleux S, Girard E, Rose M, Travagli JP, Sabbah N, Caillou B, et al. Ultrasound criteria of malignancy for cervical lymph nodes in patients followed up for differentiated thyroid cancer. J Clin Endocrinol Metab. 2007;92:3590–4.
40. Johnson JT. A surgeon looks at cervical lymph nodes. Radiology. 1990;175:607–10.
41. Greenberg JS, Fowler R, Gomez J, Mo V, Roberts D, El Naggar AK, et al. Extent of extracapsular spread: a critical prognosticator in oral tongue cancer. Cancer. 2003;97:1464–70.
42. Ahuja AT, Ying M, Ho SS, Metreweli C. Distribution of intranodal vessels in differentiating benign from metastatic neck nodes. Clin Radiol. 2001;56: 197–201.
43. Ahuja A, Ying M. Sonographic evaluation of cervical lymphadenopathy: is power Doppler sonography routinely indicated? Ultrasound Med Biol. 2003;29:353–9.
44. Na DG, Lim HK, Byun HS, Kim HD, Ko YH, Baek JH. Differential diagnosis of cervical lymphadenopathy: usefulness of color Doppler sonography. Am J Roentgenol. 1997;168:1311–6.
45. Wu CH, Chang YL, Hsu WC, Ko JY, Sheen TS, Hsieh FJ. Usefulness of Doppler spectral analysis and power Doppler sonography in the differentiation of cervical lymphadenopathies. Am J Roentgenol. 1998;171: 503–9.
46. Dangore-Khasbage S, Degwekar SS, Bhowate RR, Banode PJ, Bhake A, Choudhary MS, et al. Utility of color Doppler ultrasound in evaluating the status of cervical lymph nodes in oral cancer. Oral Surg Oral Med Oral Pathol Oral Radiol Endod. 2009;108:255–63.
47. Steinkamp HJ, Maurer J, Cornehl M, Knobber D, Hettwer H, Felix R. Recurrent cervical lymphadenopathy: differential diagnosis with color- duplex sonography. Eur Arch Otorhinolaryngol. 1994;251:404–9.
48. Furukawa MK, Furukawa M. Diagnosis of lymph node metastases of head and neck cancer and evaluation of effects of chemoradiotherapy using ultrasonography. Int J Clin Oncol. 2010;15:23–32.
49. Ho SS, Ahuja AT, Yeo W, Chan TC, Kew J, Metreweli C. Longitudinal colour doppler study of superficial lymph nodes in non- Hodgkin's lymphoma patients on chemotherapy. Clin Radiol. 2000;55:110–3.
50. Moritz JD, Ludwig A, Oestmann JW. Contrast-enhanced color Doppler sonography for evaluation of enlarged cervical lymph nodes in head and neck tumors. Am J Roentgenol. 2000;174:1279–84.
51. Rubaltelli L, Khadivi Y, Tregnaghi A, Stramare R, Ferro F, Borsato S, et al. Evaluation of lymph node perfusion using continuous mode harmonic ultrasonography with a second-generation contrast agent. J Ultrasound Med. 2004;23:829–36.
52. Rickert D, Jecker P, Metzler V, Lehmann T, Ernst E, Westhofen M. Color-coded duplex sonography of the

cervical lymph nodes: improved differential diagnostic assessment after administration of the signal enhancer SH U 508A (Levovist). Eur Arch Otorhinolaryngol. 2000;257:453–8.

53. Zenk J, Bozzato A, Steinhart H, Greess H, Iro H. Metastatic and inflammatory cervical lymph nodes as analyzed by contrast-enhanced color-coded Doppler ultrasonography: quantitative dynamic perfusion patterns and histopathologic correlation. Ann Otol Rhinol Laryngol. 2005;114:43–7.
54. Zenk J, Bozzato A, Hornung J, Gottwald F, Rabe C, Gill S, et al. Neck lymph nodes: prediction by computer-assisted contrast medium analysis? Ultrasound Med Biol. 2007;33:246–53.
55. Evans RM, Ahuja A, Rhys Williams S, Waldron C, Van Hasselt CA, King W, et al. Ultrasound and ultrasound guided fine needle aspiration in cervical lymphadenopathy. Br J Radiol. 1991;64:58.
56. Baatenburg de Jong RJ, Rongen RJ, Verwoerd CD, van Overhagen H, Lameris JS, Knegt P. Ultrasound-guided fine-needle aspiration biopsy of neck nodes. Arch Otolaryngol Head Neck Surg. 1991;117:402–4.
57. Knappe M, Louw M, Gregor RT. Ultrasonography-guided fine-needle aspiration for the assessment of cervical metastases. Arch Otolaryngol Head Neck Surg. 2000;126:1091–6.
58. Zanella AB, Meyer EL, Balzan L, Silva AC, Camargo J, Migliavacca A, et al. Thyroglobulin measurements in washout of fine needle aspirates in cervical lymph nodes for detection of papillary thyroid cancer metastases. Arq Bras Endocrinol Metabol. 2010;54:550–4.
59. Hodder SC, Evans RM, Patton DW, Silvester KC. Ultrasound and fine needle aspiration cytology in the staging of neck lymph nodes in oral squamous cell carcinoma. Br J Oral Maxillofac Surg. 2000; 38:430–6.
60. Lo CP, Chen CY, Chin SC, Lee KW, Hsueh CJ, Juan CJ, et al. Detection of suspicious malignant cervical lymph nodes of unknown origin: diagnostic accuracy of ultrasound-guided fine-needle aspiration biopsy with nodal size and central necrosis correlate. Can Assoc Radiol J. 2007;58:286–91.
61. Robinson IA, Cozens NJ. Does a joint ultrasound guided cytology clinic optimize the cytological evaluation of head and neck masses? Clin Radiol. 1999;54:312–6.
62. van den Brekel MW, Reitsma LC, Quak JJ, Smeele LE, van der Linden JC, Snow GB, et al. Sonographically guided aspiration cytology of neck nodes for selection of treatment and follow-up in patients with N0 head and neck cancer. Am J Neuroradiol. 1999;20: 1727–31.

Benign Clinical Conditions in the Adjacent Neck

11

Hok Yuen Yuen and Anil T. Ahuja

The thyroid gland is located in the anterior central part of the infrahyoid neck. During ultrasound examination of the thyroid, a large part of the neck is also included in the field of view, and unexpected incidental findings may be seen in these areas. The aim of this chapter is to review some of the more commonly encountered benign lesions that may be in the vicinity of the thyroid. This chapter does not include a discussion on lymph nodes and parathyroid glands as these are discussed in detail in other sections of the book. Please refer to other chapters for the discussion of lymph nodes and parathyroid glands.

A schematic diagram (Fig. 11.1) indicates the common lesions in the various anatomical regions of the neck in the vicinity of thyroid gland.

Branchial Cleft Cyst

Pathology

Second branchial cleft cysts (Second BCC) make up more than 90% of all the branchial cleft anomalies in teens and adults and 66–75% in children [1]. Embryologically, the branchial apparatus is the precursor of many head and neck structures [2]. The second branchial arch overgrows the second, third, and fourth clefts and results in the formation of a cavity known as the "cervical sinus." Subsequent failure of closure of this cervical sinus leads to the development of second branchial cleft remnants, which may be in the form of a cyst, a sinus, or a fistulous tract. A second branchial cleft fistula may extend from the palatine tonsil through the carotid bifurcation and along the anterior aspect of the carotid space and sternocleidomastoid muscle down to the lower neck to a skin opening in the supraclavicular fossa [3]. The most common second branchial cleft remnant is a cyst without a sinus or fistula [4]. The location of the second branchial cleft cyst is embryologically defined in the posterior submandibular region near the angle of the mandible, between the submandibular gland, carotid sheath, and sternocleidomastoid muscle [5].

These are squamous epithelial-lined cysts filled with cheesy material or serous, mucoid, or purulent fluid. Lymphoid infiltrates are present in the cystic wall often in aggregates of germinal centers [5].

First branchial cleft cyst, third branchial cleft cyst, and fourth branchial cleft anomaly may arise from failure of obliteration of other branchial apparatuses and account for 8, 3, and 1–2% of all branchial cleft remnants, respectively [3, 5–7].

The second branchial cleft cyst is the most commonly encountered branchial cleft remnant and is the major focus of discussion in the following sections.

H.Y. Yuen (✉) • A.T. Ahuja
Department of Imaging and Interventional Radiology, The Chinese University of Hong Kong, Prince of Wales Hospital, Shatin (NT), Hong Kong (SAR), China
e-mail: drhyyuen@gmail.com

R.A. Sofferman and A.T. Ahuja (eds.), *Ultrasound of the Thyroid and Parathyroid Glands*,
DOI 10.1007/978-1-4614-0974-8_11, © Springer Science+Business Media, LLC 2012

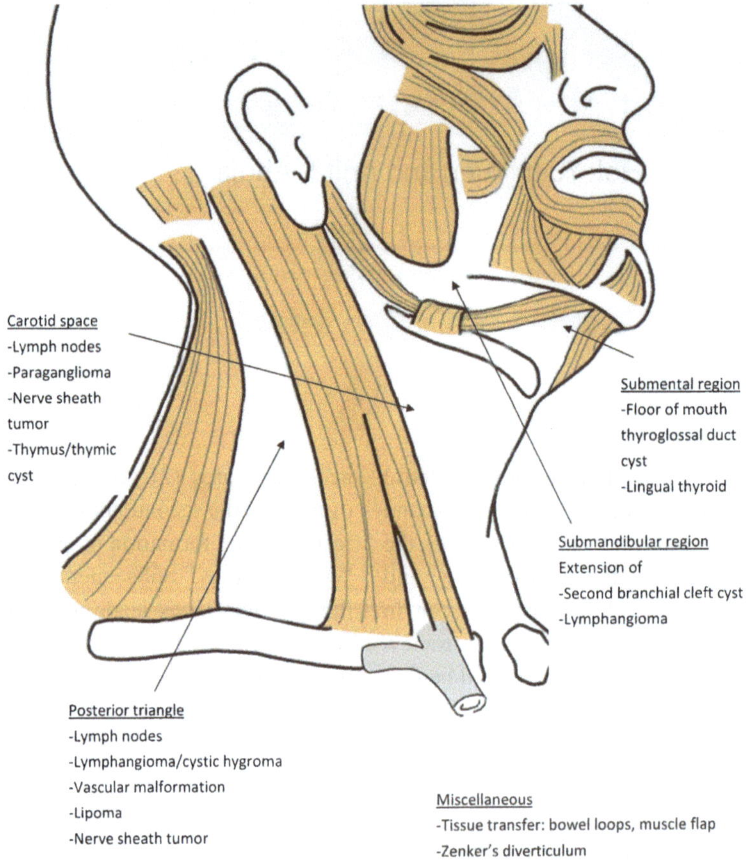

Fig. 11.1 Schematic diagram indicates the common lesions in the various anatomical regions of the neck in the vicinity of the thyroid

Clinical Presentation and Demographics

Second branchial cleft cyst typically presents as a recurrent, soft, compressible mass over the lateral upper neck in children or young adults [5]. During upper respiratory infection, it frequently becomes enlarged, probably secondary to the reactive changes in the lymphoid tissue within the cyst walls. It also enlarges and becomes painful if there is any superimposed infection, and if left untreated may become repeatedly infected and inflamed making surgical resection more difficult [8]. If there is associated fistulous tract, the skin opening is usually conspicuous since birth with intermittent discharge of mucoid secretion [9].

Most patients tend to present at an early age, usually under the age of five, but there is a second peak in the second or third decade which is less common [5].

Ultrasound Findings [5, 10]

The characteristic location of the second branchial cleft cyst in the posterior submandibular region near the angle of mandible, posterolateral to the submandibular gland, anterolateral to the carotid space, and under the medial edge of the sternocleidomastoid muscle is the main clue to its diagnosis (Figs. 11.2 and 11.3).

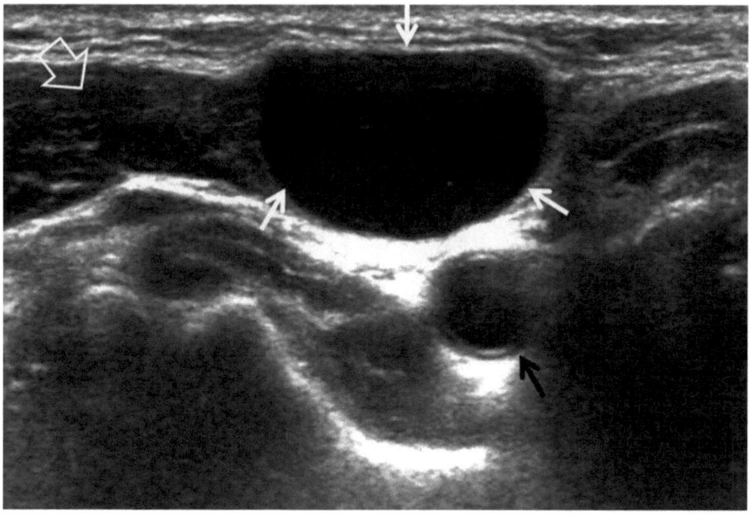

Fig. 11.2 Transverse gray-scale ultrasound shows the characteristic location of the second branchial cleft cyst (*white arrows*), anterolateral to the carotid space (*black arrow*) and under the medial edge of the sternocleidomastoid muscle (*open arrow*). Note the anechoic nature of the cyst with thin walls

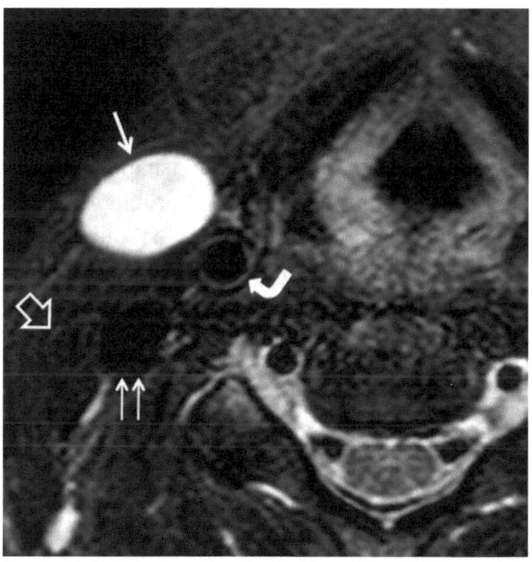

Fig. 11.3 Fat-saturated T2-weighted axial MRI of the upper neck (same patient as in Fig. 11.1). The second branchial cleft cyst appears homogeneously hyperintense (*white arrow*). Note its relationship to the common carotid artery (*curved arrow*), the internal jugular vein (*double white arrows*), and the sternocleidomastoid muscle (*open arrow*)

In the absence of associated hemorrhage or previous superimposed infection, second branchial cleft cyst appears on ultrasound as a unilocular, anechoic cyst with thin walls and posterior acoustic enhancement. Faint internal debris may also be detected (Fig. 11.4). Uncomplicated second branchial cleft cyst may also demonstrate a "pseudosolid" appearance with homogeneous internal echoes due to the presence of mucus, cholesterol crystals, epithelial cells, and debris within the cystic contents [11]. The presence of posterior acoustic enhancement, and swirling motion of the internal debris elicited by intermittent transducer pressure on real-time scanning, and color Doppler serve as valuable clues to the underlying cystic nature of these lesions. No vascularity is detected within the cyst on color Doppler in the absence of any infection (Fig. 11.5).

When second branchial cleft cysts become hemorrhagic or infected (± due to previous fine needle aspiration cytology or biopsy), ill-defined thickened walls and septa with internal debris are seen on ultrasound, associated with edema and inflammatory thickening in the surrounding soft tissues. Increased vascularity of cyst wall on color Doppler may also be detected due to inflammatory congestion.

A hemorrhagic/infected second branchial cleft cyst exactly simulates a necrotic metastatic lymph node (from squamous cell carcinoma or papillary carcinoma of thyroid) (Figs. 11.6 and 11.7), and fine needle aspiration cytology is crucial for making the diagnosis [12].

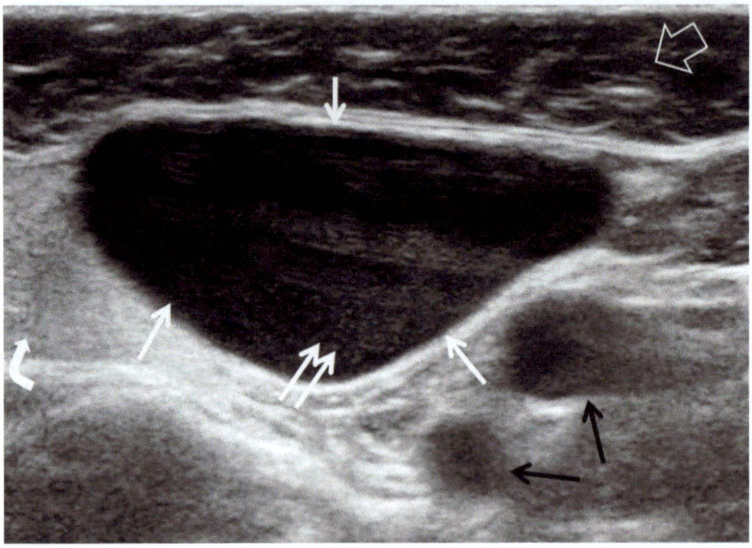

Fig. 11.4 Transverse gray-scale ultrasound shows a second branchial cleft cyst (*white arrows*) located beneath the sternocleidomastoid muscle (*open arrow*), posterolateral to the submandibular gland (*curved arrow*), and anterolateral to the carotid arteries (*black arrows*). Note the low-level echoes/debris in the dependent portion of the cyst (*double white arrows*)

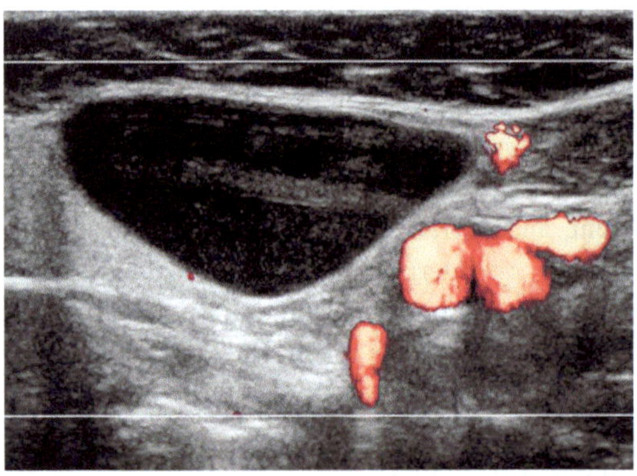

Fig. 11.5 Corresponding power Doppler examination (same patient as in Fig. 11.4) shows no vascularity in the walls or within the cyst. No vascularity should be detected within the cyst/cyst wall on Doppler in the absence of any solid component and infection

Ultrasound may be able to identify the presence of associated sinus or fistulous tract. When there is a sonographic finding of focal cystic extension/"beak" between the internal and external carotid bifurcation, it is pathognomonic of a second branchial cleft cyst [5].

It is useful to remember that these cysts may have parapharyngeal and even cranial extension beyond the reach of ultrasound visualization, and computerized tomography (CT) or magnetic resonance imaging (MRI) will then be required for a more complete assessment.

Typical locations of the first branchial cleft cyst around the pinna or extending from the external auditory canal to the angle of mandible, the third branchial cleft cyst in the posterior cervical space, and the fourth branchial cleft cyst in superolateral aspect of the left lobe of thyroid with associated thyroiditis are useful clues to the diagnosis of these other branchial cleft remnants [3, 6, 7].

Management

Symptomatic branchial cleft remnants are treated by complete surgical excision. The surgeon also resects any associated tract or fistula in order to prevent recurrence.

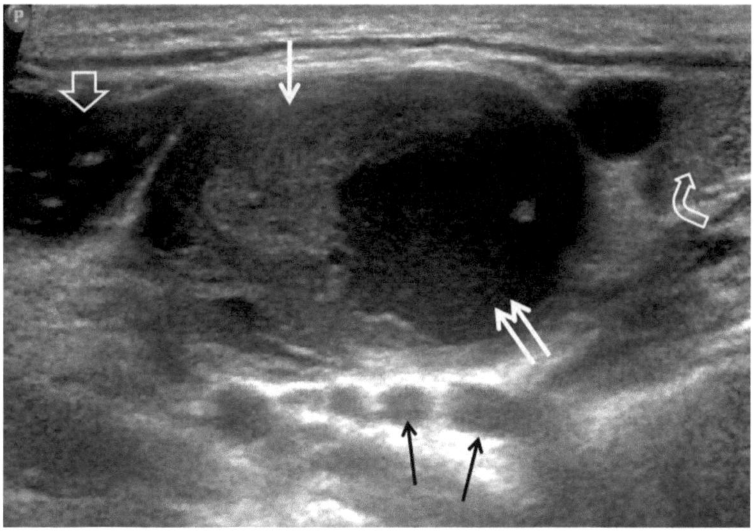

Fig. 11.6 Transverse gray-scale ultrasound shows a mass with solid (*white arrow*) and cystic elements with irregular wall and abundant internal debris (*double white arrows*). Note its characteristic location posterolateral to the submandibular gland (*curved open arrow*), anterolateral to the carotid arteries (*black arrows*), and under the medial edge of the sternocleidomastoid muscle (*open arrow*). Although the location is typical for a second BCC, the presence of a solid component (with vascularity on Doppler [not shown]) should raise the suspicion of a metastatic cystic node (commonly from an H&N SCC or papillary carcinoma thyroid), and fine needle aspiration (FNA) should be performed for differentiation. In this case, the mass was confirmed as a metastatic node from a squamous cell carcinoma

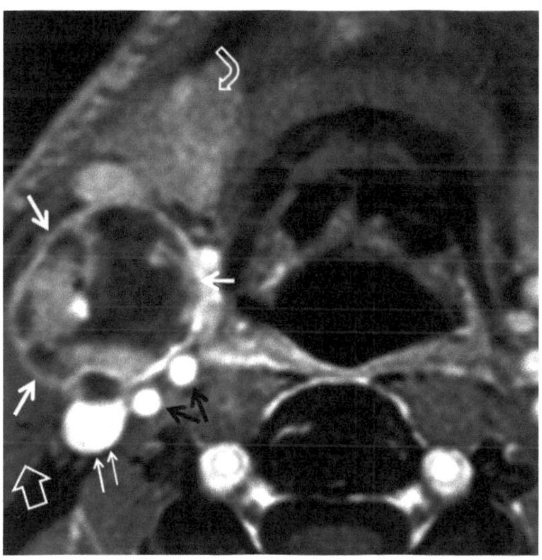

Fig. 11.7 Contrast-enhanced fat-saturated T1-weighted axial MRI of the upper neck (same patient as in Fig. 11.6) shows the mass (*white arrows*) with an irregular eccentric enhancing solid element and the non-enhancing cystic component. Note its location posterolateral to the submandibular gland (*curved open arrow*), anterolateral to the carotid arteries (*black arrows*) and internal jugular vein (*double white arrows*), and beneath the medial edge of the sternocleidomastoid muscle (*open arrow*). Confirmed metastatic node from a squamous cell carcinoma and not a second BCC

Carotid Body Paraganglioma

Pathology

Carotid body paraganglioma (also known as glomus tumor, chemodectoma) arises from the glomus bodies (paraganglia) in the carotid body and is composed of chemoreceptor cells derived from the primitive neural crest cells within the vessel wall [13]. Paragangliomas in the head and neck may also occur along the nodose ganglion of the vagus nerve (glomus vagale), along the jugular ganglion of the vagus nerve (glomus jugulare), and around the Arnold and Jacobson nerves in the middle ear over the promontory (glomus tympanicum) [14]. They may be sporadic or familial (autosomal dominant) [15].

Carotid body paraganglioma is the most common paraganglioma in the head and neck region (60–67% of all) [13, 16]. Sporadic paragangliomas are multicentric in 2–10%, while familial paragangliomas may be multicentric in up to 50–90%. Thyroid carcinoma, other visceral neoplasms, and familial multiple endocrine neoplasm

(MEN) syndromes are known to be associated with paragangliomas [13].

Clinical Presentation and Demographics

Patients most commonly present with a slow-growing, pulsatile, painless mass at the angle of mandible. Associated vagal and/or hypoglossal neuropathy may be seen in 20% of cases [15, 17]. Though carotid body paragangliomas are rarely functional [18], when they do secrete catecholamine, they may give rise to symptoms such as paroxysmal hypertension, palpitations, and flushing. These tumors are most commonly seen in middle-aged patients in their 40s to 50s.

Ultrasound Findings [13, 19]

Carotid body paraganglioma usually appears well defined, solid, and hypoechoic at the characteristic location straddling the carotid bifurcation and splaying the internal and external carotid arteries (Figs. 11.8 and 11.9). Its parenchyma shows a homogeneous echo pattern and may harbor serpiginous vessels within. There is no calcification. Large paragangliomas may occasionally demonstrate a more heterogeneous parenchymal echo pattern due to internal hemorrhage or necrosis (but necrosis is not an expected finding). Large paragangliomas may completely encase the carotid bifurcation (Figs. 11.10–11.12). Color Doppler is useful in the evaluation of paragangliomas by demonstrating the hypervascular nature of the lesion with prominent tortuous vessels within (Fig. 11.13), as well as to confirm its relationship to the carotid bifurcation with splaying of the internal and external carotid arteries.

The contralateral side must be carefully evaluated once a carotid body paraganglioma is identified, as these tumors may be bilateral

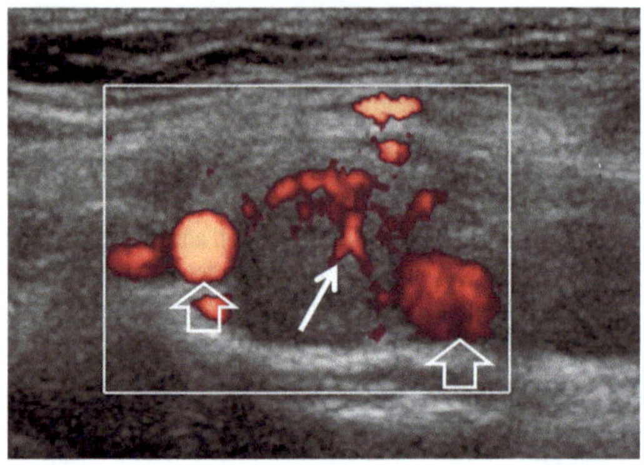

Fig. 11.9 Corresponding power Doppler of the same paraganglioma as in Fig. 11.8 demonstrates vascularity within the mass (*white arrow*) and its relationship to the carotid bifurcation with splaying of the internal and external carotid arteries (*open arrows*)

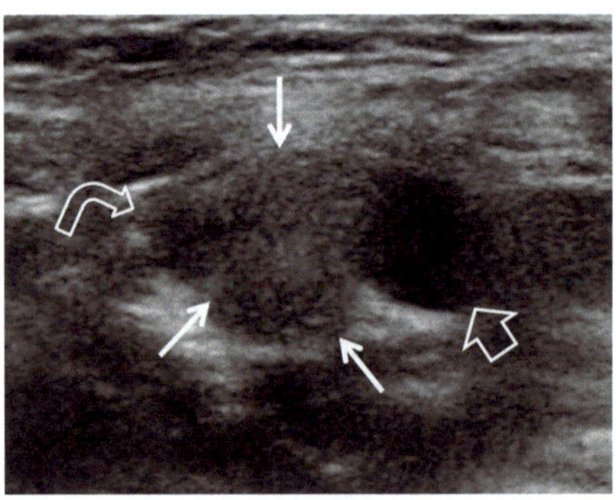

Fig. 11.8 Transverse gray-scale ultrasound shows a small carotid body paraganglioma as a well-defined, solid, and hypoechoic mass (*white arrows*) at the characteristic location straddling the carotid bifurcation and splaying the internal (*open arrow*) and external (*curved open arrow*) carotid arteries

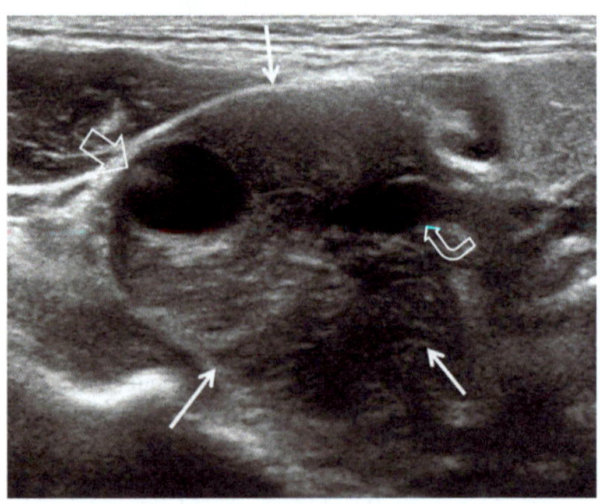

Fig. 11.10 Transverse gray-scale ultrasound shows a large carotid body paraganglioma (*white arrows*) encasing the carotid bifurcation and splaying the internal (*open arrow*) and external (*curved open arrow*) carotid arteries

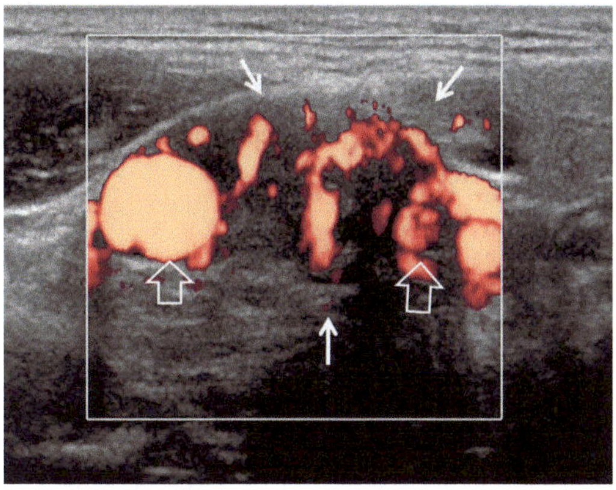

Fig. 11.11 Corresponding power Doppler of the same paragangliomas as in Fig. 11.10 demonstrates the prominent tortuous vessels within (*white arrows*) and its relationship to the carotid bifurcation with splaying of the internal and external carotid arteries (*open arrows*)

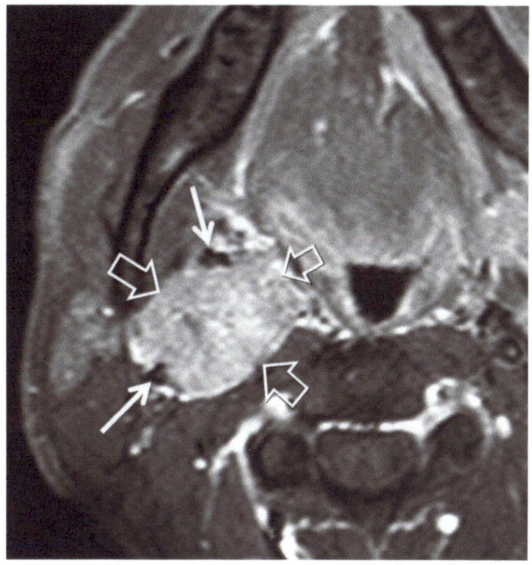

Fig. 11.12 Contrast-enhanced fat-saturated T1-weighted axial MRI of the upper neck (same patient as in Figs. 11.10 and 11.11) confirms an avidly enhancing carotid body paraganglioma (*open arrows*) straddling the carotid bifurcation and splaying the internal and external carotid arteries (*white arrows*)

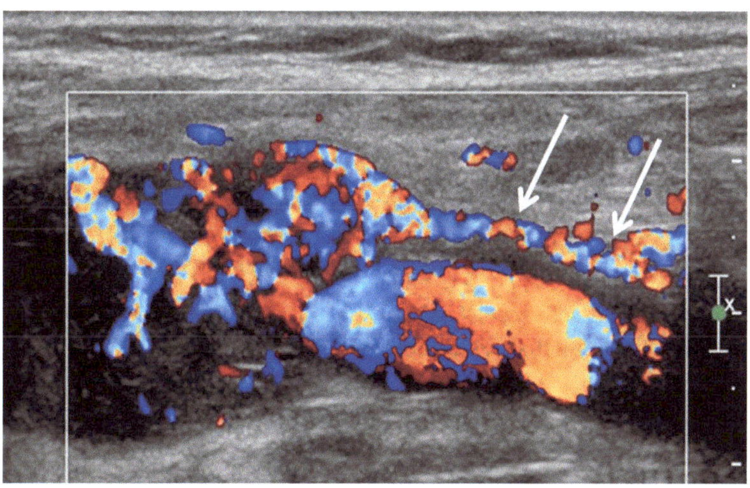

Fig. 11.13 Longitudinal color Doppler ultrasound of a carotid body tumor shows marked intratumoral vascularity and a hypertrophied ascending pharyngeal artery (*arrows*)

(approximately 10%). The other paragangliomas such as the glomus vagale and glomus jugulare, however, are not accessible by ultrasound and have to be excluded by computed tomography (CT) or magnetic resonance imaging (MRI) [20]. A diagnostic angiogram is not routinely indicated. The main role of angiography is in the preoperative embolization of these lesions.

Management

Screening of the family members of familial paraganglioma patients may begin as early as the age of 20.

Surgical resection is the treatment of choice and may benefit from preoperative embolization for prophylactic hemostasis. Radiotherapy is usually reserved for poor surgical candidates, to attain lesion control [21–24].

Dermoid Cyst

Pathology [25]

Dermoid cyst is a congenital cystic lesion, due to the inclusion of rests of epithelial elements at the site of the embryonic first and second branchial arches, resulting in sequestration of trapped surface ectoderm. Histologically, a dermoid cyst is lined by keratinizing squamous epithelium and contains dermal structures including dermal appendages such as sebaceous glands, hair follicles, blood vessels, fat, and sometimes collagen and osseo-dental structures in addition to the epithelial elements. Occasionally (20%), dermoid cysts may also contain sweat glands. There is a rare lesion of similar nature known as teratoid cysts that contain elements from all three germ layers and are epithelial-lined cysts with mesodermal or endodermal elements such as muscles, bones, teeth, and mucous membranes.

Only 7% of dermoid and epidermoid cysts occur in the head and neck region and are the rarest congenital cystic lesions in the neck [26, 27]. They are mostly located at or slightly off the midline. The floor of the mouth, including the submandibular space, sublingual space, and root of the tongue, is most commonly involved [26], though dermoid cyst may occasionally be seen at the sternal notch.

Clinical Presentation and Demographics

The mean age of presentation is in the late teens or twenties, and there is slight male preponderance of 3:1 [25]. The most common presenting symptom is that of a painless, palpable subcutaneous mass. These lesions are very slow growing and usually remain dormant for years, though there may be a rapid growth phase in the young adults [28]. Sudden growth or change may be observed after rupture, but associated significant inflammation and enlargement is a rare complication. It should be noted that dermoid and teratoid cysts have a malignant potential, the most common malignant transformation is to squamous cell carcinoma [29].

Ultrasound Findings [25, 30]

Most dermoid cysts are superficial in location which makes ultrasound an ideal initial imaging modality of choice. On ultrasound, a dermoid cyst appears as a well-demarcated lesion, with heterogeneous internal echoes due to the fatty, fluid, and mixed contents (Figs. 11.14 and 11.15), and echogenic foci from calcifications and osseo-dental structures casting dense posterior acoustic shadowing. There is sound attenuation by the fat content which tends to obscure the distal portion of the lesion. No significant vascularity is detected on color Doppler within or in the walls of dermoid cysts.

Management

Surgery is curative for dermoid and epidermoid cysts, and the entire cyst is resected in order to prevent recurrence.

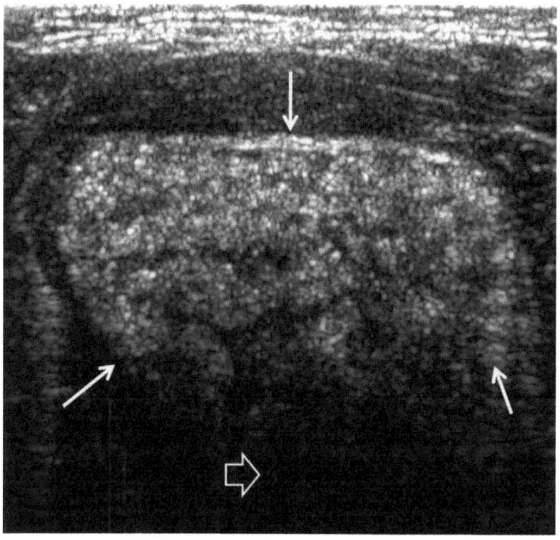

Fig. 11.14 Transverse/coronal gray-scale ultrasound shows a dermoid cyst (*white arrows*) in the floor of the mouth as a well-demarcated lesion with heterogeneous internal echoes due to the fat, fluid, and mixed contents. Note the sound attenuation posteriorly (*open arrow*) obscuring visualization of the deeper structures

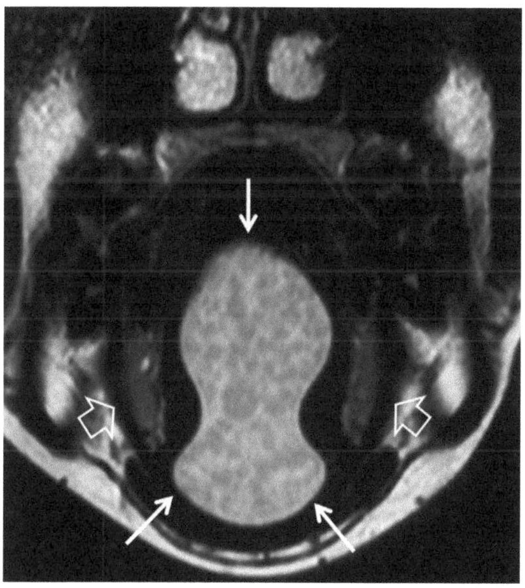

Fig. 11.15 Corresponding coronal T2-weighted MRI (same patient as in Fig. 11.14) of the floor of the mouth shows the anatomic extent of the dermoid cyst (*white arrows*). Note the "sac of marbles" appearance with the fluid content hyperintense, while the fatty and other components appear less hyperintense/hypointense. Note the mylohyoid muscles (*open arrows*)

Lipoma

Pathology

Lipomas are the most common benign mesenchymal tumors and are encapsulated lesions composed entirely of mature fat [31]. They are typically subcutaneous or submucosal in location. About 13% of all lipomas are in the head and neck region. Typical locations are adjacent to the clavicle in females and in the posterior triangle in males [32]. The other common sites include the posterior cervical space, the submandibular space, the anterior cervical space, and the parotid space. In fact, they can occur in every space in the extracranial head and neck and may be trans-spatial and involve multiple contiguous spaces [31].

Clinical Presentation and Demographics

Lipomas typically present as asymptomatic lumps in the neck. Their soft consistency may be clinically mistaken for lymphangiomas. They tend to show an initial period of discernible growth and then remain static in size. Occasionally, they may become large enough to compress adjacent structures. Lipomas are more common in males, with average age of presentation in the fifth to sixth decades [31].

Ultrasound Findings [31–33]

Typical sonographic features of lipomas are well-defined, compressible, elliptical masses. They are usually slightly hyperechoic to muscles (75%) but may be iso/hypoechoic (25%). Multiple thin linear echogenic lines parallel to the transducer are seen within the lesion irrespective of the scanning plane, producing a "feathered" or "striped" appearance (Figs. 11.16 and 11.17). No calcification, nodularity, necrosis, deep acoustic enhancement or attenuation, or significant vascularity on color Doppler should be present.

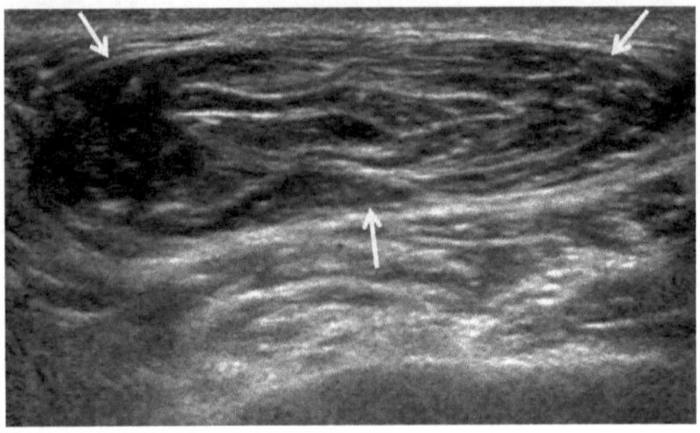

Fig. 11.16 Transverse gray-scale ultrasound shows the typical sonographic appearance of a lipoma (*white arrows*) as a well-circumscribed, elliptical lesion slightly hyperechoic to muscle with multiple thin linear echogenic lines parallel to the transducer, producing a "feathered" or "striped" appearance

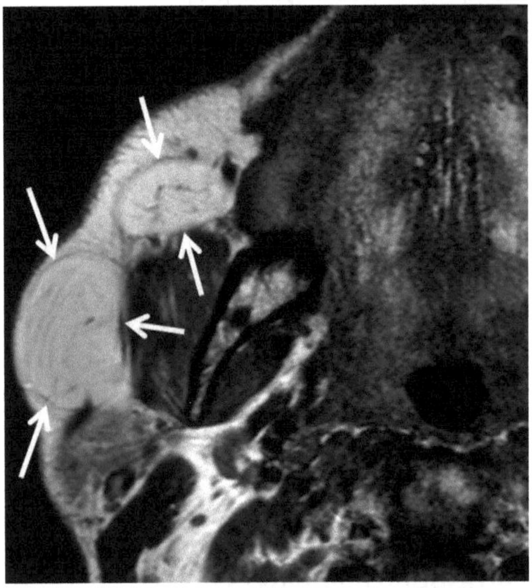

Fig. 11.17 T1-weighted axial MRI (same patient as in Fig. 11.16) shows two well-encapsulated lipomas (*white arrows*) with isointense signal to the surrounding subcutaneous fat overlying the right masseter muscle (one of which corresponds to the lipoma in Fig. 11.16). Homogeneous isointense signal to fat in all sequences in MRI including complete attenuation on fat saturation sequence is diagnostic of lipoma

Suspicion of the rare liposarcoma (instead of a lipoma) should be raised if there are sonographic findings such as infiltration stranding of the adjacent tissues, nodular mass, internal septation, increased vascularity, calcification, cystic or necrotic component detected within the lesion.

Management

Usually, no treatment is required for lipoma, but surgical resection or debulking may be indicated if the lipoma is large enough to be causing compression symptoms or is cosmetically disfiguring.

The postoperative recurrence rate for lipoma is high (50%), most likely due to microscopic infiltration of adjacent soft tissues. Infiltrating lipomas in the head and neck region are rare, but their postoperative recurrence rate is even higher and up to 62.5% [34].

Lymphangioma

Pathology

Lymphangiomas also belong to the category of vascular malformation in the Mulliken and Glowacki classification system and are dilated endothelial-lined lymphatic spaces. They are subdivided into four types according to the microscopic size of the dilated lymphatic channels. Cystic hygroma is composed of markedly dilated lymphatic spaces and is the commonest type. Cavernous lymphangioma consists of mildly dilated lymphatic spaces, while capillary lymphangioma consists of the smallest lymphatic spaces and is the least common. When both venous and lymphatic vascular malformations occur in the same lesion, it is designated as a vasculolymphatic malformation [35]. These are, however, histologic criteria and are not discernable on ultrasound.

Many theories regarding the embryogenesis of lymphangiomas have been proposed: the two more popular theories include sequestration of embryonic lymph sacs [36, 37] and failure of embryologic fusion between primordial lymph sac and the central venous system [38]. Turner syndrome is the most commonly associated syndrome [35], although association with Noonan syndrome, Klinefelter syndrome, and fetal alcohol syndrome has also been observed.

Clinical Presentation and Demographics

Lymphangioma most commonly presents as a soft, doughy, painless neck mass during the first 2 years of life (>80%, because the greatest lymphatic development occurs early in childhood [39]) and is usually an incidental finding. Cystic hygroma is most commonly seen in the posterior cervical space and the submandibular space [40]. Occasionally, large lymphangiomas may cause airway obstruction and present acutely [41]. Solitary lymphangioma may also present in young adulthood, most commonly in the submandibular region and posterior triangle. These are more likely caused by traumatic injury to the lymphatics rather than congenital in nature [42]. There is no known malignant potential in a lymphangioma.

Ultrasound Findings [39, 43, 44]

Uncomplicated lymphangiomas appear on ultrasound as well-defined, unilocular/lobulated/multilocular anechoic compressible cysts with thin walls and fine internal septa (Figs. 11.18 and 11.19). Even when they are large, there is usually no significant associated mass effect; rather, lymphangiomas are commonly indented by adjacent muscles and vessels. No vascularity should be seen on color Doppler in uncomplicated lymphangiomas. They are trans-spatial (involving more than one anatomical space) and have a tendency to insinuate between and around the neurovascular structures.

Superimposed hemorrhage or infection in lymphangiomas causes sudden increase in size and pain. The unilocular or multilocular cystic spaces become noncompressible and heterogeneous with thickened, irregular walls and septa. Internal debris and fluid–fluid levels due to sedimentation and separation of different fluid contents may be seen and are suggestive of prior

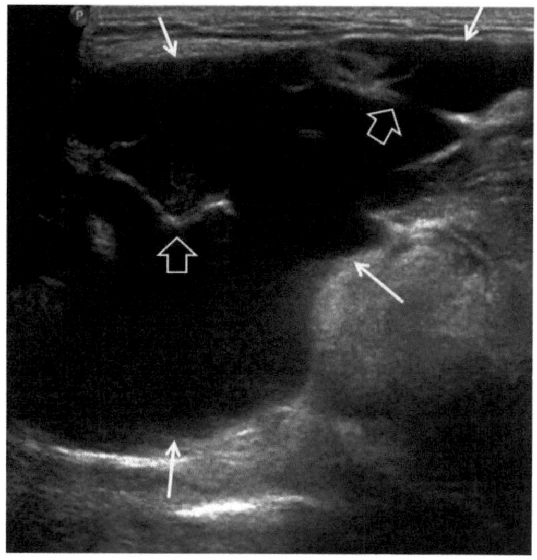

Fig. 11.18 Gray-scale ultrasound shows the typical appearance of a nonhemorrhagic/uninfected large multiloculated lymphangioma (*white arrows*) as an anechoic, compressible cystic lesion with multiple thin intervening septa (*open arrows*)

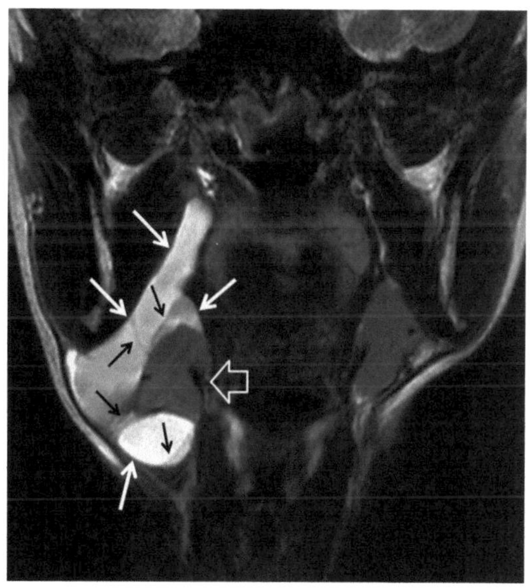

Fig. 11.19 Corresponding T2-weighted coronal MRI of the floor of the mouth shows the same lymphangioma as in Fig. 11.18. It spans the sublingual and submandibular spaces of the right side of the floor of the mouth (*white arrows*) and encases the right submandibular gland (*open arrow*). Note the low-signal thin internal septa (*black arrows*) within the high-signal lymphangioma. Although ultrasound readily identifies the lesion and suggests the diagnosis, MRI better defines its anatomical extent and relationship to adjacent structures, particularly for large and multiple lesions

hemorrhage. Mass effect may also become evident. Superimposed infection may cause increased vascularity on color Doppler, within the walls, internal septa of the lymphangiomas, and in the surrounding soft tissues.

For large neck lymphangiomas, particularly when their inferior extent cannot be defined, always examine the axilla and mediastinum, as they may extend into these areas (Figs. 11.20–11.22). Although ultrasound makes a confident diagnosis of lymphangiomas, computerized tomography (CT) or magnetic resonance imaging (MRI) is often required to delineate the full extent, particularly prior to any treatment.

Management [45–49]

When lymphangiomas are isolated and not associated with major neurovascular structures, surgical resection may be feasible. Alternatively, ultrasound-guided percutaneous injection of sclerosing agents may be performed for extensive, insinuating trans-spatial lymphangiomas.

Pyogenic Neck Abscess

Pathology

An abscess is a localized collection formed as the result of suppurative inflammation with characteristic production of pus or purulent exudate composed of leukocytes, liquefactive necrosis, and edema fluid [50]. Bacteria that produce such localized suppuration are designated as pyogenic.

Clinical Presentation and Demographics

Abscess in the neck may originate from an infective focus such as suppurative adenopathy and salivary gland infection or from direct spread through inflamed tissues as in pharyngitis and odontogenic infections [51, 52]. It is more commonly seen in the postoperative patients, patients with poor oral hygiene (particularly those after radiation therapy), drug abusers, and immunocompromised patients [52], and may be associated with a retained foreign body [53]. Diabetes mellitus is a risk factor and

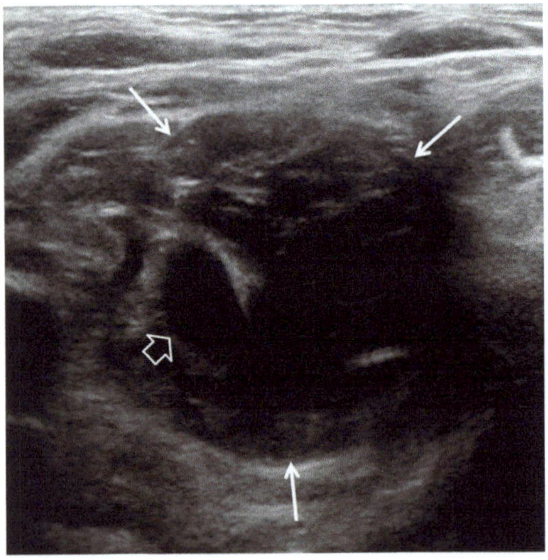

Fig. 11.20 Transverse gray-scale ultrasound shows a multiloculated lymphangioma (*white arrows*) with anechoic cystic spaces encasing the common carotid artery (*open arrow*)

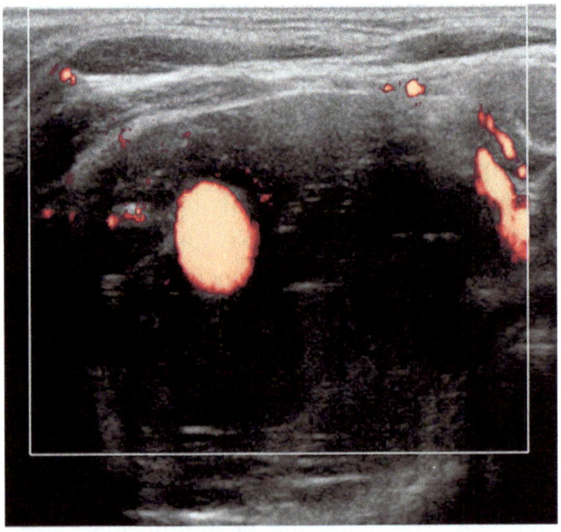

Fig. 11.21 Power Doppler ultrasound (same patient as in Fig. 11.20) confirms the location of the common carotid artery within the lymphangioma. Note the absence of vascularity within the lymphangioma

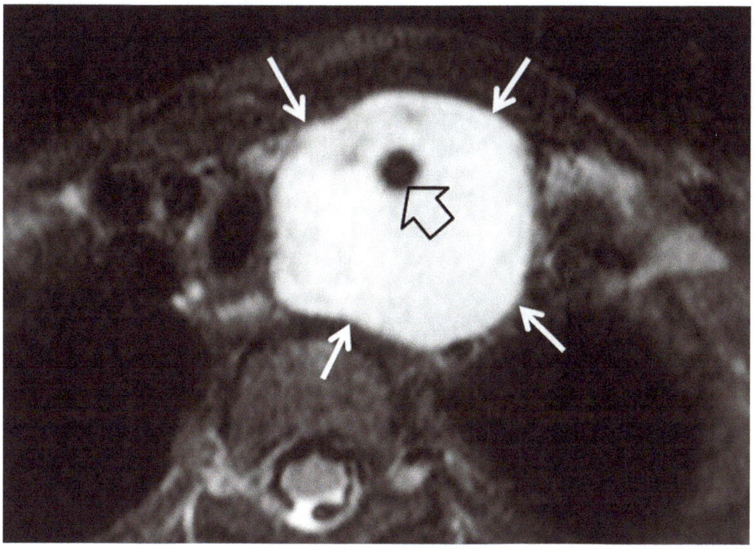

Fig. 11.22 Fat-saturated T2-weighted axial MRI shows the same lymphangioma as in Figs. 11.20 and 11.21. Note the encased common carotid artery (*open arrow*) with flow void encased by the hyperintense lymphangioma (*white arrows*)

may be seen in up to a third of the cases [54]. However, most patients with neck abscess have no known etiological cause [51, 54].

The typical presentation is of a warm, erythematous, painful swelling or fluctuant mass (Fig. 11.23). Neck abscess close to the upper aerodigestive tract may produce symptoms such as odynophagia. Constitutional symptoms like fever are often present.

Ultrasound Findings [52]

Sonographically, an abscess appears as an ill-defined, irregular, unilocular, or multilocular collection with thick walls (± septa), internal debris, and edema of adjacent soft tissues (Fig. 11.24). The abscess rim and adjacent soft tissues often demonstrate hypervascularity on color Doppler (Fig. 11.25). Prominent inflammatory lymph nodes are often present in the vicinity. Attention should be paid to possible complications such as venous thrombophlebitis or carotid involvement.

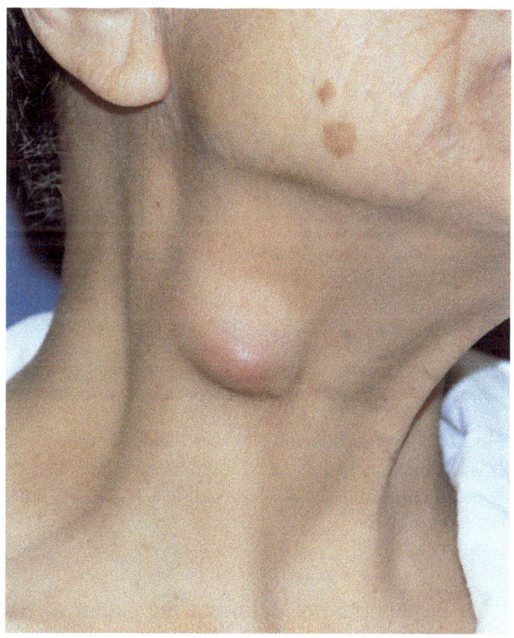

Fig. 11.23 Clinical photograph of a patient with right neck abscess shows an erythematous, painful fluctuant mass

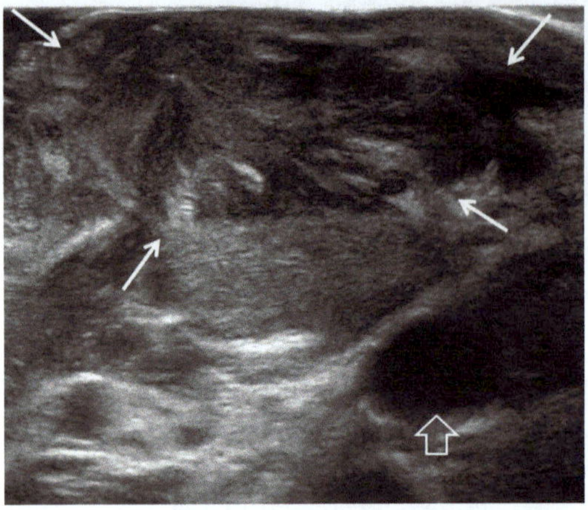

Fig. 11.24 Transverse gray-scale ultrasound of the same patient as in Fig. 11.23 shows the typical appearance of an abscess (*white arrows*) seen as an ill-defined, irregular, multilocular collection with thick walls and septa, internal debris, and edema of the adjacent soft tissues. Note its relationship to the common carotid artery (*open arrow*)

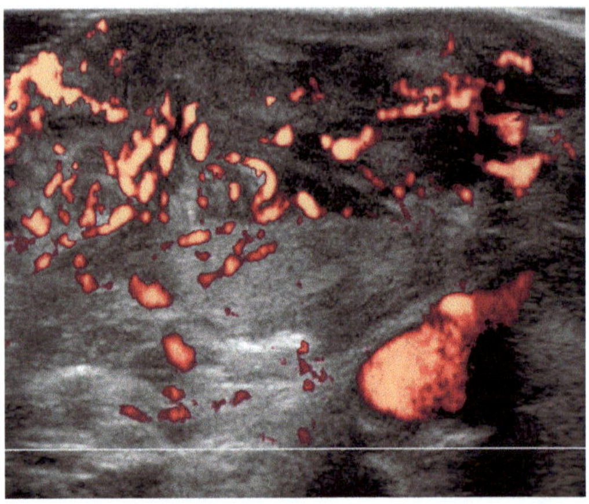

Fig. 11.25 Corresponding power Doppler ultrasound (same patient as in Figs. 11.23 and 11.24) demonstrates hypervascularity in the abscess wall and within the adjacent soft tissues

It is important to delineate the extent of the abscess and its anatomical relations before aspiration or surgery is contemplated. Deep-seated abscesses such as those in the parapharyngeal or retropharyngeal spaces and those with inferior extension into the mediastinum are beyond the visibility of ultrasound and should be further evaluated (by CT or MRI) in order to delineate their entire extent.

The differential diagnosis includes necrotic, metastatic lymphadenopathy with superimposed infection [52, 55]. Fine needle aspiration (FNA) helps to confirm the diagnosis and provides specimen for microbiology tests.

Management

The aim of treatment includes the evacuation of pus and the identification of organisms to guide subsequent antibiotic therapy. The traditional approach is open surgical drainage which carries its own risks and drawbacks [56].

Ultrasound-guided drainage for abscesses of the head and neck [57] and CT-guided aspiration of deep neck abscesses [58] have become increasingly popular as the treatment of choice.

Nerve Sheath Tumor

Pathology

Schwannomas and neurofibromas are the nerve sheath tumors most frequently detected in the head and neck [59]. Schwannomas are benign tumors composed only of Schwann cells and are encapsulated and well circumscribed. On the other hand, neurofibromas are unencapsulated tumors arising from axons and Schwann cells, with infiltration and enlargement of the nerves. Neurofibromas are often multiple and associated with neurofibromatosis type I, in which case the malignant potential of neurofibroma is much higher than that of solitary sporadic neurofibroma [60].

The vagus nerve, dorsal and ventral cervical nerve roots, the cervical sympathetic chain, and the brachial plexus are the usual sites in the neck where nerve sheath tumors are found [59].

Clinical Presentation and Demographics

A nerve sheath tumor usually presents as an asymptomatic, slow-growing, painless palpable mass in the neck. Associated symptoms of vagus schwannoma may include dysphagia, dysphonia, hoarseness, arrhythmia, and pain when the tumor is large [61]. Brachial plexus schwannoma may produce symptoms and signs of radiculopathy [62].

There is a male preponderance, and the average age of presentation is in the mid-forties.

Ultrasound Findings [59, 61, 62]

The close proximity of a nerve sheath tumor to the course of its parent nerve is the best diagnostic clue to its origin. Vagus nerve tumors are located in the anterior triangle, cervical nerve root tumors in the posterior triangle (Fig. 11.26), and tumors from the sympathetic trunk are closely related to the longus colli muscle. Tumors from the brachial plexus may be present anywhere along the course of the brachial plexus from the intra- and extradural spaces, neural foramina, perivertebral space, and posterior cervical space to the axillary apex.

Ultrasound only adequately detects and evaluates nerve sheath tumors in the infrahyoid neck.

Schwannomas are heterogeneously hypoechoic [63] (Figs. 11.27 and 11.28) and often demonstrate posterior acoustic enhancement although they are solid lesions [64, 65]. Well-defined focal cystic areas are commonly noted with schwannomas [66] (Fig. 11.29). They are usually fusiform or ovoid in shape with tapering ends, and the demonstration of continuity with adjacent

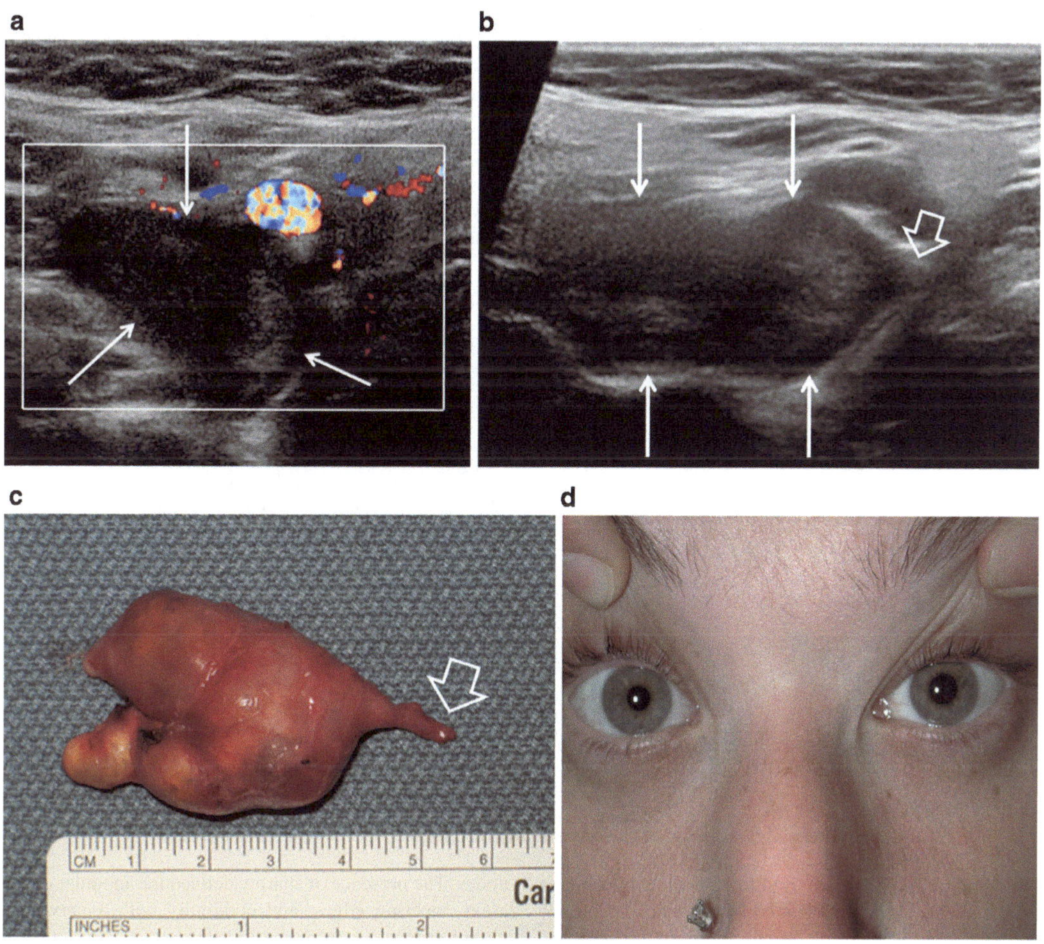

Fig. 11.26 (**a**–**d**) Transverse Doppler (**a**), longitudinal gray-scale ultrasound (**b**), and operative specimen (**c**) in a patient with a sympathetic chain schwannoma (*arrows*) presenting with Horner's syndrome (**d**). Note the marked similarity in contours and inferior tapering edge of the schwannoma as seen on the longitudinal gray-scale ultrasound and the operative specimen (*arrow heads*)

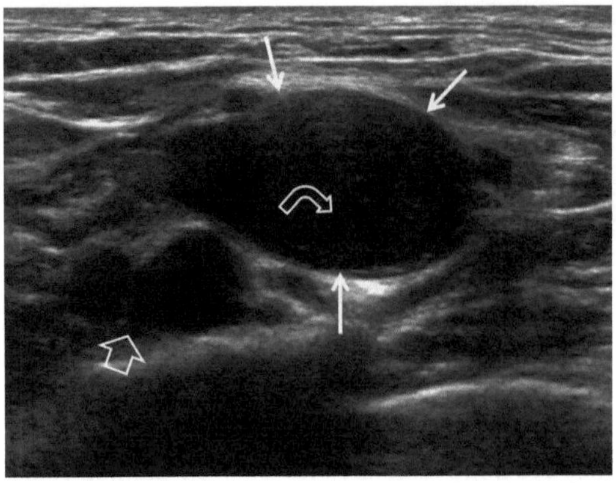

Fig. 11.27 Transverse gray-scale ultrasound shows a schwannoma which appears as a well-defined, solid, heterogeneous, hypoechoic lesion (*white arrows*) with sharply defined focal cystic areas within (*curved open arrow*). Note the adjacent carotid arteries (*open arrow*)

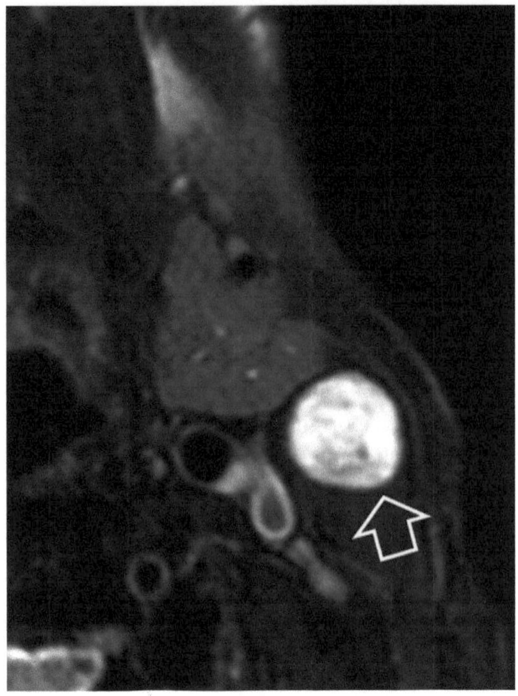

Fig. 11.28 Fat-saturated T2-weighted axial MRI shows the same schwannoma (*open arrow*) as in Fig. 11.27 appearing as a well-defined, heterogeneous hyperintense mass

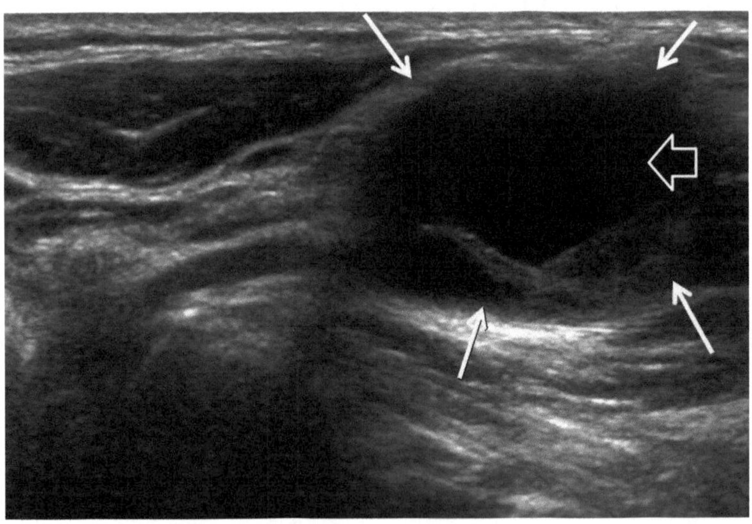

Fig. 11.29 Gray-scale ultrasound shows a schwannoma (*white arrows*) with well-defined focal cystic areas (*open arrow*). Such tumors are often mistaken for necrotic nodes. The presence of sharply defined intranodular cystic areas, tapering edges, and continuity with a nerve are clues to suggest a nerve sheath tumor

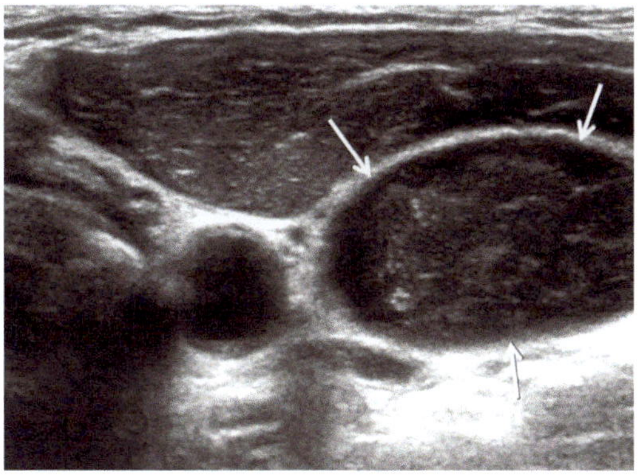

Fig. 11.30 Transverse gray-scale ultrasound image shows a neurofibroma as a well-defined, heterogeneous hypoechoic mass (*white arrows*)

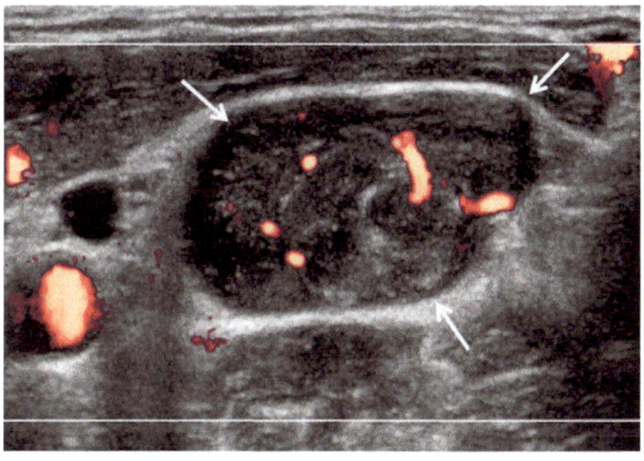

Fig. 11.31 Corresponding power Doppler (same patient as in Fig. 11.30) shows mild vascularity within the neurofibroma (*white arrows*). On Doppler, neurofibromas tend to show less vascularity compared to schwannomas

nerve (which may be thickened) is diagnostic of nerve sheath tumors.

Neurofibromas are also heterogeneously hypoechoic [63] and do not readily show posterior acoustic enhancement [66] (Fig. 11.30). On color Doppler, schwannomas are more vascular than neurofibromas and tend to show increased vascularity with prominent tortuous vessels [63] (Fig. 11.31). It should be noted that such vascularity is very sensitive to pressure and may be obliterated by increasing transducer pressure.

Despite these differences, ultrasound cannot reliably distinguish schwannomas from neurofibromas.

The normal vagus nerve is almost always visible using modern high-resolution transducers [61].

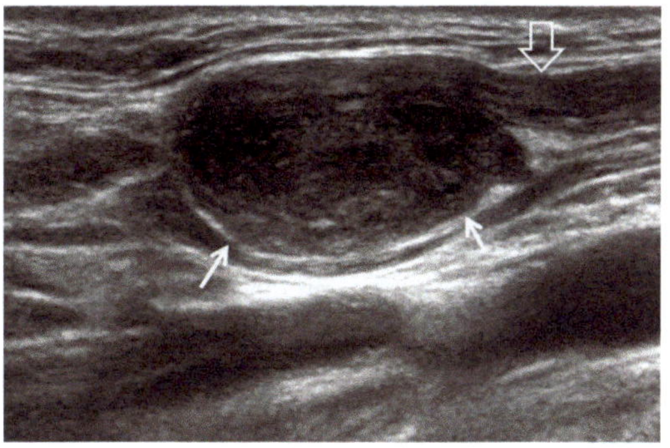

Fig. 11.32 Longitudinal gray-scale ultrasound shows a brachial plexus schwannoma (*white arrows*). Note that the continuity with a division of the brachial plexus (*open arrow*) clearly demonstrates the nature of the lesion and may prevent a painful biopsy

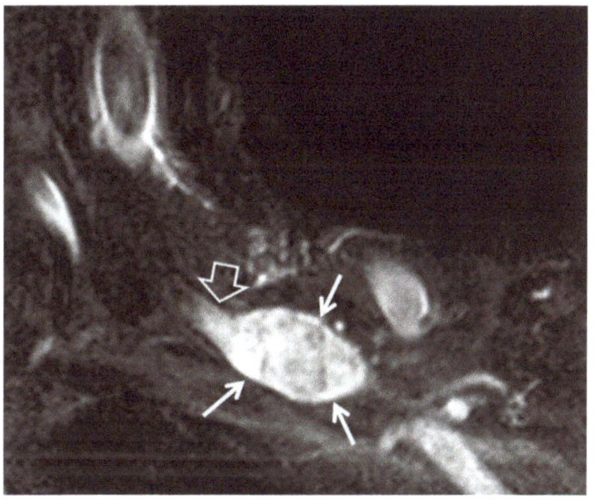

Fig. 11.33 Corresponding fat-saturated T2-weighted MRI (same patient as in Fig. 11.32) shows brachial plexus schwannoma (*white arrows*) as a well-defined heterogeneous hyperintense lesion. Again, continuity with the division of the brachial plexus (*open arrow*) provides the clue to the diagnosis

The location of vagus schwannoma in the infrahyoid carotid space in close proximity and posterior to the carotid artery and internal jugular vein and the demonstration of continuity on longitudinal scan allow a confident diagnosis to be made.

The brachial plexus trunks and divisions are delineated in the posterior cervical space between the anterior and middle scalene muscles [62]. The demonstration of continuity of brachial plexus schwannoma with these trunks and divisions is crucial in predicting the diagnosis (Figs. 11.32 and 11.33).

Fine needle aspiration or biopsy of nerve sheath tumors may elicit excruciating pain [66], and it is better to recognize these lesions before any sampling procedure is performed. If the diagnosis of a nerve sheath tumor is in doubt on sonography, magnetic resonance imaging helps in evaluating its nature, precise anatomical location, and multiplicity.

Management

Tumor resection without sacrifice of the nerve is the treatment of choice and possible in most instances. If there is nerve resection, end-to-end anastomosis or nerve graft interposition may be performed.

Thyroglossal Duct Cyst

Pathology

Thyroglossal duct cyst is the most common congenital neck lesion [67]. Embryologically, the thyroid anlage arises from the posterior tongue base and descends down to the thyroid bed along the thyroglossal duct (TGD). The TGD extends from the foramen cecum in the posterior third of the tongue, along the floor of the mouth to around the hyoid bone and anterior to the strap muscles, down to the thyroid bed anterior to the thyroid or cricoid cartilage. The thyroglossal duct usually involutes at around 5–6 weeks of gestational age. Any segment of the duct that fails to regress and subsequently differentiates into an epithelial-lined cyst with persistent secretory activity results in the formation of thyroglossal duct cyst (TGDC) [68]. It may occur anywhere along the course of the ductal remnant [69]. Ectopic thyroid tissue may also be seen anywhere along this course. Malignant degeneration (mostly into papillary carcinoma) of the epithelial lining of thyroglossal duct cyst has been reported as a rare (<1%) complication [70, 71]. However, it is believed that at least some of these lesions represent metastatic deposits from primary thyroid cancer, and some are due to direct extension from an adjacent thyroid lesion [72–78].

The majority of thyroglossal duct cysts are related to the hyoid bone. About 25–65% occur in the infrahyoid neck, 15–50% at the level of the hyoid, and 20–25% in the suprahyoid neck. Most thyroglossal duct cysts in the suprahyoid neck are located at the midline, but those in the infrahyoid neck are more likely to be off midline and paramedian in location [67, 79].

Clinical Presentation and Demographics

The typical presentation is a midline or paramedian soft, compressible, painless cystic mass in child or young adult. There may be history of recurrent, intermittent appearance or enlargement of the midline neck lesion, often triggered by upper respiratory infection or trauma. A classical clinical sign is that the thyroglossal duct cyst is supposed to elevate with tongue protrusion. Most patients are under the age of 10 at first presentation, while some may present in early adulthood.

Ultrasound Findings [67, 79]

The close relationship of the cyst to the hyoid bone and its location along the expected course of the thyroglossal duct from the foramen cecum down to the thyroid bed is the most important clue to the diagnosis.

Four sonographic patterns of thyroglossal duct cysts have been described [80]. The first group is anechoic (27.5%) and probably represents uninfected thyroglossal duct cysts (Figs. 11.34–11.36). The second group is anechoic/hypoechoic with fine internal debris (17.5%) (Fig. 11.37). The third group shows a heterogeneous echo pattern (27.5%) probably due to repeated infections and previous hemorrhage from prior aspiration (Fig. 11.38). The fourth group shows a uniformly echogenic "pseudosolid" appearance (27.5%) probably due to the proteinaceous content of the cyst secreted by the epithelial lining [69, 79]

(Fig. 11.39). Clues to the cystic nature of a "pseudosolid" thyroglossal duct cyst include posterior acoustic enhancement, swirling motion of the internal debris within the cyst seen on real-time gray-scale scan after application of intermittent transducer pressure, or with increase in power on Doppler. There should be no evidence of a mural nodule, solid mass component, or calcification. No vascularity is seen within the cyst in the absence of any infection.

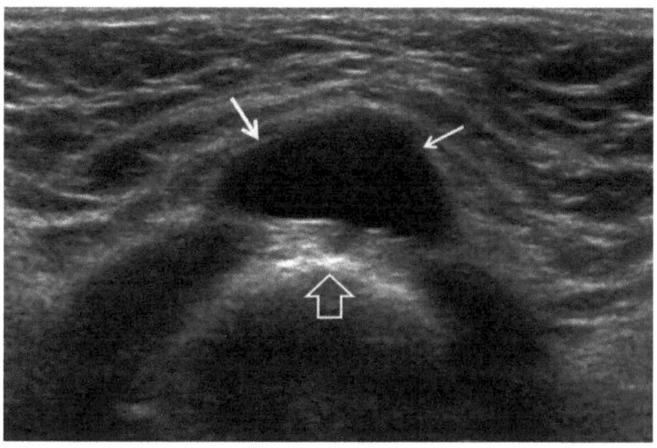

Fig. 11.34 Transverse gray-scale ultrasound shows a well-defined anechoic thyroglossal duct cyst (*white arrows*). Note its relationship to the hyoid bone (*open arrow*)

When thyroglossal duct cysts are complicated by hemorrhage or infection, they show ill-defined thick walls and septa, internal debris, and inflammatory change in the adjacent soft tissues. The walls and septa of infected cysts may demonstrate increased vascularity on color Doppler.

Usually, a confident diagnosis of thyroglossal duct cyst can often be made clinically. The aim of ultrasound is to confirm the diagnosis and to exclude the rare complication of malignant degeneration by excluding the presence of any solid component (with intranodular vascularity) or coarse, dense calcification. Ultrasound-guided fine needle aspiration cytology can be performed if suspicious. The presence of normal thyroid tissue in the thyroid bed should also be ascertained.

Management

Thyroglossal duct cysts are treated by complete surgical excision termed "Sistrunk procedure" [81] which involves resection of the entire cyst, any remaining tract, and the middle third of the hyoid bone. The tract to the foramen cecum is also dissected free in order to prevent recurrence.

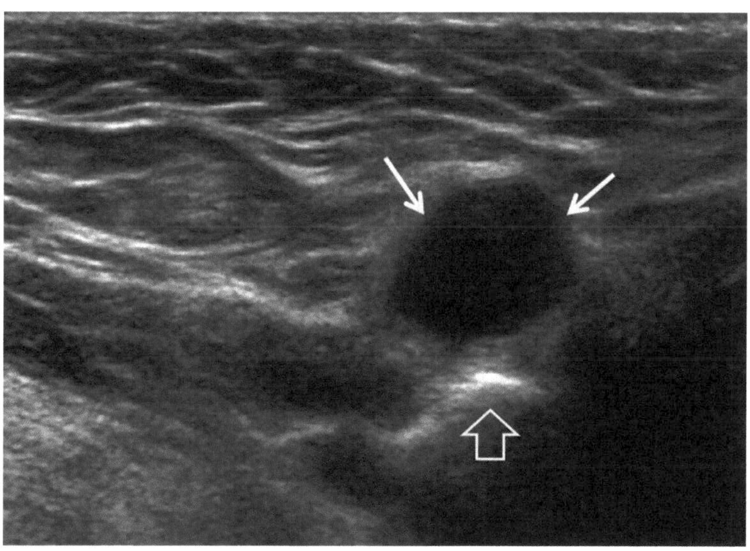

Fig. 11.35 Longitudinal gray-scale ultrasound shows the same thyroglossal duct cyst (*white arrows*) as in Fig. 11.34. Note its relationship to hyoid bone (*open arrow*)

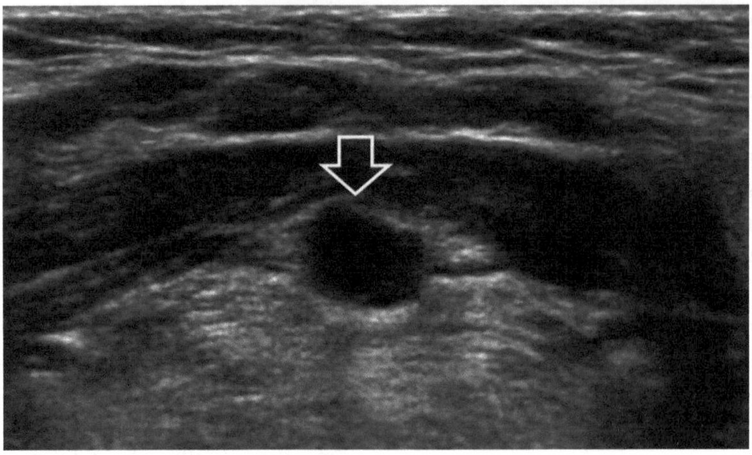

Fig. 11.36 Transverse gray-scale ultrasound shows a well-defined, anechoic thyroglossal duct cyst (*open arrow*) in the midline at the floor of the mouth. A dermoid or epidermoid in the floor of the mouth may have a similar appearance

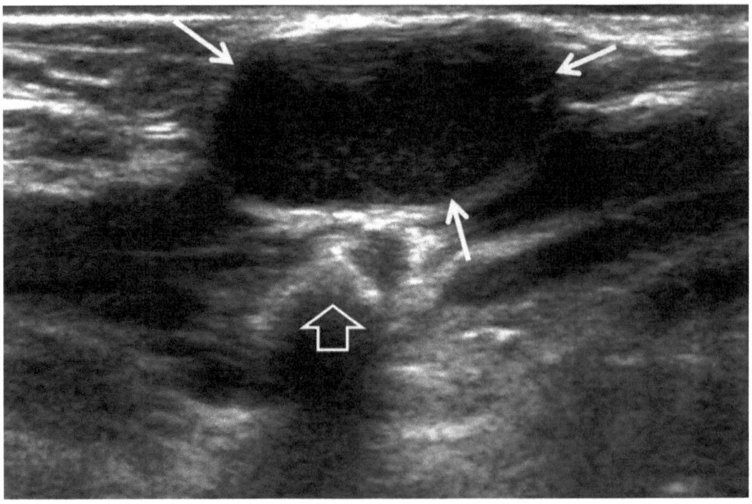

Fig. 11.37 Longitudinal gray-scale ultrasound shows an anechoic thyroglossal duct cyst (*white arrows*) with fine internal debris. Note its relationship to the hyoid bone (*open arrow*)

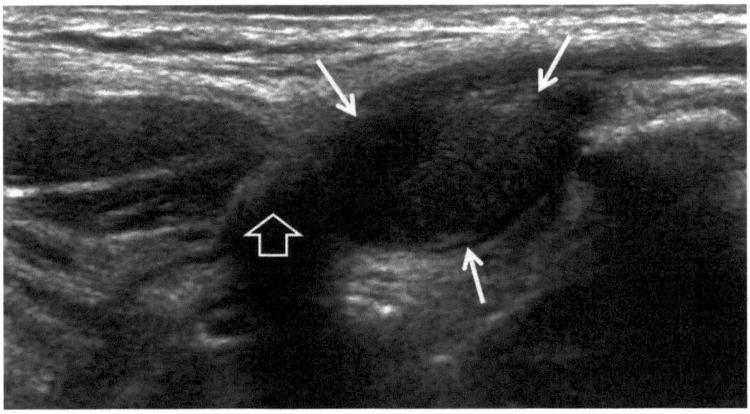

Fig. 11.38 Longitudinal gray-scale ultrasound shows a thyroglossal duct cyst (*white arrows*) with a heterogeneous echo pattern probably due to repeated infection or previous hemorrhage from prior aspiration. Note its relationship to the hyoid bone (*open arrow*)

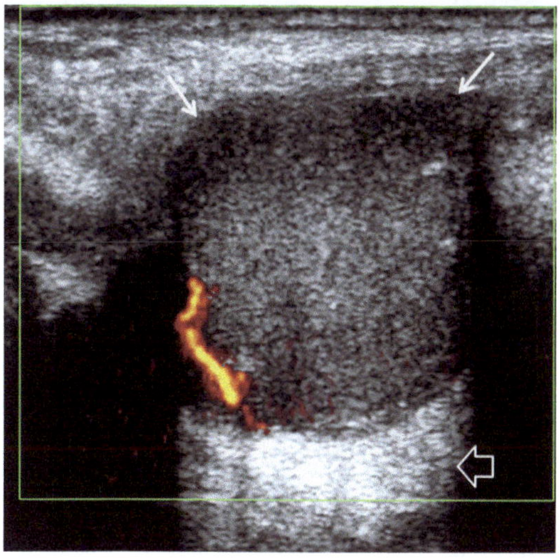

Fig. 11.39 Power Doppler ultrasound of a thyroglossal duct cyst (*white arrows*) shows the uniformly echogenic "pseudosolid" appearance due to the proteinaceous content of the cyst secreted by the epithelial lining. The cystic nature of a "pseudosolid" thyroglossal duct cyst is suggested by posterior acoustic enhancement (*open arrow*), swirling motion of the internal debris within the cyst seen on real-time gray-scale scan after application of intermittent transducer pressure, or with increase in power on Doppler

Tissue Transfer

The surgical treatment of hypopharyngeal, laryngeal, and esophageal cancers (pharyngo-laryngo-esophagectomy, PLO) and subsequent reconstruction may involve elevation of the stomach through the mediastinum, transposition of a segment of colon, interposition of a segment of jejunum, or use of a tubed free radial forearm flap. Free jejunal autotransplantation may be the most common of these reconstructive options. The bowel "signatures," the mesentery with its vascular arcades and lymph nodes, are clearly identifiable by ultrasound [82] and should not be mistaken for pathology (Figs. 11.40–11.42). Bowel-like appearance can also be seen in a Zenker's diverticulum (Fig. 11.43). Reconstruction myocutaneous flaps for replacement of portions of the trachea and cricoid cartilage for aggressive thyroid cancer may be identified on ultrasound at times long after the immediate postoperative period. These should not be mistaken for abnormal neck mass lesions or recurrence (Fig. 11.44).

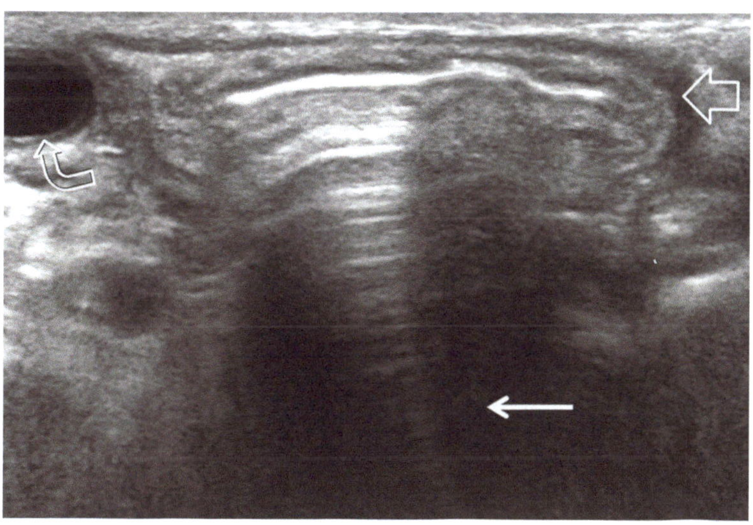

Fig. 11.40 Transverse gray-scale ultrasound shows the jejunal interposition segment (*open arrow*) in the anterior central neck and the adjacent common carotid artery (*curved arrow*). Note the bowel signature of the "mass" and reverberation artifacts (*white arrow*) from intraluminal bowel gas

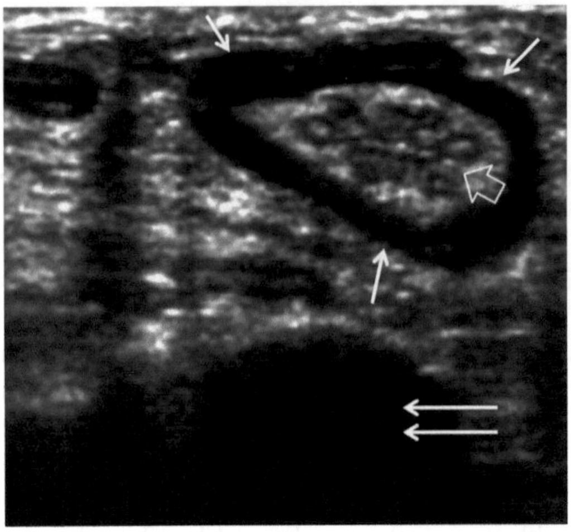

Fig. 11.41 Gray-scale ultrasound shows the hypoechoic bowel wall (*white arrows*) of the jejunal interposition segment. The mucosal folds (*open arrow*) can be clearly identified within the bowel lumen. Note its location anterior to the vertebral body with its associated shadowing (*double white arrows*)

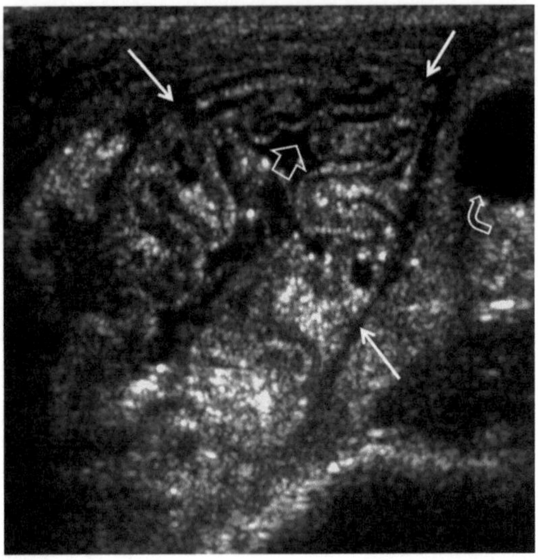

Fig. 11.42 Transverse gray-scale ultrasound shows the jejunal interposition segment (*white arrows*) in the anterior central neck adjacent to the common carotid artery (*curved arrow*). The hyperechoic mucosal folds (*open arrow*) stand out against the heterogeneous hypoechoic contents in the bowel lumen

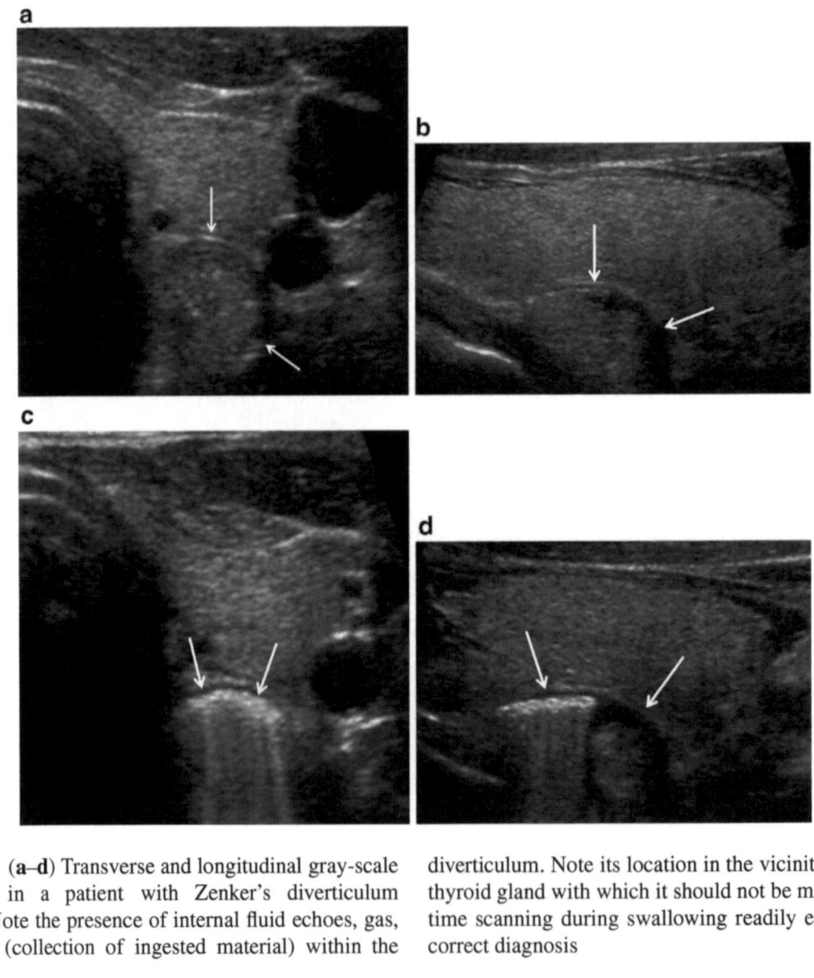

Fig. 11.43 (**a–d**) Transverse and longitudinal gray-scale ultrasound in a patient with Zenker's diverticulum (*arrows*). Note the presence of internal fluid echoes, gas, and debris (collection of ingested material) within the diverticulum. Note its location in the vicinity of the parathyroid gland with which it should not be mistaken. Real-time scanning during swallowing readily establishes the correct diagnosis

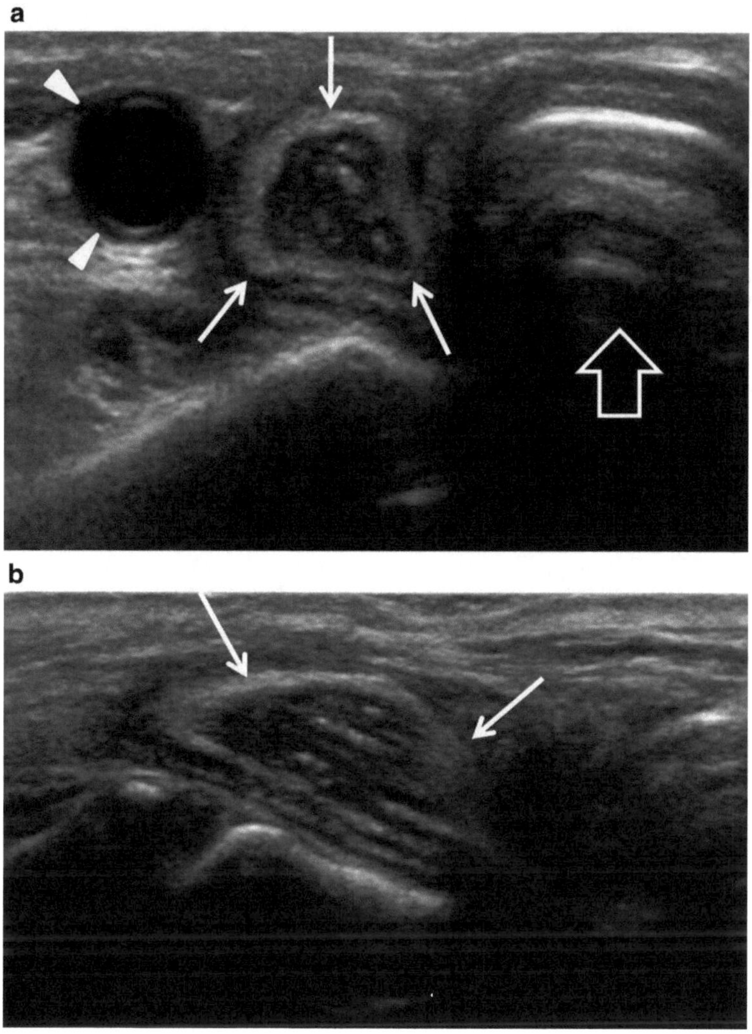

Fig. 11.44 Transverse (**a**) and longitudinal (**b**) gray scale ultrasound demonstrates the muscle fibers of an SCM myoperiosteal flap used to replace a segment of excised trachea and cricoid cartilage in tall cell variant of papillary carcinoma. In this particular instance, note its location between the common carotid artery (*arrowheads*) and trachea (*open arrow*). It should not be mistaken for recurrence or an abnormal neck mass

Thymus

The thymus is responsible for the production of T lymphocytes. It is prominent during childhood and may extend from the mediastinum to the neck. The thymus may be accessed using ultrasound via suprasternal, parasternal, or sternal approach. In adolescence and adulthood, it is difficult to visualize the thymus by ultrasound due to involution and interposition of the lungs. Typically, the normal thymus shows a characteristic echo pattern that is less echogenic than the normal thyroid gland with multiple echogenic lines and foci representing cross section of connective tissue septa or blood vessels within the septa (Fig. 11.45) [83, 84]. Rarely, because of migration anomaly, aberrant cervical thymus may be identified along the expected path of the

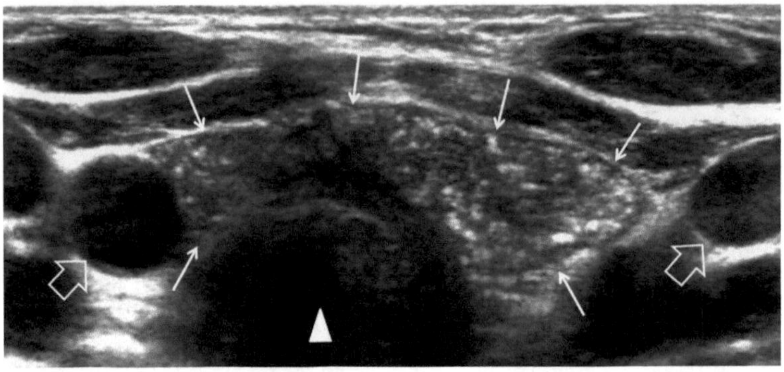

Fig. 11.45 Transverse gray-scale ultrasound of the normal thymus showing the characteristic "speckled" echo pattern. Note its location between the common carotid arteries (*open arrows*) and the trachea (*arrowhead*)

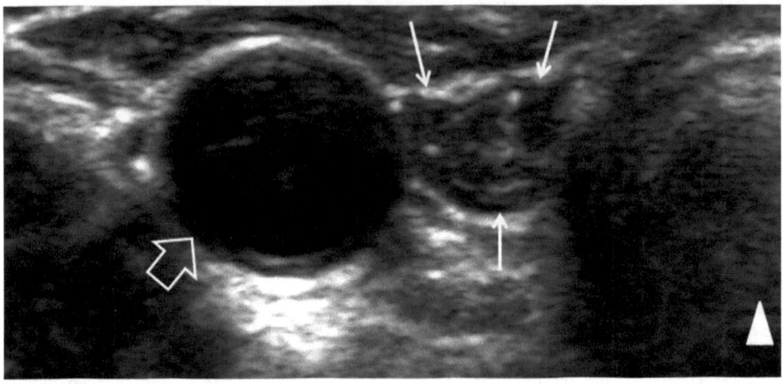

Fig. 11.46 Transverse gray-scale ultrasound shows thymic tissue (*arrows*) with speckled echogenic appearance of its Hassel's corpuscles mimicking a metastatic papillary carcinoma of thyroid. Note its relationship to the common carotid artery (*open arrow*) and the trachea (*arrowhead*)

thymopharyngeal duct from the angle of mandible to the superior mediastinum [85]. The speckled echogenic appearance, especially when the aberrant thymic tissues are multifocal, may mimic the appearance of metastatic papillary carcinoma of thyroid (Fig. 11.46). It is important to recognize this normal thymic tissue so as to avoid unnecessary investigations and biopsy. This is particularly relevant in infants and children as the thymus has not fully descended into the mediastinum.

Vascular Malformation

Pathology

In the past, vascular lesions and malformations were often described according to their morphological characteristics. This resulted in a variety of nomenclature that were interchangeably used and caused much confusion. In 1982, Mulliken and Glowacki [86] proposed a classification system of vascular anomalies in which these vascular lesions were categorized according to their endothelial cell characteristics. This classification has since gained wide acceptance. Two major categories of lesions emerged from this classification: hemangiomas and vascular malformations. Both are present since birth, but hemangiomas demonstrate rapid growth during early infancy with subsequent slow regression. Hemangiomas in the proliferating phase demonstrate endothelial hyperplasia with incorporation of [3 H]thymidine and multilaminated basement membrane formation beneath the endothelium, while hemangiomas in the involuting phase reveal histologic fibrosis and fat deposition with low to absent [3 H]thymidine labeling of endothelial cells.

On the other hand, vascular malformations grow proportionately with the growth of the child and do not involute. Vascular malformations comprise abnormal and usually combined vascular elements and may be subdivided into low-flow (venous, capillary, and lymphatic) and high-flow (arterial and arteriovenous) lesions. This classification was adopted by the International Society for the Study of Vascular Anomalies in 1996 which added the rapidly involuting congenital hemangioma, noninvoluting congenital hemangioma, Kaposiform hemangioendothelioma, tufted angioma, and pyogenic granuloma to the list of vascular tumors. Other classification systems have been developed and adopted by different specialties. However, the Mulliken and Glowacki system still serves as a simple yet comprehensive classification that incorporates histologic features and historical and physical findings to guide diagnosis and management.

Venous vascular malformation (Fig. 11.47) is the type most commonly encountered [87], and the following discussion therefore focuses on venous vascular malformation.

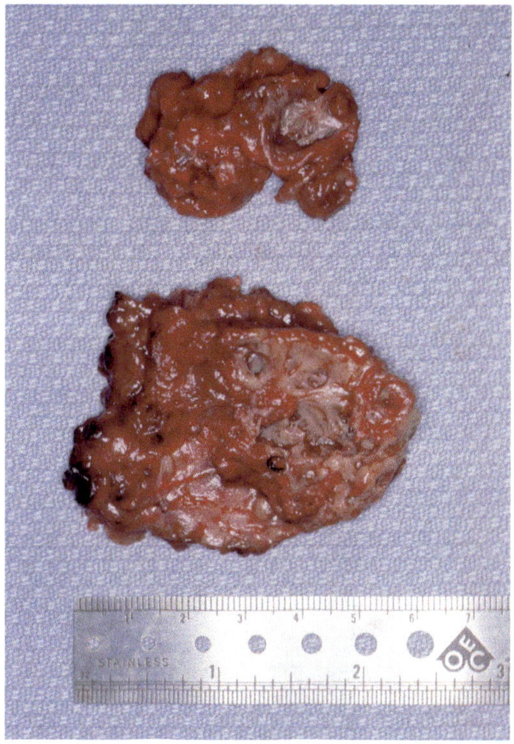

Fig. 11.47 Surgical specimen of a parotid venous vascular malformation (VVM) showing a honeycombed appearance with cystic spaces and septation within the lesion

Clinical Presentation and Demographics

Venous vascular malformation commonly presents as a soft, spongy soft tissue mass that shows proportionate growth with the patient [88]. The mass tends to increase in size with crying, Valsalva maneuver, or with the involved body part in a dependent position. Although they are usually asymptomatic, there may be pain and swelling because of venous stasis and thrombosis. Rapid enlargement or hardening may occur after trauma or superimposed infection [87]. A thrombosed venous vascular malformation may simulate the clinical signs and symptoms of thrombophlebitis. The appearance of venous malformations may be linked to times of hormonal flux, including puberty, pregnancy, and the initial use of birth control pills [88].

Venous vascular malformations in the head and neck region are most commonly seen in the buccal region, and the masticator space, sublingual space, tongue, orbit, and posterior neck are other common locations [87]. Intramuscular venous vascular malformations are commonly seen in the neck, with the masseter muscle being the most often involved [89].

Ultrasound Findings [87, 90, 91]

Venous vascular malformations may be solitary or multiple. On ultrasound, venous vascular malformations appear as soft, compressible hypoechoic masses with heterogeneous echo pattern and contain multiple serpiginous sinusoidal spaces (Figs. 11.48 and 11.49). They may be circumscribed, multilobulated or infiltrate adjacent soft tissue compartments and facial planes. The sinusoidal spaces and the lesion as a whole increase in size with crying or Valsalva. "To-and-fro" slowly moving internal echoes seen on real-time gray-scale ultrasound within the sinusoidal spaces are characteristic of internal slow vascular flow. It should be noted that

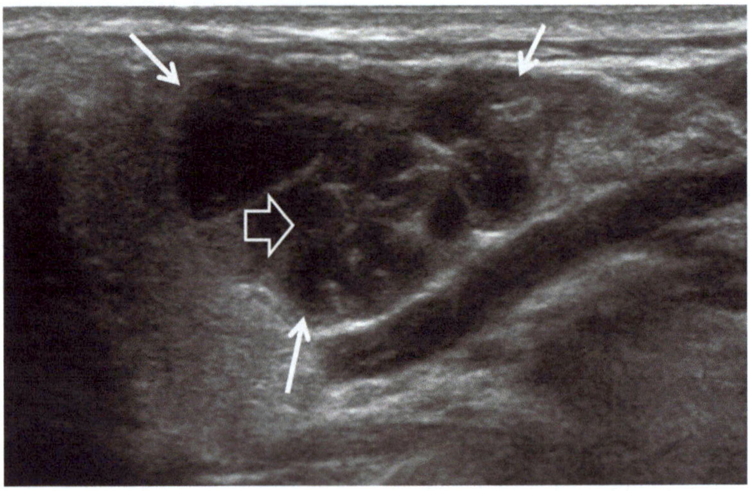

Fig. 11.48 Gray-scale ultrasound image shows a superficial mass (*white arrows*) with multiple, hypoechoic, serpiginous sinusoidal spaces. The faint internal echoes (*open arrow*) show slow "to-and-fro" movement on real-time ultrasound (gray scale or Doppler). Diagnosis: venous vascular malformation

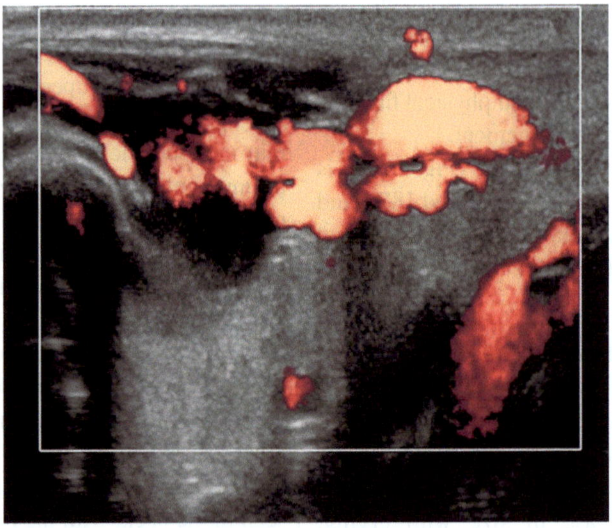

Fig. 11.49 Corresponding power Doppler ultrasound (same patient as in Fig. 11.48) shows flow within the sinusoidal/vascular spaces in the venous vascular malformation. Since the flow is usually slow, a low wall filter and pulse repetition frequency (PRF) will increase the sensitivity. However, "to-and-fro" movement on gray-scale ultrasound is also a very good clue towards the nature of the lesion

lesions with small vascular channels tend to be more echogenic (as they present multiple acoustic interfaces) and less compressible than those with large vascular lumens (Figs. 11.50 and 11.51). Phleboliths are identified as focal echogenic foci with dense posterior acoustic shadowing (Fig. 11.52). With careful search using high-frequency transducers, phleboliths can be

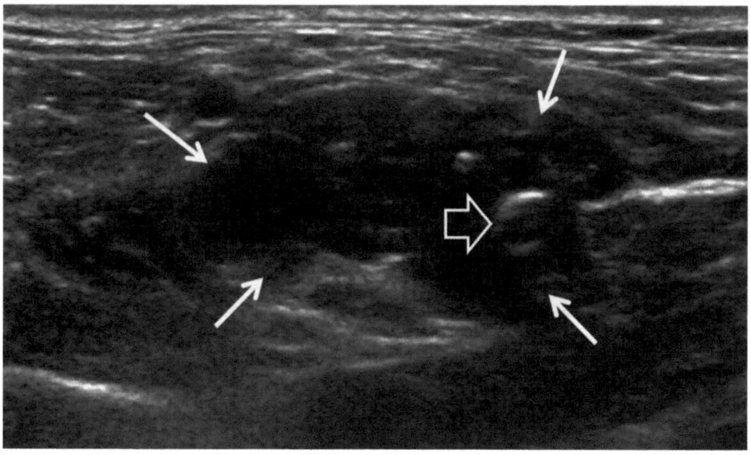

Fig. 11.50 On gray-scale ultrasound, venous vascular malformations (*white arrows*) with small vascular channels may be more echogenic (due to multiple acoustic interfaces) and less compressible than those with large vascular spaces. Note the echogenic phlebolith (*open arrow*) suggesting the nature of the lesion

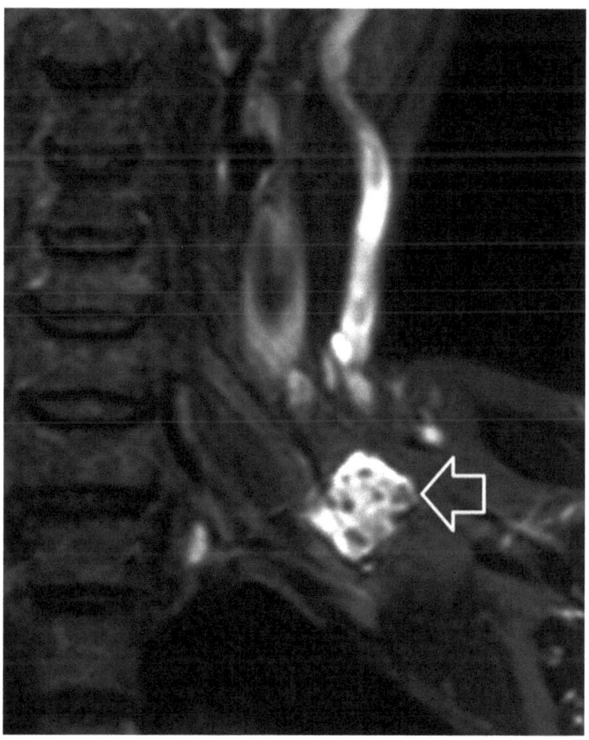

Fig. 11.51 Fat-saturated T2-weighted coronal MRI shows the same venous vascular malformation, as in Fig. 11.50, in the left supraclavicular fossa (SCF). It shows hyperintense signal (*open arrow*) with multiple phleboliths seen as round or oval signal voids within the lesion

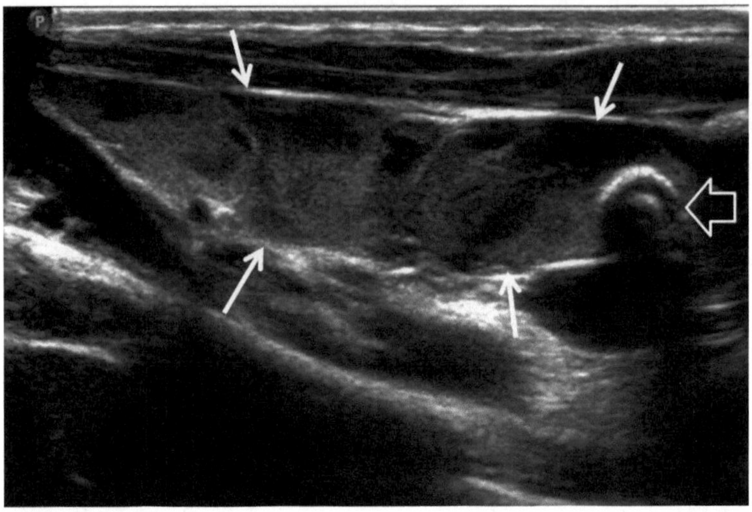

Fig. 11.52 Gray-scale ultrasound shows a venous vascular malformation (*white arrows*) with large sinusoidal spaces and uniform internal echoes which show movement on real-time gray-scale ultrasound. A phlebolith is identified as a focal echogenic focus with dense posterior acoustic shadowing (*open arrow*)

detected in up to 60% of cases, thus allowing for increased confidence in suggesting the diagnosis of venous vascular malformation. Slow venous color flow signal on color Doppler (use low wall filter and pulse repetition frequency to increase sensitivity for slow flow) and venous waveform on spectral Doppler may be detected within the sinusoidal spaces and augmented by transducer pressure. Intralesional vascularity is usually slow and better appreciated on gray scale rather than Doppler.

Ultrasound is superb in making the diagnosis. However, it often cannot detect multiplicity of lesions and cannot evaluate the entire extent of large, infiltrative, or deep-seated lesions. Magnetic resonance imaging (MRI) is the imaging modality of choice for delineating the entire extent of large lesions and detecting the presence of other lesions in the head and neck.

Management

A number of treatment options, including sclerotherapy, cryotherapy, embolization, surgery, and laser photocoagulation, are available for vascular malformations, the choice of which depends on the type of the malformation. A combined treatment is often used for best results [92–96].

References

1. Vogl T. Hypopharynx, larynx, thyroid, and parathyroid. In: Stark D, Bradley W, editors. Magnetic resonance imaging. 2nd ed. St Louis, Mo: Mosby-Yearbook; 1992. p. 1184–243.
2. Moore K. The developing human. 3rd ed. Philadelphia, PA: Saunders; 1988.
3. Benson MT, Dalen K, Mancuso AA, Kerr HH, Cacciarelli AA, Mafee MF. Congenital anomalies of the branchial apparatus: embryology and pathologic anatomy. Radiographics. 1992;12:942–60.
4. Telander R, Filston H. Review of head and neck lesions in infancy and childhood. Surg Clin North Am. 1992;72:1429–47.
5. Ahuja AT et al. Diagnostic imaging ultrasound. 1st ed. Salt Lake City: Amirsys; 2007. 11-98-101.
6. Harnsberger H, Mancuso A, Muraki A, et al. Branchial cleft anomalies and their mimics: computed tomographic evaluation. Radiology. 1984;152:739–48.
7. Cote D, Gianoli G. Fourth branchial cleft cysts. Otolaryngol Head Neck Surg. 1996;114:95–7.
8. Som P, Sacher M, Lanzieri C, et al. Parenchymal cysts of the lower neck. Radiology. 1985;157:399–406.
9. Harnsberger H. Handbook of head and neck imaging, 2nd ed. St Louis, MO: Mosby-Yearbook; 1995.
10. Ahuja AT, Evans RM, et al. Practical head and neck ultrasound. London, UK: Greenwich Medical Media Limited; 2000. p. 91–2.
11. Reynolds JH, Wolinski AP. Sonographic appearance of branchial cysts. Clin Radiol. 1993;2:109–10.
12. Ahuja AT, Ng CF, King W, Metreweli C. Solitary cystic nodal metastasis from occult papillary carcinoma of the thyroid mimicking a branchial cyst: a potential pitfall. Clin Radiol. 1998;53:61–3.

13. Ahuja AT et al. Diagnostic imaging ultrasound. 1st ed. Salt Lake City: Amirsys; 2007. 11-102-105.
14. Ahuja AT, Evans RM, et al. Practical head and neck ultrasound. London, UK: Greenwich Medical Media Limited; 2000. p. 97–8.
15. Netterville JL, Reilly KM, Robertson D, Reiber ME, Armstrong WB. Childs P carotid body tumors: a review of 30 patients with 46 tumors. Laryngoscope. 1995;105:115.
16. Capella C et al. Histopathology, cytology, and cytochemistry of pheochromocytomas and paragangliomas including chemodectomas. Pathol Res Pract. 1988;186:176.
17. Wax MK, Briant DR. Carotid body tumors: a review. J Otolaryngol. 1992;21(4):277.
18. Kumar V et al. Robbins and Cotran pathologic basis of disease. 8th ed. Philadelphia, PA: Saunders; 2010. p755.
19. Arslan H, Unal O, Kutluhan A, Sakarya ME. Power Doppler scanning in the diagnosis of carotid body tumors. J Ultrasound Med. 2000;19(6):367–70.
20. Reede DL. Nodal and non-nodal neck masses. Part II. Non-nodal neck masses. In: Som PM, Curtin HD, Holliday RA, editors. Special course in head and neck radiology. Oak Brook, IL: Radiological Society of North America; 1996. p. 75–86.
21. Zabel A, Milker-Zabel S, Huber P, Schulz-Ertner D, Schlegel W, Wannenmacher M, et al. Fractionated stereotactic conformal radiotherapy in the management of large chemodectomas of the skull base. Int J Radiat Oncol Biol Phys. 2004;58:1445–50.
22. Elshaikh MA, Mahmoud-Ahmed AS, Kinney SE, Wood BG, Lee JH, Barnett GH, et al. Recurrent head and neck chemodectomas: a comparison of surgical and radiotherapeutic results. Int J Radiat Oncol Biol Phys. 2002;52:953–6.
23. Hinerman RW, Mendenhall WM, Amdur RJ, Stringer SP, Antonelli PJ, Cassisi NJ. Definitive radiotherapy in the management of chemodectomas arising in the temporal bone, carotid body, and glomus vagale. Head Neck. 2001;23:363–71.
24. Evenson LJ, Mendenhall WM, Parsons JT, Cassisi NJ. Radiotherapy in the management of chemodectomas of the carotid body and glomus vagale. Head Neck. 1998;20:609–13.
25. Ahuja AT et al. Diagnostic imaging ultrasound. 1st ed. Salt Lake City: Amirsys; 2007. 11-124-127.
26. New G, Erich J. Dermoid cysts of the head and neck. Surg Gynecol Obstet. 1937;65:48–55.
27. New G. Congenital cysts of the tongue, the floor of the mouth, the pharynx, and the larynx. Arch Otolaryngol. 1947;45:145–58.
28. Som P. Cystic lesions of the neck. Postgrad Radiol. 1987;7:211–36.
29. Stephenson GC, Ironside JW. Squamous cell carcinoma arising in a subcutaneous dermoid cyst. Postgrad Med J. 1991;67:84–6.
30. Ahuja AT, Evans RM, et al. Practical head and neck ultrasound. London, UK: Greenwich Medical Media Limited; 2000. p. 88–9.
31. Ahuja AT et al. Diagnostic imaging ultrasound. 1st ed. Salt Lake City: Amirsys; 2007. 11-110-113.
32. Ahuja AT, Evans RM, et al. Practical head and neck ultrasound. London, UK: Greenwich Medical Media Limited; 2000. p. 90.
33. Ahuja AT et al. Head and neck lipomas: sonographic appearance. AJNR Am J Neuroradiol. 1998;19(3): 505–8.
34. Benhoff DF, Wood JW. Infiltrating lipoma of the head and neck. Laryngoscope. 1978;88:839.
35. Harnsberger HR et al. Diagnostic imaging head and neck. 1st ed. Salt Lake City: Amirsys; 2004. IV-1-30-33.
36. Dowd C. Hygroma cysticum colli. Ann Surg. 1913;58:112–32.
37. Goetch E. In discussion: Childress M, Baker C, Samson P. *Lymphangioma* of the mediastinum. J Thorac Surg. 1956;31:338–48.
38. Smith D. In discussion: Zadvinskis DP, Benson MT, Kerr HH, et al. Congenital malformations of the cervicothoracic lymphatic system: embryology and pathogenesis. RadioGraphics. 1992;12:1175–89.
39. Ahuja AT et al. Diagnostic imaging ultrasound. 1st ed. Salt Lake City: Amirsys; 2007. 11-92-97.
40. Lewin J. Imaging of the suprahyoid neck. In: Valvassori G, Mafee M, Carter B, editors. Imaging of the head and neck. 2nd ed. Stuttgart, Germany: Thieme; 1995.
41. Hartl DM, Roger G, Denoyelle F, Nicollas R. Extensive lymphangioma presenting with upper airway obstruction. Arch Otolaryngol Head Neck Surg. 2000;126:1378–82.
42. Weismann JL. Nonnodal masses of the neck. In: Som PM, Curtin HD, editors. Head and neck imaging. 3rd ed. St Louis: Mosby-Year Book; 1996. p. 794–822.
43. Sheath S, Nussbaum A, Hutchins G, Sanders R. Cystic hygromas in children: sonographic-pathologic correlation. Radiology. 1987;162:821–4.
44. Vazquez E, Enriquez G, Castellote A, et al. US, CT, and MR imaging of neck lesions in children. Radiographics. 1995;15:105–22.
45. Kennedy TL, Whitaker M, Pellitteri P. Cystic hygroma: a rational approach to management. Laryngoscope. 2001;111:1929–37.
46. Claesson G, Kuylenstierna R. OK-432 therapy for lymphatic malformation. Int J Ped Otorhinolaryngol. 2002;65:1–6.
47. Giguere CM, Bauman NM, Smith RJ. New treatment options for lymphangioma in infants and children. Ann Otol Rhinol Laryngol. 2002;111:1066–75.
48. Giguere CM, Bauman NM, Sato Y. Treatment of lymphangiomas with OK-432 sclerotherapy. Arch Otolaryngol Head Neck Surg. 2002;128:1137–44.
49. Riechelmann H, Muehlflay G, Keck T. Total, subtotal, and partial surgical removal of cervicofacial lymphangiomas. Arch Otolaryngol Head Neck Surg. 1999;12:643–8.
50. Kumar V, Abbas AK, Fausto N, Aster J, et al. Robbins and Cotran pathologic basis of disease. 8th ed. Philadelphia, PA: Saunders Elsevier; 2010. p. 68.

51. Biller JA, Murr AH. The importance of etiology on the clinical course of neck abscesses. Otolaryngol Head Neck Surg. 2004;131(4):p. 388–391.
52. Ahuja AT, Evans RM, et al. Practical head and neck ultrasound. London, UK: Greenwich Medical Media Limited; 2000. p. 89–90.
53. Lam CK, Woo KSJ, Van Hasselt CA. Esophageal perforation and neck abscess from ingested foreign bodies: treatment and outcomes. Ear, Nose Throat. 2003;82(10):786–94.
54. Mazita A, Hazim MYS, Megat Shiraz MAR, PrimuharsaPutra SHA. Neck abscess: five-year retrospective review of Hospital Universiti Kebangsaan Malaysia Experience. Med J Malaysia. 2006;61(2): 151–6.
55. Ridder GJ, Eglinger CF, Sander A, Technau-lhling K. Neck abscess as primary manifestation of head and neck carcinoma: implications for diagnostic management. Laryngorhinootologie. 2000;79(10):604–8.
56. Elliot CA, Bernard PA, Briggs VA, McDonald P. Posterolateral cervicotomy in retropharyngeal abscesses. Laryngoscope. 1992;102:585–7.
57. Chang KP, Chen YL, Hao SP, Chen SM. Ultrasound-guided closed drainage for abscesses of the head and neck. Otolaryngol-Head Neck Surg. 2005;132(1): 119–24.
58. Poe LB, Petro GR, Matta I. Percutaneous CT-guided aspiration of deep neck abscesses. AJNR. 1996;17:1359–63.
59. Ahuja AT, Evans RM, et al. Practical head and neck ultrasound. London, UK: Greenwich Medical Media Limited; 2000. p. 98–9.
60. Stull MA, Moser Jr RP, Kransdorf MJ, et al. Magnetic resonance appearance of peripheral nerve sheath tumors. Skel Radiol. 1991;20:9–14.
61. Ahuja AT et al. Diagnostic imaging ultrasound. 1st ed. Salt Lake City: Amirsys; 2007. 11-114-117.
62. Ahuja AT et al. Diagnostic imaging ultrasound. 1st ed. Salt Lake City: Amirsys; 2007. 11-118-119.
63. King AD, Ahuja AT, King W, Metreweli C. Sonography of peripheral nerve tumors of the neck. AJR. 1997;169:1695–8.
64. Hoddick WK, Callen PW, Filly RA, MAhony BS, Edwards MB. Ultrasound evaluation of benign sciatic nerve sheath tumors. J Ultrasound Med. 1984;3:505–7.
65. Chinn DH, Filly RA, Callen PW. Unusual ultrasonographic appearance of a solid schwannoma. J Clin Ultrasound. 1982;10:243–5.
66. Fornage BD. Sonography of the peripheral nerves of the extremities. Radiol Med. 1993;5:162–7.
67. Ahuja AT et al. Diagnostic imaging ultrasound. 1st ed. Salt Lake City: Amirsys; 2007. 11-106-109.
68. Noujaim S, Arpasi P, Bennett DF, Bohdiewicz P, Dworkin H. Imaging thyroglossal duct anomalies. The Radiologist. 1997;4(5):235–41.
69. Wadsworth DT, Siegel MJ. Thyroglossal duct cysts: variability of sonographic findings. AJR. 1994;163:1475–7.
70. Hayes LL, Marlow Jr SF. Papillary carcinoma arising in a thyroglossal duct cyst. Laryngoscope. 1968;78: 2189–93.
71. Boswell WC. Thyroglossal duct carcinoma. Am Surgeon. 1994;60:650–5.
72. LiVolsi VA, Perzin KH, Savetsky L. Carcinoma arising in median ectopic thyroid (including thyroglossal duct tissue). Cancer. 1974;34:1303.
73. Joseph TJ, Komorowski RA. Thyroglossal duct carcinoma. Hum Pathol. 1975;6:717.
74. Trail ML, Zeringue GP, Chicola JP. Carcinoma in thyroglossal duct remnants. Laryngoscope. 1977;87:1685.
75. Fernandez JF, Ordonez NG, Schultz PN, et al. Thyroglossal duct carcinoma. Surgery. 1991;110:928.
76. Van Vuuren PA, Balm AJ, Gregor RT, et al. Carcinoma arising in thyroglossal remnants. Clin Otolaryngol. 1994;19:509.
77. Tew S, Reeve TS, Poole AG, Delbridge L. Papillary thyroid carcinoma arising in thyroglossal duct cysts: incidence and management. Aust NZ J Surg. 1995; 65:717.
78. Hilger AW, Thompson SD, Smallman LA, Watkinson JC. Papillary carcinoma arising in a thyroglossal duct cyst: a case report and literature review. J Laryngol Otol. 1995;109:1124.
79. Ahuja AT, Evans RM, et al. Practical head and neck ultrasound. London, UK: Greenwich Medical Media Limited; 2000. p. 93–4.
80. Ahuja AT, King AD, Metreweli C. Thyroglossal duct cysts: sonographic appearances in adults. AJNR. 1999;20:579–82.
81. Pelausa EO, Forte V. Sistrunk revisited: a ten year review of revision thyroglossal duct surgery at Toronto's Hospital for Sick Children. J Otolaryngol. 1989;18:352–33.
82. Ahuja A, Zekri A, Davey IC, Mok CO, King W, Metreweli C. Ultrasound characteristics of jejunal flap used in pharyngoesophageal reconstruction. J Clin Ultrasound. 1995;23(1):38–41.
83. Fausto CSCV et al. Thymus: ultrasound characterization. Radiol Bras. 2004;7(3):207–10.
84. Han BK, Suh YL, Yoon HK. Thymic ultrasound I. Intrathymic anatomy in infants. Pediatr Radiol. 2001;31(7):474–9.
85. Han BK, Suh YL, Yoon HK. Thymic ultrasound II. Pediatr Radiol. 2001;31(7):480–7.
86. Mulliken JB, Glowacki J. Hemangiomas and vascular malformations in infants and children: a classification based on endothelial characteristics. Plast Reconstr Surg. 1982;69(3):412–22.
87. Ahuja AT et al. Diagnostic imaging ultrasound. 1st ed. Salt Lake City: Amirsys; 2007. 11-120-122.
88. Fu YS, Wenig BM, Abemayor E, Wenig BL. Head and neck pathology with clinical correlations. 1st ed. Philadelphia: Churchill Livingstone; 2001. p. 473.
89. Rai P, Setia S, Kalra N, Upreti L. Intramuscular vascular malformation of the masseter muscle presenting with turkey wattle sign. Oral Surg Oral Med Oral Pathol Oral Radiol Endod. 2006;102(5):618.

90. Ahuja AT, Evans RM, et al. Practical head and neck ultrasound. London, UK: Greenwich Medical Media Limited; 2000. p. 96–97.
91. Yang WT, Ahuja AT, Metreweli CJ. Sonographic features of head and neck hemangiomas and vascular malformations: review of 23 patients. Ultrasound Med. 1997;16:39–44.
92. Pappas DC, Persky MS, Berenstein A. Evaluation and treatment of head and neck venous vascular malformations. Ear, Nose Throat J. 1998;77(11): 914–22.
93. Tan K, Kirby J, Rajan D, Hayeems E, Beecroft J, Simons M. Percutaneous sodium tetradecyl sulfate sclerotherapy for peripheral venous vascular malformations: a single-center experience. J Vasc Interv Radiol. 2007;18(3):343–51.
94. Konosuke T, Keisuke I, Chiaya T, et al. Treatment of venous vascular malformation of the craniofacial region by ethanol injection. Jpn J Plast Reconstr Surg. 1999;42(2):133–8.
95. Cil BE, Vargel I, Geyik S, Peynircioglu B, Cavusoglu T. Venous vascular malformations of the craniofacial region: pre-operative embolisation with direct percutaneous puncture and *N*-butyl cyanoacrylate. Br J Radiol. 2008;81:935–9.
96. Derby LD, Low DW. Laser treatment of facial venous vascular malformations. Ann Plast Surg. 1997; 38(4):371–8.

Section IV

New Advances in Applied Ultrasound

Thyroid Elastography

12

Kunwar S.S. Bhatia, Darshana Dattatray Rasalkar, and Anil T. Ahuja

Introduction

Although thyroid nodules are very common, most of them are benign [1]. The aim of any imaging modality is to accurately identify the small number of nodules that are malignant so that prompt treatment can be instituted. Conventional ultrasound is very sensitive for nodule detection but may not always be able to characterize its nature. This reflects the fact that no sonographic criterion can attain sufficiently high sensitivity and positive predictive value for malignancy, while combining criteria increases specificity at the cost of lowered sensitivity [2–8]. Consequently, ultrasound is usually combined with fine needle aspiration for cytology (FNAC) to increase the accuracy. However, this approach still depends on judicious selection of nodules for FNAC. For nodules that undergo FNAC, approximately 10–20% of results are inadequate or indeterminate [9, 10]. Therefore, the quest for an accurate, non-invasive means of detecting thyroid malignancy continues.

Elasticity imaging or elastography refers to a variety of techniques used to measure and display parameters related to tissue elasticity or stiffness properties, which in turn may be used to characterize pathologies. Although elastography was initially described over two decades ago, it has undergone appreciable technological development and has only recently emerged as a real-time application on several commercially available clinical ultrasound machines [11]. For cancer detection, this technique has been most extensively evaluated not only in the breast but also in the prostate, lymph nodes, liver, cervix, pancreas, salivary glands, and thyroid [12–48].

To date, there have been approximately 20 published preliminary reports of thyroid ultrasound elastography, which have included between 34 and 309 nodules and have used either fine needle aspiration for cytology or surgery as the reference standard [12–31]. Those with accuracy data for malignancy are shown in Table 12.1. Evidently, there is considerable heterogeneity in the designs of these studies although the majority have documented promising results for the detection of malignancy. A recent meta-analysis of eight studies comprising a total of 639 nodules documented a mean sensitivity of 92% (95% confidence interval, 88–96%) and specificity of 90% (95% confidence interval 85–95%) [12–18, 20, 49].

K.S.S. Bhatia (✉)
Department of Imaging & Interventional Radiology, Prince of Wales Hospital, The Chinese University of Hong Kong, Shatin, NT, Hong Kong, People's Republic of China
e-mail: drkbhatia@cuhk.edu.hk

D.D. Rasalkar
Department of Radiology, Kokilaben Dhirubhai Ambani Hospital, Mumbai, Maharashtra, India

A.T. Ahuja
Department of Imaging and Interventional Radiology, The Chinese University of Hong Kong, Prince of Wales Hospital, Shatin (NT), Hong Kong (SAR), China

R.A. Sofferman and A.T. Ahuja (eds.), *Ultrasound of the Thyroid and Parathyroid Glands*,
DOI 10.1007/978-1-4614-0974-8_12,

Table 12.1 Selected characteristics of published thyroid ultrasound elastography studies containing accuracy data for malignancy

Author, publication year (reference)	Inclusion criteria for study[a]	No. of patients	No. of nodules (no. in final analysis if different[b])	% of nodules with surgery as reference	No. of malignant nodules (%) [phenotype]	Benign phenotype if known	Size (mm) mean [range]	Stimulus method	Elastogram generation timing	Elastogram scoring	% Sens	% Spec
Lyshchik et al. (2005) [12]	Planned for surgery	31	52	98.1	22 (42.3) [20 pc, 2 fc]	15 hy, 15 fa	CBD	Freehand	Both off-line and real time	QL, various criteria	36	88
										QT, strain of other thyroid tissue: nodule	82	96
										QT, ratio of nodule area on elastogram: sonogram	46	92
Rago et al. (2007) [13]	Solitary undergoing surgery due to symptoms or suspicious FNAC	92	92	100	31 (33.7) [28 pc, 2 fc, 1 mt]	11 hy, 48 fa, 2 ot	Mininum = 8, rest CBD	Freehand	Real time	QL, 5-point visual strain scale	97	100
Asteria et al. (2008) [14]	>10 mm and undergoing FNAC	67	86	29.1	17 (19.8) [15 pc, 1 mt, 1 ot]	61 hy, 8 fa	21 [10–50]	Freehand	Real time	QL, 4-point visual strain scale	94.1	81.1
Dighe et al. (2008) [15]	Undergoing FNAC (includes predominant cystic)	58	62	38	10 (16.1) [10 pc]	12 hy, 1 fa, 22 in, 7 ot	24 [10–60]	Carotid pulsation	Off-line	QT, ratio of highest strain near carotid artery: lowest strain in nodule	87.8	77.5
Tranquart et al. (2008) [16]	Undergoing FNAC	96	108 (107)	5.6	6 (5.6) [3 pc, 1 fc, 2 mt]	CBD	Mean CBD [9–32]	Freehand	Real time	QL, 4-point visual strain scale	100	93.1
Friedrich-Rust et al. (2009) [17]	≥10 mm and undergoing FNAC	56	59 (53)	43	7 (13.2) [6 pc, 1 fc]	CBD	20 [2–47]	Freehand	Real time	QL, 4-point visual strain scale	86	87

Hong et al. (2009) [18]	Undergoing surgery	90	145	100	49 (33.8) [44 pc, 1 fc, 1 mt, 2 ot ot]	83 hy, 8 fa, 5 ot	CBD	Freehand	Real time	QL, 6-point visual strain scale	88	90
Luo et al. (2009) [19]	Undergoing FNAC	31	34	CBD	12 (35.3) [CBD]	CBD	CBD	Carotid pulsation	Off-line	QT, 1 standard deviation of strain metric in nodule in diastole	100	82
Rubaltelli et al. (2009) [20]	Undergoing FNAC	40	51	42.5	11 (21.6) [9 pc, 2 fc]	37 hy, 3 fa	CBD	Freehand	Real time	QL, 4-point visual strain scale	81.8	87.5
Dighe et al. (2010) [21]	Undergoing FNAC or surgery	59	62 (51)	33.3	12 (23.5) [11 pc, 1 ot]	18 hy, 20 fi, 2 ot	24 [10–60]	Carotid pulsation	Off-line	QT, ratio of highest strain near carotid artery in systole: mean nodule strain in systole	100	79.4
Gietka-Czernel et al. (2010) [22]	Positive or suspicious for malignancy or undergoing surgery	52	71	56.3	22 (31) [18 pc, 3 mt, 1 ot]	CBD	CBD	Freehand	Off-line	QL, 5-point visual strain scale	86.5	97
Kagoya et al. (2010) [23]	≤40 mm undergoing FNAC	44	51	19.1	11 (21.6) [6 pc, 4 fc, 1 an, 3 ot]	CBD	19 [6–36]	Freehand	Real time	QL, 4-point visual strain scale	73	64
										QT, ratio of mean strain of nodule: sternocleido-mastoid muscle	90	50
Luo et al. (2010) [24]	Undergoing FNAC	92	98	22.4	16 (16.3) [16 pc]	CBD	23 [9–62]	Freehand	Online (30 sec delay)	QT, strain rate waveform linear discriminant analysis	100	75.6

(continued)

Table 12.1 (continued)

Author, publication year (reference)	Inclusion criteria for study[a]	No. of patients	No. of nodules (no. in final analysis if different[b])	% of nodules with surgery as reference	No. of malignant nodules (%) [phenotype]	Benign phenotype if known	Size (mm) mean [range]	Stimulus method	Elastogram generation timing	Elastogram scoring	% Sens	% Spec
Rago et al. (2010) [25]	Undergoing sugery due to indeterminate/ nondiagnostic FNAC	176	195	100	39 (20)[34 pc, 5 fc]	28 hy, 115 fa, 13 ot	CBD	Freehand	Real time	QL, 3-point visual strain scale	94.9	90.3
Sebag et al. (2010) [26]	Undergoing FNAC or surgery (includes conglomerate)	93	146	9.4	29 (19.9) [20 pc, 5 fc, 1 mt,1 an, 2 ot]	CBD	CBD	Acoustic impulse	Real time	QT, elastic modulus (kPa) calculated from shear wave velocity	85.2	93.9
Vorländer et al. (2010) [27]	Non-toxic solid dominant nodules undergoing surgery	309	309	100	50 (16.2) [35 pc, 6 fc, 9 mt]	146 hy, 110 fa, 3 ot	28 [4–83]	Freehand	Real time	QT, ratio of strain of nodule: outside nodule. Results divided by 2 cut-offs into 3 groups	70 low cut-off 100 high cut-off	82 low cut-off 37 lhigh cut-off
Wang et al. (2010) [28]	Solid solitary ≤10 mm indeterminate on US undergoing surgery	51	51	100	32 (62.7) [32 pc]	19 fa	9 (3–10)	Freehand	Real time	QL, 5-point visual strain scale	90.6	89.5
Bhatia et al. (2011) [29]	Undergoing FNAC (includes predominant cystic)	94	94 (85)	36.5	24 (28.2) [19 pc, 5 ot]	57 hy, 4 fa	21 [8–48]	Freehand	Real time	QL, 4-point visual strain scale	75 75 if solid	56 74 if solid

FNAC fine needle aspiration for cytology, *pc* papillary carcinoma, *fc* follicular carcinoma, *mt* medullary thyroid carcinoma, *an* anaplastic carcinoma, *hy* hyperplastic, *fa* follicular adenoma, *fl* follicular lesion with low–intermediate risk of malignancy on cytology, *ot* other pathologies, *QL* qualitative, *QT* quantitative, *sens* sensitivity, *spec* specificity, *CBD* cannot be determined from the available data

[a]Nodules undergoing FNAC for suspicious imaging findings; undergoing surgery for suspicious or equivocal imaging and/or cytological findings unless for symptomatic relief where stated Conglomerate or predominantly cystic nodules were excluded from studies unless stated otherwise

[b]Some nodules were excluded from final analysis due to nondiagnostic or indeterminate cytology and no available histology

Of importance, elastography has been found to be more accurate than conventional sonography in several studies that have compared both techniques [13, 14, 17, 18, 26, 28]. The elastography results are also supported by elasticity measurements obtained by direct biomechanical testing of thyroidectomy specimens, which have shown that the elastic modulus, equating to stiffness, of malignant nodules (99.7 ± 79.8 kPa) is significantly higher than benign nodules (22.5 ± 9.6 kPa) and normal thyroid parenchyma (12.3 ± 4.8 kPa) (mean ± 1 standard deviation) [12, 50].

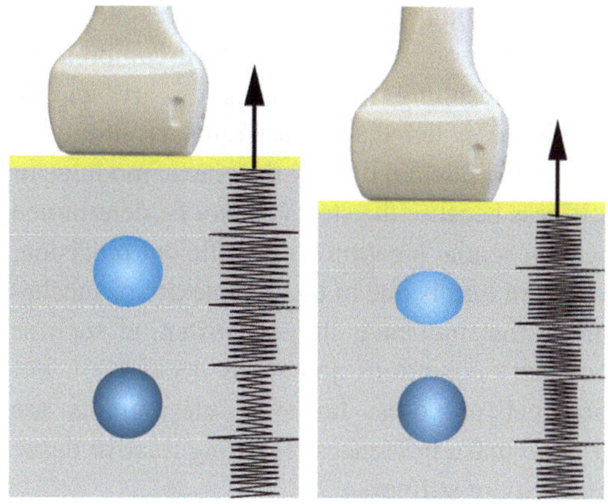

Fig. 12.1 Illustration showing compression elastography of a tissue containing two nodules of different elasticities before (*left*) and after (*right*) external compression. For the same applied force, the softer superior nodule shortens in the vertical direction much more than the stiffer lower nodule; hence, its strain (change in length divided by the original length) is greater. This can be measured by dedicated software that compares the returning ultrasound echoes from pre- and post-compression frames (*black arrows*)

Basic Physics and Practical Technique

Static Compression Elastography

Almost all published studies of thyroid ultrasound elastography to date have used a specific technique termed (quasi) static compression elastography, which measures compression or bulk waves produced by the application of a (quasi) static mechanical force [51, 52]. This technique can be performed using conventional US equipment with software modifications.

To perform compression elastography of the thyroid, a conventional linear high-frequency US transducer is initially positioned with light contact onto the anterior neck using ample coupling gel, and a field of view is selected that includes the thyroid nodule and some adjacent thyroid parenchyma. To assist in anatomic localization, it is useful to display elastograms in dual mode alongside gray scale sonograms. Subsequently, several cycles of mild freehand compression are applied via the transducer in the direction of the beam axis, or alternatively physiologic pulsations from the carotid artery are used as the sole compression source. The latter is possible because the artery expands and compresses the thyroid medially against the trachea during systole, resulting in transient thyroid lengthening in the anteroposterior direction, and vice versa. The returning ultrasound echoes before and after compression are analyzed by a dedicated software method termed cross-correlation to measure tissue displacements occurring in the direction of the ultrasound beam (Fig. 12.1) [36].

For a given force, stiff tissue deforms or displaces less than soft tissue, and accordingly, its change in length relative to its original length, or strain, is lower. The amount of strain required to perform elastography is minimal (~1%) because under these circumstances, tissues exhibit elastic properties whereby strain is linearly proportional to the force applied, according to Hooke's law [36]. This is shown by the following equations:

Stiffness = Young's elastic modulus (kPa) = stress/strain

Stress (kPa) = force/area

Strain (no units) = change in length/original length

Elastograms are maps of relative strain for each spatial location within the image frame, and are normally displayed using a color-coded scale. For this reason, it is important to have some surrounding thyroid parenchyma within the elastography window for reference. When performing compression, lateral or out-of-plane transducer motions should be avoided as these can cause misregistration of pre- and post-compression frames, resulting in decorrelation artifacts. It should be noted that elastograms produced by this method do not display the elastic modulus or stiffness because the stress cannot be determined at each spatial location with sufficient precision, which in turn is due to the complexity of mechanisms that influence stress distribution such as boundary conditions and stress decay [36]. For practical purposes, however, elastograms are used to make inferences regarding relative tissue elasticity or stiffness.

In the earliest elastography systems, elastograms could only be generated off-line due to the intensive software processing required, especially with respect to cross-correlation [36]. Fortunately, technological advances including the development of algorithms with higher computational efficiency have enabled elastograms to be generated in real time. This has the potential benefit of being used for clinical decision making during ultrasound examinations. Elastography is painless and relatively quick, taking only a few minutes to perform per nodule.

Elastogram Scoring

The majority of published studies have scored elastograms qualitatively based on a system initially described by Ueno and Ito for breast elastography [42, 53]. In this regard, the overall elasticity or strain of a nodule is graded visually using a 4–6-point scale based on the proportion of low and high strain areas present, usually with high values being assigned to nodules that have uniform low strain (high stiffness) (Fig. 12.2). Other qualitative criteria have been included into this framework including nodule conspicuity,

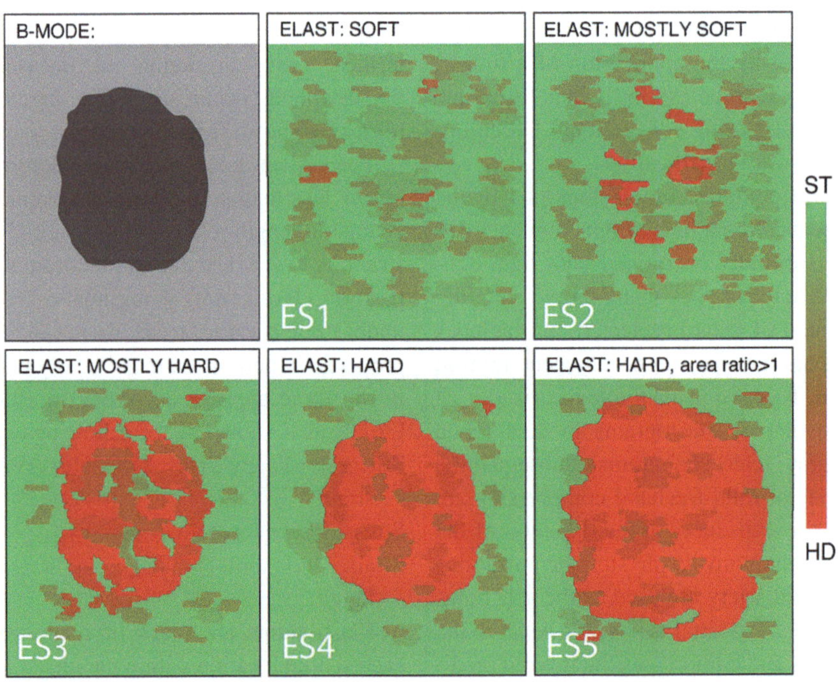

Fig. 12.2 Schematic illustration of a qualitative elastography scoring system. A B-mode US image of a nodule is shown on the *top left image*, and the corresponding elastographic appearance for progressive increases in stiffness is shown in the other images, ranging from ES 1 to ES 5. Nodules with increasing stiffness display an increasing proportion of low strain areas, shown here as *red*. The nodule classified as ES 5 has a completely low strain pattern with an area ratio (elastogram: sonogram) >1. Typically, nodules that display a predominantly low strain pattern equating to ES 3 or above suggest a higher risk of malignancy

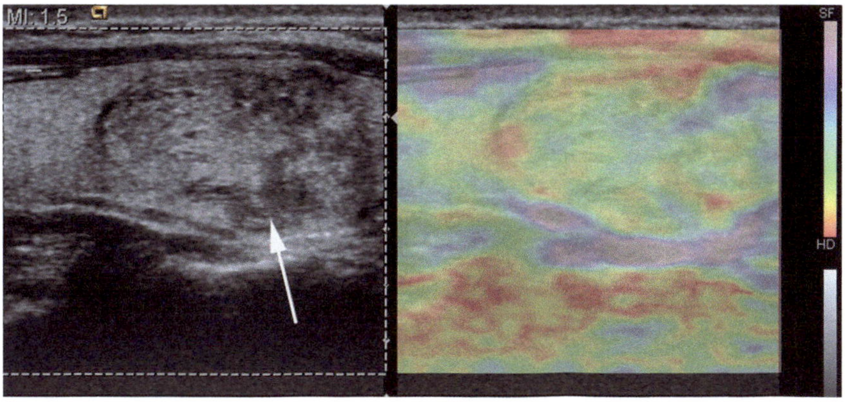

Fig. 12.3 Longitudinal gray scale US image with corresponding real-time qualitative elastogram of a hyperplastic nodule *(arrow)*. The elastogram color scale is shown on the right with "HD" indicating hard and "SF" indicating soft. The nodule displays a predominantly *green* color pattern, which suggests a soft nodule

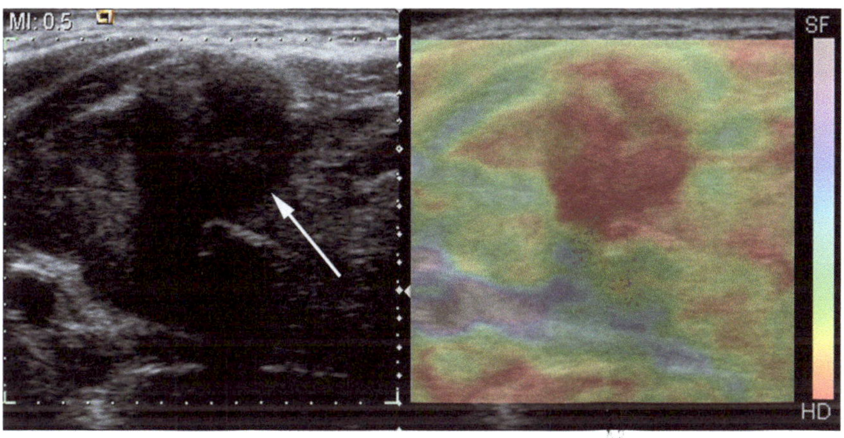

Fig. 12.4 Transverse gray scale US image with corresponding real-time qualitative elastogram of a papillary carcinoma *(arrow)*. The nodule displays a predominant *red* color pattern, which suggests a hard nodule

margin regularity, distribution of low strain areas within the nodule, and area ratios. Area ratios refer to the area of nodule visible on the elastogram divided by the area of nodule on the corresponding sonogram [12]. In breast elastography, area ratios >1.1 have been correlated with malignancy, which is attributed to a peritumoral desmoplastic response [54, 55]. In theory, area ratios may be useful in thyroid elastography because papillary thyroid cancers are unencapsulated, are infiltrative, and can incite an intense fibrotic reaction [56].

Studies utilizing qualitative elastography have shown that high scores corresponding to a predominantly or completely low strain pattern (high stiffness) within a thyroid nodule are predictive of malignancy [12–29] (Figs. 12.3–12.5). Nevertheless, false negatives and positives using any cut-off for qualitative elastography are documented (Figs. 12.6 and 12.7). The most promising results using qualitative elastography are 97% sensitivity and 100% specificity in a study of 92 solitary solid nodules scheduled for surgery due to a suspicious FNAC result or compressive symptoms [13]. Other reports document poorer results, with the lowest being 75% sensitivity and 56% specificity in 85 nodules scheduled to undergo FNAC, although this study included a high proportion of partially cystic nodules [29]. With respect to

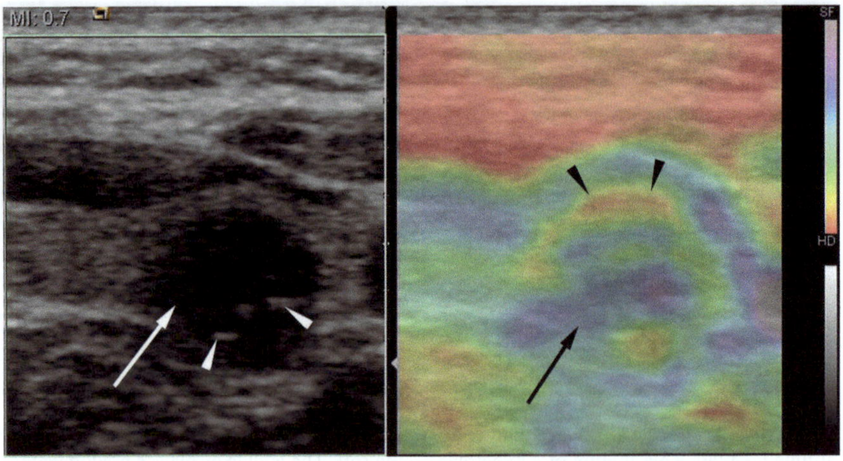

Fig. 12.5 Longitudinal gray scale US with corresponding real-time qualitative elastogram showing a hypoechoic thyroid nodule (*arrow*) with slightly irregular margins and a couple of tiny hyperreflective foci. This nodule was indeterminate on conventional US. On elastography, the majority of the nodule appears green or mauve (*black arrow*), suggesting a soft and hence benign nodule. The red margin along the superficial aspect of the nodule (*black arrowhead*) is likely to be an artifact caused by stress concentration at a tissue interface. FNA was compatible with a collapsed hemorrhagic cyst. This is a true negative for malignancy on elastography

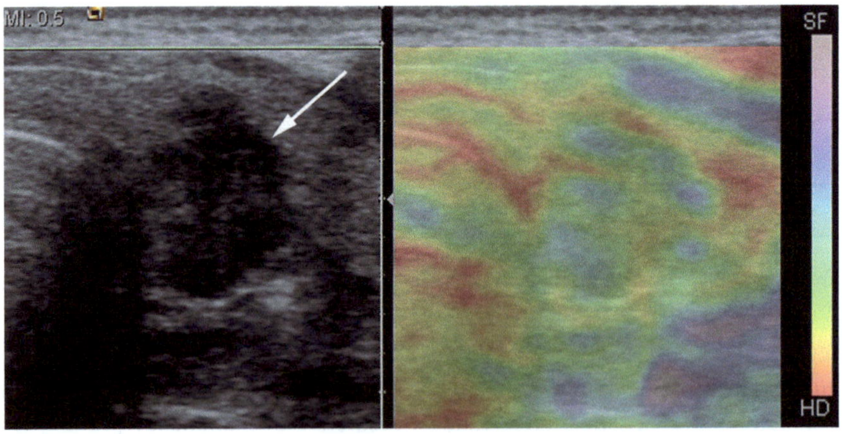

Fig. 12.6 Transverse gray scale US image with corresponding real-time qualitative elastogram showing a suspicious hypoechoic irregular nodule which is taller than wide (*arrow*). On the elastogram, it is predominantly green, suggesting a soft hence benign nodule. FNA and subsequent thyroidectomy confirmed papillary carcinoma. This is a false negative for malignancy on elastography

area ratios in thyroid elastography, Lyschik et al. found that high ratios were associated with malignancy although the discriminatory performance of this criterion was limited, achieving 46% sensitivity and 92% specificity using an area ratio cut-off >1 [12].

Until very recently, semi-quantitative analysis of elastograms could only be performed offline on customized systems, which was labor intensive and cumbersome. However, relative strain quantification is now a feature on current, second-generation, commercial elastography

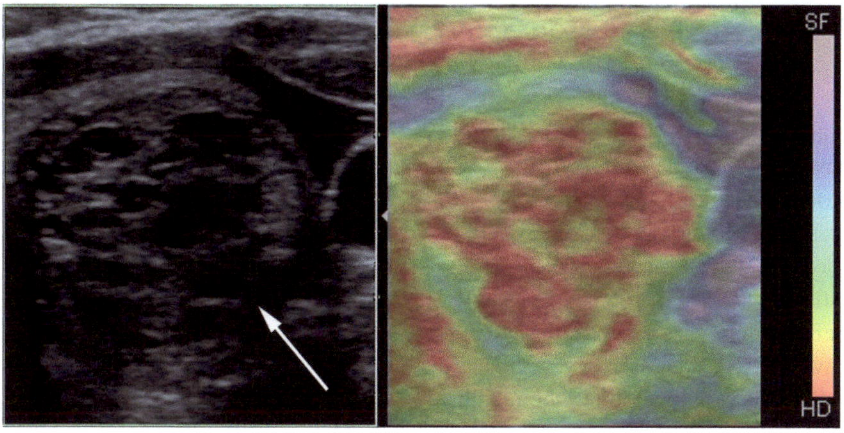

Fig. 12.7 Transverse gray scale US image with corresponding real-time qualitative elastogram of a hyperplastic nodule (*arrow*) with a classical spongiform appearance on gray scale US. On elastography, this lesion is predominantly *red*, suggesting a moderately stiff nodule. This is a false positive for malignancy on elastography

systems. Several studies have included semi-quantitative analysis of strain data [12, 15, 19, 21, 24, 27]. Lyshchik et al. performed off-line analysis of freehand compression elastograms to generate a metric termed the strain index, which referred to the strain value in normal thyroid tissue divided by the strain value in the nodule [12]. A strain index >4 achieved 82% sensitivity and 96% specificity for malignancy and was found to be the strongest independent predictor of malignancy when compared to qualitative and other semi-quantitative elastography criteria. Dighe et al. performed thyroid elastography using carotid artery pulsations and devised a metric termed the thyroid stiffness index, which referred to the highest strain near the carotid artery divided by the lowest strain in the nodule [15]. A value of >18.0 achieved 87.8% sensitivity and 77.5% specificity for malignancy. They later refined their method to utilize strain data acquired only during systole and reported improved results, 100% sensitivity and 79.4% specificity, using a larger sample [21]. Luo et al. measured the standard deviation of strain in the nodule during diastole, and using this criterion, they documented 100% sensitivity and 82% specificity for malignancy [19]. Subsequently, Luo et al. documented results of 100% sensitivity and 75.6% specificity for elastography using linear discriminant analysis of strain rate waveforms produced by carotid pulsations [24]. Vorländer et al. performed quantitative elastography on a commercial system in 309 solitary, dominant, non-toxic nodules undergoing surgery and measured the ratio of the strain in the nodule to adjacent thyroid tissue. Nodules were divided into soft, medium, and hard groups based on two strain ratio cut-offs, and using the lower cut-off achieved 70% sensitivity and 82% specificity for malignancy [27]. Kagoya et al. performed semi- quantitative elastography in 51 nodules undergoing FNAC and documented 90% sensitivity and 50% specificity when using the ratio of strain in the thyroid nodule compared to the sternocleidomastoid muscle [23]. It should be stressed that accuracy results from semi-quantitative studies using off-line processing may not be applicable to those from real-time processing, as the former has the benefit of allowing more sophisticated albeit time-intensive software algorithms to be used, whereas the latter needs to computationally efficient. In this respect, Lyschik et al. compared real-time and off-line elastograms generated in their study and documented that the former had lower image quality (i.e., lower spatial and contrast resolution, and higher noise) and were less accurate for detecting malignancy [12].

Limitations of Thyroid Elastography

Despite the encouraging data, there are several limitations as well as questions regarding thyroid elastography that need to be addressed:

1. Operator dependence
   Compression elastography is highly operator dependent for several reasons.

   Firstly, the amount of force applied to tissues before compression (preload) and during active compression (afterload) influences the resultant elastograms due to the fact that the elastic modulus (stiffness) of a tissue is not fixed but rises nonlinearly with increases in stress [36]. As a consequence, if excessive force is applied inadvertently or otherwise, tissues will appear spuriously stiff (Fig. 12.8a, b).

   Secondly, cross-correlation algorithms measure tissue displacements occurring in the beam axis, while lateral or out-of-plane motions produce decorrelation artifacts on elastograms that may be indistinguishable from genuine strain information. In breast elastography, most nodules are surrounded

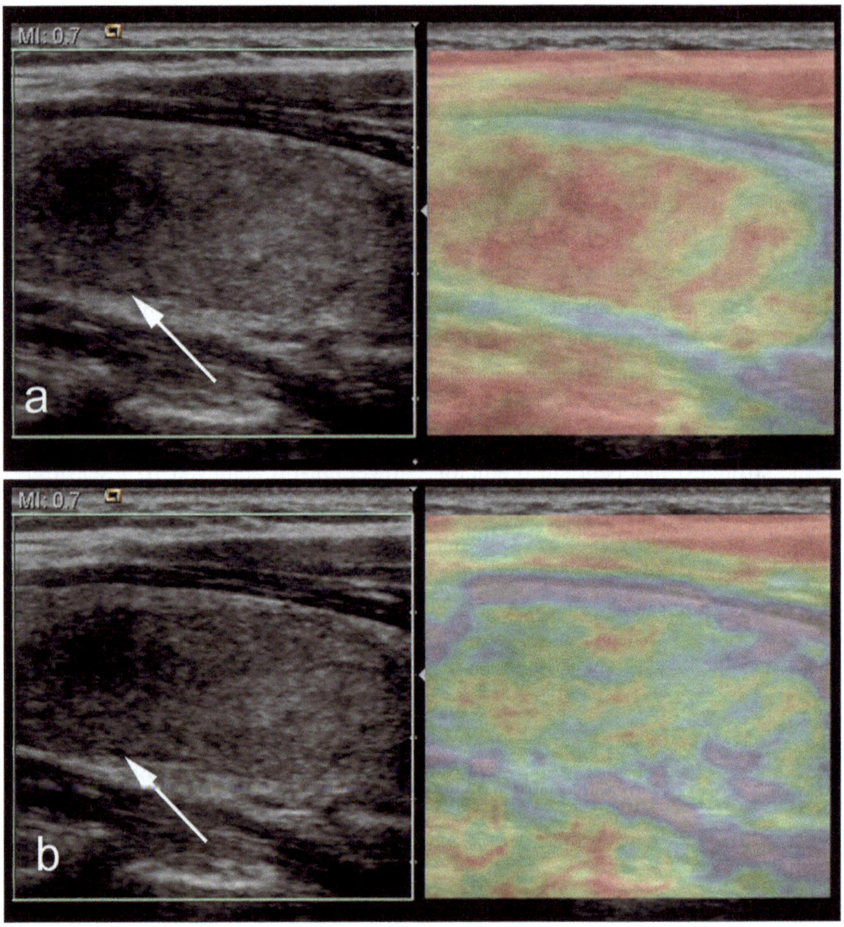

Fig. 12.8 (**a, b**) Longitudinal gray scale US image with corresponding real-time qualitative elastogram of a hyperplastic thyroid nodule (*arrow*), with a time interval of less than 0.5 s. In (**a**), the nodule predominantly red suggesting low strain (high stiffness), whereas in (**b**), it appears mostly green suggesting high strain (low stiffness). This discrepancy reflects minor differences in stress applied by the operator with excessive compression thought to have been applied at the time that (**a**) was generated. This nodule was finally graded as soft after review of the entire elastogram video segment. This illustrates the challenges in real-time qualitative elastography in terms of operator technique and selection of static images from a dynamic series

by ample tissue of uniform stiffness, and thus they can compress uniformly against the chest wall. In thyroid elastography, however, the differing stiffness and mobility of tissues bordering the thyroid, namely, the mobile soft vessels laterally and immobile stiff trachea medially, make it more difficult to apply uniform thyroid compression along the beam axis. Furthermore, even with meticulous technique, patient breathing and carotid artery pulsations generate non-axial motions that can detrimentally affect elastograms.

Thirdly, selection of a representative static image from a dynamic series of elastograms is a subjective process. This is made more difficult by the fact that elastograms continually fluctuate depending on the stress field that can vary during compression cycles (Fig. 12.8a, b). Furthermore, artifacts and image noise may fluctuate temporally and be selected unintentionally in static images, although their appearance may be reduced by software temporal averaging [57].

To assist operators in optimizing their compression technique and to select representative elastograms for analysis, more recent commercially available elastography systems analyze the quality of compression technique and display this either as a numerical score or graphic scale beside elastograms in real time.

2. Unsuitable nodules
   As compression elastography produces a map of relative strain, nodules that cannot be compared against normal thyroid within the elastography window are unsuitable. This includes large, coalescent or exophytic nodules with minimal normal surrounding thyroid parenchyma, although these may be suitable for elastography performed using other methods such as shear wave elastography. In addition, nodules that cannot be penetrated by ultrasound such as those obscured by rim calcifications are unsuitable for any elastographic technique.
3. Elastographic artifacts
   Artifacts in elastography differ in type and conspicuity depending on software used as well as the properties of the tissue being imaged [58]. While artifacts have been documented in breast elastography [46], to date they have received little attention in thyroid elastography. In our experience, we observed low strain areas mainly along the superficial margin of 15% of solid or partially cystic thyroid nodules on real-time qualitative elastography, which were postulated to represent artifacts caused by stress concentration at the tissue interface [29] (Fig. 12.5). We also documented another type of elastographic artifact in 11% of nodules that corresponded to reverberation artifacts on gray scale sonography [29]. Familiarity with the types and frequency of artifacts occurring in thyroid elastography is important to avoid systematic errors in image interpretation.
4. Limited sample size
   Published studies of thyroid elastography have been relatively small (mean 96.7 nodules; range 34–309 nodules), with only five studies containing more than 100 nodules. Furthermore, the numbers of malignant nodules have been low (mean 22.2 nodules; range 6–50 nodules) [12–30, 44, 59]. Consequently, the accuracy data for thyroid elastography still needs to be determined in larger studies.
5. Selection bias
   Published studies of thyroid elastography have included nodules that have been preselected for FNAC due to suspicious gray-scale sonographic appearances, or for surgery on the basis of compressive symptoms or a suspicious or positive malignant FNAC result [12–30, 44]. Additionally, several studies have restricted their samples to nodules of a specific size, or solitary nodules, or have excluded predominantly cystic or moderately calcified nodules [13, 14, 17, 23, 25, 27, 28]. As a result, most published studies contain a much higher proportion of malignant nodules (mean 24%, range 5.6–62.7%) than is present in the general population (~5%) [12–15, 17–29]. Clearly, published accuracy results from these studies cannot be applied to all nodules encountered in the general population.

6. Mixed solid-cystic nodules
   There is currently limited evidence regarding the accuracy of elastography for mixed solid-cystic nodules. While the risk of malignancy in a thyroid nodule is much lower if it is cystic [7, 60], it is not nil and mixed nodules are very common in the general population [60]. Lyshchik et al. included a small number of nodules with <20% cystic components (which by definition would be "predominantly solid") and noted that this did not adversely influence the accuracy of thyroid elastography [12]. In our experience, cystic change was a confounding factor for elastography, as solid tissue appeared stiffer in benign nodules that were predominantly cystic than slightly cystic [29] (Fig. 12.9). This may be explained by the fact that solid components of mixed nodules may deform relatively little during compression elastography because they can displace the fluid surrounding them.
7. Course calcifications
   Benign nodules containing coarse calcifications (>2 mm) appeared to be stiff on elastography, and it was postulated that these false positive results were caused by the calcification [12, 14, 28]. While this may be the case, more detailed studies are required to assess the precise influence of different types and degrees of calcification. This is important as calcified thyroid nodules (benign and malignant) are often seen in the general population.
8. Minimum nodule size
   The accuracy of thyroid elastography appears to be independent of nodule size for nodules greater than 1 cm in maximum diameter [13]. With respect to smaller nodules, in a study by Rago et al., all nine papillary cancers with a maximum diameter between 8 and 10 mm were classified correctly by elastography [13]. Hong et al. reported 88% sensitivity and 93% specificity using elastography for 68 nodules measuring ≤1 cm in maximum diameter compared to 87% sensitivity and 87% specificity for 77 nodules measuring >1 cm [18]. Wang et al. evaluated 51 nodules between 3 and 10 mm with indeterminate sonographic features and documented a sensitivity of 90.6%, a specificity of 89.5%, and an accuracy of 90.2% using elastography [28]. There are also documented examples of papillary microcarcinomas between 2 and 8 mm in maximum diameter that displayed high strain (low stiffness) on elastography [15, 18]. Therefore, although not definitive, there is likely to be a minimum size threshold for accurate cancer detection [15, 18].

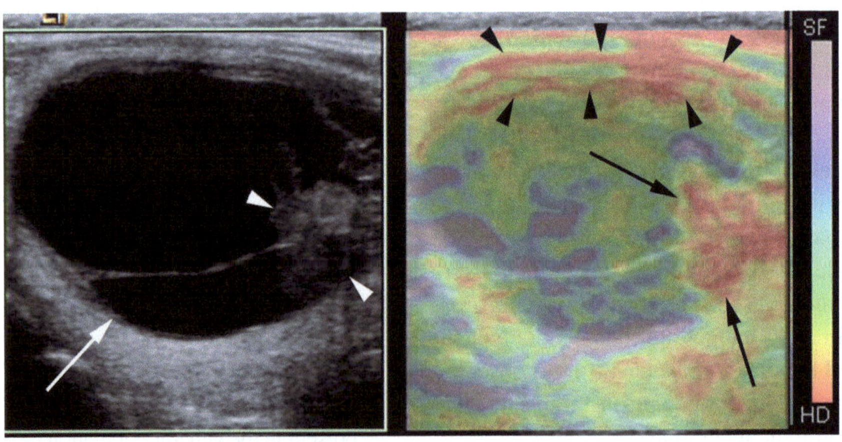

Fig. 12.9 Transverse gray scale US image with corresponding real-time qualitative elastogram showing a hyperplastic nodule with cystic degeneration (*white arrow*). On the elastogram, the superficial margin of the nodule is displayed as a double red line (*black arrowheads*), which is likely to be artifactual in view of the obviously cystic content of the nodule at this location. While the cystic component displays colors corresponding to a soft pattern, the small solid component protruding into the cavity (*white arrowheads*) displays as red (*black arrows*), suggesting it is stiff. This is a false positive for malignancy on elastography

9. Nodule position
   The precise influence of nodule position on elastography has not been evaluated thoroughly. This may be relevant because of local inhomogeneities in the stress field caused by boundary conditions and stress decay [43]. In a recent study of 51 subcentimeter thyroid nodules, 2 out of 3 nodules that were false negative for cancer using qualitative elastography were located within the thyroid isthmus [28]. This finding may be explained by the shallow depth of normal isthmic thyroid tissue over the relatively stiff trachea which may have been inadvertently overcompressed, thereby causing an underestimation of nodule stiffness [28].
10. Non-papillary cancers
    The vast majority of malignant nodules in published studies have been papillary carcinomas, while sparse numbers of primary cancers such as follicular, medullary, or anaplastic carcinoma have been evaluated. Consequently, the accuracy of elastography for non-papillary cancers is unknown. Using direct biomechanical testing of resected specimens, Lyshchik et al. documented that the elastic modulus of follicular carcinomas (3 of 3) was significantly lower than papillary carcinoma and comparable to normal tissue [50]. Rago et al. documented that of 32 nodules with an indeterminate diagnosis of follicular lesion on cytology, all benign adenomas (25 of 25) and most (6 of 7) cancers were correctly classified by qualitative elastography in terms of low and high elastographic scores, respectively. In other studies, follicular or follicular variant carcinomas could not be discriminated from benign nodules using strain ratios or qualitative scoring of the entire nodule [12, 14, 16–18]. Another report documented that follicular carcinomas displayed low strain (high stiffness) only in the peripheral margin, which was in contrast to the uniform low strain (high stiffness) observed in papillary carcinomas and uniform high strain (low stiffness) observed in adenomatous nodules [30]. Although this finding has not been correlated pathologically, if genuine, it may reflect differences related to increased tumor cellularity or thickness of the capsule in follicular cancers compared to adenomas [30, 56, 61]. As many follicular carcinomas are microinvasive and can only be reliably distinguished from adenomas by careful microscopic analysis [56], doubts remain as to whether elastography can reliably discriminate follicular lesions [13].
11. Thyroiditis
    Currently, there is no clear evidence whether elastography is reliable in the presence of diffuse parenchymal diseases such as thyroiditis or subtle multinodular goiter. Theoretically, these conditions may alter the overall stiffness of the thyroid parenchyma and thus result in erroneous estimations of nodule stiffness [50]. Interestingly, one study of real-time elastography documented the presence of Hashimoto's thyroiditis (diagnosed biochemically) in 12 of 22 of papillary cancers (55%), and 11 of these were correctly diagnosed as cancer on elastography [22]. Other workers have documented cases of focal fibrotic nodules and subacute thyroiditis that were false positive on elastography [15, 18].

    Scacchi et al. found that a high proportion of thyroid nodules in patients with acromegaly appeared stiff on elastography (56.8%) although all of these were benign. This finding suggests that these nodules may be of a more fibrous nature than in the general population, and that elastography is of limited value for detecting cancer in these patients [31].
12. Reproducibility
    There are several potential sources of variation that may influence the reproducibility of elastography including compression technique, software processing, elastogram selection, and interpretation. Several studies of qualitative thyroid elastography have documented >90% agreement between reviewers who interpreted the same prerecorded elastograms [14, 18, 25, 28], although as alluded to earlier, these results may be falsely reassuring as they do not account for variation in the factors leading up to image interpretation. In a study specifically addressing this issue, no statistically significant correlation was found between the elastography scores of three operators who independently performed and

scored real-time qualitative elastography (on the same nodule), which was in contrast to a high correlation for their scores using conventional sonographic criteria [45]. These discrepant findings highlight the need for properly conducted reproducibility studies that include all aspects of the technique. It should also be noted that even for quantitative elastography, subjective assessment may still be required in terms of selecting regions for strain calculations [55]. This source of interobserver variation has been documented in breast elastography with respect to estimating nodule margins for the calculation of area ratios [55].

It has been shown that elastograms produced using carotid artery pulsations are of higher quality and more reproducible than by freehand compression because the former effectively reduces errors and variations caused by operator compression technique [44].

Elastography of Thyroid Lymph Node Metastases

Several preliminary studies have shown that malignant infiltration of lymph nodes is associated with lower strain (higher stiffness) than benign nodes [34, 35, 37, 38]. Two of these have included cervical nodal metastases from thyroid malignancy [35, 37]. Lyshchik et al. performed conventional sonography and off-line freehand compression elastography for 141 cervical nodes, in which 39 of 60 metastatic nodes were from thyroid papillary cancer [37]. Several qualitative and quantitative elastographic criteria were tested, of which an index of strain in adjacent neck muscle (lymph node >1.5) was the most accurate predictor of malignancy, achieving 85% sensitivity, 98% specificity, and 92% accuracy. Nine false negatives on elastography were documented (including from thyroid cancer) in nodal metastases that were either incompletely infiltrated or had central necrosis. By comparison, the best conventional sonographic criterion, a short-to-long axis diameter ratio >0.5, achieved 81% specificity, 75% sensitivity, and 79% accuracy. Alam et al. performed B-mode sonography and qualitative real-time elastography of 85 lymph nodes, in which 13 of 53 metastatic nodes were from thyroid cancer [35]. Differing from the study by Lyschik et al., qualitative analysis of different patterns of strain was performed that could account for incomplete nodal infiltration and central necrosis. In their series, elastography achieved 83% sensitivity, 100% specificity, and 89% accuracy for malignancy, which was superior to B-mode sonography. When both B-mode sonography and elastography were combined, sensitivity increased to 92%, specificity to 94%, and accuracy to 93%. Although these results are encouraging, they need to be validated in larger studies.

Current Directions

A recent refinement of elastography termed acoustic radiation force impulse (ARFI) imaging is now available on commercial clinical ultrasound machines. In ARFI imaging, transient pushing pulses of acoustic radiation (ultrasound) generated by a modified transducer are used to produce tissue displacements instead of mechanical compressions by the operator or a physiologic source. The tissue displacements (~10 μm) can be tracked with the same transducer using ultrasonic correlation-based methods [62, 63]. Pushing pulses can be focused to different spatial locations and can stimulate tissues at depths relatively distant from the skin surface. Preliminary evidence indicates that ARFI images have more uniform stress distribution and higher signal-to-noise ratio than elastograms produced by freehand compression, as they are less susceptible to artifacts associated with boundary conditions and stress decay [63].

Shear wave elastography is an emerging elasticity imaging technique that uses a different method to static elastography for measuring tissue elasticity. Shear waves are transient tissue displacements produced by tangential sliding of adjacent tissue layers in response to a loading and are propagated transversely within tissues.

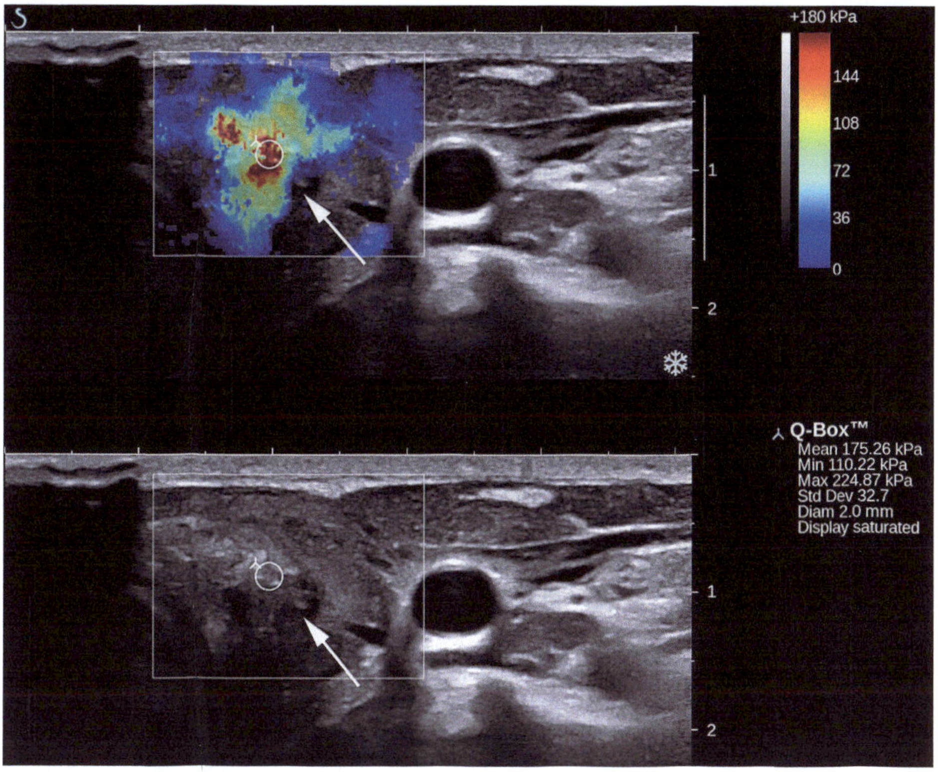

Fig. 12.10 Transverse gray scale US image with corresponding shear wave elastogram showing a papillary carcinoma (*arrow*). Differing from relative strain estimates used in compression elastography, the color scale shown here (*right top corner*) displays in absolute kilopascal units. A region of interest in nodule has a mean elasticity index of 175.26 kPa, indicating a firm nodule, and thus highly suspicious of malignancy

Tissue stiffness or elasticity and shear wave speed are directly related through a simple formula:

$$E = 3pc^2.$$

E = stiffness = Young's elastic modulus, p = density of the tissue (kg/m^3), c = shear wave speed (m/s).

Soft tissues have a density similar to water, 1,000 kg/m^3, hence the elasticity of tissues can be estimated from the shear wave velocity. This differs from static elastography, which only estimates tissue strain.

Although the principles underlying shear wave measurement have been known for decades, there have been significant technical obstacles in terms of shear wave generation and measurement by ultrasound. This may be due to the fact that shear waves have extremely small amplitudes (a few microns) and travel only very short distances before dissipating. Current ultrasound systems using shear wave imaging have tried to overcome these challenges by utilizing specifically focused acoustic radiation impulses to generate shear waves and amplify their propagation, as well as an ultrafast ultrasound imaging method to detect the propagated shear waves in real time. Shear wave imaging is claimed to be superior to static elastography in terms of reduced operator dependence, higher reproducibility, and ability to produce quantitative measurements more directly related to tissue stiffness (Figs. 12.10–12.12) [64]. In addition, it can be performed in nodules lacking normal surrounding thyroid parenchyma such as large or conglomerate nodules. A recent study evaluated this technique in the thyroid, which included 146 nodules of which 29 were malignant and in which an elasticity index >65 kPa achieved 85% sensitivity and 94% specificity [26].

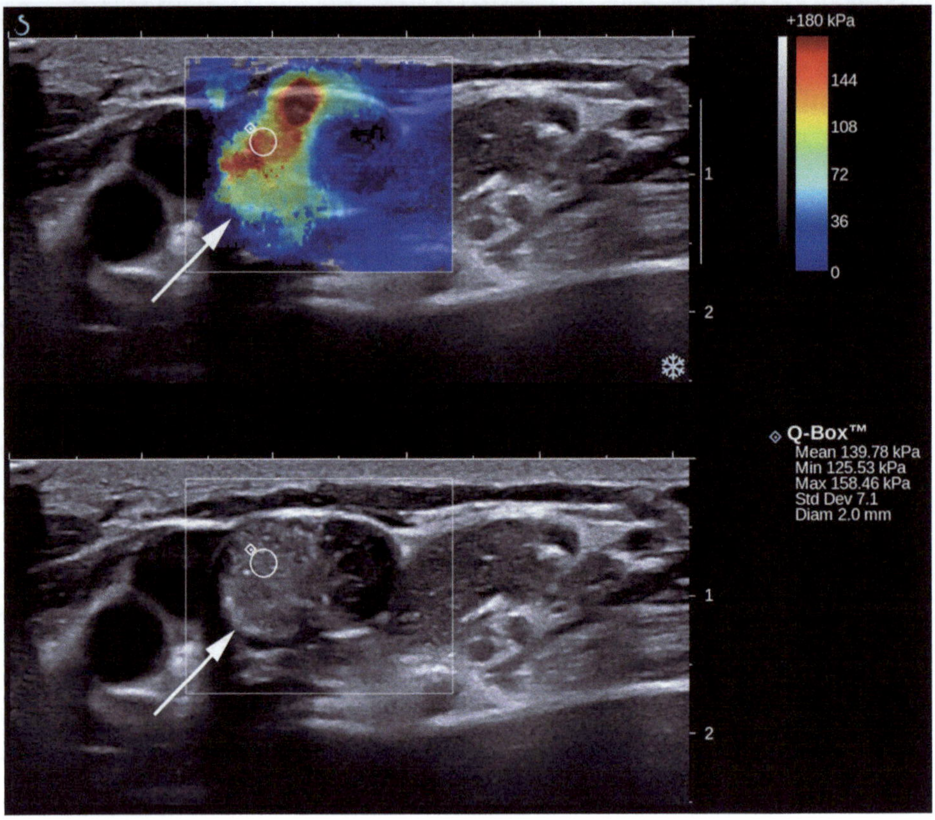

Fig. 12.12 Transverse gray scale US image with corresponding shear wave elastogram showing a metastatic cervical lymph node from papillary thyroid carcinoma (*arrow*). The node is clearly metastatic on gray scale US in view of its abnormal shape heterogeneously increased echotexture, foci of punctate calcification and necrosis. A region of interest within a more solid component of the nodule has a mean elasticity index of 139.78 kPa, which is high and may be predictive of metastatic infiltration

Role of Elastography in Routine Practice

The issue that all investigators are trying to address is the definitive role of elastography in the diagnostic algorithm of evaluating a thyroid nodule. Clearly, this depends on the emerging accuracy data for malignancy. Given the high prevalence of nodules in the general population yet low incidence of malignancy, one approach would be for it to identify nodules that are benign, including nodules that would have otherwise been biopsied on the basis of their conventional sonographic appearances. This approach would require elastographic criteria with high negative predictive value, i.e., approaching 100% and sufficiently high sensitivity to be of practical use. Alternatively, elastography could be used to identify nodules that are likely to be malignant and therefore require biopsy or further follow up. This approach may identify malignant nodules that were previously unsuspected on sonography or equivocal but not biopsied due to their small size.

Another potential role for elastography is to highlight areas within nodules to target or avoid

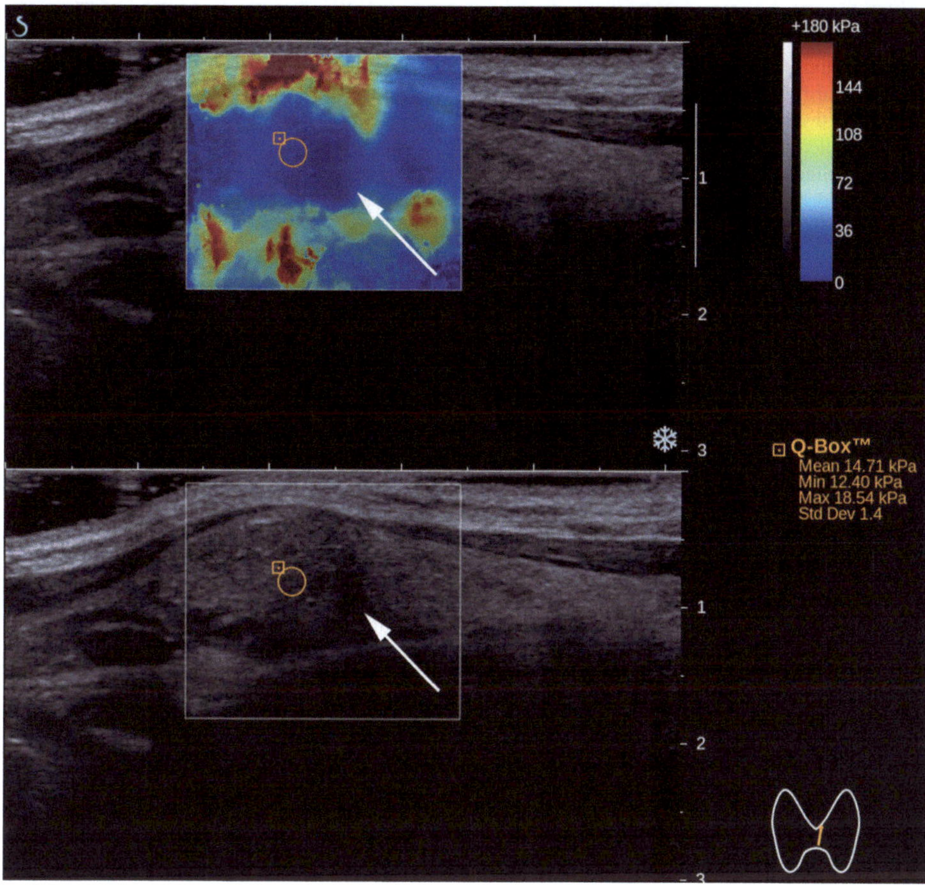

Fig. 12.11 Transverse gray scale US image with corresponding shear wave elastogram showing a follicular adenoma (*arrow*). A region of interest in the nodule has a mean elasticity index of 14.71 kPa, which is comparable to normal parenchyma, and hence suggestive of benignity

for FNAC in order to reduce nondiagnostic or inadequate cytology. Despite further improvements in equipment/technology, technique and familiarization with elastography, we believe it is unlikely that elastography will entirely replace a FNAC in the near future.

References

1. Yassa L, Cibas ES, Benson CB, et al. Long-term assessment of a multidisciplinary approach to thyroid nodule diagnostic evaluation. Cancer. 2007;111:508–16.
2. Cappelli C, Castellano M, Pirola I, et al. The predictive value of ultrasound findings in the management of thyroid nodules. QJM. 2007;100:29–35.
3. Frates MC, Benson CB, Charboneau JW, et al. Management of thyroid nodules detected at US: Society of Radiologists in ultrasound consensus conference statement. Radiology. 2005;237:794–800.
4. Rago T, Vitti P, Chiovato L, et al. Role of conventional ultrasonography and color flow-doppler sonography in predicting malignancy in 'cold' thyroid nodules. Eur J Endocrinol. 1998;138:41–6.
5. Cerbone G, Spiezia S, Colao A, et al. Power Doppler improves the diagnostic accuracy of color Doppler ultrasonography in cold thyroid nodules: follow-up results. Horm Res. 1999;52:19–24.
6. Kim EK, Park CS, Chung WY, et al. New sonographic criteria for recommending fine-needle aspiration biopsy of nonpalpable solid nodules of the thyroid. Am J Roentgenol. 2002;178:687–91.
7. Kim JY, Lee CH, Kim SY, et al. Radiologic and pathologic findings of nonpalpable thyroid carcinomas detected by ultrasonography in a medical screening center. J Ultrasound Med. 2008;27:215–23.

8. Moon WJ, Jung SL, Lee JH, et al. Benign and malignant thyroid nodules: US differentiation–multicenter retrospective study. Radiology. 2008;247:762–70.
9. Chow LS, Gharib H, Goellner JR, van Heerden JA. Nondiagnostic thyroid fine-needle aspiration cytology: management dilemmas. Thyroid. 2001;11:1147–51.
10. Gharib H, Goellner JR. Fine-needle aspiration biopsy of the thyroid: an appraisal. Ann Intern Med. 1993;118:282–9.
11. Ophir J, Cespedes I, Ponnekanti H, Yazdi Y, Li X. Elastography: a quantitative method for imaging the elasticity of biological tissues. Ultrason Imaging. 1991;13:111–34.
12. Lyshchik A, Higashi T, Asato R, et al. Thyroid gland tumor diagnosis at US elastography. Radiology. 2005;237:202–11.
13. Rago T, Santini F, Scutari M, Pinchera A, Vitti P. Elastography: new developments in ultrasound for predicting malignancy in thyroid nodules. J Clin Endocrinol Metab. 2007;92:2917–22.
14. Asteria C, Giovanardi A, Pizzocaro A, et al. US-elastography in the differential diagnosis of benign and malignant thyroid nodules. Thyroid. 2008;18:523–31.
15. Dighe M, Bae U, Richardson ML, Dubinsky TJ, Minoshima S, Kim Y. Differential diagnosis of thyroid nodules with US elastography using carotid artery pulsation. Radiology. 2008;248:662–9.
16. Tranquart F, Bleuzen A, Pierre-Renoult P, Chabrolle C, Sam Giao M, Lecomte P. [Elastosonography of thyroid lesions]. J Radiol. 2008;89:35–9.
17. Friedrich-Rust M, Sperber A, Holzer K, et al. Real-time elastography and contrast-enhanced ultrasound for the assessment of thyroid nodules. Exp Clin Endocrinol Diabetes. 2009;118(9):602–9.
18. Hong Y, Liu X, Li Z, Zhang X, Chen M, Luo Z. Real-time ultrasound elastography in the differential diagnosis of benign and malignant thyroid nodules. J Ultrasound Med. 2009;28:861–7.
19. Luo S, Kim EH, Dighe M, Kim Y. Screening of thyroid nodules by ultrasound elastography using diastolic strain variation. Conf Proc IEEE Eng Med Biol Soc. 2009;2009:4420–3.
20. Rubaltelli L, Corradin S, Dorigo A, et al. Differential diagnosis of benign and malignant thyroid nodules at elastosonography. Ultraschall Med. 2009;30:175–9.
21. Dighe M, Kim J, Luo S, Kim Y. Utility of the ultrasound elastographic systolic thyroid stiffness index in reducing fine-needle aspirations. J Ultrasound Med. 2010;29:565–74.
22. Gietka-Czernel M, Kochman M, Bujalska K, Stachlewska-Nasfeter E, Zgliczynski W. Real-time ultrasound elastography – a new tool for diagnosing thyroid nodules. Endokrynol Pol. 2010;61:652–7.
23. Kagoya R, Monobe H, Tojima H. Utility of elastography for differential diagnosis of benign and malignant thyroid nodules. Otolaryngol Head Neck Surg. 2010;143:230–4.
24. Luo S, Kim EH, Dighe M, Kim Y. Thyroid nodule classification using ultrasound elastography via linear discriminant analysis. Ultrasonics. 2011;51(4):425–31.
25. Rago T, Scutari M, Santini F, et al. Real-time elastosonography: useful tool for refining the presurgical diagnosis in thyroid nodules with indeterminate or nondiagnostic cytology. J Clin Endocrinol Metab. 2010;95(12):5274–80.
26. Sebag F, Vaillant-Lombard J, Berbis J, et al. Shear wave elastography: a new ultrasound imaging mode for the differential diagnosis of benign and malignant thyroid nodules. J Clin Endocrinol Metab. 2010;95:5281–8.
27. Vorlander C, Wolff J, Saalabian S, Lienenluke RH, Wahl RA. Real-time ultrasound elastography–a noninvasive diagnostic procedure for evaluating dominant thyroid nodules. Langenbecks Arch Surg. 2010;395:865–71.
28. Wang Y, Dan HJ, Dan HY, Li T, Hu B. Differential diagnosis of small single solid thyroid nodules using real-time ultrasound elastography. J Int Med Res. 2010;38:466–72.
29. Bhatia KSS, Rasalkar DD, Yim PL, et al. Cystic change in thyroid nodules: a confounding factor for real-time qualitative thyroid ultrasound elastography. Clin Radiol. 2011;66(9):799–807.
30. Fukunari N. More accurate and sensitive diagnosis for thyroid tumours with elastography. In: MEDIX Suppl2007; 2007.
31. Scacchi M, Andrioli M, Carzaniga C, et al. Elastosonographic evaluation of thyroid nodules in acromegaly. Eur J Endocrinol. 2009;161:607–13.
32. Ginat DT, Destounis SV, Barr RG, Castaneda B, Strang JG, Rubens DJ. US elastography of breast and prostate lesions. Radiographics. 2009;29:2007–16.
33. Janssen J, Schlorer E, Greiner L. EUS elastography of the pancreas: feasibility and pattern description of the normal pancreas, chronic pancreatitis, and focal pancreatic lesions. Gastrointest Endosc. 2007;65:971–8.
34. Janssen J, Dietrich CF, Will U, Greiner L. Endosonographic elastography in the diagnosis of mediastinal lymph nodes. Endoscopy. 2007;39:952–7.
35. Alam F, Naito K, Horiguchi J, Fukuda H, Tachikake T, Ito K. Accuracy of sonographic elastography in the differential diagnosis of enlarged cervical lymph nodes: comparison with conventional B-mode sonography. Am J Roentgenol. 2008;191:604–10.
36. Garra BS. Imaging and estimation of tissue elasticity by ultrasound. Ultrasound Q. 2007;23:255–68.
37. Lyshchik A, Higashi T, Asato R, et al. Cervical lymph node metastases: diagnosis at sonoelastography–initial experience. Radiology. 2007;243:258–67.
38. Saftoiu A, Vilmann P, Hassan H, Gorunescu F. Analysis of endoscopic ultrasound elastography used for characterisation and differentiation of benign and malignant lymph nodes. Ultraschall Med. 2006;27:535–42.

39. Zhi H, Ou B, Luo BM, Feng X, Wen YL, Yang HY. Comparison of ultrasound elastography, mammography, and sonography in the diagnosis of solid breast lesions. J Ultrasound Med. 2007;26:807–15.
40. Thomas A, Kummel S, Gemeinhardt O, Fischer T. Real-time sonoelastography of the cervix: tissue elasticity of the normal and abnormal cervix. Acad Radiol. 2007;14:193–200.
41. Taylor LS, Rubens DJ, Porter BC, et al. Prostate cancer: three-dimensional sonoelastography for in vitro detection. Radiology. 2005;237:981–5.
42. Itoh A, Ueno E, Tohno E, et al. Breast disease: clinical application of US elastography for diagnosis. Radiology. 2006;239:341–50.
43. Thomas A, Fischer T, Frey H, et al. Real-time elastography–an advanced method of ultrasound: first results in 108 patients with breast lesions. Ultrasound Obstet Gynecol. 2006;28:335–40.
44. Bae U, Dighe M, Dubinsky T, Minoshima S, Shamdasani V, Kim Y. Ultrasound thyroid elastography using carotid artery pulsation: preliminary study. J Ultrasound Med. 2007;26:797–805.
45. Park SH, Kim SJ, Kim EK, Kim MJ, Son EJ, Kwak JY. Interobserver agreement in assessing the sonographic and elastographic features of malignant thyroid nodules. Am J Roentgenol. 2009;193: W416–23.
46. Raza S, Odulate A, Ong EM, Chikarmane S, Harston CW. Using real-time tissue elastography for breast lesion evaluation: our initial experience. J Ultrasound Med. 2010;29:551–63.
47. Bhatia KS, Cho CC, Yuen YH, Rasalkar DD, King AD, Ahuja AT. Real-time qualitative ultrasound elastography of cervical lymph nodes in routine clinical practice: interobserver agreement and correlation with malignancy. Ultrasound Med Biol. 2010;36: 1990–7.
48. Bhatia KS, Rasalkar DD, Lee YP, et al. Evaluation of real-time qualitative sonoelastography of focal lesions in the parotid and submandibular glands: applications and limitations. Eur Radiol. 2010;20:1958–64.
49. Bojunga J, Herrmann E, Meyer G, Weber S, Zeuzem S, Friedrich-Rust M. Real-time elastography for the differentiation of benign and malignant thyroid nodules: a meta-analysis. Thyroid. 2010;20:1145–50.
50. Lyshchik A, Higashi T, Asato R, et al. Elastic moduli of thyroid tissues under compression. Ultrason Imaging. 2005;27:101–10.
51. Ophir J, Garra B, Kallel F, et al. Elastographic imaging. Ultrasound Med Biol. 2000;26 Suppl 1:S23–9.
52. Hall TJ. AAPM/RSNA physics tutorial for residents: topics in US: beyond the basics: elasticity imaging with US. Radiographics. 2003;23:1657–71.
53. Ueno E, Ito A. Diagnosis of breast cancer by elasticity imaging. Eizo Joho Med. 2004;36:2–6.
54. Hall TJ, Zhu Y, Spalding CS. In vivo real-time freehand palpation imaging. Ultrasound Med Biol. 2003;29:427–35.
55. Regner DM, Hesley GK, Hangiandreou NJ, et al. Breast lesions: evaluation with US strain imaging–clinical experience of multiple observers. Radiology. 2006;238:425–37.
56. DeLellis RA, Guiter G, Weinstein BJ. Pathology of the thyroid and parathyroid glands. In: Gnepp DR, editor. Diagnostic and surgical pathology of the head and neck. Philadelphia: W.B. Saunders; 2001.
57. Havre RF, Elde E, Gilja OH, et al. Freehand real-time elastography: impact of scanning parameters on image quality and in vitro intra- and interobserver validations. Ultrasound Med Biol. 2008;34:1638–50.
58. Ophir J, Cespedes I, Garra B, Ponnekanti H, Huang Y, Maklad N. Elastography: ultrasonic imaging of tissue strain and elastic modulus in vivo. Eur J Ultrasound. 1996;3:49–70.
59. Friedrich-Rust M, Schwarz A, Ong M, et al. Real-time tissue elastography versus FibroScan for noninvasive assessment of liver fibrosis in chronic liver disease. Ultraschall Med. 2009;30:478–84.
60. Frates MC, Benson CB, Charboneau JW, et al. Management of thyroid nodules detected at US: Society of Radiologists in Ultrasound consensus conference statement. Ultrasound Q 2006;22:231–8; discussion 9–40.
61. Evans HL. Follicular neoplasms of the thyroid. A study of 44 cases followed for a minimum of 10 years, with emphasis on differential diagnosis. Cancer. 1984;54:535–40.
62. Nightingale K, Soo MS, Nightingale R, Trahey G. Acoustic radiation force impulse imaging: in vivo demonstration of clinical feasibility. Ultrasound Med Biol. 2002;28:227–35.
63. Melodelima D, Bamber JC, Duck FA, Shipley JA. Transient elastography using impulsive ultrasound radiation force: a preliminary comparison with surface palpation elastography. Ultrasound Med Biol. 2007;33:959–69.
64. Tanter M, Bercoff J, Athanasiou A, et al. Quantitative assessment of breast lesion viscoelasticity: initial clinical results using supersonic shear imaging. Ultrasound Med Biol. 2008;34:1373–86.

Percutaneous Ethanol Injection for Thyroid and Parathyroid Disorders

13

Daniel S. Duick

Introduction

The initial utilization of percutaneous ethanol injection (PEI) in thyroid and parathyroid diseases was adapted from earlier work in renal cysts, hepatic cysts, and the treatment of hepatocellular carcinoma [1–3]. Early initial reports for thyroid were in hyperfunctioning thyroid nodules and in parathyroid disease for the treatment of enlarged parathyroid glands due to secondary hyperparathyroidism and renal failure [4, 5].

The sclerosing capability of 95–98% ethanol, directly injected into nodular tissue or cysts, is induced through denaturation of protein, coagulative necrosis, cellular dehydration, microcirculatory thrombosis, and local hemorrhage. All of these lead to reactive fibrosis.

In the recent past, PEI was further investigated for the treatment of hyperfunctioning nodules and, eventually, isofunctioning nodules and cold nodules [6–9]. All were delineated by isotopic scanning and fine needle aspiration-derived benign diagnoses. Today, solid thyroid nodule ablation is more of historical interest rather than practical application since these types of solid lesions may require as many as eight to ten visits and injection treatments to attain a satisfactory reduction in a 2–4-cm solid mass. Additionally, premedication and sedation is required as well as postprocedure pain medication and glucocorticoids depending on the volume of injection, size and number of nodules, and the amount of reaction in the nodules and surrounding tissue.

Currently, the primary thyroid applications for PEI are for the reduction of cystic nodules, thyroid cysts [10, 11]; and isolated, residual metastatic thyroid cancer lymph nodes [12]. In parathyroid disease, PEI is utilized for tumor mass reduction in chronic renal failure patients with secondary parathyroid hyperplasia or occasionally for treatment of primary hyperparathyroidism due to single adenoma in patients who decline or are not suitable candidates for parathyroid surgery [5, 13]. In incidentally discovered parathyroid cysts, postaspiration frequently recurs, and, similar to thyroid cysts, these can be successfully ablated with PEI [14].

Indications and outcome goals for PEI will differ for various types of thyroid and parathyroid tumors and cysts. However, contraindications for all are essentially the same and include (1) an uncooperative patient for any reason (e.g., severe anxiety, uncontrollable swallowing, uncontrolled respirations, inability to lie recumbent); (2) uncontrolled bleeding or clotting disorder, poorly controlled anticoagulation, or antiplatelet therapy with increased bleeding tendency; (3) lack of a safe needle access path, or unsafe juxtaposition of major blood vessels; and (4) inability to sonographically visualize in an optimal manner the planned treatment lesion for PEI. Table 13.1

D.S. Duick (✉)
Staff Physician, Endocrinology Associates, Third Ave., 3522 N, PA 85013, Phoenix, PA, Arizona
e-mail: aduick@aol.com

Clinical Professor of Medicine, College of Medicine, University of Arizona, Phoenix, Arizona

R.A. Sofferman and A.T. Ahuja (eds.), *Ultrasound of the Thyroid and Parathyroid Glands*, DOI 10.1007/978-1-4614-0974-8_13, © Springer Science+Business Media, LLC 2012

Table 13.1 Percutaneous ethanol injection (PEI) therapy for thyroid and parathyroid disorders

A. Historical perspective of PEI – hyperfunctioning adenoma, nonfunctioning adenoma, multinodular goiter
B. Current utility of PEI ablation therapy
1. Thyroid PEI procedures:
Thyroid cyst
Thyroid cystic adenoma
DTC or MTC cervical residual lymph node disease – palliative only in patients who are not candidates or refuse further surgery for enlarging node(s)
2. Parathyroid procedures – FNA and PEI:
Parathyroid adenoma FNA – occasionally utilized for verification
Parathyroid cyst and parathyroid cystic adenoma (nonfunctioning and hyperfunctioning)
Parathyroid adenoma – palliative for rare patient who is not able to tolerate a mini-invasive procedure or refuses surgery
3. Parathyroid hyperplasia diseases:
Palliative for secondary hyperparathyroidism (SPH)
Palliative for tertiary hyperparathyroidism (TPH) in patients intolerant or not controlled by Cincalcet and nonsurgical candidates
Palliative for forearm implantation tissue or residual hyperplastic gland when hyperparathyroidism recurs after multigland resection for primary parathyroid hyperplasia (PPH)

outlines both the historical as well as the current utilization of PEI for endocrine neck disorders.

Overview

Percutaneous Ethanol Injection for Thyroid Cysts and Cystic Thyroid Nodules

The great majority of thyroid cysts are actually thyroid nodules with only a small fraction, on the order of 1% being true cysts of the thyroid [15]. Approximately one third of all thyroid nodules have some component of cystic degeneration or hemorrhagic degeneration [16]. They are occasionally symptomatic when associated with acute hemorrhage and rapid expansion of tissue in the thyroid and the thyroid capsule. However, the majority do not present in this manner but rather as an indolent process over a protracted period of time. Larger cystic nodules may be visible on external examination of the neck especially when located anteriorly within a thyroid lobe or centrally over the trachea in the isthmus of the thyroid gland. Additionally, large cysts may produce compressive symptoms including fullness, dysphagia, or hoarseness.

Drainage and fine needle aspiration biopsy of the residual solid component of a cystic thyroid lesion is important to rule out malignancy and the need for surgery [17]. Postdrainage, more than three fourths of cystic nodules recur either completely or to a significant degree over time [18]. Since cystic fluid is degenerative, colloidal, or old hemorrhagic fluid, liquid-based cytopathology studies of the aspirated fluid are of virtually no benefit. Cysts, which develop from nodular tissue containing colloidal material, may or may not undergo degenerative change. The colloidal material itself may have variable consistency and viscosity including liquid, oil, or a thickened, gel-like matrix. The latter is often very difficult to reduce in size by aspiration alone, even with large-bore needles after the utilization of a local anesthetic.

The main indications for percutaneous ethanol injection (PEI) are compressive symptoms or cosmetic appearance. The efficacy of percutaneous ethanol injection for the management of thyroid cysts has been well documented for more than 15 years [10, 11, 19–21, 53]. The results of PEI are based on the ratio of cystic to solid portion of a given nodule. In a nearly pure cystic lesion, PEI can achieve 85–95% plus volume reductions, and there are occasional cysts that completely disappear [20]. However, in mixed or complex, cystic and solid nodules (depending on the amount of solid tissue and the complexity of the cystic compartment), PEI achieves volume reductions on the order of less than 50% to as high as 75% [19–21]. It is important to note that the recurrence rate of thyroid cysts is reduced to less than 20% after PEI therapy [19]. Any recurrence should also suggest the need in a mixed nodule for rebiopsy to exclude the potential of a previously missed malignancy.

Although an overwhelming number of cystic nodules are benign tumors, an occasional cystic nodule with only a mural component or a complex nodule (cystic and solid by ultrasonography criteria) may be a malignancy. Thus, it is the author's practice to perform a single initial drainage procedure on all cystic nodules, and if there is a significant solid component, an FNA is performed at the same procedure. This provides initial information concerning the cytologic status of the nodule, the viscosity of the cystic fluid, and some thyroid cysts and cystic thyroid nodules may not recur after the aspirate and biopsy procedure, thus avoiding the need for subsequent PEI.

Technique

Percutaneous Ethanol Injection for Thyroid Cysts and Cystic Thyroid Nodule

Cyst drainage and PEI are performed by sterile technique utilizing sterile gloves for the operator and an imaging assistant, skin sterilization, and the utilization of sterile gel and a sterile probe cover. Use of a local anesthetic is desirable since a larger needle may be utilized, and patient cooperation is mandatory during the performance of the aspiration and the reinstillation of ethanol. The selection of needle size is important to evacuate the cystic component. A collection of shorter, spinal-type needles (e.g., needle with stylus) varying in size from 18 to 25 gauge should be available. The use of more costly, ultrasound-echoic needles is not necessary since this is a superficial and not a deep visceral procedure. The assistant holding and performing the ultrasound transducer visualization and needle localization during the procedure must be an experienced and skilled imaging technologist or physician. Imaging is performed in the longitudinal plane of the transducer (midsagittal axis) to monitor the needle in its path and needle tip location. Needle tip imaging is enhanced by introducing the needle with the bevel facing upward or toward the transducer during the procedure. During real-time ultrasound imaging, the hypoechoic cyst contrasts well with the bright reflectance of the needle which allows for ready visualization throughout the procedure.

Additional setup material should include a three-way stopcock to utilize one port for direct aspiration and the second port for reinstillation of ethanol. Usually, cystic nodules less than 15–20 ml in volume do not require a pistol grip syringe holder and can be performed freehand. Very large cysts (20 mL volume to 75 mL or greater) may require the utilization of a larger aspirating syringe (e.g., a 30- or 50-mL syringe) for drainage. For larger fluid volumes, a short-length extension tubing can be connected to the stopcock port, and an additional assistant can aid in the drainage procedure. Cysts should be slowly evacuated of as much fluid as possible without traumatizing the cyst wall with the needle tip of the syringe. This may require partial needle withdrawal while staying within the cyst during the procedure to be sure the needle tip remains free during the aspiration phase. Leaving 1–3 ml of residual fluid in a cyst allows for immediate identification of the needle tip prior to the instillation of ethanol. The total withdrawal volume is monitored, and approximately 50% of that volume is utilized to calculate the amount of ethanol for instillation.

Ethanol infusion creates a hyperechoic fluid blush as the previously drained cyst is gradually refilled with ethanol. Usually, there is no significant discomfort or pain during the ethanol instillation, and if such does occur, it suggests that the needle has either penetrated or been partially withdrawn from the cyst or ethanol may have refluxed. The ethanol instillation should be immediately terminated and the needle withdrawn. This may be associated with transient mild but sometimes intense pain 10–20% of the time radiating in the

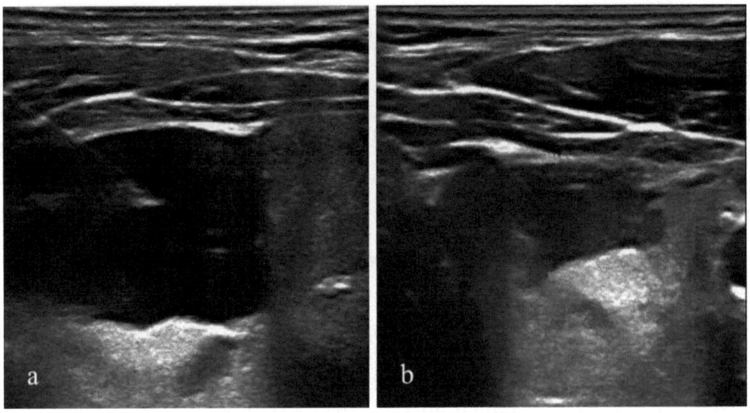

Fig. 13.1 Thyroid cystic nodule. 57-year-old male with thyroid cyst and compressive symptoms. (**a**) Pre-PEI volume of 22.7 mL. (**b**) Partial drainage volume of 11.8 mL

anterior neck, lateral neck, and also to the ear or the jaw [20]. Immediate application of a small ice pack for 10–15 min can help alleviate pain. During the instillation of ethanol, inadvertent penetration through the cystic nodule or the posterior thyroid capsule may be associated with pain and transient dysphonia. Fortunately, this is usually transient, unless the nerve is accidentally penetrated and directly injected, or, if there is a significant amount of perineural ethanol deposited from cyst leakage that occurs from puncturing through the cyst. Cyst penetration, leakage and injury is usually associated with a large 16–18-gauge needle [22].

Normally, there may be some discomfort at the skin level which is momentary during the needle withdrawal due to a small amount of ethanol residual on the external surface of the needle. Occasionally, when a larger needle is used (16–18 gauge), a small amount of alcohol may reflux from the nodule into the perinodular tissue after needle withdrawal. This may also be associated with transient discomfort in the anterior neck and lateral neck and radiate to the ear or the jaw. This is usually self-limiting and may last for a few seconds to as long as 1 min. Rarely, if the pain persists, an ice pack may be applied to reduce the pain or discomfort. As noted above, serious adverse events are rare in the drainage and installation of ethanol in thyroid cysts under ultrasound guidance. Transient dysphonia or possible recurrent laryngeal nerve paralysis is extremely rare and anecdotal with a less than 1% occurrence [22]. In marked contrast, PEI of solid thyroid nodules requires many sessions, a proportionate increase in risk, and has multiple reported serious adverse events including and up to a 3.9% risk of unilateral recurrent laryngeal nerve paralysis; and other rare complications including permanent ipsilateral facial dysesthesia or ipsilateral jugular vein thrombosis [9, 22, 23] (Figs. 13.1 and 13.2).

PEI: Consent and Complications

All patients should have an informed consent for a PEI procedure, and it is imperative that all minor side effects and potential serious adverse events should be listed and carefully explained to the patient prior to the consent signature. The patient should also be advised that these side effects and complications are uncommon but may occur more frequently when there is utilization of a large-bore needle [24].

Overview

PEI of Metastatic Thyroid Cancer Lymph Nodes

Differentiated thyroid cancer (DTC) comprises approximately 90% of all thyroid cancer cases.

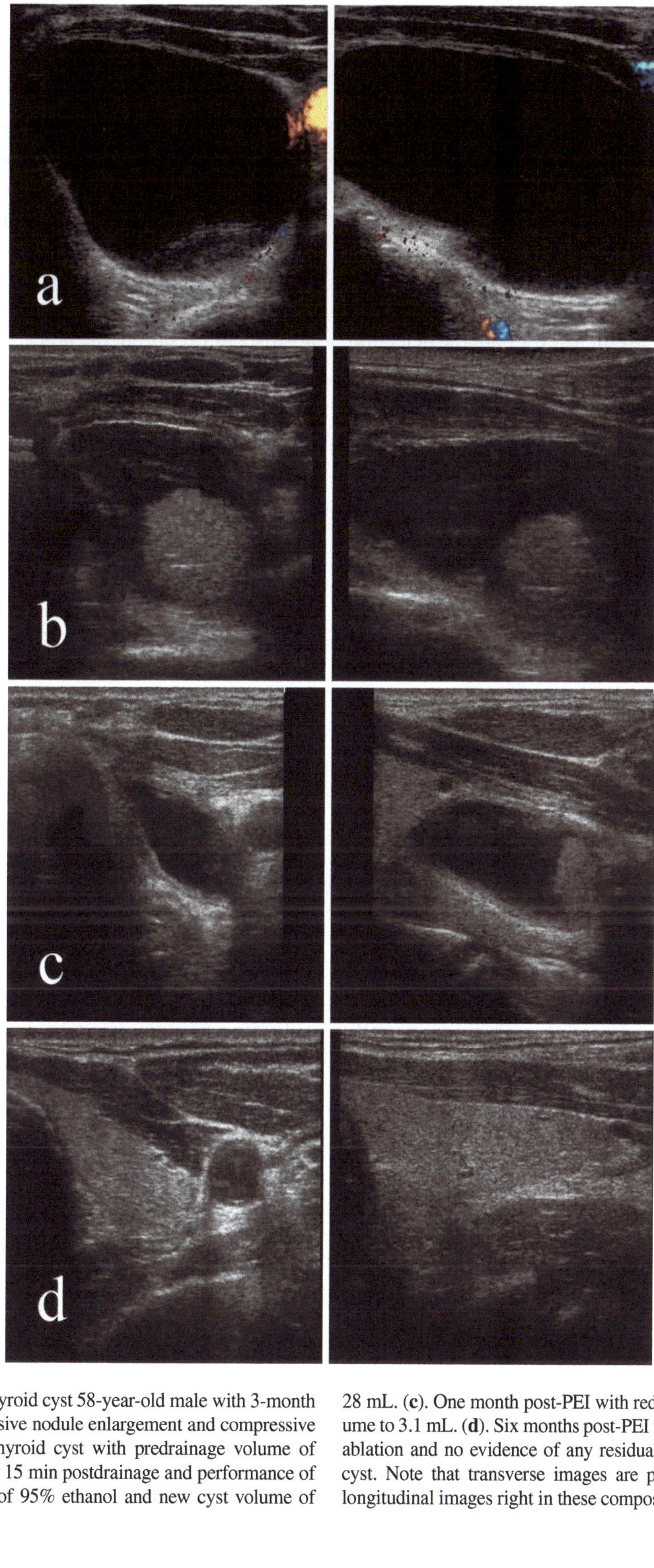

Fig. 13.2 True thyroid cyst 58-year-old male with 3-month history of progressive nodule enlargement and compressive symptoms. (**a**) Thyroid cyst with predrainage volume of 53.2 mL. (**b**) Cyst 15 min postdrainage and performance of PEI with 25 mL of 95% ethanol and new cyst volume of 28 mL. (**c**). One month post-PEI with reduction of cyst volume to 3.1 mL. (**d**). Six months post-PEI with complete cyst ablation and no evidence of any residual nodular tissue or cyst. Note that transverse images are positioned left and longitudinal images right in these composite views

Surgery, radioactive iodine ablation, radioactive iodine therapy and, when necessary, external beam radiation therapy (EBRT) are the time-tested mainstays for local–regional primary and recurrent DTC. Ultrasonography of the postoperative neck is an ideal technology for the detection of persistent or recurrent DTC in the central or lateral neck lymph nodes or the thyroid bed [25, 26]. Serum thyroglobulin has also been demonstrated to be a useful test for both the detection as well as the prediction of risk due to residual DTC [27–29].

As a result of these above modalities, monitoring of thyroid cancer patients after initial treatment is primarily via ultrasound and serum thyroglobulin [30]. Ultrasonographic detection of recurrent or persistent metastatic thyroid lymph nodes may indicate the need for some form of potential further intervention such as surgery, radioactive iodine, alternative ablation therapy, or external beam radiation therapy. When additional therapy is deemed necessary, and more surgery, radioactive iodine, or EBRT are either declined or not indicated, nor appropriate, PEI is an efficacious, palliative, and/or occasionally curative procedure for the ablation of a single or small number of pathologically involved lymph nodes [12].

Previous series have revealed the efficacy of PEI for locally recurrent differentiated thyroid cancer, primarily papillary thyroid cancer [12, 31–33]. Indications for PEI are for one to three ultrasonographically suspicious lymph nodes, previously biopsied and demonstrating metastatic tumor [12, 32].

Technique

PEI for Differentiated Thyroid Cancer Metastatic Lymph Node

The technique has been well described, and outcomes have been demonstrated due to its rapid efficacy over a short period of time (e.g., a few weeks to a few months) to assess reduction or occasional total ablation of metastatic lymph nodes. One to three sessions may be required to optimize reduction in nodal size [12, 32, 33].

The percutaneous ethanol injection of a metastatic cervical lymph node or less commonly a small, central recurrent tumor mass is performed in a sterile manner. One percent or 2% lidocaine is utilized to anesthetize the skin. Subcutaneous tissue and the area immediately adjacent to the lymph node can also be anesthetized to reduce any discomfort during the procedure. As a rule, a metastatic lymph node is less sensitive to injection of ethanol with engorgement of the node versus a thyroid nodule. A 25- or 27-gauge needle is utilized for this technique, and it is attached to a 1-cc tuberculin syringe, which is then filled with 95–98% ethanol.

It is optimum to perform the procedure with the transducer in the longitudinal axis in order to visualize the needle throughout the procedure. The freehand technique is utilized due to the size of the syringe and the sensitive need to administer very small amounts of ethanol in the small volume lesion. Usually increments of 0.05–0.1 ml are introduced in the most distal portion of the node. This allows for slow withdrawal of the needle back through the node and the repositioning of the needle tip to deliver repeated, small injections of ethanol. There is a hyperechogenic blush with each injection, which gradually clears over a few minutes and leaves a variable or mixed hyperechogenic image after 5–10 min (Figs. 13.3 and 13.4).

Postinjection, intranodular vascularity can be rechecked by Doppler flow to evaluate the efficacy of treatment. If remaining intranodular vascularity is present, retreatment can be performed within 24–48 h or delayed a few weeks. For smaller lymph nodes, usually one or two sessions are all that is required to induce necrosis, thrombosis, and eventually sclerotic injury. Lymph nodes with larger diameters (e.g., greater than 20 mm) in two planes may require more sessions. Premeasurement of the lymph node sonographic volume often allows for assessment of the required volume of ethanol injection. Over time (1–2 years), there is gradual sclerosis and nodal

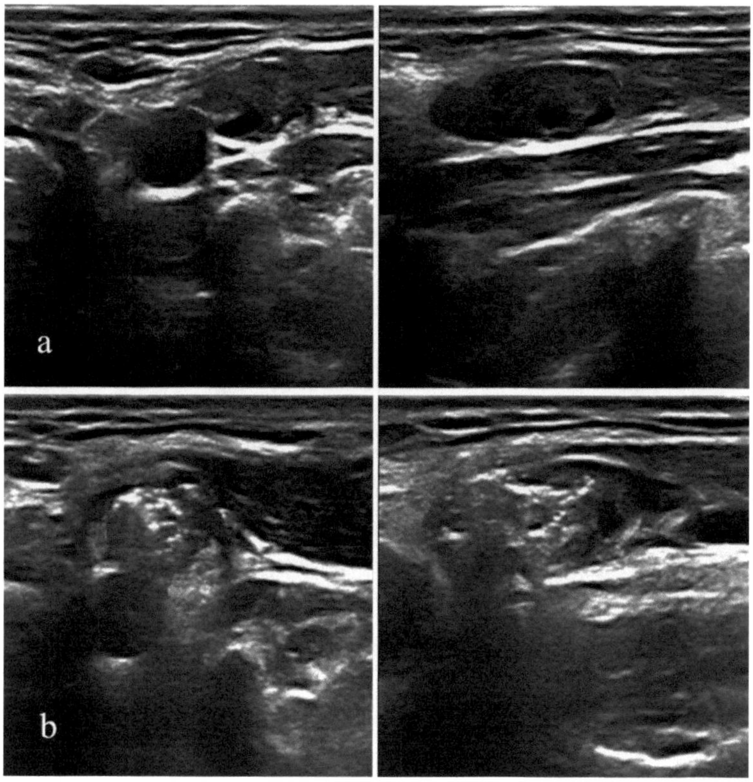

Fig. 13.3 PTC lymph node metastases. 30-year-old female with PTC 8 months postthyroidectomy and radioiodine ablation. Left level IV lymph node: FNA cytopathology and thyroglobulin positive for PTC diagnosis. (**a**) Left level IV pathologic lymph node: pre-PEI volume of 0.290 mL. (**b**) Lymph node 10 min post-PEI (0.5 ml of 95% ethanol) volume of 0.506 mL. Note that transverse images are positioned left and longitudinal images right in these composite views

or mass size reduction which ranges from 50 to >75% [12, 31–33]. Some patients will have complete obliteration of their lymph nodes, and only a few will have minimal regression of volume size. Consideration can be given to retreatment of these nodes at 6 or 12 months or longer pending lack of size reduction, initial regression followed by some regrowth, or the recurrence of Doppler flow in the node [12, 31]. In patients who have minimal residual disease, serologic marker for differentiated thyroid cancer (thyroglobulin) is relatively low. When there are only one or two residual, significant lymph nodes detected by ultrasound and no other evidence of disease in the neck (assuming no systemic metastases) by ultrasound or CT scan, the serum thyroglobulin may become negative after successful nodal ablation. By following a protocol of successful Doppler flow ablation over one or two initial sessions, patients who are considered nonoperative, or refuse surgery, can have a successful outcome.

In the central compartment, caution should be utilized, and it is imperative that cytology be obtained from small lymph nodes to exclude the ablation of a small or hypertrophied remaining parathyroid gland. With the thyroid gland removed, ultrasonographically, a residual, hypertrophied parathyroid gland appears similar to a

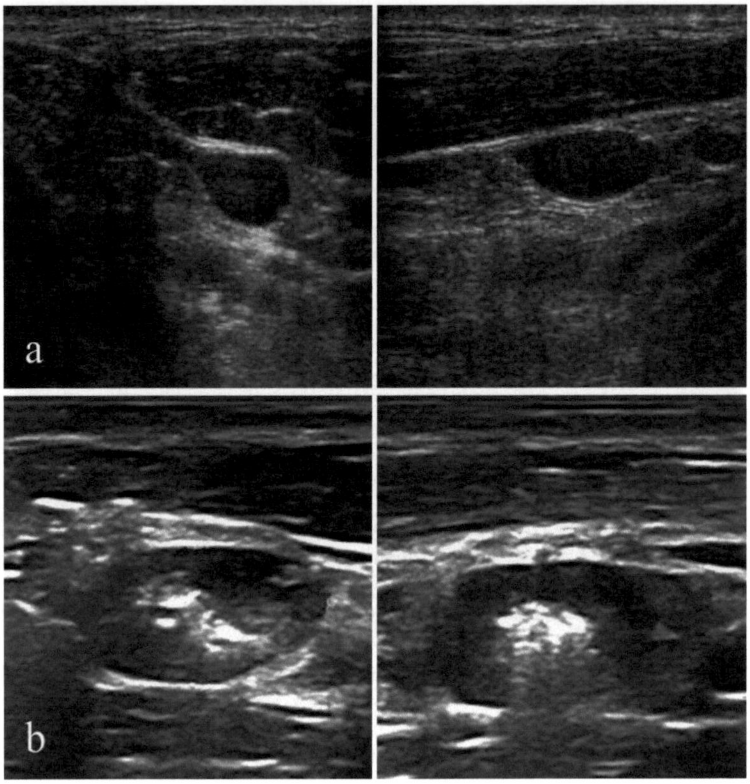

Fig. 13.4 PTC metastatic lymph node. 42-year-old male, 9 years postsurgery and radiodine with 18 months observation of an enlarging right level III lymph node. FNA revealed positive cytopathology and thyroglobulin for PTC. (**a**) Pre-PEI volume of 0.330 mL. (**b**). Five minutes postinjection volume of 0.600 mL. Note that transverse images are positioned left and longitudinal right in these composite views

small lymph node against the hyperechogenic background of scar tissue.

Side effects occur and include transient local pain in 50–75% at the time and site of the injection. Serious adverse events include occasional, transient dysphonia, and rarely permanent recurrent laryngeal nerve paralysis (<1%) has been reported [31, 33] (Fig. 13.5).

Percutaneous Ethanol Injection for Parathyroid Adenoma and Parathyroid Hyperplasia

Overview

Ultrasound-guided percutaneous ethanol injection (PEI) has been utilized for the treatment of multiple forms of parathyroid disease including primary hyperparathyroidism [34, 35], secondary hyperparathyroidism [5, 36, 37], tertiary hyperplasia due to chronic renal failure [38], and parathyroid autografts [39]. Indications and target end points in primary and tertiary hyperparathyroidism are normalization of hypercalcemia and reduction of tumor mass and the level of parathyroid hormone (PTH) in the circulation [40, 41]. Similarly, in secondary hyperparathyroidism, indications and end points are reductions of parathyroid mass and serum PTH level to less than 300 ng/ml [36, 37]. One to four or more sessions may be required to achieve the above end points in all forms of parathyroid disease [37, 38, 41, 42].

Currently, alcohol ablation is not used routinely in the treatment of patients with primary hyperparathyroidism due to parathyroid adenoma. In the United States, over the past 15–20 years, the parathyroid sestamibi scan, ultrasonography,

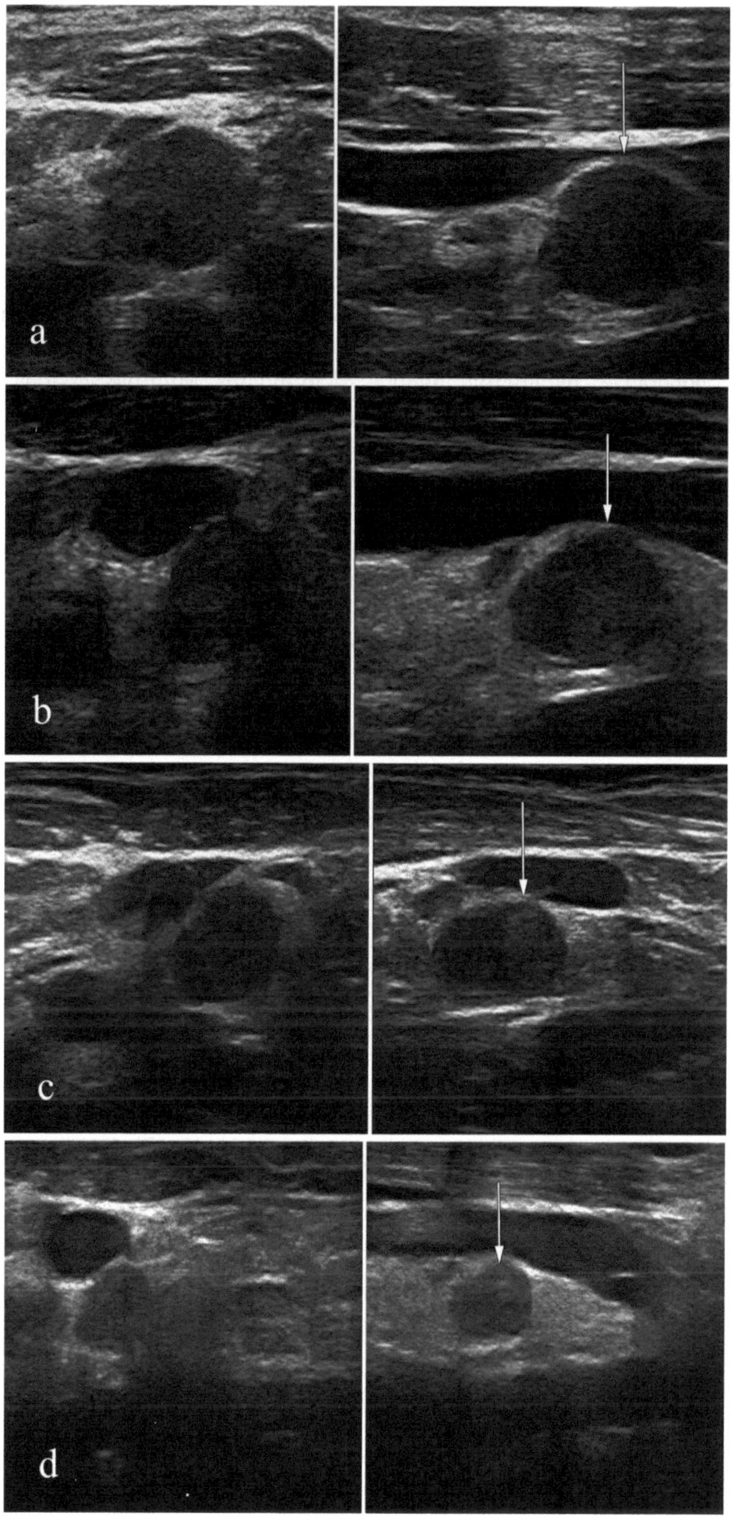

Fig. 13.5 Sequential images pre- and post-PEI of a follicular variant PTC (FVPTC). 64-year-old male with prior surgery and radioiodine FVPTC with left level IV nodal recurrence after 2 years. Arrows demonstrate indentation of the internal jugular vein in sagittal orientation and progressive reduction after alcohol ablation. (**a**) Pre-PEI lymph node volume is 1.10 mL PEI performed with 0.5 ml of 95% ethanol. (**b**). One month post-PEI: lymph node volume is 0.627 mL. (**c**). Three months post-PEI: lymph node volume is 0.368 mL. (**d**) Six months post-PEI: lymph node volume is 0.202 mL equaling a 6-month post-PEI volume reduction of 82%. Note that transverse images are positioned left and longitudinal right in these composite views

multiple microsurgical techniques, and the rapid intraoperative parathyroid hormone assay have all contributed to enhanced preoperative localization of parathyroid tumors as well as more rapid, shorter surgical procedures and successful, definitive outcomes. However, in patients who are unsatisfactory candidates for surgery or refuse surgery, PEI can be successfully applied [42].

In primary hyperparathyroidism, which has been deemed nonoperative, parathyroid tumor tissue should be evident by ultrasound and may require sestamibi scan confirmation prior to a PEI procedure. Occasionally, with uncertain or nondiagnostic imaging, an ultrasound-guided FNA biopsy of a suspect tumor nodule can be safely performed with a 25- or 27-gauge needle in a single pass with minimal negative aspiration pressure. The aspirated material can be suspended in 1 cc of normal saline, and a parathyroid hormone level can be measured for verification.

The results of PEI for treatment of primary hyperparathyroidism vary and, in general, have improved over 20 years. Results for less than 2 years show control of hypercalcemia in 56–92% of patients. Longer-term results vary, and permanent "cures" vary and range from 12 to 25%. Side effects include local transient pain in 80% at the time of injection and transient dysphonia in 4–12%. One to three sessions may be required to achieve successful outcome. The primary serious adverse event is recurrent laryngeal nerve paralysis in 2–8% [34, 35, 40–45].

Results for PEI in the treatment of secondary hyperparathyroidism range for reduction in PTH and tumor mass from 44 to >90%. Outcomes are predicated on the technique and skills of the interventionalist performing the procedure as well as appropriate selection of larger and more active parathyroid glands. Successful reductions in PTH are correlative with the volume of the tissue mass reduction. Similar to primary hyperparathyroidism, over the past 20 years, side effects have been reduced and results have steadily improved. Serious injury to the recurrent laryngeal nerve is reported with less frequency in the last decade and ranged from as high as 4 to 16% and more recently from 0 to 4%. One to four or more sessions may be required to achieve a successful outcome [36, 37, 46–50].

The outcomes for tertiary hyperparathyroidism reveal a more refractory condition for prolonged success. Initial control of hypercalcemia and reductions in PTH and tumor mass are on the order 45–55%. More than half experience recurrent hypercalcemia and rising PTH levels in 6–36 months. Multiple sessions are required to achieve a successful outcome. In the majority of patients, alternative therapies and surgery may ultimately be required to control the disease. Transient pain at the time injection occurs in 90% or more of patients with secondary or tertiary hyperparathyroidism who undergo PEI. Recurrent laryngeal nerve paralysis occurs at a rate of 4–8% [38, 43, 51].

Technique

Percutaneous Ethanol Injection for Parathyroid Tumors

PEI technique includes sterile setup and local anesthesia. A 23–25-gauge needle is inserted into multiple regions of the tumor mass under real-time visualization. Pre- and postprocedure intranodular Doppler vascularity is utilized for all three forms of hyperparathyroidism as criteria for optimal ethanol instillation and obliteration of tumor perfusion [41, 46, 47]. Additionally, the serum calcium value is measured on a daily basis, and PEI may be repeated every day or every other day until the serum calcium level normalizes. Occasionally, up to three to five sessions of PEI may be required to accomplish this goal [38, 40]. The amount of alcohol injected is usually calculated to be one half of the volume of the preinjection tumor nodule in both primary hyperparathyroidism and in secondary hyperparathyroidism. This is usually performed with deliberately slow injection technique to avoid extravasation and potential injury to the immediately adjacent recurrent laryngeal nerve or its branches.

Overview

Percutaneous Ethanol Injection for Parathyroid Cyst

Parathyroid cysts occur in the neck and superior mediastinum relatively infrequently. Over the past 15 years, however, there has been a movement toward utilizing diagnostic ultrasound on all palpable neck masses, thyroid nodules, and ultrasound guidance for the fine needle aspiration of thyroid nodules. This activity has led to an increasing frequency in the incidental discovery of parathyroid tumors and parathyroid cysts than previously suspected [22].

Parathyroid cysts differ from thyroid cysts by the fact that they appear to be primarily nonfunctional cysts which arise from parathyroid embryologic remnants. Parathyroid cysts almost invariably have water-clear fluid on aspiration, and assay of the fluid within the cyst reveals high levels of parathyroid hormone. Parathyroid cysts are seldom functioning, but occasionally represent a cystic functioning parathyroid tumor and need observation over time. Similar to thyroid cysts, the majority of parathyroid cysts tend to recur after fine needle aspiration, and like thyroid cysts, they are ideal for the application of PEI. Preliminary results of PEI of parathyroid cysts have yielded this technique to be safe and effective with greater than an 80% cure rate being reported [14, 22, 52] (Fig. 13.6).

Technique

Percutaneous Ethanol Ablation for Parathyroid Cyst

The technique of parathyroid cyst injection is identical to that of thyroid cyst injection with the only difference being the absence of any need for a large-bore needle since fluid extraction from a parathyroid cyst is almost invariably liquid and water-clear. The reader is referred to the above technique described for the PEI of thyroid cyst treatment. The outcomes for parathyroid cyst are nearly identical to that of pure, low-viscosity cystic lesions of the thyroid with greater than 80% being ablated in one session [22, 43]. The complication rate is exceedingly low in parathyroid cysts since fluid extraction

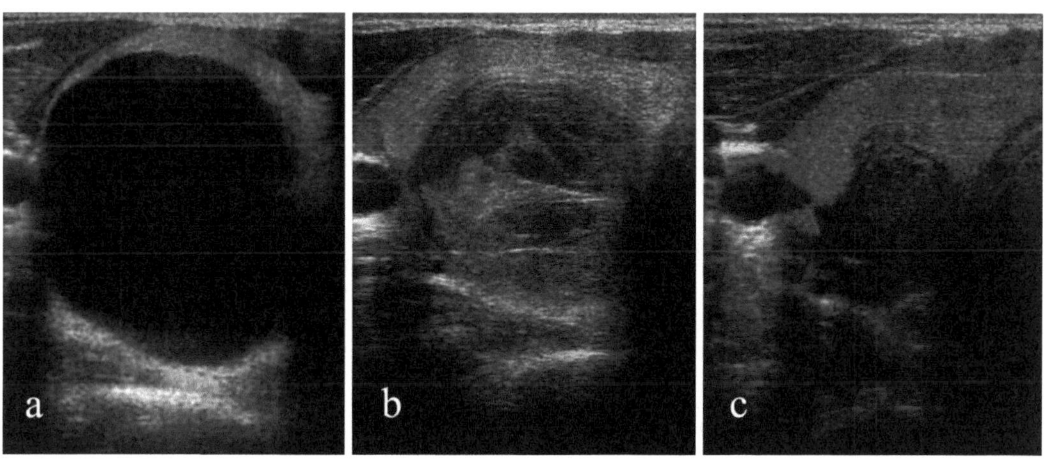

Fig. 13.6 Parathyroid cyst (intrathyroidal, transverse view) 22-year-old male with an asymptomatic mass of right neck discovered during preemployment physical exam. Patient had a negative evaluation for primary hyperparathyroidism. (**a**) Rare intrathyroidal, parathyroid cyst with a pre-PEI volume of 25.16 mL. Previous aspirate revealed "water-clear" fluid with >25,000 pg/ml parathyroid hormone determination. (**b**) One month post-PEI with 12 ml of 95% ethanol; cyst volume is reduced to 10.84 mL. (**c**) Three months post-PEI volume has regressed to 2.71 mL which represents an 89% volume reduction in the intrathyroidal parathyroid cyst

and subsequent alcohol instillation can be easily monitored against the hypoechoic background of the cyst.

References

1. Bean WJ. Renal cysts: treatment with alcohol. Radiology. 1981;138(2):329–31.
2. Bean WJ, Rodan BA. Hepatic cysts: treatment with alcohol. Am J Roentgenol. 1985;144(2):237–4.
3. Livraghi T, Festi D, Monti F, et al. US-guided percutaneous alcohol injection of small hepatic and abdominal tumors. Radiology. 1986;161(2):309–12.
4. Livraghi T, Paracchi A, Ferrari C, et al. Treatment of autonomous thyroid nodules with percutaneous ethanol injection: preliminary results. Work in Progress. Radiology. 1990;175(3):827–9.
5. Solbiati L, Giangrande A, De Pra L, et al. Percutaneous ethanol injection of parathyroid tumors under ultrasound guidance: treatment for secondary hyperparathyroidism. Radiology. 1985;155(3):607–10.
6. Martino E, Murtas ML, Loviselli A, et al. Percutaneous intranodular ethanol injection for treatment of autonomously functioning thyroid nodules. Surgery. 1992;112(6):1161–4.
7. Papini E, Panunzi C, Pacella CM, et al. Percutaneous ultrasound-guided ethanol injection: a new treatment of autonomously functioning thyroid nodules? J Clin Endocrinol Metab. 1993;76(2):411–6.
8. Bennedbaek FN, Hegedüs L. Alcohol sclerotherapy for benign solitary solid cold thyroid nodules. Lancet. 1995;346(8984):1227.
9. Bennedbaek FN, Hegedüs L. Percutaneous ethanol sclerotherapy in benign solid cold thyroid nodules: a randomized trial comparing one injection with three injections. Thyroid. 1999;9(3):225–33.
10. Monzani F, Lippi F, Goletti O, Del Guerra P, Caraccio N, Lippolis PV, et al. Percutaneous aspiration and ethanol sclerotherapy for thyroid cysts. J Clin Endocrinol Metabol. 1994;78(3):800–2.
11. Verde G, Papini E, Pacella CM, Gallotti C, Delpiano S, Strada S, et al. Ultrasound guided percutaneous ethanol injection in the treatment of cystic thyroid nodules. Clin Endocrinol. 1994;41(6):719–24.
12. Lewis BD, Hay ID, Charboneau JW, McIver B, Reading CC, Goellner JR. Percutaneous ethanol injection for treatment of cervical lymph node metastases in patients with papillary thyroid carcinoma. AJR Am J Roentgenol. 2002;178(3):699–704.
13. Charboneau JW, Hay ID, Van Heerden JA. Persistent primary hyperparathyroidism: successful ultrasound-guided percutaneous ethanol ablation of an occult adenoma. Mayo Clin Proc. 1988;63(9):913–7.
14. Zingrillo M, Ghiggi MR, Liuzzi A. A large, nonfunctioning parathyroid cyst recurring after aspiration and subsequently cured by percutaneous ethanol injection. J Clin Ultrasound. 1996;24(7):378–82.
15. Sheppard MC, Franklyn JA. Management of the single thyroid nodule. Clin Endocrinol (Oxf). 1992;37(5):398–401.
16. de los Santos ET, Keyhani-Rofagha S, Cunningham JJ, Mazzaferri EL. Cystic thyroid nodules. The dilemma of malignant lesions. Arch Intern Med. 1990;150(7):1422–7.
17. Bellantone R, Lombardi CP, Raffaelli M, Traini E, De Crea C, Rossi ED, et al. Management of cystic or predominantly cystic thyroid nodules: the role of ultrasound-guided fine-needle aspiration biopsy. Thyroid. 2004;14(1):43–7.
18. Jensen F, Rasmussen SN. The treatment of thyroid cysts by ultrasonically guided fine needle aspiration. Acta Chir Scand. 1976;142(3):209–11.
19. Bennedbaek FN, Hegedus L. Treatment of recurrent thyroid cysts with ethanol: a randomized double-blind controlled trial. J Clin Endocrinol Metab. 2003; 88(12):5773–7.
20. Valcavi R, Frasoldati A. Ultrasound-guided percutaneous ethanol injection therapy in thyroid cystic nodules. Endocrine Pract. 2004;10(3):269–75.
21. Lee SJ, Ahn I-M. Effectiveness of percutaneous ethanol injection therapy in benign nodular and cystic thyroid diseases: long-term follow-up experience. Endocrine J. 2005;52(4):455–62.
22. Frasoldati A, Valcavi R. Pecutaneous ethanol injection (PEI): Thyroid cysts and other neck lesions, Chapter 11. In: Baskin HJ, Duick DS, Levine RA, editors. Thyroid ultrasound and ultrasound-guided FNA. Heidelberg: Springer; 2004. p. 182–5.
23. Lippi F, Ferrari C, Manetti L, Rago T, Santini F, Monzani F, et al. Treatment of solitary autonomous thyroid nodules by percutaneous ethanol injection: results of an Italian multicenter study. J Clin Endocrinol Metabol. 1996;81(9):3261–4.
24. Pacini F. Role of percutaneous ethanol injection in management of nodular lesions of the thyroid gland. J Nucl Med. 2003;44(2):211–2.
25. Ahuja AT, Ying M, Yuen HY, Metreweli C. Power Doppler sonography of metastatic nodes from papillary carcinoma of the thyroid. Clin Radiol. 2001; 56(4):284–8.
26. Frasoldati A, Pesenti M, Gallo M, Caroggio A, Salvo D, Valcavi R. Diagnosis of neck recurrences in patients with differentiated thyroid carcinoma. Cancer. 2003;97(1):90–6.
27. Pacini F, Fugazzola L, Lippi F, Ceccarelli C, Centoni R, Miccoli P, et al. Detection of thyroglobulin in fine needle aspirates of nonthyroidal neck masses: a clue to the diagnosis of metastatic differentiated thyroid cancer. J Clin Endocrinol Metab. 1992;74(6):1401–4.
28. Frasoldati A, Toschi E, Zini M, Flora M, Caroggio A, Dotti C, et al. Role of thyroglobulin measurement in fine-needle aspiration biopsies of cervical lymph nodes in patients with differentiated thyroid cancer. Thyroid. 1999;9(2):105–11.
29. Cignarelli M, Ambrosi A, Marino A, Lamacchia O, Campo M, Picca G, et al. Diagnostic utility of thyroglobulin detection in fine-needle aspiration of cervical

cystic metastatic lymph nodes from papillary thyroid cancer with negative cytology. Thyroid. 2003;13(12):1163–7.
30. Baskin HJ. Detection of recurrent papillary thyroid carcinoma by thyroglobulin assessment in the needle washout after fine-needle aspiration of suspicious lymph nodes. Thyroid. 2004;14(11):959–63.
31. Lim CY, Yun J-S, Lee J, Nam K-H, Chung WY, Park CS. Percutaneous ethanol injection therapy for locally recurrent papillary thyroid carcinoma. Thyroid. 2007;17(4):347–50.
32. Monchik JM, Donatini G, Iannuccilli J, Dupuy DE. Radiofrequency ablation and percutaneous ethanol injection treatment for recurrent local and distant well-differentiated thyroid carcinoma. Ann Surg. 2006;244(2):296–304.
33. Kim BM, Kim MJ, Kim E-K, Park SI, Park CS, Chung WY. Controlling recurrent papillary thyroid carcinoma in the neck by ultrasonography-guided percutaneous ethanol injection. Eur Radiol. 2008;18(4):835–42.
34. Charboneau JW, Hay ID, Van Heerden JA. Persistent primary hyperparathyroidism: successful ultrasound-guided percutaneous ethanol ablation of an occult adenoma. Mayo Clinic Proc. 1988;63(9):913–7.
35. Karstrup S, Hegedus L, Holm HH. Ultrasonically guided chemical parathyroidectomy in patients with primary hyperparathyroidism: a follow-up study. Clin Endocrinol. 1993;38(5):523–30.
36. Takeda SI, Michigishi T, Takazakura E. Successful ultrasonically guided percutaneous ethanol injection for secondary hyperparathyroidism. Nephron. 1992;62(1):100–3.
37. Kitaoka M, Fukagawa M, Ogata E, Kurokawa K. Reduction of functioning parathyroid cell mass by ethanol injection in chronic dialysis patients. Kidney Int. 1994;46(4):1110–7.
38. Cintin C, Karstrup S, Ladefoged SD, Joffe P. Tertiary hyperparathyroidism treated by ultrasonically guided percutaneous fine-needle ethanol injection. Nephron. 1994;68(2):217–20.
39. Takeda S, Michigishi T, Takazakura E. Ultrasonically guided percutaneous ethanol injection to parathyroid autografts for recurrent hyperparathyroidism. Nephron. 1993;65(4):651–2.
40. Verges BL, Cercueil JP, Jacob D, Vaillant G, Brun JM, Putelat R. Results of ultrasonically guided percutaneous ethanol injection into parathyroid adenomas in primary hyperparathyroidism. Acta Endocrinologica. 1993;129(5):381–7.
41. Cercueil JP, Jacob D, Verges B, Holtzmann P, Lerais JM, Krause D. Percutaneous ethanol injection into parathyroid adenomas: Mid- and long-term results. Eur Radiol. 1998;8(9):1565–9.
42. Harman CR, Grant CS, Hay ID, Hurley DL, van Heerden JA, Thompson GB, et al. Indications, technique, and efficacy of alcohol injection of enlarged parathyroid glands in patients with primary hyperparathyroidism. Surgery. 1998;124(6):1011–20.
43. Bennedbæk FN, Karstrup S, Hegedüs L. Percutaneous ethanol injection therapy in the treatment of thyroid and parathyroid diseases. Eur J Endocrinol. 1997;136(3):240–50.
44. Tomić Brzac H. Ultrasonography-guided therapeutic procedures in the neck region. Acta Medica Croatica. 2009;63 Suppl 3:21–7.
45. Stratigis S, Stylianou K, Mamalaki E, et al. Percutaneous ethanol injection therapy: a surgery-sparing treatment for primary hyperparathyroidism. Clin Endocrinol. 2008;69(4):542–8.
46. Chen HH, Lu KC, Lin CJ, Wu CJ. Role of the Parathyroid Gland Vascularization Index in predicting percutaneous ethanol injection efficacy in refractory uremic hyperparathyroidism. Nephron Clin Pract. 2010;117(2):120–6.
47. Kakuta T, Kunimatsu K, Tadaki F, Fujisaki T, Noguchi M, Abe Y, et al. Long-term prognosis of parathyroid function after successful percutaneous ethanol injection therapy (PEIT) guided by color Doppler flow mapping in chronic dialysis patients. Biomed Pharmacother. 2000;54 Suppl 1:60s–5s.
48. Douthat WG, Orozco SE, De Arteaga J, Massari PU. Treatment of refractory secondary hyperparathyroidism with ethanol injection: the importance of glandular volume. Kidney Int. 2003;63(85):S101–4.
49. Tanaka M, Itoh K, Matsushita K, Fukagawa M. Efficacy of percutaneous ethanol injection therapy for secondary hyperparathyroidism in patients on hemodialysis as evaluated by parathyroid hormone levels according to K/DOQI guidelines. Ther Apher Dial. 2005;9(1):48–52.
50. Kitaoka M. "Changes in interventional treatment – From the viewpoint of percutaneous ethanol injection therapy. Therap Apher Dial. 2008;12 Suppl 1:S16–20.
51. Fletcher S, Kanagasundaram NS, Rayner HC, Irving HC, Fowler RC, Brownjohn AM, et al. Assessment of ultrasound guide percutaneous ethanol injection and parathyroidectomy in patients with tertiary hyperparathyroidism. Nephrol Dial Transplant. 1998;13(12):3111–7.
52. Akel M, Salti I, Azar ST. Successful treatment of parathyroid cyst using ethanol sclerotherapy. Am J Med Sci. 1999;317(1):50–2.
53. Zingrillo M, Torlontano M, Chiarella R, Ghiggi MR, Nirchio V, Bisceglia M, et al. Percutaneous ethanol injection may be a definitive treatment for symptomatic thyroid cystic nodules not treatable by surgery: five-year follow-up study. Thyroid. 1999;9(8):763–7.

14 Contrast Enhanced Ultrasound and Ultrasound-Guided Minimally Invasive Therapy for the Diagnosis and Treatment of Focal Thyroid Lesions

Hok Yuen Yuen and Anil T. Ahuja

Introduction

Although the role of non-invasive diagnostic and therapeutic procedures such as contrast enhanced ultrasound (CEUS), ethanol/radiofrequency/laser/high intensity focused ultrasound (HIFU) ablation is established in other parts of the body, their routine applications in the head and neck remain limited. Therefore, despite their experience with such techniques in other parts of the body, the authors' own experience with the use of these techniques in the head and neck is also very limited. The information in this chapter is based on what is already known and published in medical literature in the form of research papers, texts, and the subsequent discussion will review:

- Microbubble contrast in ultrasound and contrast enhanced ultrasound (CEUS) for the assessment of thyroid nodules.
- Ultrasound guided minimally invasive therapy for focal thyroid lesions.
  - Ultrasound guided percutaneous ethanol injection therapy.
  - Ultrasound guided radiofrequency and laser ablation procedures.
  - High Intensity Focused Ultrasound (HIFU) ablation therapy.

H.Y. Yuen (✉) • A.T. Ahuja
Department of Imaging and Interventional Radiology, The Chinese University of Hong Kong, Prince of Wales Hospital, Shatin (NT), Hong Kong (SAR), China
e-mail: drhyyuen@gmail.com

Microbubble Contrast in Ultrasound and Contrast Enhanced Ultrasound for the Assessment of Thyroid Nodules [1–5]

Soon after the advent of cross-sectional imaging modalities such as computed tomography (CT) and magnetic resonance imaging (MRI), the use of intravenous contrast quickly found wide clinical applications to rapidly become an integral imaging protocol. However, ultrasound (US) contrast agents were not readily available for clinical use until recently; this was due to the unique properties required of these ultrasound contrast agents. Ultrasound contrast is now routinely used for a wide variety of clinical conditions (particularly non-head and neck) in many parts of the world (Asia, Europe). However, it still remains to be approved for routine clinical use in the United States of America.

Basic Principles of Microbubble Contrast Agents and Contrast Enhanced Ultrasound Imaging

Conventional ultrasound makes use of gray scale imaging to assess tissue architecture, and color/power Doppler to assess vascular flow within large and medium sized vessels with high velocity blood flow. As such the slow blood flow within the microvasculature is beyond the reach of conventional color/power Doppler imaging.

R.A. Sofferman and A.T. Ahuja (eds.), *Ultrasound of the Thyroid and Parathyroid Glands*,
DOI 10.1007/978-1-4614-0974-8_14, © Springer Science+Business Media, LLC 2012

Ultrasound microbubble contrast agents with their superior scattering properties compared to blood cells, improve the detection of Doppler signals from small volumes of blood flow and better delineate the vascular architecture. This allows sonographic visualization of organs and lesion perfusion in real time.

Ultrasound microbubble contrast agents are encapsulated microbubbles. In order to be suitable for clinical use, they have to fulfill a number of requirements and should be:

- Easily introducible into the venous system.
- Small enough to pass through the pulmonary and systemic capillary system.
- Stable and durable enough to recirculate for at least several minutes.
- Non-toxic, and subsequently dissolve or be metabolized without accumulating in the body and
- Bear desirable modification effects on the acoustic properties of tissues.

Several commercially available ultrasound contrast agents have used different gases, and encapsulating agents to produce suitable ultrasound contrast agents.

Levovist (Schering AG, Berlin, Germany) consists of galactose microparticles with irregular surfaces for adhesion of microbubbles and palmitic acid coating to increase stability. SonoVue (Bracco, Inc., NJ) is a sulfur hexafluoride filled phospholipid shell; the perfluorocarbon has low solubility and thus low diffusion rate which prolongs the survival of the contrast agent in blood. Some contrast agents, including Levovist, are also taken up by the reticuloendothelial system after being cleared from the blood producing late phase enhancement in the liver and spleen.

The peak pressure of the incident ultrasound field affects the scattering behavior of microbubbles, and forms the basis of clinical contrast enhanced ultrasound imaging techniques.

At low incident pressures (low transmit power), the agents demonstrate linear backscatter enhancement to enhance the echo from blood. This is used clinically for Doppler signal enhancement. When the incident pressure is increased to above 50–100 kPa, the contrast agents demonstrate non-linear harmonic backscatter which is employed for contrast specific imaging modes including harmonic and pulse inversion imaging and Doppler. At about 1 MPa (near the maximum intensity emitted by most commercially available ultrasound machines), the backscatter of the contrast agents shows a transient, non-linear pattern because of their physical destruction. This phenomenon forms the basis for triggered imaging and the most sensitive perfusion imaging.

The harmonic signals generated by the microbubbles, particularly the second harmonic, can be preferentially received while the echoes from background solid tissues are suppressed. With this second harmonic imaging, it is possible to only detect the contrast agent, with better signal to noise ratio, and no interference from the adjacent anatomic structures. This allows visualization of extremely small vessels (down to 40 μm) with very slow flow.

In pulse inversion imaging, two pulses are transmitted in rapid succession, the second pulse being an inverse of the first. The returning two successive signals are then summated. The signals from soft tissues behave in a linear manner, and the two inverted pulses cancel out each other. However, the harmonic echoes from contrast comprise non-linear components, therefore the two returning pulses are not mirror images of each other and thus their sum is not zero. Hence, signal is detected only from contrast but not from tissue. This returning signal also contains the non-linear harmonic components (including the second harmonic). Compared with harmonic imaging, pulse inversion imaging better suppresses linear echoes, is effective over the full bandwidth and results in better resolution.

Information acquired from time-intensity curves from dynamic imaging of the region of interest generates various parameters for quantitative analysis. Commonly used parameters include the peak value (PEAK), the time to peak (TTP), the regional blood volume (RBV), the mean transit time (MTT), the regional blood flow (RBF), the refilling time (RT) and the refilling velocity (beta).

Clinical Applications of Contrast Enhanced Ultrasound in the Evaluation of Thyroid Nodules

Although contrast ultrasound is used for the evaluation of a variety of clinical conditions, characterization of liver mass is the most established and successful indication for contrast enhanced ultrasound [6–8]. The other applications for contrast enhanced ultrasound in evaluating focal lesions [6, 9–11] include kidney, pancreas, spleen, breast, ovary and prostate. In addition to characterization of focal lesions, contrast ultrasound is also used for evaluating the efficacy of guided minimally invasive ablation procedures. The absence of demonstrable vascularity on a contrast enhanced ultrasound is often considered a gold standard to assess the effectiveness or completion/adequacy of such procedures.

The data in the literature on thyroid imaging using contrast enhanced ultrasound is relatively scanty and its efficacy debatable.

In 2001 Spiezia et al. [12] reported a series of 54 patients with thyroid nodules evaluated by contrast enhanced ultrasound using Levovist. Their results suggested that analysis of the time-intensity curves can allow differentiation among thyroid carcinomas, hyperplastic benign nodules and follicular adenomas. In this study the carcinomas showed an early arrival time and time to peak and a very delayed and irregular return to baseline. Hyperplastic benign nodules showed a delayed arrival time and time to peak, with a progressive and regular return to baseline while adenomas showed an early arrival time and time to peak, with a regular and progressive return to baseline. On the other hand, a report in 2002 by Argalia et al. [13] on analysis of the time-intensity curves, in 61 patients undergoing contrast enhanced ultrasound assessment of solitary cold thyroid nodules using Levovist showed different results. In this group all malignant and benign nodules showed similar rapid wash-in curves with no difference in the time of appearance of the contrast enhancement. However, the wash-out curves were regular and monophasic in most benign nodules but were irregular and polyphasic in most malignant nodules.

In 2006, Bartolotta et al. [14] reported their results from a short series of 18 patients assessed by gray scale contrast enhanced ultrasound with SonoVue, and pulse inversion technique using low mechanical index. In this group benign nodules showed a diffuse pattern of either homogeneous or inhomogeneous enhancement, whereas most malignant nodules showed an absent or faint dotted pattern of enhancement. Furthermore, irrespective of the histological diagnosis, all nodules with detectable intranodular vascular signals on the baseline power Doppler assessment demonstrated diffuse contrast enhancement, while all nodules with a perinodular vascular pattern at baseline demonstrated an absent or faint contrast enhancement.

Friedrich-Rust et al. [15] recently (2010) reported a series of 50 patients with 53 thyroid nodules, evaluated by real-time elastography, and contrast enhanced ultrasound with SonoVue for the differentiation between benign and malignant thyroid nodules. Contrast enhanced ultrasound video clips were digitally recorded and analysed using time-intensity-curves within selected regions-of-interest. In this study no specific contrast enhanced ultrasound pattern could be identified to differentiate between benign and malignant nodules.

Recently (2011), Zhang et al. [16] reported a prospective study of 95 patients undergoing gray scale contrast enhanced ultrasound for the evaluation of thyroid nodules. Altogether 104 thyroid nodules (47 papillary carcinomas, 3 medullary carcinomas, 1 metastatic carcinoma, 44 hyperplasia nodules, 7 follicular adenomas, 1 suture granuloma and 1 Hashimoto's disease) were assessed. The nodules were scanned after intravenous injection of a 1.2 ml bolus of SonoVue, with real time gray scale pulse inversion harmonic imaging ultrasound for at least 3 min at low mechanical index (MI) (0.05–0.08). The enhancement patterns of the nodules were classified into one of four patterns: homogeneous, heterogeneous, ring-enhancing and no enhancement. The results showed that in both mixed and solid nodules ring-enhancement correlated highly with a benign diagnosis (sensitivity 83.0%, specificity 94.1%, positive predictive value 93.6%, negative predictive value 84.2% and accuracy 88.5%) while heterogeneous enhancement correlated highly with a malignant diagnosis (sensitivity 88.2%, specificity 92.5%, positive predictive value 91.8%, negative predictive value 89.1% and accuracy 90.4%).

The varied and sometimes contradictory findings from these studies may in part be due to the difference in agents used, equipment settings, imaging protocols and the heterogeneous disease groups. With refinements in contrast and technology, standardization of imaging protocols, further prospective studies may help to better define the definitive role of contrast enhanced ultrasound in the evaluation of thyroid nodules.

Ultrasound Guided Minimally Invasive Therapy for Focal Thyroid Lesions

Ultrasound Guided Percutaneous Ethanol Injection Therapy

Thyroid cancer is the most common malignancy of the endocrine system, of which papillary carcinoma comprises more than 80% of all thyroid cancers and is the commonest histological subtype [17]. Well-differentiated papillary thyroid carcinomas are indolent in nature and tend to bear good prognosis with prolonged survival. In fact the 10-year cause-specific survival rate is up to 93% for patients with any stage [18].

The standard treatment for papillary thyroid cancer includes total or near-total thyroidectomy with selective removal of adjacent involved metastatic lymph nodes. The extent of the neck dissection required is still controversial [19]. Post-operative radio-iodine therapy usually follows to ablate any remnant thyroid tissue. Despite this vigorous approach, residual or recurrent neck nodal metastatic disease is common and found in 9–20% of patients during long term follow-up [20, 21]. Patients with recurrent papillary thyroid cancer are commonly poor candidates for re-operation due to neck scarring and higher risks of surgical complications, and are also often reluctant to have repeated neck dissections.

In this context ultrasound guided minimally invasive therapy for recurrent papillary thyroid cancer in the neck was developed. Ultrasound guided percutaneous ethanol injection (PEI) is now a well-accepted and popular technique. It was initially used for treatment of hyperfunctioning thyroid nodules [22] and sclerosing cystic thyroid nodules [23], and was first reported by Lewis et al. [24] as a treatment option for patients with limited cervical lymph node metastases from papillary thyroid cancer. Its mechanism of action is based on the fact that ethanol ablation is thought to cause ischemic tumor necrosis by inducing intralesional vessel thrombosis [22].

Lewis et al. [24] and Kim et al. [25] have previously described similar inclusion criteria and technique for percutaneous ethanol injection (PEI). The inclusion criteria include: (1) the presence of no more than three to five neck recurrence of papillary thyroid carcinomas (NR-PTCs) and absence of recurrence outside the neck at the PEI point in time; (2) the NR-PTCs were not in close proximity to vessels in order to avoid the potential risk of ethanol intravasation; (3) the patients with NR-PTCs were poor surgical candidates and/or preferred to refrain from further surgery.

Ultrasound guided percutaneous ethanol injection therapy is usually an out-patient procedure which usually does not require pre-procedure preparation, premedication or hospitalization. The anteroposterior, transverse and craniocaudal diameters of each NR-PTC are precisely measured to obtain the baseline tumor volume for future reference. A high frequency ultrasound transducer is used for guiding free hand approach of needle insertion. Careful infiltration of local anesthetics around the lesion serves to minimize the localized pain associated with the procedure. A fine needle (25 G) is used through which 95% or 99% ethanol is delivered from a 1 ml syringe. The injection starts from one end of the edge of the lesion and progresses toward the opposite end. Injection is slow and under real time ultrasound monitoring to prevent inadvertent over-spillage. Immediately following injection, the injected area becomes hyperechogenic due to the formation of microbubbles obscuring the needle tip.

This diminishes shortly and allows re-positioning of the needle tip to the adjacent site for further ethanol injection. Ethanol injection is then repeated until the entire volume of the lesion appears to be ablated.

Follow-up ultrasound is done at 3–6 month intervals after the procedure to assess effectiveness of the PEI. Decrease in size of the lesion and absence of intralesional color or power Doppler signal particularly on contrast enhanced ultrasound are signs of a successful procedcure. Successfully treated lesions are routinely followed up and if there is persistence/recurrence of intralesional Doppler signals and/or increase in size of the lesion indicating treatment failure, further PEI can be performed until successful ablation is attained.

Both Lewis et al. [24] and Kim et al. [25] reported very satisfactory results with effective local control achieved in all subjects. There were also only minor complications such as localized pain and transient hoarseness which were self-limiting and resolved spontaneously. Similarly encouraging results were also reported in the series by Lim et al. [26] and Monchik et al. [27].

Other sonographically guided percutaneous ablative procedures for effective and less invasive treatment of focal thyroid lesions have also been described, among which is radiofrequency ablation (RFA). RFA induces focal coagulative necrosis to ablate tissue in a controlled manner. Continuous real time ultrasound monitoring with both gray scale and color Doppler imaging is required to ensure proper electrode positions and to assess microbubble formation during the actual RF ablation [27]. The formation of microbubbles is due to the water vapour which forms when the RF energy boils the tissue within the treatment region. The temperature within the lesion is measured to ensure attainment of the cytotoxic threshold temperature of 50°C. The immediate loss of color Doppler signal within the treated lesion that was previously hypervascular is regarded as adequate indication of appropriate thermocoagulation.

The series reported by Monchik et al. [27] showed no recurrent disease detectable at the RFA treatment site in 14 of 16 patients with neck recurrent well-differentiated thyroid cancer at a mean follow-up of 40.7 months. 1 minor skin burn and 1 permanent vocal cord palsy occurred in this RFA treatment group as well.

A recent (2010) study by Beak et al. [28] suggested that radiofrequency ablation is effective for reducing benign solid thyroid nodule volume and relieving nodule-related clinical problems. In another earlier (2009) study reported by Beak et al. [29], RFA seemed to be effective and safe for the treatment of autonomously functioning thyroid nodules (AFTN).

Kim et al. [30] also reported RF ablation may be an effective and safe nonsurgical technique to treat benign cold thyroid nodules.

However, percutaneous ethanol injection (PEI) has potential advantages over radiofrequency ablation (RFA). PEI is less expensive, the volume of ethanol injected can be closely monitored and controlled under ultrasound visualization and PEI can be performed under local anesthesia for adequate pain control. On the other hand, RFA requires expensive electrodes, has a higher risk of collateral damage to the adjacent structures because the exact extent of ablation cannot be identified on ultrasound, and is more painful often requiring heavy IV sedation. Also, the use of large needle electrodes (14–18 G), multiple needles or hooked needles are also considered to be too invasive for the thyroid gland.

The use of ultrasound guided laser ablation of thyroid tissue has also been described as a safe and effective alternative.

Papini et al. [31] proposed the use of laser ablation therapy for the shrinkage of benign cold nodules in patients with local pressure symptoms who are poor surgical candidates. However, laser ablation does not appear to be consistently effective in achieving long-term control of hyperfunctioning thyroid nodules, and is not an alternative treatment to 131I therapy. Laser ablation may be useful for reduction of tumor tissue before external radiation therapy, or chemotherapy of local or distant recurrences of thyroid malignancy that are not amenable to surgical or radioiodine treatment.

Valcavi et al. [32] reported a series of 122 patients in which the percutaneous laser ablation (PLA) technique was able to achieve shrinkage of about 50% of the initial volume in a wide size range of benign cold thyroid nodules, with satisfactory local symptom control.

Other than providing imaging guidance for ablative procedures, ultrasound itself may be employed for therapeutic purposes. High intensity focused ultrasound (HIFU) is a special technique of power ultrasound to deliver a large amount of heat energy even at a distance to a confined region to coagulate tissue. The acoustic energy is produced by a piezoelectric transducer and emitted as a beam of convergent ultrasound wave towards a tissue target to be treated. As the beam converges into the target, the energy heats the tissue target to therapeutic temperature and produces necrosis by thermal effect, sparing the superficial and surrounding structures [33].

Potential applications of HIFU are being investigated for prostatic carcinoma, benign prostatic hypertrophy, hepatomas, breast cancer, uterine leiomyoma, gynecological tumors and renal cell carcinoma.

Recently (2010) the first case of successful ablation of a toxic thyroid nodule by HIFU was reported [34]. Normalizations of TSH and radioiodine scan were achieved with no complication and maintained for 18 months.

Conclusion

The increasing use of high frequency ultrasound in the neck has resulted in an explosion in the number of incidental nodules detected in the thyroid. It may be impossible/even unethical to "surgically" deal with this epidemic of thyroid nodules. Therefore the search for alternative/innovative ways to manage this crisis continues and ranges from a "wait and see" approach to alternative non-invasive means of treating such lesions (some of which have been discussed in this chapter). Some of these techniques may well have no future use in the routine management of head and neck lesions whereas others may become well established in clinical practice. Continuing development of technology and research into its clinical application is necessary for such techniques to find a well-accepted role in the routine clinical management of thyroid, parathyroid and other head and neck abnormalities.

References

1. Chapter 1 Practical physics In: Middleton WD, Kurtz AB. Ultrasound: the requisites. 2nd ed. St. Louis: Mosby; 2003.
2. Burns PN. Chapter 3 Microbubble contrast for ultrasound imaging: where, how and why? In: Rumack C, Wilson S, Charboneau JW, Johnson J, editors. Diagnostic ultrasound. 3rd ed. St. Louis: Mosby; 2004.
3. Papini E, Bizzarri G, Bianchini A, Guglielmi R, Graziano F, Lonero F, et al. Chapter 10 Contrast-enhanced ultrasound in the management of thyroid nodules. In: Baskin HJ, Duick DS, Levine RA, editors. Thyroid ultrasound and ultrasound guided FNA. 2nd ed. New York: Springer; 2008.
4. Stride E, Saffari N. Microbubble ultrasound contrast agents: a review. Proc Inst Mech Eng H. 2003; 217(6):429–47.
5. Calliada F, Campani R, Bottinelli O, Bozzini A, Sommaruga MG. Ultrasound contrast agents: basic principles. Eur J Radiol. 1998;27 Suppl 2:S157–60.
6. Wilson SR, Greenbaum LD, Goldberg BB. Contrast-enhanced ultrasound: what is the evidence and what are the obstacles? AJR Am J Roentgenol. 2009; 193:55–60.
7. Leen E, Ceccotti P, Kalogeropoulou C, Angerson WJ, Moug SJ, Horgan PG. Prospective multicenter trial evaluating a novel method of characterizing focal liver lesions using contrast-enhanced sonography. AJR Am J Roentgenol. 2006;186:1551–9.
8. Ding H, Wang WP, Huang BJ. Imaging of focal liver lesions low-mechanical index real-time ultrasonography with SonoVue. J Ultrasound Med. 2005;24:285–97.
9. Robbin ML, Lockhart ME, Barr RG. Renal imaging with ultrasound contrast: current status. Radiol Clin North Am. 2003;41:963–78.
10. Correas JM, Claudon M, Tranquart F, Helenon O. Contrast-enhanced ultrasonography: renal applications. J Radiol. 2003;84(12 Pt 2):2041–54.
11. Fleischer AC, Lyshchik A, Jones Jr HW, et al. Contrast-enhanced transvaginal sonography of benign versus malignant ovarian masses: preliminary findings. J Ultrasound Med. 2008;27:1011–8. quiz, 1019–21.
12. Spiezia S, Farina R, Cerbone G, Assanti AP, Iovino V, Siciliani M, et al. Analysis of color Doppler signal intensity variation after Levovist injection. A new approach to the diagnosis of thyroid nodules. J Ultrasound Med. 2001;20:223–31.
13. Argalia G, De Bernardis S, Mariani D, et al. Ultrasonographic contrast agent: evaluation of time intensity curves in the characterization of solitary thyroid nodules. Radiol Med. 2002;103:407–13.
14. Bartolotta TV, Midiri M, Galia M, et al. Qualitative and quantitative evaluation of solitary thyroid nodules with contrast-enhanced ultrasound: initial results. Eur Radiol. 2006;16:2234–41.
15. Friedrich-Rust M, Sperber A, Holzer K, Diener J, Grunwald F, Badenhoop K, et al. Real-time elastography

and contrast enhanced ultrasound for the assessment of thyroid nodules. Exp Clin Endocrinol Diabetes. 2010;118(9):602–9. Epub 2009 Oct 23.
16. Zhang B, Jiang YX, Liu JB, Yang M, Dai Q, Zhu QL, et al. Utility of contrast-enhanced ultrasound for evaluation of thyroid nodules. Thyroid. 2010;20(1):51–7.
17. Greenlee RT, Hill-Harmon MB, Murray T, Thun M. Cancer statistics. Cancer J Clin. 2001;51:15–36.
18. Hundahl SA, Fleming ID, Fremgen AM, Menck HR. A national cancer data base report on 53,856 cases of thyroid carcinoma treated in the U.S., 1985–1995. Cancer. 1998;83:2638–48.
19. Grebe SK, Hay ID. Thyroid cancer nodal metastases: biologic significance and therapeutic considerations. Surg Oncol Clin N Am. 1996;5:43–63.
20. Hay ID. Papillary thyroid carcinoma. Endocrinol Metab Clin North Am. 1990;19:545–76.
21. Hay ID, Bergstralh EJ, Grant CS, et al. Impact of primary surgery on outcome in 300 patients with pathologic tumor-node-metastasis stage III papillary thyroid carcinoma treated at one institution from 1940 through 1989. Surgery. 1999;126:1173–82.
22. Tarantino L, Giorgio A, Mariniello N, et al. Percutaneous ethanol injection of large autonomous hyperfunctioning thyroid nodules. Radiology. 2000; 214:143–8.
23. Cho YS, Lee HK, Ahn IM, et al. Sonographically guided ethanol sclerotherapy for benign thyroid cysts: results in 22 patients. AJR Am J Roentgenol. 2000;174:213–6.
24. Lewis BD, Hay ID, Charboneau JW, McIver B, Reading CC, Goellner JR. Percutaneous ethanol injection for treatment of cervical lymph node metastases in patients with papillary thyroid carcinoma. AJR Am J Roentgenol. 2002;178:699–704.
25. Kim BM, Kim MJ, Kim EK, Park SI, Park CS, Chung WY. Controlling recurrent papillary thyroid carcinoma in the neck by ultrasonography-guided percutaneous ethanol injection. Eur Radiol. 2008;18:835–42.
26. Lim CY, Yun JS, Lee J, Nam KH, Chung WY, Park CS. Percutaneous ethanol injection therapy for locally recurrent papillary thyroid carcinoma. Thyroid. 2007;17(4):347–50.
27. Monchik JM, Donatini G, Iannuccilli J, Dupuy DE. Radiofrequency ablation and percutaneous ethanol injection treatment for recurrent local and distant well-differentiated thyroid carcinoma. Ann Surg. 2006;244:296–304.
28. Baek JH, Kim YS, Lee D, Huh JY, Lee JH. Benign predominantly solid thyroid nodules: prospective study of efficacy of sonographically guided radiofrequency ablation versus control condition. AJR Am J Roentgenol. 2010;194:1137–42.
29. Baek JH, Moon WJ, Kim YS, Lee JH, Lee D. Radiofrequency ablation for the treatment of autonomously functioning thyroid nodules. World J Surg. 2009;33(9):1971–7.
30. Kim YS, Rhim H, Tae K, Park DW, Kim ST. Radiofrequency ablation of benign cold thyroid nodules: initial clinical experience. Thyroid. 2006;16(4): 361–7.
31. Papini E, Bizzarri G, Pacella CM. Percutaneous laser ablation of benign and malignant thyroid nodules. Curr Opin Endocrinol Diabetes Obes. 2008; 15(5):434–9.
32. Valcavi R, Riganti F, Bertani A, Formisano D, Pacella CM. Percutaneous laser ablation of cold benign thyroid nodules: a 3-year follow-up study in 122 patients. Thyroid. 2010;20(11):1253–61. Epub 2010 Oct 7.
33. Esnault O, Leenhardt L. Chapter 13 high intensity focused ultrasound (HIFU) ablation therapy for thyroid nodules. In: Baskin HJ, Duick DS, Levine RA, editors. Thyroid ultrasound and ultrasound guided FNA. 2nd ed. New York: Springer; 2008.
34. Esnault O, Rouxel A, Le Nestour E, Gheron G, Leenhardt L. Minimally invasive ablation of a toxic thyroid nodule by high-intensity focused ultrasound. AJNR Am J Neuroradiol. 2010;31:1967–8.

Index

R.A. Sofferman and A.T. Ahuja (eds.), *Ultrasound of the Thyroid and Parathyroid Glands*,
DOI 10.1007/978-1-4614-0974-8, © Springer Science+Business Media, LLC 2012

MIX
Papier aus verantwortungsvollen Quellen
Paper from responsible sources
FSC® C105338

If you have any concerns about our products,
you can contact us on
ProductSafety@springernature.com

In case Publisher is established outside the EU,
the EU authorized representative is:
Springer Nature Customer Service Center GmbH
Europaplatz 3, 69115 Heidelberg, Germany

Printed by Libri Plureos GmbH
in Hamburg, Germany